UROLOGIC DISORDERS

Adult and Pediatric Care

UROLOGIC DISORDERS
Adult and Pediatric Care

MIKEL GRAY

PhD, FNP, PNP, CUNP, CCCN, FAANP, FAAN

Professor and Nurse Practitioner
Department of Urology
School of Nursing
University of Virginia
Charlottesville, Virginia

KATHERINE N. MOORE

PhD, RN, CCCN

Professor
Associate Dean Graduate Studies
Faculty of Nursing;
Adjunct Professor
Faculty of Medicine/Division of Urology
University of Alberta
Edmonton, Alberta, Canada

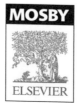

MOSBY

ELSEVIER

11830 Westline Industrial Drive
St. Louis, Missouri 63146

UROLOGIC DISORDERS: ADULT AND PEDIATRIC CARE
ISBN: 978-0-323-01912-5

Notice

Knowledge and best practice in this field are constantly changing. As new research and experience broaden our knowledge, changes in practice, treatment and drug therapy may become necessary or appropriate. Readers are advised to check the most current information provided (i) on procedures featured or (ii) by the manufacturer of each product to be administered, to verify the recommended dose or formula, the method and duration of administration, and contraindications. It is the responsibility of the practitioner, relying on their own experience and knowledge of the patient, to make diagnoses, to determine dosages and the best treatment for each individual patient, and to take all appropriate safety precautions. To the fullest extent of the law, neither the Publisher nor the Authors assume any liability for any injury and/or damage to persons or property arising out of or related to any use of the material contained in this book.

The Publisher

Library of Congress Cataloging-in-Publication Data
Gray, Mikel.
  Urologic disorders : adult & pediatric care / Mikel Gray, Katherine N. Moore. – 1st ed.
    p. ; cm.
  Includes bibliographical references and index.
  ISBN 978-0-323-01912-5 (hardcover : alk. paper)
1. Genitourinary organs–Diseases. 2. Urology. 3. Pediatric urology. I. Moore, Katherine N. II. Title.
  [DNLM: 1. Urologic Diseases. WJ 140 G781u 2009]
  RC871.G73 2009
  616.6–dc22
                                                                        2008028799

Executive Publisher: Darlene Como
Developmental Editor: Charlene Ketchum
Publishing Services Manager: John Rogers
Senior Project Manager: Doug Turner
Designer: Amy Buxton

Printed in the United States of America

Last digit is the print number: 9 8 7 6 5 4 3 2 1

Reviewers

....

Patricia Bates, RN, BSN, CURN
Staff Nurse
Kaiser Permanente
Portland, Oregon
Chapters 1, 2, 4, 8, and 11

Fern Campbell, RN, MSN, FNP
Pediatric Urology Nurse Practicner
Department of Urology
University of Virginia
Charlottesville, Virginia
Chapters 13 and 14

Jane Hawks, DNSc, RN, BC
Associate Professor
Midland Lutheran College
Fremont, Nebraska
Chapters 1, 2, 4, 5, 6, and 8

Jean Lewis, BSN, RN, CNP
Urology Nurse Practitioner
Coordinator, Erectile Dysfunction Clinic
Veterans Affairs Medical Center
Minneapolis, Minnesota
Chapter 9

Dana Overstreet, RN, MSN, FNP
Nurse Practitioner
Department of Urology
University of Virginia
Charlottesville, Virginia
Chapter 11

Jonathan Roth, MD
Attending Pediatric Urologist
Philadelphia, Pennsylvania
Chapter 13, 16, and 17

Preface

Comprehensive and accessible, *Urologic Disorders: Adult and Pediatric Care* is ideal for use in acute adult or pediatric care, long-term care, outpatient, and home care settings—anywhere patients with urologic disorders are found. This book includes information on assessment, diagnostic procedures, and pharmacology that is specifically aimed at advanced practice nurses, including clinical nurse specialists and nurse practitioners. Chapters on urinary incontinence will appeal to urologic nurses; wound, ostomy, and continence (WOC) nurses; continence advisers; and physical therapists with an interest in pelvic floor and voiding disorders. This book will also be a valuable reference for WOC (enterostomal therapy) nurses because of its emphasis on urologic cancers and the continent and incontinent urinary diversions that are frequently used to treat specific urologic cancers. It is the only text for nurses and other urologic providers that incorporates extensive information about pediatric and adult urologic disorders, and it is the only textbook that incorporates detailed information for expert and advanced practice urologic nurses. All material presented can easily be adapted to patient teaching materials and individual care plans. Presentation is greatly enhanced by inclusion of many original color plates and drawings.

The book, divided into 3 sections, is organized into 18 chapters. Chapters 1 through 4 provide the fundamentals to urologic care: embryology, anatomy and physiology, assessment, and diagnostic procedures. Chapters 5 through 11 cover topics related to adult urology, and Chapters 12 through 18 address specific pediatric urology issues.

Chapter 1, *Embryology and Congenital Defects of the Urinary System*, establishes the fundamentals of urology, allowing the reader to integrate a solid foundation in the core issues of urology and apply these to pathophysiologic states. Easy-to-follow tables and boxes assist in learning complex embryologic details

and understanding congenital anomalies. Chapter 2, *Atlas of Genitourinary Anatomy and Physiology*, features clinically relevant illustrations and clear, accessible explanations of complex anatomical concepts, which greatly assists with the understanding of pharmacotherapeutics in later chapters. The color plates are particularly valuable supplements for material covered in Chapters 1 and 2. Chapter 3, *Signs and Symptoms in the Urologic Patient: Basic Principles of Screening and Assessment*, offers the principles of a systematic nursing assessment and several validated assessment tools. This chapter emphasizes assessment of the whole patient and family within the context of a urologic disorder and provides direction for both the novice and expert practitioner to ensure that the patient is part of the process. Chapter 4, *Diagnostic Procedures,* itemizes the approaches to obtain a differential diagnosis, describing for each test the patient preparation, possible side effects, and nursing care. Photographs of equipment, urodynamic tracings, and interpretation provide a unique level of detail to this chapter. From these foundational chapters, the discussions of urologic disorders in adults and children are built.

Chapters 5 through 7 discuss the etiology, nursing diagnoses, nursing care, and treatment of individuals with urologic infections, urinary incontinence, and urinary tract obstructions. Detailed boxes highlight key points, pharmacologic management, and features specific to nurse practitioners or those in advanced practice roles.

Chapters 8 through 11 provide comprehensive detail on etiology and management of urologic cancers, sexual health, trauma to the urinary tract, and surgical procedures. The level of detail provided on the oncologic procedures in Chapter 8 is unique to this book, and care that is comprehensive and collaborative within the whole health care team is emphasized. Similarly, Chapter 9 addresses the psychosocial consequences of sexual health issues and the need for specialized and informed care. Chapter 10, *Genitourinary Trauma*, addresses common urologic emergencies, including renal, pelvic, and lower urinary tract injuries and the residual effects of such trauma on the patient's quality of life. Chapter 11 provides details on nursing care of the individual undergoing urologic surgery—preoperative preparation, postoperative care in hospital, and after discharge.

Chapters 12 through 16 are pediatric specific. The principles of embryology from Chapter 1 are reflected in Chapter 12, *Congenital Anomalies of the Genitourinary System,* and Chapter 13, *Multisystem Anomalies.* Emphasis is placed on the impact on both the child and the family of a chronic health challenge and the psychological cost that can ensue if care is not comprehensive. Urinary tract infections, voiding dysfunction, and enuresis comprise Chapters 14 through 16, and details are provided on both etiology and patient teaching. Pediatric uro-oncology, specifically neuroblastoma, rhabdomyosarcoma, and Wilm's tumor, is the focus of Chapter 17, with particular emphasis on the treatment side effects endured by children and their families. Chapter 18, the final chapter, addresses many surgical procedures in the child, preoperative and postoperative care, informed consent, and pain control. Highlights inclued patient teaching points for nurses and families.

Urologic Disorders: Adult and Pediatric Care addresses urologic nursing care in a comprehensive and evidence-based manner. We hope that the book will contribute to the advancement of professional knowledge for students and practitioners alike.

ACKNOWLEDGMENTS

In particular, we thank Mr. Gary Mawyer and Mr. Wayne Day for their timely attention to our requests for library searches, editing, formatting, and reviewing all of our drafts. Without their assistance this project would not have been possible. We are sincerely grateful to all the reviewers for taking the time to read and critique each chapter. Their insightful and thoughtful comments greatly improved the final product. Jeanne Robertson's drawings certainly added skillful presentation of some difficult concepts. Finally, we thank our Elsevier publishing team, Darlene Como, Charlene Ketchum, and Doug Turner, for bringing this book to print.

Mikel Gray
Katherine Moore

Contents

Embryology and Congenital Defects of the Urinary System

Embryology is the study of prenatal development. Its significance is apparent to the pediatric urology nurse who participates in the management of congenital defects affecting the urinary system. Understanding the fundamental principles of embryology is no less important for the urologic nurse who cares for adults or elders, since their management may also be influenced by birth defects that have been forgotten or remain unrecognized or untreated. In addition, novel research techniques, such as polymerase chain reaction, in-situ hybridization, and genetic sequencing, have given researchers new insights into the genetic processes governing embryogenesis, and research seeking ways to reverse the processes leading to embryologic defects has begun. This chapter will review basic principles of the prenatal development of the urinary system (i.e., kidneys, ureters, and bladder) and the genital systems of both the female and the male.

FERTILIZATION AND EMBRYONIC DEVELOPMENT

Fertilization occurs when genetic materials contained within the nucleus of the oocyte and spermatid merge.[1] Each of these cells contains a haploid number of chromosomes (i.e., one half the number contained in other cells of the body). The union of these cells restores the normal chromosomal count (i.e., diploid number). The resulting diploid number comprises 22 pairs of autosomal genes and a single pair of chromosomes that determine chromosomal (i.e., genetic) gender. Following fertilization, the embryo travels down the fallopian tube to a site within the uterus; this migration requires approximately 5 days. During this initial journey, rapid cell division and growth occur, resulting in a 32-cell embryo at about the time of implantation by day 4. On about day 5, the embryo resembles a spherical structure called a blastocyst. The blastocyst implants into the uterus, establishing pregnancy.

Subsequent embryonic development in the human occurs over a period of approximately 38 weeks or 9 months. For clinical purposes, pregnancy is subdivided into three trimesters.

Development of the urinary system starts relatively early during pregnancy, with the most primitive excretory structure appearing early in the fourth week.[1] Urinary system embryogenesis not only progresses throughout prenatal development but also continues into the neonatal period, as evidenced by the comparatively poor concentrating function of the kidneys observed when attempting to complete intravenous urography during the first weeks of life. Development of the genital system also has its roots at the moment of fertilization, when X and Y sex chromosomes merge to create a genotypic male or when two X sex chromosomes merge to create a chromosomal female. The evolution of the internal and external genital organs occurs later during embryogenesis, with the earliest stage of gonadal development occurring at about week 5 and distinguishable testes or ovaries appearing at the eighth and tenth weeks of prenatal development, respectively. Table 1-1 summarizes major events in the development of the genitourinary system.

Kidneys and Ureters

More than any other aspect of the genitourinary system, the prenatal development of the kidneys reflects a historic rule of embryogenesis, "ontogeny recapitulates phylogeny" (i.e., development of the human embryo reflects earlier stages of human evolution). Specifically, three structures more or less capable of excretory function are observed during prenatal development, but only the last structure (i.e., the metanephros) ultimately develops into the mature functioning kidneys of the adult. The pronephroi are transient structures that appear early in the fourth week of prenatal development (Plate 1).[2,3] Pronephroi are clusters of cells near the cervical

TABLE I-I Development of the Genitourinary System

STRUCTURE	EMBRYONIC COURSE
Kidneys and Ureters	
Pronephros	Appears early in wk 4, regresses by wk 8
Mesonephros	Appears later in wk 4, regresses by wk 16
Metanephros	Appears early in wk 5; nephrogenesis requires additional 30 wk
Ureter	Contact with ureteric bud day 32 (early wk 5)
	Urine production wk 9-12
	Recognizable pelvicalyceal system wk 11-14
	Ureteral ampullae formation ceases wk 14-22
	Nephrogenesis completed wk 36
	Contact with metanephroi early wk 5
	Distal ureter incorporated into evolving bladder base wk 5
Bladder and Urethra	Embryonal folding creates cloacal sinus wk 4
	Anterior urethral plate forms wk 4
	Tourneux's fold divides into anterior urogenital and posterior anorectal compartment wk 5-6
	Cannulization of the anterior urethra wk 11-12
	Detrusor smooth muscle develops wk 7-13
	Skeletal muscle of sphincter mechanism appears wk 12
	Urethral closure by wk 15
Reproductive System	Genotypic (chromosomal) gender determined at fertilization
	Primordial germ cells migrate from yolk sac to genital ridge wk 5
	Differentiation into female or male begins wk 6
	Sertoli cells in male secrete MIS at wk 7
	Testosterone synthesis begins wk 9
	Epididymis, vas deferens, rete testes, and seminal vesicles wk 8-12
	Prostate appears wk 12-15
	Testes enter inguinal canal wk 8-15
	Septation of vagina wk 10-20
	Vagina canalized wk 20
	Testes enter scrotum wk 25-30

MIS, Müllerian inhibiting substance.

region of the embryo that resemble the urinary system of primitive fishes. They form tubules that empty into the cloaca through a structure called the pronephric duct. Although a pronephros may superficially resemble the functioning urinary system of primitive fish, it is not capable of efficient filtration or excretion in the human. Instead, the pronephroi undergo a process called apoptosis (programmed cellular death) soon after development. The remaining debris is rapidly ingested or removed by growing cells and does not lead to an inflammatory response. The pronephric duct also degenerates, but its caudal portion evolves into the wolffian duct that will play a role later in the prenatal development of the urinary system.[4]

Mesonephroi appear late during the fourth week of prenatal development, at about day 24 to 26 (see Plate 1).[5] The mesonephric kidneys arise from the nephrogenic ridge (located at the caudal aspect of the midline) to join the cloaca by week 8. Whereas mesonephroi are only transient in the developing human embryo, such structures persist in modern fish and amphibians to form mature kidneys. In the human, the mesonephroi have glomeruli and tubules that excrete hypotonic urine, but they lack the loop of Henle and are incapable of concentrating urine, as are the nephrons of mature human kidneys. The glomeruli of the mesonephroi are comparatively large but relatively few in number (ranging from 4 to 16 in the human). Nevertheless, the mesonephric kidneys are

TABLE 1-2 Molecular Signaling Factors Critical to the Development of the Kidneys and Ureters[4-9,20]

SIGNALING FACTOR	ACTION
Wnt*	Six Wnt ligands (signaling molecules capable of attaching to a receptor and stimulating growth and development) influence multiple aspects of renal development, including ureteral branching, tubule induction and formation, renal vesicle formation; they may play a yet undefined role in renal maintenance in the adult
Glial cell line–derived neurotropic factor (GDNF)	Ligand (signaling molecule capable of attaching to a receptor and stimulating growth and development) activates formation of the ureteric bud from the mesonephric duct
Proto-oncogene *c-Ret*	Gene that produces receptors critical for nephron growth when metanephroi interact with divisions of the ureteric bud; this gene is not expressed in either of the intermediary kidneys (pronephros or mesonephros)
Wilms' tumor suppressor gene	Gene that releases WT-1, a transcription factor (signaling protein) that promotes ureteric bud development and growth
Pax-2 gene *Emx2* gene	Transcription factor genes critical for formation of mesonephric tubules, müllerian ducts, ureters, and nephrons
Cysteine-rich protein 61 (CCN1; Cyr61)	Extracellular matrix–associated ligand found in human podocytes, hypothesized to influence glomerular modeling and maintenance during embryogenesis and glomerular maintenance in adults
Retinoic acid (vitamin A) Epidermal growth factor (EGF) Fibroblast growth factor (FGF) Hepatocyte growth/scatter factor (HGF/SF) Transforming growth factor–beta (TGF-β)	Growth factors that influence multiple aspects of embryogenic growth and development in kidney and ureter formation; maternal vitamin A deficiency has been linked to low parenchymal volume at birth
Matrix metalloproteinase	Promotes ureteral branching by degrading extracellular matrix proteins
Receptor tyrosine kinases Sprouty1	Promote ureteral branching and development of glomeruli

*Family of glycoprotein ligands important to embryogenesis of multiple organs; Wnt ligands exist on at least four genes within the human genome.

important to the developing embryo. Specifically, they produce hypotonic urine that adds to the amniotic fluid, and recent evidence suggests that they produce erythropoietin (leading to fetal red blood cell production), contribute to the development of the gonads and adrenals, and promote limb development. Although the mesonephroi are an important intermediary organ system, they also undergo apoptosis and degenerate by the sixteenth week of embryogenesis. In the female the mesonephroi regress significantly, although their remnants are observed as vestigial structures including Gartner's ducts. Regression is only partial in the male, and the caudal portion evolves into the vas deferens, seminal vesicles, and epididymis.

Unlike the pronephros and mesonephros that evolve and deteriorate during prenatal development, the metanephros is the basis of the mature kidney of the adult human.[1-5] The metanephroi appear early in the fifth week of embryonic development (Plate 2). They are derived from mesoderm located near the tail of the embryo and flanking the midline. The development of functioning nephrons from the metanephros requires approximately 30 weeks and depends on complex interactions involving multiple genes, protein signaling, and growth factors (Table 1-2).[4-9] Initially, metanephric growth requires a signal from the surrounding mesenchyme. Although the precise mechanism and signaling substances that initiate renal organogenesis are not yet known, it is known that the ureteric bud (the tissue that grows into the calyces, renal pelvis, and ureter) contains growth receptors critical to the growth and proliferation of nephrons.[6] In addition, interaction between the ureteric bud and metanephric cap is essential for growth of the renal parenchyma, development of its drainage system, and migration from the pelvis to the retroperitoneum.

As they grow and ascend from the pelvis to the retroperitoneum, the metanephroi assume some of the functions of mature kidneys. For example, both the mesonephric and metanephric kidneys produce erythropoietin. The metanephric kidney, in particular, plays a larger role in stimulating early red blood cell production than was once postulated.[4] Also, the renin-angiotensin hormone system develops and functions during prenatal development. It is primarily responsible for maintaining adequate glomerular filtration in the fetus, and it probably stimulates further development of the metanephric caps.

The ureteric buds arise from mesoderm within the wolffian duct and make first contact with the metanephroi at about day 32. This contact leads to three phases of evolution resulting in the mature human kidney. Cannulization of the primitive ureter occurs with an ampullary tip that will divide and branch to form a recognizable pelvicalyceal system between the eleventh and fourteenth weeks of gestation. The ureter will undergo repeated cannulization and obstruction during embryogenesis before evolving into the mature urinary tract as a functionally continuous tract connecting nephron and urethral meatus.

Formation and division of the ureteric bud ampullae are also critical to maturation of the renal parenchyma since their division directly stimulates nephron production (Figure 1-1). As the ureteric bud grows, nephrons attach themselves directly to newly branching ampullae. However, between weeks 14 and 22, the formation of new ureteral ampullae and directly attached nephrons ceases. Nevertheless, the process of nephron proliferation is far from over. Instead, three to seven additional nephrons develop from each ampulla attached to the collecting ducts branching from the various ampullae. This final stage of nephrogenesis (formation of *new* nephrons) continues until about the thirty-sixth week of gestation, although the kidneys begin manufacturing urine between weeks 9 and 12. Although the nephrons within the kidneys continue to grow and mature beyond week 36, the human body does

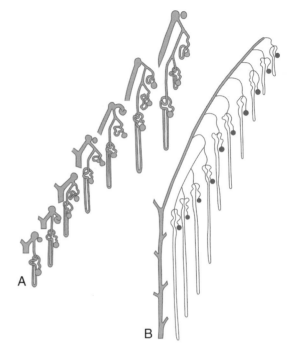

Fig. 1-1 Successive generations of ureteral bud branching lead to formation of mature nephrons. **A,** Early generations bud directly from newly formed ampullae. **B,** During later phases of nephrogenesis, collecting ducts branch from the ampullae, leading to successive branches of nephrons. (From Carlson B: Human Embryology & Developmental Biology, 3rd edition. St Louis: Mosby, 2005.)

not generate new nephrons following this period of intense nephrogenesis.

Whereas the ampullary portion of the ureters interacts with the metanephric cap to generate the nephrons and renal parenchyma and pelvicalyceal system, the distal ureter becomes tubular and develops the epithelium and smooth muscle needed to connect the upper and lower urinary tracts for transport of urine from kidney to bladder by means of peristalsis. Traditionally the ureteric bud has been hypothesized to give rise to the renal pelvis and entire ureteral course, but more recent observations challenge this belief.[5-7] Although it remains unclear whether the embryonic origins of the distal ureter are identical to those of its proximal segment, it is known that the distal ureter incorporates a portion of the wolffian duct and that it initially drains into the urogenital sinus. The epithelium of the ureter develops first, followed by differentiation of mesenchyme into the smooth muscle that lines the mature ureter and

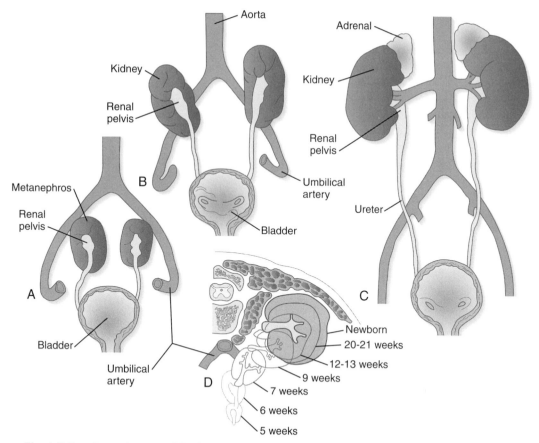

Fig. 1-2 Rotation and ascent of the developing kidneys. **A** to **C,** Cross-sectional views demonstrate ascent from the pelvis to their final location in the retroperitoneum and rotation from ventral to lateral orientation with respect to spine. **D,** Cross-sectional view shows progressive development from 5 weeks to newborn. (From Carlson B: Human Embryology & Developmental Biology, 3rd edition. St Louis: Mosby, 2005.)

ensures the transport of urine from kidney to bladder by peristalsis.[7] As with the growth and development of the kidneys and proximal ureters, the genetic and protein substances that trigger development in the distal ureter are not completely understood.

As the kidneys and ureters grow, they ascend from the pelvis to a final location in the retroperitoneum (Figure 1-2). The kidneys also rotate approximately 90 degrees from a parallel orientation until the pelvicalyceal systems face one another across the centrally located spine. The molecular signaling that governs this migration remains to be completely elucidated.

Bladder, Urethra, and Trigone

The bladder, trigone, and proximal urethra trace their origins to the development of the neural tube

and subsequent embryonal folding that occurs during week 4 of prenatal development.[1,6] Like the upper urinary tract, their embryogenesis is based on complex interactions involving multiple growth factors that act by way of autocrine, paracrine, or endocrine pathways (Table 1-3).[10-12] As the embryo folds, the cloacal membrane is reoriented so that its terminal portion becomes the cloacal sinus (a space that will ultimately evolve into the urogenital and anorectal organs) (Plate 3). During weeks 5 and 6, a wedge of mesenchyme called Tourneux's fold or the urorectal septum divides the cloacal sinus. Tourneux's fold is lined by endoderm, and it bisects the cloacal sinus into a urogenital sinus and an anorectal canal by the end of week 6. This process is aided by growth of Rathke's folds. The cloacal membrane itself degenerates by week 7, but the anorectal canal goes on to form the rectum and anus while the urogenital sinus evolves into the lower urinary tract. At the end of week 4 (i.e., about day 28), one portion of the mesonephric duct fuses with the cloaca and is incorporated into the urogenital sinus. The entrance of this duct further subdivides the urogenital sinus into the vesicourethral canal (located cephalad or toward the head) and the caudal sinus (located closer to the tail).

The vesicourethral canal evolves into the bladder and proximal urethra, and the caudal sinus evolves into the distal urethra in the male or labia minora in the female. The smooth muscle of the bladder wall (i.e., detrusor) develops from mesoderm within

the vesicoureteral canal between weeks 7 and 13 of gestation. In contrast, the trigone muscle arises from distinctive embryonic sources; it evolves from incorporation of left and right common excretory ducts that are incorporated into the base of the developing bladder (Figure 1-3). Early in the fifth week of prenatal development the distal ureter is brought into the bladder. It migrates to its location at the lateral portions of the bladder base to assume the position seen in the mature human. The orifice of the mesonephric duct subsequently deteriorates in females, but it is incorporated into the developing urethra in males and forms the verumontanum. Ultimately, the smooth muscles of the distal ureter

TABLE I-3 Growth Factors Critical to the Development of the Bladder[10-12]

GROWTH FACTOR	ACTION
Transforming growth factor–beta$_2$ (TGF-β_2) Transforming growth factor–beta$_3$ (TGF-β_3)	Development of detrusor smooth muscle bundles from mesenchymal cells
Transforming growth factor–alpha (TGF-α)	Peaks during postnatal period; stimulates growth of epithelium, fibroblasts, and smooth muscle
Keratinocyte growth factor (KGF)	Promotes growth of urinary epithelium, postulated to promote smooth muscle development by paracrine activity

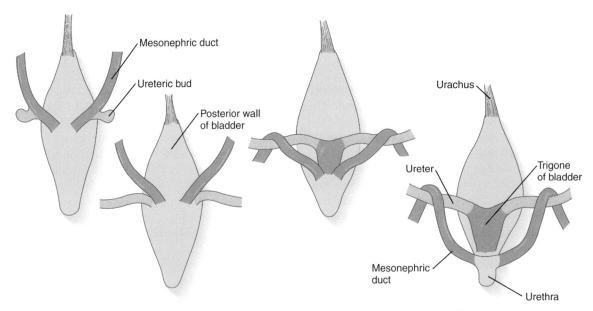

Fig. 1-3 Dorsal view of the prenatal development of the ureterovesical junction including the trigone and distal ureters. Note that portions of the mesonephric duct are incorporated into the trigone. (From Carlson B: Human Embryology & Developmental Biology, 3rd edition. St Louis: Mosby, 2005.)

and trigone become contiguous and interact with the adjacent detrusor muscle to allow efflux of urine while preventing urinary reflux from lower to upper urinary tracts.

The vesicourethral canal gives rise to the proximal urethra in males and the entire urethra of females.[1,2] From a functional perspective, the proximal urethra of the male and the entire female urethra contain elements of a sphincter mechanism preventing uncontrolled urine loss during bladder filling and storage and relaxing to allow unimpeded outflow during urination. This sphincter mechanism contains both smooth muscle bundles and skeletal muscle fibers. The smooth muscle of the sphincter mechanism consists of circular and longitudinal smooth muscle, particularly in the male urethra. The skeletal muscles of the sphincter mechanism develop at about week 12 in both genders, arising from mesenchymal tissue that is detectable as early as week 9.[12] It does not arise as a circular muscle surrounding the urethra; instead, it develops as an omega (Ω)–shaped structure with muscle fibers at its anterior aspect and connective tissue at the posterior aspect of the urethra.

The anterior urethra in the male is embryologically distinctive from the proximal segment.[13,14] The penile urethra arises as an epithelial seam from the anterior part of the cloaca and by means of fusion of urogenital swellings. During fusion, an epithelial plate is formed. The middle portion of this plate narrows and forms the urethra, while additional cells evolve into the corpus spongiosum, albuginea, and ventral skin of the penis (Figure 1-4). Embryogenesis of the glandular portion of the anterior urethra is not entirely understood. It is thought to evolve from an epithelial plate that develops within the genital tubercle during week 4, with complete tubularization occurring much later, probably at about weeks 11 to 12. The development of the glandular and penile urethra occurs simultaneously, ensuring an anatomically continuous urethral course originating at the bladder neck and terminating at the meatus at the distal tip of the glans penis.

The urothelium of the proximal urethra, bladder, and ureter arises from three distinctive embryonic origins.[15] Differences in the embryonic origins of the bladder, urethra, and ureters, in combination with cell migration and replacement, may account for squamous metaplasia in the adult.

GENDER, EXTERNAL GENITALIA, AND REPRODUCTIVE ORGANS

The embryology of the reproductive system can be approached by differentiating the concepts of genetic gender, phenotypic gender, and sexuality.[1,2] Genotypic or chromosomal gender is determined by the union of XX or XY sex chromosomes. Phenotypic gender is the outcome of embryonic development from common structures at the end of week 6 to readily distinguishable internal and external reproductive organs by the end of pregnancy. Secondary sexual characteristics continue to develop throughout childhood and particularly during adolescence. In contrast to these primarily physiologic events, sexuality is the aggregate of an individual's sexual behaviors and tendencies; it incorporates physiologic determinants of gender as well as psychosocial, cultural, and spiritual values.[16] This chapter reviews basic embryologic principles that determine genotypic (chromosomal) and phenotypic gender.

Genotypic gender is determined at the time of conception. This union of the paired sex chromosomes initiates a cascade of events that lead to the development of the reproductive system of a male or female. The external genitalia and reproductive organs of both genders trace their origins to primitive germ cells arising from an undifferentiated genital ridge located in the lumbar region (Plate 4). These primordial germ cells migrate from the yolk sac to the genital ridges during week 5. The origin of the genital ridge is not completely understood; it is hypothesized to evolve during week 5 from coelomic epithelial cells arising from the medial border of the mesonephroi.[1,2] In addition to the mesonephroi, paramesonephric ducts play a role in phenotypic gender. These are derived from condensation of epithelium located lateral to the mesonephric ducts and fuse distally to the urogenital canal. By week 6, primitive sex cords appear. Under the right genetic and hormonal influences, they evolve into the germ cells of the testis or ovary (Table 1-4).[16-18]

No distinctive hormone or growth factor primarily responsible for stimulating differentiation of primitive genital tissues into ovarian tissue has been identified.[13] Nevertheless, it is known that, in the absence of testosterone, the primitive sex cords in the female deteriorate while secondary germ cells from adjacent genital ridge mesoderm evolve into primitive follicles that will ultimately be incorporated into the ovaries. The germ cells within these follicles

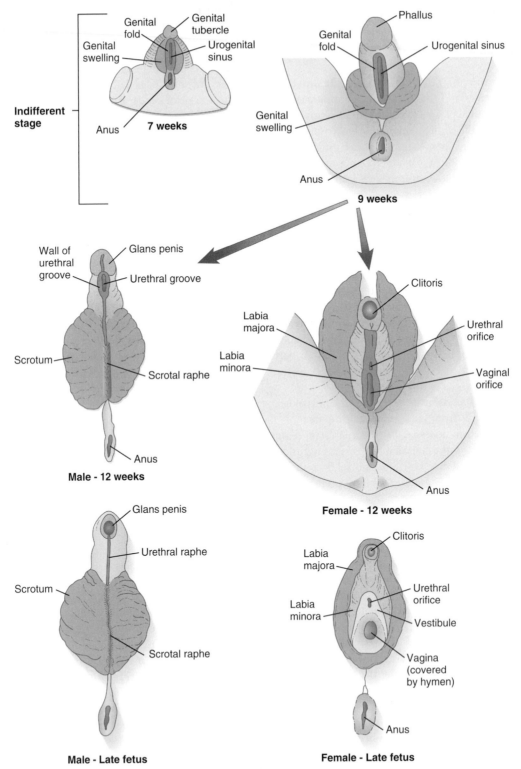

Fig. 1-4 Prenatal development of the male and female external genitalia. (From Carlson B: Human Embryology & Developmental Biology, 3rd edition. St Louis: Mosby, 2005.)

TABLE 1-4 Hormones Influencing Reproductive System Development in Males[16-18]

HORMONE	ACTIONS
Müllerian inhibiting substance (MIS)	Regression of müllerian and paramesonephric ducts Production of fetal testosterone Initial phase of testicular descent
Testosterone (T)	Differentiation of wolffian ducts into epididymis, vas deferens, seminal vesicles
Dihydrotestosterone (DHT)	Penile growth; requires presence of the enzymes 5α-reductase 1 and 2

undergo initial cell division to form primary oocytes (containing a haploid chromosomal count) during embryonic development. Further division of the primary oocytes within the ovaries is arrested until after the onset of puberty. The distal mesonephric ducts degenerate into vestigial structures, but the paramesonephric ducts grow into the fallopian tubes and upper two thirds of the vagina. Separation of the proximal vagina and urethra occurs between weeks 10 and 20 of prenatal development because of growth of the sinovaginal bulb. The distal third of the vagina arises from endoderm of the urogenital sinus. Initially, the sinus is a solid organ, but the lumen characteristic of the mature female develops by week 20. The external female genitalia arise from a number of sources. The clitoris arises from the genital tubercle, the vestibule of the vagina arises from the urogenital sinus, the urogenital folds (that contribute to the distal urethra in males) form the labia minora, and the labioscrotal folds evolve into the labia majora.

A single testis-determining gene (i.e., *SRY* gene) located on the Y chromosome is primarily responsible for development of a male reproductive system.[17] This gene acts as an instigator, stimulating other genes within the genital ridge to differentiate into Sertoli cells and secrete müllerian inhibiting substance (MIS), at about week 7. MIS then provokes a cascade of events leading to the development of the testes and accessory organs. The timing of these events is important; otherwise, the genital ridge will proceed toward development of ovaries and a female phenotypic gender orientation. Important actions of the MIS include regression of the paramesonephric ducts, embryonic production of testosterone, and initial descent of the testes by means of action on the gubernaculum.

Unlike the female embryonic development that leads to production of primary oocytes, primitive germ cells are generated in the male, but further division is arrested until puberty. Like the ovaries, the testes arise from the genital ridges. During weeks 6 to 7 the seminiferous tubules appear, but they remain solid until puberty. The stroma cells that support spermiogenesis, including the Leydig cells, assume a location outside the tubule, and the Sertoli cells appear. Synthesis of fetal testosterone begins at 9 weeks. By week 12 the testis has assumed its characteristic spherical shape and is covered by the tunica albuginea.[17]

Gametogenesis, the process that leads to production of ova in females and spermatids in males, differs significantly from the processes that lead to development and differentiation of somatic cells.[19] When compared with other cells in the body, reproductive tissues produce higher levels of transcription factors, and these transcription factors are used in unique ways when compared with developing somatic cell lines. Germ cells also develop and use new DNA packaging factors and differing patterns of chromatin organization when compared with somatic cell lines. The reasons for these differences are not known, but it is hypothesized that these differences may allow the germ cells in both genders to develop at their own rate, ultimately producing the unique cells essential to the union of a mature spermatid and ovum and the formation of a new human being.

Portions of the mesonephric ducts evolve into the epididymis, vas deferens, ejaculatory ducts, rete testis, and seminal vesicles between the eighth and twelfth weeks of prenatal development.[17] The testes continue to develop during this period, and the seminiferous tubules arise from endoderm within the primitive genital ridge. The prostate develops around week 12 from a condensation of mesenchyme on the fetal pelvis. Endodermal buds sprout and develop from the developing urethra. These buds evolve into the ducts and acini of the prostate by the fifteenth week of gestation. While the ductal system of the prostate is developing, local mesenchymal tissue differentiates into the prostatic smooth muscle and capsule.

Both the testes and ovaries are held in place by a suspensory ligament adjacent to the tenth thoracic vertebra. This ligament is formed as the mesonephroi regress. In the female the suspensory ligament elongates, thus allowing the ovary to assume its position at the pelvic brim by week 12. The ovary remains in this position, which is ideally suited for transport of an oocyte into the fallopian tube.

Like the kidneys, which rise from a pelvic to a retroperitoneal position during embryonic development, the testes must complete a more extensive journey as they move from a retroperitoneal position to the scrotum (Plate 5).[18] Similar to the female embryo, a suspensory ligament is formed as the mesonephros deteriorates; it is called the gubernaculum in the male. The first phase of testicular descent occurs under the influence of MIS; it is characterized by growth of the distal portion of the gubernaculum that fixes the testis within the inguinal canal between weeks 8 and 15. The second phase is primarily modulated by fetal testosterone; it is characterized by contraction of the gubernaculum, guiding the testis from the proximal aspect of the inguinal canal to the inguinal ring, just above the scrotum between weeks 25 and 30. The third and final phase of testicular descent transports the testes into the scrotum. Like phase 2, it is primarily mediated by testosterone, but the mechanical descent occurs as the result of the presence of the gubernaculum. Whether changes in the gubernaculum itself deliver the testes into the scrotum or it acts to anchor the testes as the scrotum develops and surrounds the testes is not known.

The scrotum develops from labioscrotal swellings that grow toward one another and fuse at the centrally locate raphe (see Plate 5). Before the testes descend, a saclike protrusion of the peritoneum, called the processus vaginalis, enters the developing scrotum. This sac closes before delivery or during early infancy.

Prenatal development of the penis depends on conversion of testosterone to dihydrotestosterone in the presence of 5α-reductase (the family enzymes responsible for this conversion). During the twelfth to fourteenth weeks of prenatal development the penis begins to assume a characteristic shape and extend from the pelvis. Urethral closure is typically complete by the end of week 15, and the penis and foreskin evolve from ectodermal structures soon afterward. The prepuce (foreskin) begins to appear around weeks 9 to 10 when fusion of the glandular urethra is completed. It arises from a double layer of ectoderm that differentiates into skin that will engulf the entire glans penis.[13]

SUMMARY

Although many urologic clinicians consider embryogenesis difficult or even esoteric, an understanding of the basic processes that regulate the growth and development of the genitourinary system is increasingly important. This knowledge is critical to caring for both children with newly discovered defects and older patients with forgotten or undiscovered anomalies. In addition, knowledge of genitourinary embryogenesis is critical as genetic therapies designed to prevent or alleviate the sometimes devastating effects of these disorders move from possibility to reality.

REFERENCES

1. Thomas DFM: Embryology. In Mundy AR, Fitzpatrick JM, Neal DE, George NJR (eds): The Scientific Basis of Urology. Oxford: Isis Medical, 1999; pp 407-20.
2. Moore KL, Persaud TVN: The Developing Human, 8th edition. Philadelphia: Saunders, 2008.
3. Pole RJ, Qi BQ, Basley SW: Patterns of apoptosis during degeneration of the pronephros and mesonephros. Journal of Urology, 2002; 167:269-71.
4. Moritz KM, Wintour EM: Functional development of the meso- and metanephros. Pediatric Nephrology, 1999; 13:171-8.
5. Baker LA, Gomez RA: Embryonic development of the ureter. Seminars in Nephrology, 2000; 18:569-84.
6. Herzlinger D: Inductive interactions during kidney development. Seminars in Nephrology, 1995; 15:255-62.
7. Baker LA, Gomez AR: Embryonic development of the ureter and bladder: acquisition of smooth muscle. Journal of Urology, 1998; 160:545-50.
8. Basson MA, Akbulut S, Watson-Johnson J, Simon R, Carroll TJ, Shakya R, Gross I, Martin GR, Lufkin T, McMahon AP, Wilson PD, Costantini FD, Mason IJ, Licht JD: Sprouty1 is a critical regulator of GDNF/RET-mediated kidney induction. Developmental Cell, 2005; 8(2):229-39.
9. Scholz H, Kirschner KM: A role for the Wilms' tumor protein WT1 in organ development. Physiology, 2005; 20:54-9.
10. Baskin LS, Sutherland RS, Thomson AA, Hayward SW, Cunha GR: Growth factors and receptors in bladder development and obstruction. Laboratory Investigation, 1996; 75:157-66.
11. Baskin LS, Hayward SW, Sutherland RA, DiSandro MJ, Thomson AA, Goodman J, Cunha GR: Mesenchymal-epithelial interactions in the bladder. World Journal of Urology, 1996; 14:301-9.
12. Ludwikowski B, Oesch H, Brenner E, Fritsch H: The development of the external urethral sphincter in humans. BJU International, 2001; 87:565-8.
13. Van der Werf JFA, Nievelstein RAJ, Brands E, Luijsterburg AJM, Vermeij-Keers C: Normal development of the male anterior urethra. Teratology, 2000; 61:172-83.

14. Baskin LS, Erol A, Jegatheesan P, Yingwu L, Wenhui L, Cunha GR: Urethral seam formation and hypospadias. Cell Tissue Research, 2001; 305:379-87.

15. Liang FX, Bosland MC, Huang H, Romih R, Baptiste S, Deng FM, Wu XR, Shapiro E, Sun TT: Cellular basis of urothelial squamous metaplasia: roles of lineage heterogeneity and cell replacement. Journal of Cell Biology, 2005; 171(5):835-44.

16. MacLaughlin DT, Teixeira J, Donahoe PK: Perspective: reproductive tract development—new discoveries and future directions. Endocrinology, 2001; 142:2167-72.

17. Coplen DE, Orgtenberg J: Early development of the genitourinary tract. In Gillenwater JY, Grayhack JT, Howards SS, Mitchell ME: Adult and Pediatric Urology, 4th edition. Philadelphia: Lippincott Williams & Wilkins, 2002; pp 2027-40.

18. Carlson BM: Human Embryology and Developmental Biology, 2nd edition. St Louis: Mosby, 1999.

19. DeJong J: Basic mechanisms for the control of germ cell gene expression. Gene, 2006; 366(1):39-50.

20. Merkel CE, Karner CM, Carroll TJ: Molecular regulation of kidney development: is the answer blowing in the Wnt? Pediatric Nephrology, 2007; 22(11):1825-38.

21. Grieshammer U Le Ma, Plump AS, Wang F, Tessier-Lavigne M, Martin GR: SLIT2-mediated ROBO2 signaling restricts kidney induction to a single site. Developmental Cell, 2004; 6(5):709-17.

22. Goodyer P, Kurpad A, Rekha S, Muthayya S, Dwarkanath P, Iyengar A, Philip B, Mhaskar A, Benjamin A, Maharaj S, Laforte D, Raju C, Phadke K: Effects of maternal vitamin A status on kidney development: a pilot study. Pediatric Nephrology, 2007; 22(2):209-14.

23. Sawai K, Mukoyama M, Mori K, Kasahara M, Koshikawa M, Yokoi H, Yoshioka T, Ogawa Y, Sugawara A, Nishiyama H, Yamada S, Kuwahara T, Saleem MA, Shiota K, Ogawa O, Miyazato M, Kangawa K, Nakao K: Expression of CCN1 (CYR61) in developing, normal, and diseased human kidney. American Journal of Physiology - Renal Physiology 2007; 293(4):F1363-72.

Atlas of Genitourinary Anatomy and Physiology

The urinary system consists of the paired kidneys, renal pelves, and ureters, as well as the urinary bladder and urethra. Urologic nursing care focuses on urine transport, storage, and elimination, in contrast to nephrologic nursing, which emphasizes care related to changes in urine production.

KIDNEYS AND ADRENALS

The kidneys are a pair of dark reddish brown organs located in the retroperitoneal space adjacent to spinal levels T12, L1, L2, and L3 (Figure 2-1 and Plate 6). The convex surface of each kidney faces away from the spine at a 90-degree angle, and its concave surface faces the spine. The kidney's concave surface contains the renal hilus and the point where the renal artery, veins, and ureter exit the organ.

The weight of the adult kidney varies from 115 to 175 g; women typically have slightly smaller kidneys than do men.[1,2] The normal adult kidney is 11 cm long from upper to lower pole, 5 to 7 cm wide, and up to 3.5 cm thick. Normally an adult's kidneys are symmetric in shape and size, although the right kidney is situated slightly lower than the left because of the presence of the liver.

The cross-sectional anatomy of the kidney is important, because it helps explain how urine is transported from the nephron to the renal pelvis. Two distinct sections are noted, the pelvis and the parenchyma. The renal parenchyma comprises a cortex and medulla that are visible to the unaided eye. The renal medulla contains the pyramids, cone-shaped structures with bases oriented toward the lateral border of the kidney and apices approaching the renal hilus. The renal cortex surrounds the medulla, forming columns and lobules that surround and fill the space between pyramids.

The coverings of the kidney support and protect the organ from physical stress or trauma (Plate 7). A capsule of dense connective tissue loosely adheres to the renal cortex. It is surrounded by a layer of perirenal fascia and enclosed within a layer of perinephric fat. The entire kidney and the superiorly located adrenal gland are covered in another layer of dense connective tissue, called Gerota's fascia. The kidneys are further protected by the abdominal muscles, diaphragm, quadratus lumborum muscles, and overlying ribs. Collectively, these structures form a shock absorber and protective shields that guard against damage to the urinary system from blunt or penetrating trauma.

The blood supply of the kidneys arises from the renal arteries that branch directly from the abdominal aorta (Plate 8). Normally an adult has one renal artery, but pairing is not unusual. The renal arteries bifurcate (split) in subsequent generations to form segmental, lobar, interlobar, and intralobular arteries before dividing to form the afferent arteriole for individual nephrons. Bifurcation tends to be at a nearly 90-degree angle; this configuration helps to slow flow and promote filtration of the blood in the nephron. The postglomerular capillaries drain into interlobular veins, which merge into arcuate, interlobar, lobar, and segmental veins. Ultimately, venous blood drains into the right or left renal vein. The shorter right renal vein enters directly into the vena cava. In contrast, the left renal vein is three times as long as the right and it crosses anterior to the aorta before merging with the inferior vena cava. Lymphatic channels drain into paraaortic and para–vena caval node chains.

The adrenal glands lie superior to each kidney and measure approximately 3 to 5 cm in height, 2 to 3 cm in width, and 1 cm in thickness.[3] They are divided into two regions: an outer cortex and an inner medulla (Figure 2-2). The adrenal cortex is the largest portion of the gland. It originates from the mesoderm of an embryo and produces essential life hormones. Without the necessary hormones produced by the cortex, fatal dehydration and electrolyte imbalance can occur. Three layers make up the adrenal cortex: the zona glomerulosa, the zona fasciculata, and the zona reticularis. The zona glomerulosa is the outermost layer of the cortex, and its cells are

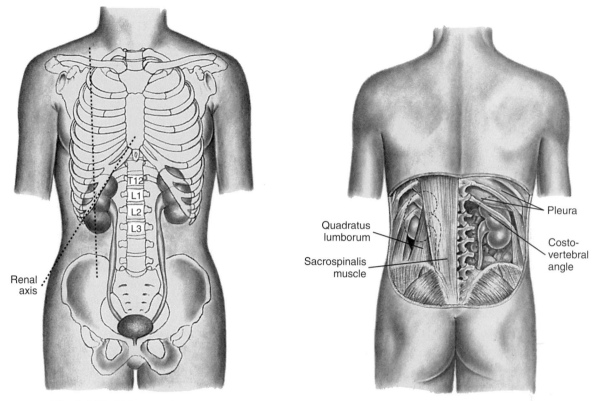

Fig. 2-1 The kidneys in their retroperitoneal location. Note the relationships with the spinal column, ribs, and muscles of the lower back. (From Thompson J, McFarland G, Hirsch J, Tucker S: *Mosby's Clinical Nursing*, 5th edition. Philadelphia: Mosby, 2002.)

arranged in round balls or arched loops. The zona glomerulosa is responsible for producing the mineralocorticoid aldosterone, which helps maintain sodium and potassium levels. The middle layer, the zona fasciculata, has a long cord cell arrangement and synthesizes glucocorticoids, particularly cortisol, necessary for carbohydrate and protein metabolism. The zona reticularis produces adrenocortical androgens and estrogens in small amounts.

The adrenal medulla consists of chromaffin cells that produce the hormones epinephrine and norepinephrine. Chromaffin cells are controlled by the autonomic nervous system, allowing hormone release to occur at a rapid pace. Epinephrine and norepinephrine act as coping mechanisms for possible stressors and are largely responsible for the *fight-or-flight* reaction.

Microscopic Anatomy of the Kidney

The functional unit of the kidney is the nephron, which consists of a glomerulus, proximal convoluted tubule (twisted section of the nephron that is located closest to the glomerulus), loop of Henle, distal convoluted tubule, and collecting duct (Plate 9).[4-6] The collecting duct of a single nephron joins other ducts to empty into a minor calyx. The minor calices empty into major calices that drain into the renal pelvis. Because of its role in blood filtration and urine formation, the nephron is intimately related to local blood vessels. Each nephron is associated with afferent and efferent arterioles found at either end of Bowman's capsule, glomerular capillaries, peritubular capillaries, and the vasa recta. These relationships are critical to filtration of the blood by the glomerulus, the reabsorption of needed water and electrolytes, and urine formation.

The glomerulus is a network of capillaries stored in a fibrous capsule enclosed in a spherical covering called Bowman's capsule. Hydrostatic blood pressure within the glomerular capillaries, when combined with the low filtrate pressures found in the tubules

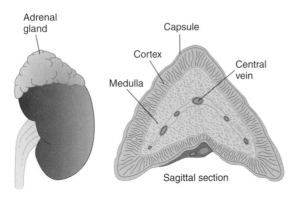

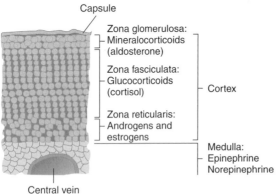

Fig. 2-2 Adrenal gland, sagittal and cross-sectional views demonstrating cortex, medulla, and histologic zones. (From Thompson J, McFarland G, Hirsch J, Tucker S: Mosby's clinical nursing, 5th edition. Philadelphia: Mosby, 2002.)

of the nephron and special features of the glomerulus, allows fluid and electrolytes (solutes) to filter into the space created by Bowman's capsule before the blood exits the glomerulus by way of the efferent arteriole. This filtrate then enters the proximal convoluted tubule, where approximately 64% of it is reabsorbed by way of the peritubular capillaries. The fluid filtrate remaining in the nephron then enters the loop of Henle, a specialized portion of the nephron that dips into the renal parenchyma. This loop is divided into ascending and descending limbs that allow finely tuned reabsorption or excretion of water and sodium. This exchange of water and sodium involves both the loop and vasa recta (looped capillaries adjacent to the course of the loop of Henle). After passing through the loop of Henle, the filtrate enters the distal convoluted tubule and finally the collecting duct. It is only at this point that the renal filtrate can truly be called urine.

Two types of nephrons are observed in the kidneys. Cortical nephrons are found near the surface of the kidney; they have relatively short loops of Henle that travel only a small distance into the renal cortex. Juxtamedullary nephrons, in contrast, extend more deeply into the renal cortex; they have long loops of Henle and are particularly suited for reabsorbing water and sodium during periods when intake of these essential nutrients is low.

Physiology of the Kidney

The kidneys perform a number of functions that are essential to life, including filtration of metabolic waste and toxins from the blood and maintenance of internal homeostasis. They also function as endocrine and paracrine organs affecting blood pressure, fluid and electrolyte balance, production of red blood cells (erythrocytes), and bone growth and maintenance. The most important function of the kidneys is filtration of the blood and production of urine. They filter water and solutes from the bloodstream and then selectively reabsorb or excrete fluids and solutes. Renal function requires a low-pressure transport and storage system extending from the collecting duct to the urethral meatus. Disorders of urinary transport, storage, or expulsive functions endanger filtration and urine formation, particularly when they produce obstruction, resulting in elevated pressure within the tract, and urinary stasis.

Urine Formation. Urine formation is an essential component of renal function by which the kidneys maintain internal homeostasis and rid the body of metabolic waste products and toxins.[4-6] The efficiency of filtration and urine formation is a result of blood flow to the kidneys. In the normal adult, approximately 1200 ml of blood, or 25% of the heart's output, reaches the paired kidneys each minute. However, during periods of intense physical exertion the proportion of heart output reaching the kidneys can vary greatly, ranging from 30% of cardiac output to as little as 12%. Periods of acute and profound physical distress may cause blood flow to the kidneys to fall even lower, leading to acute renal insufficiency or failure unless renal flow is promptly reestablished.

The glomerular capillaries have porous walls that ensure filtration of a large amount of fluid (approximately 180 L/day). Fortunately, this filtration is followed by reabsorption of all but 1 to 2 L per day, representing approximately four times as much fluid as is reabsorbed by all the other capillary beds in the body combined. Several histologic features of the glomerular capillary membrane contribute to this unique ability to filter the blood without allowing excessive fluid loss.[7] The epithelial cells lining the glomerular capillaries have three layers: an inner capillary endothelium, a basement membrane, and an outer epithelial layer made up of specialized cells often called podocytes. The inner epithelium of the glomerular capillary is penetrated with small slitlike openings called fenestrae. The basement membrane that lies adjacent to the podocytes is negatively charged and highly permeable to small molecules such as fluids and electrolytes found in serum. The podocytes of the outer layer, the glomerular epithelium, have footlike processes that adhere to the negatively charged basement membrane. These feet interlock, forming a network of intercellular clefts called filtration slits. Although these features render the glomerular capillaries 100 to 500 times more permeable than capillary beds in the body, they are highly selective in the type of substances they filter. As a result, smaller molecules such as water, electrolytes, and waste products including urea are readily filtered from the blood whereas larger molecules (e.g., proteins) or blood cells are not filtered. Because of this selectivity, the composition of the filtrate present in Bowman's capsule is approximately the same as that in plasma with the exception of most proteins and blood cells.

The volume of fluid filtered by the kidneys over a given period of time is referred to as the glomerular filtration rate (GFR).[8] The GFR is determined by a balance among three primary forces: hydrostatic pressure, filtration pressure, and plasma oncotic pressure. Hydrostatic pressure arises from blood flow within the glomerular capillaries and promotes the process of filtration. Filtration pressure is the pressure within Bowman's capsule. It acts to restrict the GFR. Plasma oncotic pressure is the osmotic pressure that promotes movement of water and solutes from an area of high concentration to one of lower concentration until equilibrium is achieved; it usually promotes filtration since the filtrate contains fewer large molecules as compared with the blood flowing through the glomerular capillaries. In the normal individual, hydrostatic pressure and plasma oncotic pressure (i.e., the forces favoring GFR) are greater

than the pressure found in Bowman's space, favoring filtration of the blood and removal of toxins and unneeded fluid and electrolytes.

A number of factors can alter the hydrostatic pressure favoring filtration or the pressure within Bowman's space (opposing filtration), leading to significant changes in the GFR and rate of urine formation.[4-7] For example, dilation of the afferent arteriole or simultaneous dilation of both afferent and efferent arterioles will significantly increase renal blood flow and GFR, and constriction of these arterioles reduces both flow and GFR. However, although selective constriction of the *efferent* arteriole transiently increases pressure in the glomerular capillaries, the resulting increase in GFR is slight and brief because any initial gain is soon offset by increased plasma colloid osmotic pressure as blood moves slowly though the glomerular capillaries.

Extrinsic factors affecting renal blood flow and GFR include sympathetic nervous system tone and systemic blood pressure. Sympathetic nervous stimulation causes constriction of the afferent arteriole, resulting in reduced blood flow to the nephron and a diminished GFR. With massive stimulation (e.g., that seen with severe physical distress) the GFR can fall to 0 ml/min for a period of 5 to 10 minutes or longer. In contrast, changes in systemic blood pressure do not affect renal blood flow as profoundly because of the kidney's ability to *autoregulate* blood flow despite variation in overall blood pressure.

After the initial filtrate is collected in the glomerulus, it moves into the proximal convoluted tubule (Figure 2-3).[7] Cells with a special brush border line the proximal convoluted tubule that reabsorbs the vast majority of the filtrate. This process uses both active (energy requiring) and passive (osmotic) mechanisms. Sodium (as well as chloride and some urea) is actively reabsorbed by the proximal tubule, which leads to passive reabsorption of water along its osmotic gradient. The proximal tubule also uses energy to reabsorb glucose, bicarbonate, potassium, calcium, phosphate, uric acid, and amino acids. By the time the filtrate enters the loop of Henle, 60% to 70% of the filtered sodium and water as well as 50% of the urea has been reabsorbed. In addition, 90% or more of the potassium, glucose, bicarbonate, calcium, and phosphate has been reabsorbed. Each of these substances is reabsorbed from the proximal convoluted tubule according to its *transport*

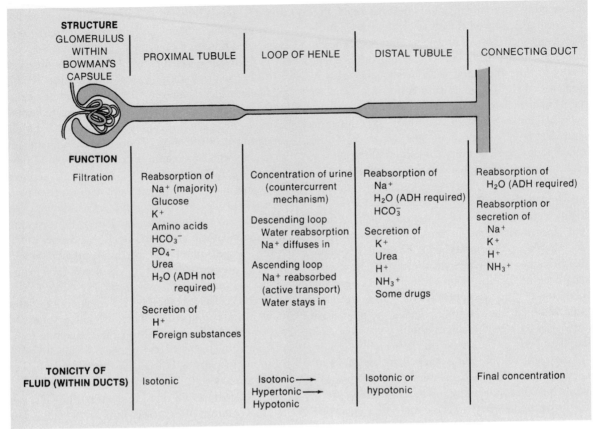

Fig. 2-3 Process of urine formation. (From Thompson J, McFacland F, Hirsh J, Tucker S: Mosby's Clinical Nursing, 5th edition. Philadelphia: Mosby, 2002.)

maximum (TM). The TM is the highest volume of a given substance that can be reabsorbed by means of active transport over a given period of time. When the TM is exceeded, the remaining portion of that substance will remain in the filtrate to be excreted with the urine. This is an important concept in the assessment and management of diabetes mellitus since a plasma glucose of 180 mg/dl or greater will exceed the TM for this substance, causing glucosuria that can be detected by dipstick urinalysis.

In addition to reabsorbing the majority of water and solutes filtered by the glomerulus, the proximal tubule also exchanges hydrogen ions for sodium. A similar process of secretion exists for creatinine and other organic bases, as well as exogenous organic acids including penicillin and other drugs. These secretory pathways are important because they allow the body to rid itself of metabolic waste products or drugs and regulate the body's pH (acid-base balance).

As the filtrate enters the loop of Henle, sodium and water are selectively excreted and reabsorbed, profoundly affecting the concentration of the urine and the body's hydration (Figure 2-4).[9,10] The fluid that enters the loop of Henle is approximately equal to the plasma with respect to its osmotic pressure. However, within the loop, sodium and water are secreted or reabsorbed by means of a complex process that allows the urine to be more or less dilute than the plasma. This ability to concentrate or dilute the urine is affected by the length of the loop and by the varying permeabilities of the loop's cells to sodium and water. This process is called the *countercurrent exchange system* and involves both the loop and the vasa recta (adjacent blood vessels).[11]

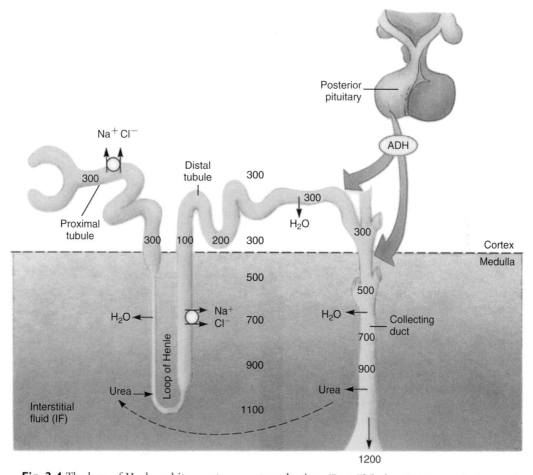

Fig. 2-4 The loop of Henle and its countercurrent mechanism. (From Thibodeau G, Patton K: Anatomy and Physiology, 6th edition. St Louis: Mosby, 2007.)

After the loop of Henle adjusts the concentration of water within the filtrate according to the homeostatic needs of the body, further addition of water may occur as the filtrate enters the distal convoluted tubule and collecting duct.[7] Specialized epithelial cells within these segments are impermeable to urea and therefore favor excretion of urea in the urine. They are also able to reabsorb large volumes of sodium, allowing further concentration of the urine and preservation of water if needed. However, unlike the loop of Henle, reabsorption of sodium from this portion of the nephron is regulated by aldosterone and antidiuretic hormone. After the filtrate has passed from the collecting duct and encounters the epithelium of the calyx it can be truly labeled urine. At this point it will enter the pelvicalyceal system, ureters, and bladder with little or no alteration.

The goals of this vastly complex process are to rid the body of water-soluble waste products and toxins and maintain homeostasis of the body's internal environment. Although the vast majority of the filtrate that enters the glomerulus on a daily basis is reabsorbed, most of the urea and nitrogenous water-soluble waste products are excreted with the urine, lest they build up in the body and create toxic effects.

Homeostatic Functions of the Kidney. Through the parallel processes of filtration of the blood and urine formation, the kidneys regulate the body's internal (homeostatic) environment. The kidneys balance proper concentrations of water and multiple electrolytes, including hydrogen, needed to maintain pH while they selectively excrete water-soluble metabolic end products and toxic substances.

Water and hydration (Box 2-1). The human body primarily consists of water, which accounts for 57% to 75% of its total weight.[5] The majority (25 L) is contained within the intracellular space, and 15 L is contained in the extracellular space (including 3 L in the plasma). Each day, the human body loses approximately 2.3 L of water through the urine, feces, lungs, and skin. Since the kidneys filter 180 L of plasma per day, they must also reabsorb the vast majority of the fluids and solutes comprising the filtrate in order to prevent rapid dehydration and death. The process of water reabsorption begins in the proximal tubule, and it is continued throughout the loop of Henle. The magnitude of water permeability throughout the renal tubule varies significantly and is regulated by a group or a family of aquaporin water channels.[12] The proximal tubule and loop of Henle contain an abundance of aquaporin-1 channels that are highly water permeable, and they are the principal sites of water reabsorption in the nephron. In the distal tubule, aquaporin-2 channels act under the influence of antidiuretic hormone (ADH), a substance formed in the pituitary that influences both the volume of water excreted as urine and the individual's thirst or desire to consume fluids. As the total water volume drops, the plasma becomes hyperosmotic (the concentration of solutes to water rises), which stimulates the release of ADH from the posterior pituitary gland. This leads to conservation of water through reabsorption of water that would otherwise be excreted. In contrast, if a person drinks enough fluids to render the plasma slightly hypoosmotic, ADH secretion is inhibited, which in turn reduces thirst and increases water excretion within the urine until a state of internal homeostasis is restored. A number of diuretic medications may be administered that affect one or more mechanisms of water reabsorption and excretion (Table 2-1).[13] In addition to water, the kidneys regulate multiple electrolytes essential to normal metabolic function. These include sodium, chloride, potassium, bicarbonate, calcium, and magnesium.

BOX 2-1 Fluid Requirements of Adults

Adequate fluid intake is necessary for health. A person requires 100 ml of water per 100 calories metabolized; thus a person who expends 1800 calories for energy requires about 1800 ml of fluid intake (or approximately 30 ml/kg body weight). The metabolic rate increases with fever, rising about 12% for every 1° C. Fever also increases the respiratory rate, resulting in further loss of water vapor through the lungs. Fat is essentially water free so obesity decreases the percentage of water that the body contains.

TABLE 2-1 Diuretics and Their Actions in the Nephron

TYPE OF DIURETIC	ACTION	SITE OF ACTION	COMMON NAMES
Osmotic diuretics	Increase osmolarity of tubular fluid by inhibiting water and solute reabsorption	Proximal tubules	Urea Mannitol Sucrose
Loop diuretics	Inhibit the cotransport of Na and Cl in the luminal membrane	Thick ascending loop of Henle	Furosemide Ethacrynic acid Bumetanide
Thiazide diuretics	Inhibit Na and Cl cotransport in luminal membrane	Early distal tubules	Chlorothiazide
Carbonic anhydrase inhibitors	Inhibit H^+ secretion and HCO_3^- reabsorption, which reduces Na^+ reabsorption	Proximal tubules	Acetazolamide
Competitive inhibitors of aldosterone	Inhibit action of aldosterone on tubular receptor, decrease Na^+ reabsorption, and decrease K^+ secretion	Collecting tubules	Spironolactone
Sodium channel blockers	Block entry of Na^+ into Na^+ channels of luminal membrane, decrease Na^+ reabsorption, and decrease K^+ secretion	Collecting tubules	Amiloride Triamterene

Modified from Guyton A, Hall J: Textbook of Medical Physiology, 9th edition. Philadelphia: Saunders, 1996; p 409.

Sodium. Sodium is the most abundant cation (positively charged ion) in the body.[4,5] Most is contained in the extracellular fluid space (135 to 145 mEq/L), and only a small amount is found in the intracellular fluid compartment (10 to 14 mEq/L). Excretion and reabsorption are primarily regulated by the kidneys in response to fluid volume and sodium concentrations in the plasma. Other factors responsible for sodium regulation include the sympathetic nervous system, the renin-angiotensin-aldosterone hormone mechanism, and atrial natriuretic peptide (a hormone released from cells in the atria of the heart in response to atrial stretch). Sodium excretion and reabsorption are closely related to the fate of water. Sodium is reabsorbed both passively and by active (energy-requiring) mechanisms. Most sodium is reabsorbed from the proximal tubule as $NaHCO_3$ or $NaCl$. Sodium is used by the loop of Henle to concentrate urine and preserve water using active mechanisms. In addition, it is reabsorbed from the distal tubule and collecting duct, primarily under the influence of aldosterone.

Potassium. Like sodium, most potassium entering the glomerular filtrate is reabsorbed in the proximal convoluted tubule, although the ascending loop of Henle also reabsorbs a significant proportion.[14] Fine tuning of the remaining potassium concentration, essential for meeting the metabolic needs of cardiac muscle and many other cells in the body, is accomplished in the late distal tubule and collecting duct using an active process. Potassium balance is primarily regulated by dietary intake, serum levels of adrenal mineralocorticoids (primarily aldosterone), hydrogen ion balance, and certain diuretics. The significance of renal-mediated potassium is seen in renal failure. Initially, the nephrons increase their potassium excretion to adjust for a reduced GFR. This compensatory mechanism is adequate until the GFR falls to less than 5 ml/min, a value seen only in advanced or end-stage renal failure. At this point, fatal hyperkalemia occurs unless it is promptly corrected.

A growing body of evidence demonstrates racial differences in sodium sensitivity, resulting in a rise in blood pressure linked to dietary intake of sodium.[15] When compared with whites, African Americans are at higher risk for salt sensitivity, and this risk has been linked to racial differences in sodium–potassium chloride cotransport in the thick ascending limb of the loop of Henle. This difference in renal function is hypothesized to result in an increased ability to conserve sodium and water, as well as higher glomerular capillary hydraulic pressure and a predilection to glomerular injury, particularly in the presence of hypertension.

Calcium, phosphate, and magnesium. Calcium, phosphate, and magnesium are primarily eliminated in the urine.[16] The majority (60% to 65%) is passively reabsorbed in the proximal convoluted tubule, and up to 20% is reabsorbed in the loop of Henle. Fine-tuning of calcium occurs in the distal convoluted tubule; reabsorption in this portion of the nephron is an active process influenced by several hormones, including parathormone, calcitonin, and glucagon. Magnesium, phosphorus, and calcium reabsorption are influenced by dietary intake, hydrogen ion (acid-base) balance, and a metabolic form of vitamin D (cholecalciferol). Loop diuretics decrease calcium reabsorption in the loop of Henle.[10]

Acid-base balance. Maintaining long-term hydrogen ion balance is one of the kidney's most important functions.[17] The pH of the internal environment must be maintained within a relatively tight range, as reflected in the serum pH, which varies between 7.37 and 7.42. An ongoing threat to this balance occurs when we produce CO_2 or consume inorganic acids from dietary sources such as meat. If production of naturally occurring acidic substances were left unchecked, the body's pH would rapidly fall below its usual mildly alkaline state, interrupting metabolic processes and leading to death. The body controls pH by a number of mechanisms. They are typically divided into short- and long-term regulators. The short-term regulators of pH are the lungs that rid the body of excess CO_2 by way of respiration (expiration), the rapid binding of hydrogen ions entering the blood by way of special buffering properties of hemoglobin, and our substantial store of the bicarbonate ions. The kidneys contribute to long-term regulation of pH by excreting excessive hydrogen ions in exchange for bicarbonate (thus ensuring the bicarbonate stores needed for rapid buffering) and by excreting ammonium ions and exogenous acids consumed in our diet.

Endocrine Functions of the Kidney. The kidneys also produce or secrete paracrine or endocrine substances including erythropoietin, renin, angiotensin, and cholecalciferol. These substances affect both adjacent tissues and distant organs.

Erythropoietin. Erythropoietin is a hormone produced by cells lining capillaries adjacent to the renal tubules.[6] It stimulates the bone marrow to produce erythrocytes (red blood cells). The kidneys produce 90% to 95% of the body's erythropoietin. It is secreted in response to hypoxia and reduction in renal blood flow and inhibited as the body's oxygen and renal blood flow are restored. Renal failure compromises the production of erythropoietin, leading to a decline in hematocrit and profound anemia; in this case recombinant human erythropoietin (r-HuEPO) or a erythropoietin receptor activator is administered to restore and maintain an adequate hematocrit level.[18]

Renin-angiotensin. Renin is an enzyme produced in the juxtaglomerular apparatus (JGA), a group of specialized cells that lie adjacent to the glomerulus.[8] It is released in response to several stimuli, including decreased plasma sodium concentration, systemic blood pressure, and stimulation of β-adrenergic nerve receptors in the JGA of the kidney. Secretion of renin converts angiotensinogen to angiotensin I. When angiotensin I interacts with the angiotensin-converting enzyme (ACE), manufactured primarily in the small blood vessels of the lung, it is further converted to angiotensin II. This metabolically active hormone is a powerful vasopressor that stimulates sodium reabsorption by constricting the afferent arteriole of the glomerulus, thereby decreasing GFR and slowing sodium filtration. Activation of the renin-angiotensin system also leads to the secretion of aldosterone from the adrenal glands (Figure 2-5).

Aldosterone. Aldosterone is produced by the adrenal cortex.[3] Secretion is stimulated by the presence of angiotensin II, an increase in the serum concentration of potassium, and a decrease in the concentration of sodium in the extracellular fluid or the secretion of adrenocorticotropic hormone (ACTH). Aldosterone acts on nephrons in conjunction with angiotensin II to increase sodium reabsorption within the distal convoluted tubule into the blood. In contrast to its effect on sodium, aldosterone acts to *increase* the elimination of potassium in the urine. In addition to its primary role in the regulation of fluid and electrolyte balance, aldosterone has been shown to create oxidative stress, endothelial dysfunction, and inflammation and fibrosis in the vasculature, heart, and kidney.[19] Although these negative effects are avoided when aldosterone binds to mineralocorticoid receptors, ongoing research is needed

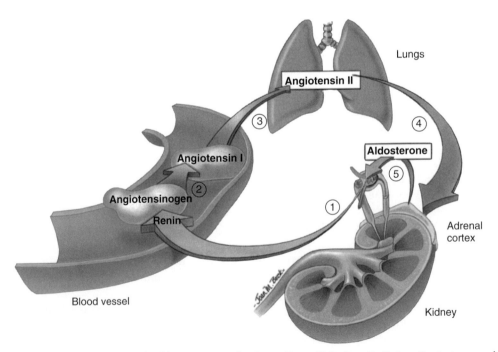

Fig. 2-5 The renin-angiotensin-aldosterone mechanism. (From Thibodeau F, Patton K: Anatomy and Physiology, 6th edition. St. Louis: Mosby, 2007.)

to better understand the effects of aldosterone that is not bound to mineralocorticoid receptors and its potential contribution to cardiovascular and renal disease.

Vitamin D (cholecalciferol). The kidney also plays a central role in the production of 1,25-dihydroxycholecalciferol.[20] Exogenous (dietary) sources of vitamin D include fortified dairy products, margarine, fish oils, and egg yolk. Whether consumed in its dietary form (7-dehydrocholesterol) or taken as a vitamin supplement (ergocalciferol), vitamin D is ultimately altered into its metabolically active form (1,25-dihydroxycholecalciferol), first in the liver and finally in the kidneys. Metabolically active vitamin D regulates calcium absorption from the gastrointestinal system and calcium deposition in the bone. In its metabolic formulation, vitamin D increases intestinal absorption of calcium and promotes ossification of bones and teeth. Vitamin D deficiency is uncommon in the United States, Canada, and other countries where multiple foods are fortified, but it may occur in strict vegetarians or in frail elders as a result of poor nutrition or age-related intestinal malabsorption problems. Vitamin D deficiency related to impaired renal function is called renal rickets and occurs when the kidney is unable to manufacture the metabolically active substance 1,25-dihydroxycholecalciferol.

RENAL PELVIS AND URETER

Each of the paired renal pelvis and ureter transports urine from the kidney to the bladder in an antegrade fashion called efflux (Figure 2-6).[21] The two structures form a continuous tube extending from the renal hilus to the trigone of the bladder. The renal pelvis is funnel shaped with a larger end draining the major calices before it tapers to a diameter of approximately 2 mm (6F) at the ureteropelvic junction (UPJ). The tube-shaped ureter is approximately 24 to 30 cm long. The left ureter is slightly longer than the right because of the difference in the location of the kidneys. The ureter follows a course from the renal pelvis to the bladder that resembles an inverted S traveling medially from the UPJ to pass over the psoas muscle to the sacroiliac joint of the bony pelvis. It then turns laterally toward the ischial spine of the pelvis and curves back toward the base of the bladder, where it inserts into the trigone of the bladder (Figure 2-7).

The lumen (interior) of the ureter varies in diameter from 0.2 to 1 cm. Three areas of the lumen are particularly narrow and susceptible to obstruction by calculi (urinary stones): the UPJ, the point where the

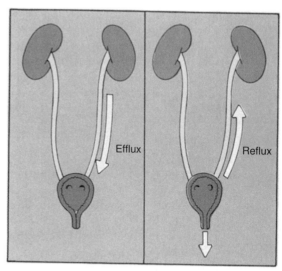

Fig. 2-6 The normal ureters allow antegrade movement of urine (efflux) while preventing its retrograde movement (reflux).

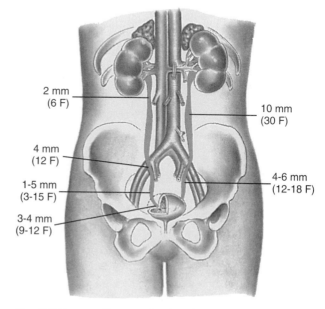

Fig. 2-7 Course of ureter showing three areas with relatively narrow internal radii. (From Thompson J, McFarland G, Hirsch J, Tucker S: Mosby's Clinical Nursing, 5th edition. Philadelphia: Mosby, 2002.)

ureter crosses the iliac arteries, and the ureterovesical junction (UVJ) (Figure 2-8).

Four histologic layers characterize the microscopic anatomy of the ureters: the mucosa, submucosa, muscular tunic, and adventitia. The innermost layer contains transitional-cell epithelium that is resistant to secretion or reabsorption of urine contents. A submucosal lamina propria contains nerves, a rich vascular network, and lymphatic drainage channels. It lies between the mucosa and the muscular tunic. Ureteral smooth muscle bundles are arranged into a complex network that contracts to transport urine from the kidneys to the bladder in response to neural, chemical, or mechanical influences.

The arterial blood supply of the ureters varies among individuals. Upper ureteral segments may receive blood from branches of the renal, gonadal, or adrenal arteries, and lower (pelvic) segments may receive blood from branches of the obturator artery, deferential artery (men), or uterine artery (women). Venous blood drains into a venous plexus and leaves the ureter by way of vessels that parallel the arterial supply. Lymphatic drainage is provided by paraaortic or renal node chains and common or external iliac nodes.

Ureteral Function

The primary function of the ureter and renal pelvis is to transport urine by coordinated smooth muscle contractions (peristalsis) that originate in the renal pelvis, terminate at the UVJ, and push a bolus of urine from upper to lower urinary tracts.[22] Nevertheless, some evidence exists that while the osmolality and pH of the urine remain unchanged as it travels through the ureters, sodium and potassium levels are higher than urine entering the renal pelvis from the collecting ducts.[23] These findings indicate that the ureteral epithelium acts as more than a barrier to reabsorption of urinary constituents, but the clinical relevance of these findings (if any) is not yet known.

The renal pelvis stores only a small amount of urine (15 to 20 ml) before distention propagates a peristaltic wave. Ureteral peristalsis was traditionally hypothesized to be controlled by an as yet unidentified pacemaker cell similar to those seen in the heart; more recent evidence now suggests that contractions are coordinated by the activity of interstitial Cajal–like cells found in the renal pelvis, ureter, and ureteropelvic junction.[23a] A peristaltic contraction creates a propulsive wave that opens the ureteropelvic junction and propels a bolus of urine from the pelvis through the entire ureteral course and into the bladder by way of the UVJ. A peristaltic contraction raises the resting intraluminal pressure from 0 to 5 cm H_2O to 20 to 80 cm H_2O and pushes the bolus of urine before it. The smooth muscle of the ureter contains gap junctions (areas of cytoplasm allowing electrochemical communication between muscle cells), allowing it to act as a single unit. Thus a single peristaltic wave causes a continuous contraction that pushes the urine through the entire ureteral course and into the bladder, even if the ureter has been denervated or transplanted from donor to recipient.

In addition to mechanical distention, neurologic, endocrine, and pharmacologic factors modulate ureteral peristalsis. Stimulation of α-adrenergic receptors in the ureteral wall increases the number and amplitude (strength) of contractions, whereas stimulation of β-adrenergic receptors causes ureteral relaxation. Stimulation of cholinergic receptors by the administration of epinephrine or catecholamines is thought to cause more vigorous ureteral peristalsis through the release of catecholamines. Tachykinins and calcitonin gene-related peptide (CGRP) also act as neurotransmitters within the ureter. Tachykinins stimulate peristalsis, and CGRP inhibits this activity. The neurotransmitter glutamate stimulates ureteral smooth muscle contraction by activating N-methyl-D-aspartic acid (NMDA) receptors.[23b] Sensory nerves containing the tachykinins substance P, neurokinin A, and neuropeptide K are particularly abundant in the renal pelvis. In contrast, inhibitory nerves

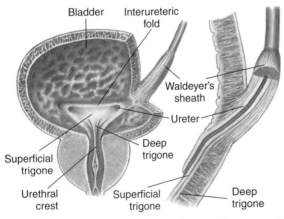

Fig. 2-8 Ureterovesical junction. (From Thompson J, McFarland G, Hirsch J, Tucker S: Mosby's Clinical Nursing, 5th edition. Philadelphia: Mosby, 2002.)

containing CGRP are more abundant in the distal ureter. Interactions between these factors are postulated to produce the renal colic seen with an obstructive urinary calculus. Several drugs are known to influence ureteral peristalsis. For example, administration of epinephrine or catecholamines enhances peristalsis whereas administration of antimuscarinic agents exert a modest effect on ureteral peristalsis. Administration of α-adrenergic blocking agents such as terazosin, doxazosin, or tamsulosin enhances peristalsis. Hormonal changes related to pregnancy indirectly influence ureteral dilation and peristaltic waves, allowing physiologic dilation of their lumina during parturition.

Ureteropelvic Junction and Trigone. The UVJ is particularly important to urinary system function because it allows efflux of urine from upper to lower urinary tracts while preventing reflux from the lower to upper tract (see Figure 2-6).[21,24] It is formed by the terminal ureter, adjacent bladder wall, and trigone. The distal ureter pierces the bladder wall near its base; it does not enter at a right angle as it is sometimes depicted. Instead, it tunnels through the bladder wall and trigone over a length of approximately 1.5 cm. This arrangement promotes ureteral closure with contraction of the detrusor or the trigone. The adventitia of the intramural ureter includes three sheaths. A superficial sheath is continuous with the bladder wall, a deep sheath is continuous with the distal ureter, and a middle element is composed of a loose plane of connective tissue called Waldeyer's sheath. The three sheaths allow limited mobility of the distal ureter while preserving its integrity with the bladder and upper ureter. The bladder wall adjacent to the intramural ureter is composed of smooth muscle bundles arranged in a circular and longitudinal fashion. These smooth muscle bundles provide additional anatomic integrity between ureter and bladder and promote closure of the intramural ureter during micturition. The trigone is a triangular-shaped muscle located in the base of the bladder, divided into superficial and deep elements. Although it arises from a distinct embryogenic source as compared with the ureter and bladder, its superficial segment is anatomically contiguous with the intravesical ureter and its deep portion is anatomically contiguous with Waldeyer's sheath. The apex of the trigone extends to the bladder neck in women and the verumontanum in men.

During bladder filling and urine storage, the UVJ allows the efflux of urine from ureter to bladder in response to peristalsis, while it prevents reflux (backward flow) of urine from the bladder to the upper urinary tract. Because the vesicle of the bladder maintains a low pressure, a peristaltic contraction easily overcomes the low resistance mounted by the UVJ allowing the upper urinary tracts to regularly transport urine into the bladder for storage and elimination. However, in the absence of a peristaltic wave, the UVJ mounts sufficient passive resistance (created by the tunneling of the intravesical ureter, the resting tone of the trigone, and tension from the adjacent bladder wall) to prevent urinary reflux. In addition, when micturition occurs, the trigone contracts several seconds before micturition and remains contracted for as long as 20 seconds after voiding is completed. This contraction, along with increased tension from the detrusor muscle, provides the additional resistance needed to prevent reflux during micturition.

Lower Urinary Tract. In the normal adult, the lower urinary tract consists of the bladder, urethra, and pelvic floor. These organs function as a coordinated unit to store and evacuate urine in order to ensure continence.

Urinary bladder. The urinary bladder is a hollow organ designed to store and expel the urine produced by the kidneys.[21,25,26] From a functional perspective, it is divided into two portions, a fixed base and a distensible body (Figure 2-9). Often misrepresented in anatomic illustrations, the size and shape of the bladder vary according to its state of fullness. An air bubble is not normally present in the bladder dome. When empty, the bladder assumes an approximate tetrahedron shape as the walls of the body collapse against the fixed base. As it fills, the body of the bladder assumes the nearly spherical shape typically depicted in anteroposterior drawings as it rises toward the umbilicus. The bladder also contains two inlets, the orifices of the UVJs described previously, and a single outlet, the bladder neck or urethrovesical junction.

The microscopic anatomy of the bladder wall consists of four histologic layers. Its lumen is lined by a transitional-cell epithelium that prevents the reabsorption of urine. This layer is arranged in a distinctive supportive matrix, allowing the cells to thin from five to seven deep to a single cell deep as the bladder

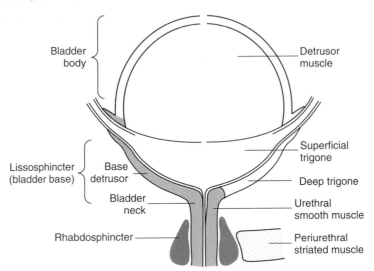

Fig. 2-9 Bladder is divided into two regions: the fixed base (sometimes called the lissosphincter) and the flexible body containing the detrusor muscle. (From Doughty D: Urinary and Fecal Incontinence: Nursing Management, 3rd edition. St Louis: Mosby, 2006.)

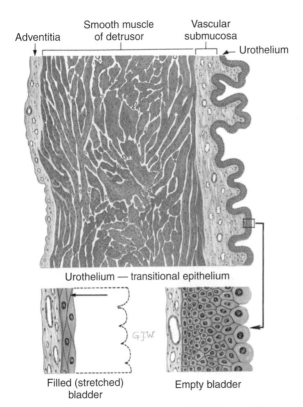

Fig. 2-10 Microscopic anatomy of bladder epithelium illustrates ability of lining to narrow from multiple cellular thickness to as little as one cell with vesical filling.

fills with urine (Figure 2-10). The uroepithelium also manufactures glycosaminoglycans (polysaccharides that form a thick mucoidlike substance) that protect the mucosa from potentially irritating components of the urine. Immediately underneath the uroepithelium is a loosely attached lamina propria. It contains connective tissues, arteries, and veins. It also contains interstitial cells that are extensively linked by gap junctions.[27] The gap junctions allow the interstitial cells to communicate electrically, although the purpose of this communication is not entirely understood.

Smooth muscle bundles, collectively called the detrusor muscle, are arranged in a complex meshwork rather than longitudinal or circular layers characteristic of the bowel or other hollow viscera. The detrusor muscle also contains interstitial cells that communicate by way of gap junctions and are hypothesized to act as pacemaker cells, modulating the bladder's response to urine filling, storage, and micturition.[27] Collagen and elastin provide structural integrity to the detrusor muscle and bladder wall. Deposition of excessive collagen occurs in certain disorders of the lower urinary tract, including obstruction and specific types of denervation. As a result, the bladder becomes trabeculated and its contractility is compromised. Deposits of large amounts of collagen cause marked trabeculation and loss of the distensibility of the bladder wall, compromising upper urinary

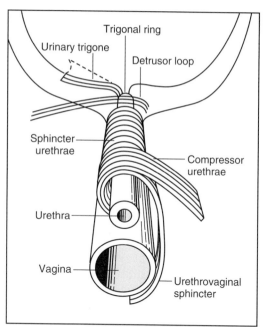
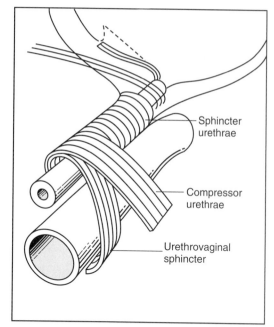

Fig. 2-11 Female urethra and muscular components of the female rhabdosphincter and periurethral muscle: sphincter urethrae, urethrovaginal sphincter, and compressor urethrae. (From Doughty D: *Urinary and Fecal Incontinence: Nursing Management*, 3rd edition. St Louis: Mosby, 2006.)

tract drainage and urine production. Like the ureters, the outermost layer of the bladder is an adventitia composed of fibroelastic connective tissues.

The bladder receives arterial blood from a number of sources including the superior, inferior, and medial vesical arteries, as well as branches of the obturator, inferior gluteal, or internal iliac arteries. Branches of the uterine and vaginal arteries also provide arterial blood to the female bladder. Unlike the kidney, renal pelvis, and ureter, the venous drainage of the bladder does not mirror its arterial supply. Instead, bladder veins drain into Santorini's plexus and ultimately into the inferior hypogastric vein. Lymphatic channels in the bladder drain into the external iliac, hypogastric, and common iliac nodes.

Urethra. In women the urethra follows a relatively short, straight course compared with the male (Figure 2-11).[28,29] It originates at the bladder neck and travels at an approximate 16-degree angle for a distance of 3.5 to 5.5 cm to its termination just above the vaginal vestibule. Like the bladder, epithelium and glands that manufacture and secrete glycosaminoglycans line the urethral lumen. The urethral submucosa contains a rich network of arteries, veins, and lymphatics, and varying amounts of striated and

smooth muscle densest at its middle third. The lower two thirds of the female urethra are anatomically contiguous with the vagina, and the striated and smooth muscle in this area is closely shared with the vagina. From a physiologic perspective, the entire length of the female urethra acts as a sphincter mechanism that provides continence during bladder filling while serving as a conduit for urine expulsion during micturition.

The male urethra is approximately 23 cm long and divided into two portions, proximal and distal (Figure 2-12).[30] The proximal urethra is functionally comparable to the entire length of the female urethra with its sphincter mechanism. The distal urethra does not contribute to continence; instead, it acts as a conduit for urine or semen. The proximal urethra originates at the bladder neck and travels through the prostate. The floor of the prostatic urethra is elevated because of the verumontanum before it tapers into its membranous segment. The membranous urethra is approximately 2 to 2.5 cm in length. It extends from the prostatic apex and pierces the pelvic floor at a point often called the urogenital diaphragm. The distal urethra begins at the termination of the membranous urethra. It includes the bulbous urethra, pendulous urethra, fossa navicularis,

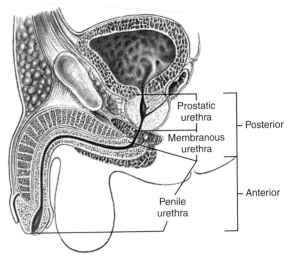

Prostatic
urethra

Posterior

Membranous
urethra

Anterior

Penile
urethra

Fig. 2-12 Male urethra is divided into two functional portions: the posterior or sphincteric urethra containing the bladder neck and prostatic and membranous urethra, and the anterior or distal urethra containing the penile urethra, fossa navicularis, and meatus. (From Thompson J, McFarland G, Hirsch J, Tucker S: Mosby's Clinical Nursing, 5th edition. Philadelphia: Mosby, 2002.)

and meatus. The microscopic anatomy of the male urethra includes an epithelial lining, submucosal vascular and lymphatic networks (lamina propria), and outer adventitia. The proximal urethral wall also contains varying amounts of striated and smooth muscle that contribute to the male sphincter mechanism. No such muscle is found in the wall of the distal urethra.

The arterial blood supply of the urethra arises from branches of the pudendal artery in men and the vaginal artery in women.[21] Venous blood drains by way of the deep dorsal vein in the male and by way of the pelvic venous plexus in the female. Lymphatic channels of the urethra empty into the superficial and deep nodes, as well as the hypogastric, obturator, and internal and external nodes.

Pelvic floor. A detailed description of the entire pelvic floor, including the rectal gutter and female reproductive system, is beyond the scope of this chapter. However, a review of the portion of the pelvic floor that supports the bladder base and urethra and contributes to urethral sphincter function is provided because of its significance to urinary continence.

Female pelvic floor. Several structures within the female pelvic floor contribute to continence by providing support to the lower urinary tract. They are the endopelvic fascia, levator ani, perineal membrane, and external anal sphincter.[28,29] The endopelvic fascia connects the various pelvic organs to the bony pelvis. It is distinct from other fascia within the body in that it contains collagen, elastin, *and* smooth muscle. Because the entire endopelvic fascia is not visible during surgery, portions have been named as if they were true ligaments. Although these condensations of endopelvic fascia clearly have significance from a surgical perspective, it is important to remember that this aspect of the pelvic floor is a functional unit compared with the network of true ligaments that lends flexible support to the bladder and urethra of both women and men (Table 2-2).

The primary supportive structure of the female pelvic floor is the levator ani muscle (Plate 10). The levator ani is a U-shaped muscle that attaches anteriorly to the paired pubic bones and laterally to the ischial spines and the arcus tendineus. Like the endopelvic fascia, the levator ani may be subdivided into smaller muscles including the iliococcygeus and the pubococcygeus, but it is best conceptualized as a single functional muscle from the perspective of continence nursing. The levator ani is the primary supportive structure for the bladder base and urethra. It is often misrepresented in anatomic depiction as a bowl or hammock that hangs loosely when supporting the pelvic viscera including the lower urinary tract. However, the levator ani is better represented as a floor that does not sag or bulge as the viscera move down on it when the woman assumes a standing position.

The anal sphincter and the perineal membrane also provide support to the lower urinary tract. The perineal membrane is a triangular fibrous structure that attaches the perineal body to the pubic bones and thereby limits descent of the pelvic viscera. This triangular membrane spans the anterior pelvis, with the exception of a central hole through which the vagina and urethra pass. Like the endopelvic fascia, the perineal membrane plays a secondary role in support of the lower urinary tract.

Male pelvic floor. The male pelvic floor also contains endopelvic fascia, the levator ani, and the anal sphincter that contribute to continence.[30,31] Less is known about the histology of endopelvic fascia in men compared with women; but it is clear that it also contains collagen, elastin, and smooth muscle. The endopelvic fascia in the male also consists of a reflection of retroperitoneal fascia. Its outer stratum

TABLE 2-2 Condensations of the Female Endopelvic Fascia

LIGAMENT	DESCRIPTION
Pubourethral ligaments	Condensations of endopelvic fascia that bridge lower, inner surface of symphysis pubis and middle of urethra
Urethropelvic ligaments	Endopelvic fascia providing support for bladder neck and proximal urethra
Vesicopelvic ligaments	Fascial condensations that attach to pelvic side walls providing lateral support to bladder base and pelvic side wall; loss of this fascial support creates a paravaginal wall defect
Cooper's ligaments	Condensation of connective tissue at the top of the crural arch from the inferior iliac to the pubic bone; provides support and structure for the floor of the inguinal canal
Broad ligament	Triangular fold of the peritoneum; supports uterus and fallopian tube
Round ligament	Passes from superior lateral angle of the uterus to the internal inguinal ring and supports uterus and fallopian tube
Uterosacral ligament (sacrouterine ligament, or cardinal-uterosacral complex)	Two short cords that pass from cervix toward sacrum; holds the cervix upward and backward and provides slant of uterus
Mackenrodt's ligament (cardinal ligament)	Condensation of uterosacral fascial complex; contributes to support of upper vagina, cervix, and uterus
Sacrospinous ligaments	Attach ischial spine to lateral aspect of sacrum and coccyx; used for repair of severe uterine prolapse
Arcus tendineus fasciae pelvis "white line"	Linear condensation extending from the pubic bone to the ischial spine; acts as important surgical landmark

From Doughty D: Urinary and Fecal Incontinence: Current Management Concepts, 3rd edition. St Louis: Mosby, 2006; p 30.

enfolds the inner surface of the pelvic muscles, its intermediate stratum embeds the pelvic organs in a protective layer of compressible fat, and its inner stratum enfolds part of the gastrointestinal tract and the bladder dome. As in the female, the levator ani (often subdivided into pubococcygeus and iliococcygeus) provides the primary support for the lower urinary tract. This muscle assumes a U shape similar to that seen in women, but it is larger and thicker, probably because of differing physiologic demands placed on the male pelvis compared with the female pelvis. The anal sphincter and perineal membrane contribute to pelvic support in men, but the existence of a distinct urogenital diaphragm remains controversial.

Continence in the adult. Urinary continence can be defined as the ability to postpone urination and to void based on physiologic, social, and cultural norms. Specifically, the individual should be able to postpone urination for at least 2 hours while awake and arise from sleep no more than once (if under 65 years of age) or twice (if over 65 years of age) to urinate. The continent person also should be able to engage in

physical activity without appreciable urine loss and to postpone urination despite a perceived urge to void. Deferral of micturition should be sustained until a socially appropriate location for urination is found.

A brief summary of continence physiology will help the reader synthesize the multiple, complex factors needed to maintain continence (Figure 2-13). As the bladder begins to fill after an episode of micturition, the detrusor is relaxed and the sphincter mechanism is closed. These events occur under neurologic modulation of the brain and brainstem micturition center; appropriate signals are carried to the bladder by sympathetic nuclei arising from spinal roots at T10 to L2. Further bladder filling stretches the bladder wall, stimulating afferent pathways in the pelvic and pudendal nerves within the detrusor and signaling the first urge to urinate. The processing of these afferent impulses within the brainstem and brain is not entirely understood, but it is likely that the thalamus and detrusor motor center play important roles. Continued filling leads to an increase in both the frequency and amplitude

NEURAL CONTROL OF THE BLADDER

Neural control of urinary bladder requires integration of central and peripheral nervous system and detrusor muscles.

The following brain centers act as a unit to provide stability (voluntary control) of urination. Dysfunction of any one brain center is likely to cause instability (loss of detrusor muscle control):
• Cerebral cortex
(location of detrusor motor center)
• Thalamus
• Hypothalamus
• Basal ganglia
• Cerebellum

In the brainstem, the dorsal tegmentum of pons is the origin of the detrusor reflex and the coordination center between the detrusor and sphincter muscles.

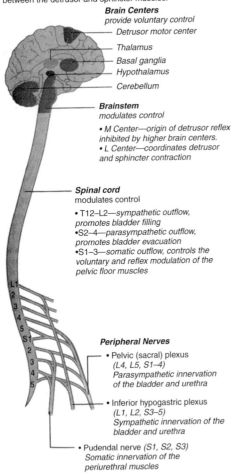

Brain Centers
provide voluntary control
— *Detrusor motor center*
— *Thalamus*
— *Basal ganglia*
— *Hypothalamus*
— *Cerebellum*

Brainstem
modulates control
• *M Center—origin of detrusor reflex inhibited by higher brain centers.*
• *L Center—coordinates detrusor and sphincter contraction*

Spinal cord
modulates control
• *T12–L2—sympathetic outflow, promotes bladder filling*
•*S2–4—parasympathetic outflow, promotes bladder evacuation*
•*S1–3—somatic outflow, controls the voluntary and reflex modulation of the pelvic floor muscles*

Peripheral Nerves
• *Pelvic (sacral) plexus (L4, L5, S1–4) Parasympathetic innervation of the bladder and urethra*
• *Inferior hypogastric plexus (L1, L2, S3–5) Sympathetic innervation of the bladder and urethra*
• *Pudendal nerve (S1, S2, S3) Somatic innervation of the periurethral muscles*

Fig. 2-13 Neurologic control of the detrusor muscle.

(intensity) of afferent signals, causing a growing perception of urinary urgency. In addition to bladder volume, the perception of urinary urgency is influenced by emotions such as anxiety or fear. Stimulation of spinal interneurons also impacts perceptions of urgency. For example, stroking the perineal skin facilitates urgency (and micturition) whereas stimulation of the genitalia is inhibitory.

Based on multiple factors including the intensity of urinary urgency and the availability of a toileting facility, the continent adult ultimately makes the decision to empty the bladder by micturition. The micturition reflex pathway is best described as spinobulbospinal (spine to brainstem to spine).[32] Voiding begins with relaxation of the pelvic muscles and by activation of the sacral parasympathetic pathways that reflexively inhibit the urethral sphincter mechanism while activating a contraction of the detrusor. The brain temporarily reverses its typically inhibitory influence on the brainstem by means of unknown mechanisms, and the brainstem stimulates a detrusor contraction by means of activation of parasympathetic (muscarinic) receptors in the bladder wall. The brainstem also inhibits urethral sphincter tone by means of spinal reflex pathways. Voiding ensues and continues until the bladder is completely emptied of its contents and the cycle starts again. If the individual wishes to discontinue voiding before complete bladder emptying, the sensorimotor cortex is activated, leading first to interruption of the urinary stream owing to contraction of the periurethral and pelvic floor muscles and ultimately because of inhibition of the detrusor contraction and micturition reflex.

Three main processes are responsible for continence in the adult: anatomic integrity of the urinary system, control of the detrusor, and competence of the urethral sphincter mechanism.[21,33]

From a urodynamic perspective, the entire urinary system, from glomerulus to urethral meatus, can be regarded as a single tube. In order to maintain continence, this tube must remain anatomically intact so that urine is expelled only by way of the urethra and only during voluntary micturition. Two conditions, ectopia and fistula, occasionally violate this integrity, allowing urinary leakage from an extraurethral source. Chapter 6 discusses these two conditions in detail.

Control of the detrusor muscle. Urinary continence also requires control of the detrusor muscle.

The term *stable detrusor* has been used to describe voluntary control over bladder contractions necessary for the maintenance of continence.[34] Detrusor control represents the effect of multiple modulating areas of the brain, spinal cord, and peripheral nervous system. It also reflects aspects of the detrusor smooth muscle that distinguish it from the upper urinary tracts or gastrointestinal system (Plate 11).

Advances in positron emission tomography (PET) and single-photon emission computed tomography (SPECT) scans have dramatically enhanced our understanding of how the brain modulates lower urinary tract function and continence.[35] PET and SPECT scans provide a noninvasive method for imaging blood flow (indicating metabolic activity) during bladder filling and storage and during micturition. In most instances, insights gained from PET or SPECT scans have confirmed prior research using animal models, but these techniques have also led to new insights about phenomena such as urgency, a perception that is difficult to measure in an animal model. These scans have revealed that several areas of the brain modulate bladder function.[32] A detrusor motor area is located within the superomedial area of each frontal lobe. It is active during bladder filling, but its activity is diminished as the individual experiences stronger desires to urinate.[36] The cingulate gyrus, which regulates sensory input and emotions and emotional responses to pain, and the thalamus are thought to act as a relay center for sensory afferents from the bladder. Components of the extrapyramidal nervous system (basal ganglia and cerebellum), the limbic system (insula), and the hypothalamus are also involved with motor function of the bladder and hypothesized to exert a net inhibitory influence on the detrusor reflex, possibly preventing premature (overactive) detrusor contractions until the individual voluntarily prepares for urination.

PET and SPECT scans also provide insights into the influence of modulating centers in the brain on micturition.[37] Despite clear and consistent evidence from animal model and human studies revealing that the brain is actively involved in inhibition of detrusor contractions in the continent adult, little is known about its role in micturition. It was previously thought that modulating centers in the brain somehow removed inhibitory influence over the brainstem, resulting in a micturition reflex, but more recent studies in humans demonstrate activity in multiple areas of the brain, including the cerebral cortex, cingulate gyrus, thalamus, and cerebellum. Although the full significance of these findings is not known, they do support speculations arising from animal models that the brain is involved in the activation and maintenance of the detrusor contraction essential for effective evacuation of urine.

The brainstem is particularly significant to bladder function.[38] The periaqueductal gray matter is active during bladder filling/storage and micturition.[35] It has multiple connections to higher brain structures, including the cerebral cortex and cingulate gyrus, and to the other structures in the brainstem known to modulate lower urinary tract function. These centers include the pontine micturition center. It was originally described by Barrington in 1921 using an animal model,[39] and newer research findings tend to strengthen the accuracy of this original research. A micturition center is located in the dorsolateral region of the pons. It coordinates detrusor and striated sphincter responses to bladder filling and micturition. Under the influence of the pontine micturition center, the striated muscle of the urethral sphincter mechanism reflexively relaxes during micturition and contracts during bladder filling/storage, promoting urethral closure. The clinical significance of the pontine micturition center is illustrated in patients who experience a complete spinal cord injury causing neurogenic detrusor overactivity and uncoordinated contraction of the striated sphincter muscle during voiding (detrusor sphincter dyssynergia).

The spinal cord influences detrusor control through neurons located within the sympathetic and parasympathetic nervous systems.[34] Sympathetic neurons located at spinal levels T10 to L2 promote bladder storage. Stimulation of these nerves, under the influence of modulating centers in the brainstem and brain, excites β_3-adrenergic receptors in the detrusor muscle that promote relaxation and further filling and storage. In addition, excitation of α-adrenergic receptors in the proximal urethra and bladder neck causes urethral closure. This effect is postulated to inhibit detrusor contractions via reflex pathways within the spine. Stimulation of the parasympathetic nervous system promotes micturition. Parasympathetic neurons are located within sacral spinal segments 2 to 4; stimulation of these neurons under the influence of modulating areas in the brain and brainstem causes detrusor contraction and sphincter relaxation. Damage to these neurons arrests the nervous stimulus for detrusor contraction and leads to areflexia (paralysis) of this muscle with subsequent urinary retention.

Directions from the brain and brainstem micturition center are transmitted to the bladder via peripheral nerves. Sympathetic stimuli reach the bladder primarily through lumbar sympathetic nerves, and parasympathetic stimuli reach the bladder primarily through the pelvic plexus. Each of these nerves contains afferent (sensory) as well as efferent (motor) axons transmitting critical information to the central nervous system concerning the volume of urine within the bladder and the status of the bladder wall.

Afferent and efferent signals rely on neurotransmitters to relay messages to and from the bladder spine, brainstem, and brain.[32,34] These neurotransmitters facilitate the ongoing communication needed for the individual to sense bladder filling, the desire to urinate, and act on this desire by micturition or postponing micturition until a socially acceptable time and location. Relatively little is known about neurotransmitters in the brain and their influence on bladder function. Research using animal models indicates that glutamic acid may act as the primary neurotransmitter in the brain. Other transmitters thought to influence these modulating areas include serotonin, γ-aminobutyric acid (GABA), dopamine, acetylcholine, adenosine triphosphate (ATP), and nitric oxide. Within the spinal cord and periphery, preganglionic nerve synapses respond to acetylcholine. These receptors are distinguished from peripheral cholinergic receptors as nicotinic rather than muscarinic. This distinction is important from both pharmacologic and clinical perspectives since drugs capable of blocking nicotinic cholinergic receptors, such as curare, produce respiratory paralysis as a side effect, whereas muscarinic cholinergic blockers, such as oxybutynin, reduce overactive contractions without compromising respiratory or cardiac functions.

In addition to the modulating centers in the central and peripheral nervous systems, the detrusor muscle itself contributes to continence. Because most smooth muscle within the body is not under volitional control, it is often called an "involuntary muscle." While this description is accurate of smooth

muscle of the small bowel, ureter, or renal pelvis, it is fortunately not accurate when applied to the detrusor. Several characteristics account for our ability to control this unique smooth muscle.[33,34] The smooth muscle of the bladder contains many more nerve receptors than do smooth muscle bundles within the ureter or gastrointestinal system. In addition, the smooth muscle bundles of the bladder lack the large number of close (gap) junctions characteristic of the ureter or gastrointestinal tract. Gap junctions in visceral smooth muscle allow rapid propagation of a peristaltic contraction independent of nervous stimulation. A similar situation in the bladder would render continence impossible because it would not allow the person to postpone a detrusor contraction after the bladder wall stretched in response to bladder filling. Fortunately, the small number of gap junctions in the detrusor smooth muscle, in combination with the high ratio of nerve endings to muscle cells (nearly 1:1), ensures that a detrusor contraction sufficient for micturition occurs *only* under voluntary control.

Neurotransmitters within the bladder wall are the final messengers ensuring detrusor control (Table 2-3).[32,34] The primary excitatory neurotransmitter of the detrusor is acetylcholine, which acts on specific receptors within the bladder wall to cause muscle contraction under nervous control. Acetylcholine acts on two principal types of receptors: muscarinic and nicotinic. Muscarinic receptors are found in smooth muscle throughout the body, including the gastrointestinal tract, cardiovascular system, eyes, and salivary glands.[38] Five types of muscarinic receptors have been identified, but the detrusor muscle contains only two types: M_2 and M_3. M_3 comprises only 20% of the cholinergic receptors within the bladder wall, but stimulation of these receptors leads to the sustained and forceful phasic contraction needed for micturition. Approximately 80% of the cholinergic receptors in the bladder wall are M_2, but their influence on detrusor muscle tone is subtler. Excitation of M_2 receptors does not cause a forceful contraction; instead, it increases detrusor muscle tone by partially inhibiting the relaxing effects of adrenergic stimulation.

Other neurotransmitters influence detrusor control.[32,34] Norepinephrine acts on β$_3$-adrenergic receptors in the bladder wall to promote detrusor relaxation and bladder filling. ATP is found in nonadrenergic,

TABLE 2-3 Major Postganglionic Neurotransmitters of the Lower Urinary Tract

NEUROTRANSMITTER	LOCATION/RECEPTOR TYPE	PHYSIOLOGIC EFFECT
Acetylcholine	Detrusor/muscarinic	Contraction (voiding)
Norepinephrine	Detrusor/β-adrenergic	Relaxation (filling/storage)
	Proximal urethra/α-adrenergic	Contraction (sphincter closure, filling/storage)
Adenosine triphosphate	Detrusor/nonadrenergic, noncholinergic (NANC)	Contraction (acts as cotransmitter with acetylcholine)
Vasoactive intestinal polypeptide, substance P, calcitonin gene-related peptide (CGRP), nitric oxide synthase		Afferent transmission of lower urinary tract sensations

noncholinergic (NANC) receptors. Stimulation of these purinergic receptors facilitates detrusor muscle contraction, but it must be remembered that cholinergic receptors remain the predominant neurologic stimulus in the bladder. Other substances that are postulated to act as neurotransmitters in the lower urinary tract include vasoactive intestinal polypeptide (VIP), substance P, CGRP, and nitric oxide synthase. These substances are thought to be involved with bladder sensations, including urgency, pressure, pain, or temperature.

Sphincter mechanism competence. The urethral sphincter is traditionally defined only in terms of its muscular components.[21,33,40] An internal sphincter is described at the bladder neck, and an external sphincter is located within the mid and distal urethra in women and the membranous urethra in men. However, such conceptualizations fail to recognize the significance of compressive elements of the sphincter and the relevance of the rhabdosphincter. Because of these limitations, the urethral sphincter should be conceptualized as a unified mechanism, comprising elements of compression, elements of tension, and supportive structures (Box 2-2). During bladder filling and storage, these factors interact to produce a watertight seal against leakage. Even more remarkably, this flexible structure rapidly reverses its role during micturition, serving as a conduit for the expulsion of urine.

The compressive elements of the sphincter mechanism include a soft urethral mucosa, glycosaminoglycans produced by this epithelium, and the vascular cushion formed by the lamina propria (Figure 2-14).[40,41] The epithelial mucosa of the

BOX 2-2 Elements of the Urethral Sphincter Mechanism

Elements of Compression
Softness of the urethral epithelium
Mucosal secretions
Submucosal vascular cushion

Elements of Tension
Smooth muscle of bladder neck and proximal urethra
Rhabdosphincter
Periurethral striated muscle

Supportive Structures
Endopelvic fascia
Levator ani muscle
Perineal membrane

urethra must be soft and flexible to maintain the watertight seal needed for continence. The remarkable flexibility of this mucosa is demonstrated by the passage of a catheter, which allows urine to pass through its lumen while preventing leakage of urine *around* the catheter, even though the urethra has been significantly deformed by the passage of this relatively stiff instrument. Mucoidlike secretions contribute to sphincter compression because they raise the surface tension of the urethral wall, filling in microscopic gaps left when the epithelium closes between urination episodes. The concept of the glycosaminoglycan and its contribution to surface tension is illustrated by unrolling a nonlubricated condom and trimming its closed end. When shaken, the walls of the condom fall apart. However, when the condom is immersed in a water-soluble lubricant analogous to the secretions of the

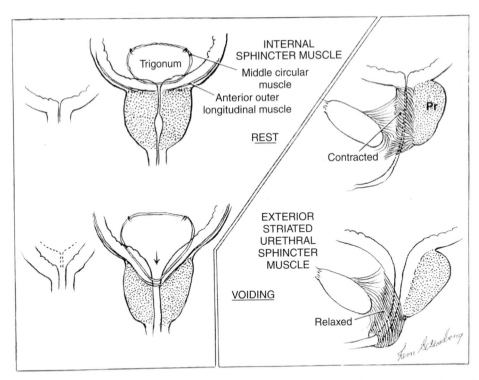

Fig. 2-14 Smooth and striated muscles of the male urethral sphincter mechanism. (From O'Donnell P: *Urinary Incontinence.* St Louis: Mosby, 1997.)

human urethra, increased surface tension causes the walls to cling together. The third compressive element of the urethral sphincter mechanism is the vascular cushion of the lamina propria. This rich network of arteries and veins provides a noncompressible cushion of blood that transmits closing forces acting on the urethra, including abdominal pressure and tension from the muscular elements of the sphincter.

Although elements of urethral compression are necessary for maintaining a watertight seal, they alone will not prevent urinary leakage in the presence of gravity or physical exertion. Instead, sphincter closure under stress is achieved by active contraction of smooth and striated (i.e., skeletal) muscle within the urethral wall.

In men smooth muscle bundles encircle the bladder neck, forming what is traditionally referred to as the internal sphincter.[34] Smooth muscle tone of the bladder neck contributes to continence and prevents retrograde movement of semen into the bladder during ejaculation. Additional smooth muscle bundles arranged in a longitudinal fashion extend into the prostatic urethra and also contribute to sphincter closure. The rhabdosphincter is a set of specialized

Ω-shaped skeletal muscle fibers located within the membranous urethra.[42] The fibers of the rhabdosphincter are notably small and exclusively slow twitch (type 1), two characteristics that render them ideal for maintaining prolonged periods of tone needed to ensure continence between episodes of urination.[43] In addition to the smooth and striated muscle intrinsic to the urethral wall, periurethral striated muscle contributes to urethral closure in men and women.[44] Unlike the rhabdosphincter, the periurethral striated muscles represent a combination of slow and rapid twitch fibers that provide additional protection in response to intense physical exertion or a sudden increase in abdominal pressure (Figure 2-15).

Smooth muscle and skeletal muscle combine to form tension elements of the female urethral sphincter as well.[28,29,40] Longitudinal smooth muscle bundles observed at the base of the bladder extend nearly the entire length of the urethra. In addition, circularly arranged smooth muscle is found at the bladder neck, but its contribution to continence remains controversial. A rhabdosphincter is located in the middle third of the female urethra; it is also called the

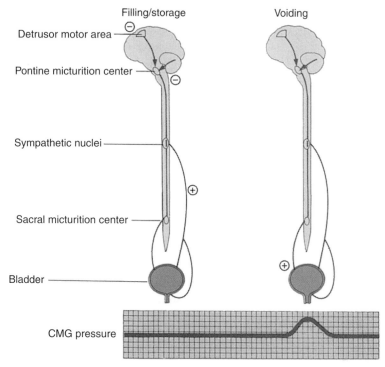

Fig. 2-15 Phases of bladder function (i.e., filling, storage, and micturition) are represented by a cystometrogram. Note the varying influences of major modulating centers in the brain, brainstem, and spine.

sphincter urethrae. Two other muscles, comprising primarily slow twitch fibers but containing some fast twitch elements, also contribute to sphincter function in the female. The compressor urethrae originates at the perineal membrane, and the urethrovaginal sphincter extends further to encircle the vaginal wall.

The structures that support the urethra and bladder base are critical to continence, particularly in the female.[28,29] The levator ani, endopelvic fascia, perineal membrane, and anal sphincter each provide support to the bladder base and urethra, maintaining the bladder base in an intraabdominal position. This position is significant because it ensures optimal position for urethral closure under the influence of the muscular elements of the sphincter mechanism and because it promotes transmission of abdominal forces to the urethral lumen. Descent of this bladder base is associated with sphincter incompetence (stress urinary incontinence), even in the absence of detectable deficiency of the intrinsic muscular elements of the sphincter.[40]

Like the detrusor, the urethral smooth muscle is primarily under neurologic control, and individual muscle cells respond to excitation from local nerve receptors (see Table 2-3).[34] The smooth muscle of the bladder neck and proximal urethra in both genders contains an abundance of α-adrenergic receptors. However, in contrast to the detrusor, stimulation of these receptors causes contraction of these muscle bundles and urethral sphincter closure. It has also been postulated that cholinergic innervation of urethral smooth muscle may contribute to urethral funneling during micturition. The rhabdosphincter (sphincter urethrae in women) receives triple innervation in certain animals, but it is dually innervated in humans, with somatic innervation from the pudendal nerve and sympathetic receptors arising from the inferior hypogastric plexus. The periurethral and pelvic floor muscles, including the levator ani, receive somatic innervation from the levator ani nerve. The roots of this nerve arise from the sacral spinal cord at levels S2 to S4. Reflexive responses (contraction during bladder filling and relaxation during urination) occur under the influence of the brainstem micturition center but can be overridden as demonstrated by abrupt interruption of micturition caused by contraction of the pelvic floor and periurethral striated muscles when a person is startled during urination. Voluntary control of the periurethral and pelvic floor muscle is mediated by the sensorimotor nucleus of the brain. It sends signals to the pelvic muscles by way of the pyramidal tracts of the spine.

MALE GENITALIA AND REPRODUCTIVE SYSTEM

The male reproductive system comprises the penis, scrotum, testis, epididymis, vas deferens, prostate, seminal vesicles, and ejaculatory ducts (Plate 12). These organs are responsible for procreation, including generation of an erection for vaginal penetration, production of sperm-containing semen capable of fertilizing the ovum, and ejaculation of sperm and semen into the woman's reproductive tract.

Penis

The penis is a cylindrical organ attached to the body by its root, which inserts into the pelvic floor beneath the symphysis pubis.[45] The root of the penis is attached to the pubic rami and abdomen wall by a reflection of Scarpa's fascia and the suspensory ligament. The internal architecture of the penis is characterized by three elongated structures: the paired corpora cavernosa and the corpora spongiosum that surrounds the urethra (Figure 2-16). These bodies contain a system formed

of small sinuses (vascular spaces) capable of engorging with blood during tumescence. The sinusoids are lined with endothelium, and their walls are made of smooth muscle bundles, elastin fibers, and collagen. Within these erectile bodies are numerous arterioles, venules, and nerves needed to control blood flow during an erection. At their proximal ends, the corpora cavernosa begin at the crura. These relatively noncompliant structures gradually change into compliant corporal tissue capable of erection as they extend below the pubic arch and into the pendulous portion of the penis. The paired corpora cavernosa do not extend the entire length of the penis; instead, they terminate within the glans penis, before the urethra ends at its meatus.

Each of the three cavernosal bodies is enclosed within a strong fibrous membrane, called the tunica albuginea, and all three are encased within a fibrous structure called Buck's fascia. The tunica albuginea consists mainly of collagen that surrounds the paired corpora cavernosa, and it forms a complete septum at the level of the crura. However, this septum becomes incomplete distal to the pubic arch. A loose covering of skin that lacks any subcutaneous fat surrounds Buck's fascia. Redundant integument, called the foreskin, covers the glans penis, which remains moist unless the foreskin is removed by circumcision.

Two skeletal (striated) muscles are significant for erectile and ejaculatory function, the ischiocavernosus and the bulbocavernosus. The ischiocavernosus covers

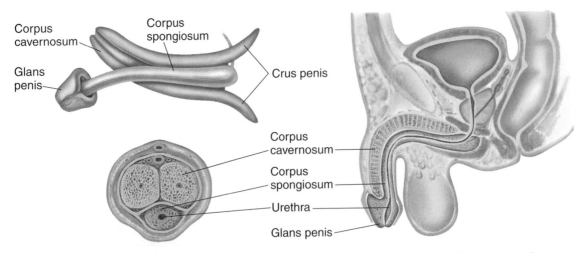

Fig. 2-16 Anatomy of penis showing corporal bodies and urethra. (From Seidel H, Ball J, Dains J, Benedict GW: Mosby's Guide to Physical Examination, 6th edition. St Louis: Mosby, 2006.)

the crura and attaches to the ischial tuberosity and to the pubic rami. The bulbocavernosus arises from the median raphe and the perineal body, encircles the urethral bulb and the adjacent corpus spongiosum, and attaches to the tunica albuginea.

Branches of the internal pudendal artery primarily supply arterial blood for the penis (Plate 13).[45,46] One of these branches, the bulbourethral artery, supplies the proximal urethral bulb and adjacent mucus-producing glands. Another branch, the dorsal artery, traverses the dorsal aspect of the penis just beneath Buck's fascia. Branches from this artery are primarily responsible for the blood needed for penile erection, although it usually shares this responsibility with the circumflex arteries. The cavernous (deep) artery also participates in erectile function and provides for nutritional needs of local tissues. It traverses the dorsomedial aspect of the paired corpora cavernosa before diving into the center of these bodies. Throughout its intracavernous course, branches of the cavernosal artery form the tortuous helicine arteries that empty into the sinusoidal spaces of the erectile tissues.

The venous system of the penis is typically divided into three functional units: superficial, intermediate, and deep (see Plate 13). The superficial system comprises multiple veins that run on the dorsolateral surface of the penis, just superficial to Buck's fascia.

They drain blood from the penile skin and underlying fascia. The intermediate venous system includes two sets of veins important to erectile function, the deep dorsal and the circumflex. The deep drainage system includes the cavernous and crural veins, which unite to form one or two larger main cavernous veins, found in the penile hilum, that are also important to erectile function. Deoxygenated blood is ultimately drained by way of the internal pudendal vein that empties into the internal vein.

Erectile Physiology. Recent advances in our understanding of the physiology of penile erections have significantly changed our understanding and management of erectile dysfunction (impotence).[47] These advances primarily involve our understanding of the local events that occur during penile erection. During the flaccid state, the smooth muscle of local arterioles and the sinusoids of the cavernosal bodies are in a mildly contracted state under the influence of sympathetic nervous modulation (Figure 2-17, A). Psychological or other stimuli trigger the release of specific neurotransmitters from nerve receptors within the corpora cavernosa. Release of these neurotransmitters causes relaxation of the smooth muscle within local arterioles and the sinusoidal spaces of the corporal bodies. As a result, arterial blood flow increases, which fills the sinusoids and causes an increase in penile length and circumference. At a certain point,

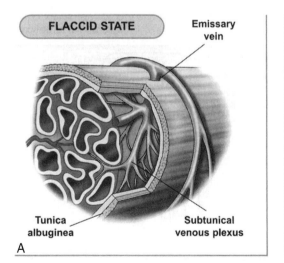
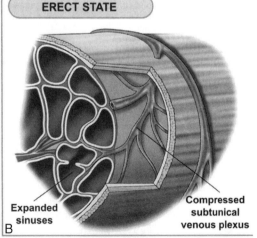

Fig. 2-17 A, Subtunical plexus, flaccid state. **B,** Compression of veins with erection. (**A,** From Wein A, Kavonssi L, Novick K: Campbell-Walsh Urology, 9th edition. Philadelphia: Saunders, 2007; **B,** From Lue TF, Guiliano F, Khoury S, Rosen R: Clinical Manual of Sexual Medicine: Sexual Dysfunction in Men. Paris, France, Health Publications, 2007. In Wein A, Kavoussi L, Novick A: Campbell-Walsh Urology, 9th edition. Philadelphia, Saunders, 2007.)

sinusoidal filling is limited by compression of the sub-tunical venous plexuses between the tunica albuginea and peripheral sinusoids. This causes further engorgement of blood that compresses the emissary veins (see Figure 2-17, B). At this point, the penis becomes rigid (erect) and intracavernous pressure reaches approximately 100 mm Hg as the erectile tissue fills the limited space allowed by its fascial coverings. Intracavernous pressure may rise to suprasystolic levels (as high as 200 mm Hg) with contraction of the ischiocavernous muscle, although this rigid erection state is more transient than the usual erect state achieved without contraction of this accessory muscle.

Detumescence (return to the flaccid state) occurs in three phases. In the first phase, a brief rise in intracavernosal pressure occurs as the smooth muscles of the arterioles and sinusoids regain some of their tone. This is followed by a longer, second phase characterized by a slow decline in intracavernosal pressure as the venous channels open and arterial blood flow returns to baseline values. At some point, venous outflow reaches its baseline state, and intracavernosal pressure rapidly falls to pre-erection values.

Since these events rely on the release of local neurotransmitters, it follows that the nervous system modulates erectile function.[48] In the human, both autonomic (i.e., sympathetic and parasympathetic) and somatic nerves modulate penile erections. Sympathetic innervation arises from neural roots from the tenth thoracic to the second lumbar spinal segments. These fibers reach the penis by way of the superior hypogastric, inferior mesenteric, and splanchnic nerve plexuses. Parasympathetic innervation arises from neural roots at sacral spinal segments 2, 3, and 4, and it reaches the penis by way of the pelvic plexus. Afferent somatic pathways originate from sensory nerves in the penile skin, glans penis, urethra, and corpora cavernosa. They reach the central nervous system by way of the dorsal nerve that joins other local nerves to form the pudendal nerves before entering the spine at Onuf's nucleus, located at sacral segments 2 to 4. In addition to somatic sensations (e.g., touch, temperature, and pain), the dorsal nerve also carries autonomic impulses to and from the central nervous system, explaining its modulating role in both penile erection and ejaculation.

Similar to the bladder, erectile function is modulated by specific areas of the brain. In the human, elements of the limbic system, including the medial preoptic area and areas of the hypothalamus, including the amygdala and paraventricular nuclei, act as the primary integrative centers for sexual drive and penile erection.[47-49] Functional scans of the brain reveal that areas within the cerebral cortex and cerebellum are involved in sexual arousal, and the cerebral cortex and limbic system are involved in the maintenance of an erection. The hypothalamus was also found to be involved with the maintenance of a penile erection, demonstrating physiologic differences in arousal and maintenance (plateau) phases of male sexual response.[49a] These physiologic responses support psychologic observations that male sexual response involves both cognitive and emotional responses and provide evidence contradicting cultural myths that sexual arousal is a merely mechanical response to specific stimuli.

Several central and peripheral neurotransmitters are significant to erectile function (Table 2-4).[48,50] In the brain and brainstem, stimulation of dopaminergic and adrenergic receptors appear to promote sexual drive while serotonergic receptors appear to inhibit erectile activity. At the level of the penis, norepinephrine increases smooth muscle tone in the sinusoids and local arterioles, promoting flaccidity. Endothelin, a potent vasoconstrictor produced by the endothelial cells of the corpora cavernosa, also plays a role in detumescence. Although acetylcholine is released from parasympathetic (muscarinic) receptors in the corporal bodies and local arteries, it is not the neurotransmitter primarily responsible for initiating or maintaining an erection. Instead, it appears to play an important but secondary role as a stimulus for the release of nitric oxide from endothelial cells. It is the release of nitric oxide from NANC receptors that increases the production of cyclic guanosine monophosphate (cGMP), which is primarily responsible for the smooth muscle relaxation essential for penile erection.

Other substances are known to play a modulating role in erectile activity. Testosterone was once postulated to play an essential role in penile erection. However, more recent data show that while testosterone promotes libido and enhances erectile activity, it is not essential for erections in adult men with otherwise mature and functioning reproductive organs.[50] Additional hormones can affect erectile activity. For example, excess production of prolactin, a hormone present in both genders but particularly

TABLE 2-4 Major Neurotransmitters Modulating Erectile Function in the Male

NEUROTRANSMITTER	LOCATION	PHYSIOLOGIC EFFECT
Norepinephrine	Erectile tissue of corpora cavernosa	Smooth muscle contraction, reduced blood flow, and flaccidity
Acetylcholine	Erectile tissue of corpora cavernosa	*Indirectly* promotes erection by stimulating production of nitric oxide and endothelin
Vasoactive intestinal polypeptide	Erectile tissue of corpora cavernosa	*Indirectly* promotes erection by stimulating production of nitric oxide and endothelin
Nitric oxide*	Erectile tissue of corpora cavernosa	Smooth muscle relaxation directly promotes erection
Endothelin	Erectile tissue of corpora cavernosa	Smooth muscle contraction promotes detumescence
Dopamine	Brain, brainstem	Promotes sexual drive, erectile function
Serotonin	Brain, brainstem	Inhibits sexual drive, erectile function

*Primary postganglionic neurotransmitter for erection.

significant for women during lactation, suppresses erectile function in men.[51]

Based on this understanding of erectile physiology, it is possible to describe three types of erections.[48] Psychogenic erections occur when sexually provocative stimuli from higher brain centers are integrated into erectile activity in the medial preoptic area and paraventricular nucleus of the hypothalamus, leading to inhibition of sympathetic tone and activation of the smooth muscle relaxation under the indirect influence of acetylcholine and the direct influence of nitric oxide. Psychogenic erections are independent of testosterone, although this androgenic hormone enhances libido and subsequent sexual drive. In contrast, a reflexogenic erection is caused by tactile stimulation of the genitalia sending afferent signals to the brainstem and brain, directly activating autonomic nuclei within the spine to initiate the cascade of events leading to an erection. Unlike the psychogenic erection, these erections rely on the presence of testosterone. A third type of erection, the nocturnal erection occurring during rapid eye movement (REM) sleep, results from imperfectly understood mechanisms. Nocturnal erections are reduced in frequency, but not obliterated, when testosterone levels are diminished.[50]

Scrotum and Testes

The scrotum is a cutaneous sac that extends below the pubic bone and houses the testes, epididymis, and terminal portion of the testicular cord.[52] The skin of the scrotum is darker than surrounding integument;

it contains rugae (wrinkles), hair, and abundant sebaceous and sweat glands. A median raphe (ridge) divides the organ into two hemispheres, each containing a testis, epididymis, and terminal portion of the spermatic cord. Beneath the skin of the scrotum is the dartos muscle. This specialized muscle consists of smooth muscle bundles and elastin. Contraction of this muscle elevates the testes toward the abdomen. The primary purpose of the scrotum is to house the testes and to provide an environment favorable to spermatogenesis.

The paired testes are oval organs that lie in the cavity formed by the scrotum (Figure 2-18).[53,54] However, they originate in the abdomen and descend into the scrotum during embryogenesis. As a result, their arterial and venous blood supply and their lymphatic drainage arise from abdominal rather than perineal origins. A fibrous capsule with three layers (i.e., the outer tunica vaginalis, intermediate tunica albuginea, and inner tunica vasculosa) covers each testis. Its posterior border is distinguished by the C-shaped epididymis.

A cross section of the testis shows that it is divided into compartments. Each compartment contains many seminiferous tubules (the functional unit of the testis) and supporting interstitial tissue. The 600 to 1200 seminiferous tubules are quite long; if laid end to end they would stretch for approximately 250 m. The two ends of these U-shaped tortuous tubules are connected to shorter, straighter structures, the tubuli recti, which open into the rete testis. The rete testis, in turn, combines to form 6 to 15 ductuli

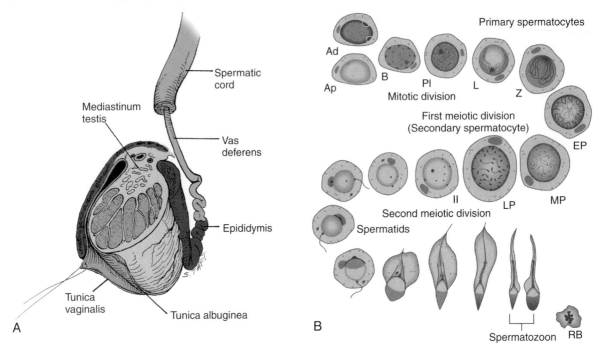

Fig. 2-18 A, Cross-sectional anatomy of testis. **B,** Cutout demonstrates process of spermatogenesis. (**A,** From Wein A, Kavoussi L, Novick A: Campbell-Walsh Urology, 9th edition. Philadelphia.: Saunders, 2007; **B,** from Hermo L, Clemant Y: How germ cells produce and what factors control their production. In Robaine B, Pryor J, Trasler J [eds]: Handbook of Andrology. New York: America Handbook of Andrology, 1995, pp. 13-15. Taken from Foldman L, Ausiello D: Cecil Medicine, 23rd edition. Philadelphia: Saunders, 2008.)

efferentes. These ductuli ultimately end in the epididymis. The interstitial tissue of the testis contains the local vascular and lymphatic network for the testis and specialized cells including Leydig cells, mast cells, and macrophages. Collectively, 85% of the testicular tissue is dedicated to sperm production.

The blood supply of the testis is unique, because the temperature of arterial blood must be cooled several degrees to support spermatogenesis. Cooling is attributable to several processes, including a countercurrent heat loss mechanism that exists between veins and arteries contained within the spermatic cord, and a slowing of blood flow within the dependent testes within their scrotal housing. The internal spermatic, deferential, and external spermatic arteries provide arterial blood to the testes. The internal spermatic artery arises from a branch of the abdominal aorta just below the renal artery. The veins of the testes are unusual because they do not travel with the corresponding arteries as they do in most organs. Instead, they are drained by the pampiniform venous plexus, which is found within the spermatic cord.

The testes are also characterized by their prominent lymphatic drainage that exits the organs by way of the spermatic cord. Lymphatic capillaries are abundant throughout the intertubular spaces of the testis. Because of its intraabdominal origin, lymphatic drainage from the testes empties into the preaortic as compared with the inguinal or pelvic nodes.

Testicular Physiology: Spermatogenesis

Spermatogenesis is defined as the production of spermatozoa within the seminiferous tubules of the testes.[53,54] It is regulated by a hormonal axis incorporating the hypothalamus, pituitary, testicular interstitium, and accessory, androgen-sensitive organs within the male reproductive tract (Figure 2-19). The process begins in the hypothalamus where luteinizing hormone–releasing hormone (LHRH) is produced and travels a short distance to the pituitary by way of a venous portal system. LHRH stimulates the secretion of follicle-stimulating hormone (FSH) and luteinizing hormone (LH). They enter the general circulation and act at receptor sites within the testis to produce

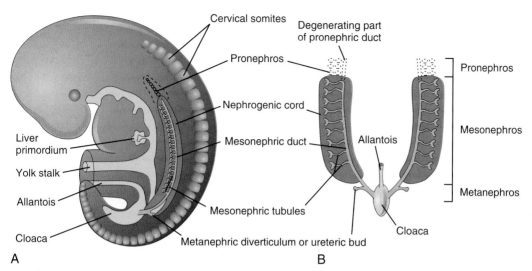

Cervical somites

Degenerating part
of pronephric duct

Pronephros

Pronephros

Nephrogenic cord

Mesonephros

Liver
primordium

Mesonephric duct

Allantois

Yolk stalk

Allantois

Metanephros

Mesonephric tubules

Cloaca

Cloaca

Metanephric diverticulum or ureteric bud

A

B

Plate 1 By the fifth week of embryogenesis, pronephroi have appeared and are beginning to degenerate. Mesonephric tubules provide some renal function, and the ureteric bud and metanephroi are beginning to develop into the mature upper urinary tracts. **A,** Lateral view demonstrates the location of the pronephroi in the cervical region, the mesonephroi adjacent to the developing spine, and the ureteric bud. **B,** Ventral view highlights the relative locations of the pronephros, mesonephros, and metanephros. (From Moore K, Persaud TVN: The Developing Human, 8th ed. Philadelphia: Saunders, 2008.)

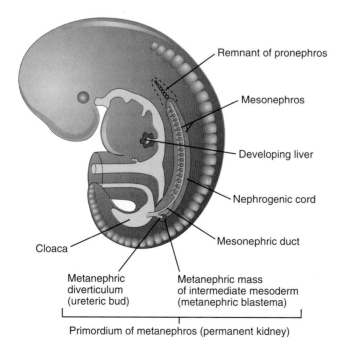

Remnant of pronephros

Mesonephros

Developing liver

Nephrogenic cord

Mesonephric duct

Cloaca

Metanephric
diverticulum
(ureteric bud)

Metanephric mass
of intermediate mesoderm
(metanephric blastema)

Primordium of metanephros (permanent kidney)

Plate 2 Metanephric ridge and ureteric bud around week 6 to 8. Note the remnant of the now degenerated pronephroi. (From Moore K, Persaud TVN: The Developing Human, 8th ed. Philadelphia: Saunders, 2008.)

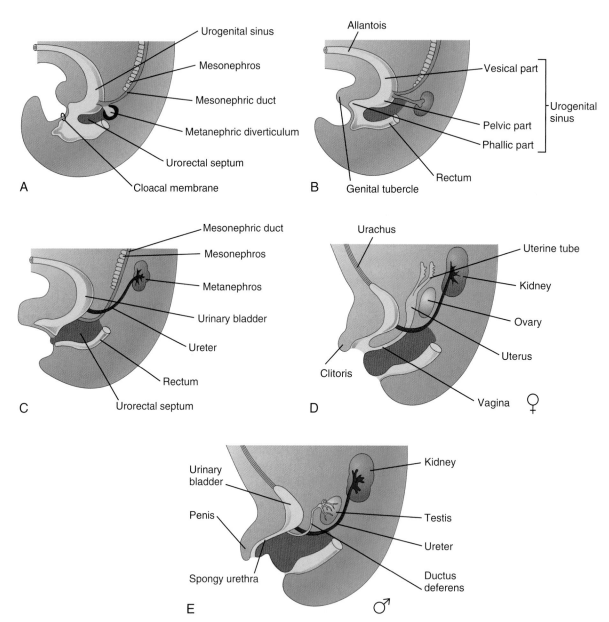

Plate 3 Prenatal development of the lower urinary tract. **A,** Lateral view of embryo around week 5, prior to differentiation of urogenital sinus and rectum. **B** and **C,** Further division and separation of anterior structures (lower urinary tract) and posterior rectum. **D,** Twelve-week female embryo demonstrates bladder and developing urethra, vagina, and rectum. **E,** Twelve-week male embryo demonstrates bladder and urethra, developing penis, and posterior rectum. (From Moore K, Persaud TVN: The Developing Human, 8th ed. Philadelphia: Saunders, 2008.)

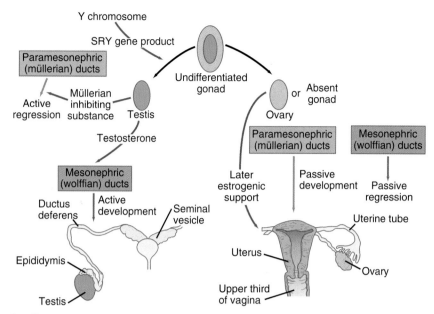

Plate 4 Differentiation of the male and female reproductive systems is determined by genetic gender (presence of X or Y chromosome with SRY gene product) and is influenced by specific substances including müllerian inhibiting substance, testosterone, and estrogen. (From Carlson B: Human Embryology & Developmental Biology, 3rd ed. St. Louis: Mosby, 2005.)

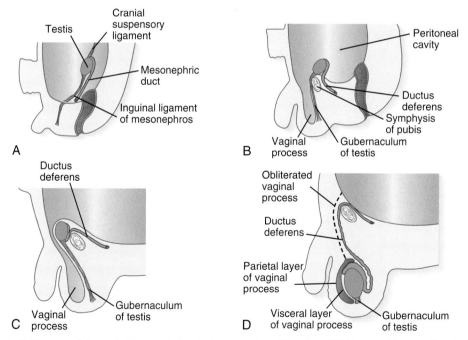

Plate 5 Descent of the testis from an abdominal to scrotal position. **A** and **B** illustrate Phase 1 of testicular descent. **A,** Around 8 weeks, the testis is in its primitive retroperitoneal location. **B,** Around week 12, note the extension of the vaginal process into the developing scrotum. **C,** Phase 2 (around month 7). The testis is at the inguinal ring just above the scrotum. **D,** Phase 3 (around term). The testis has moved into the scrotum. (From Carlson B: Human Embryology & Developmental Biology, 3rd ed. St. Louis: Mosby, 2005.)

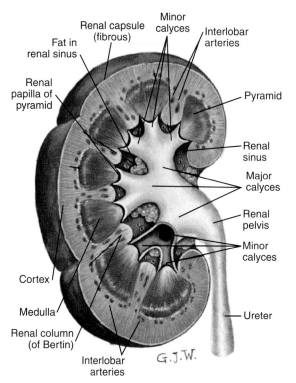

Fat in renal sinus
Renal capsule (fibrous)
Renal papilla of pyramid
Minor calyces
Interlobar arteries
Renal capsule (fibrous)
Pyramid
Renal sinus
Major calyces
Renal pelvis
Minor calyces
Cortex
Medulla
Renal column (of Bertin)
Ureter
Interlobar arteries

G.J.W.

Plate 6 Cross-section of the kidney showing basic structures. (From Brundage D: Renal Disorders. St. Louis: Mosby, 1992.)

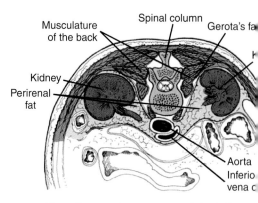

Musculature of the back
Spinal column
Gerota's fa
Kidney
Perirenal fat
Aorta
Inferio
vena c

Plate 7 Protective coverings of the kidneys.

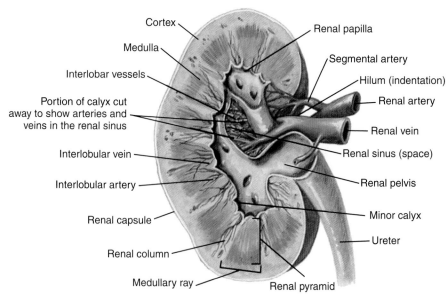

Cortex
Medulla
Renal papilla
Interlobar vessels
Segmental artery
Hilum (indentation)
Portion of calyx cut away to show arteries and veins in the renal sinus
Renal artery
Renal vein
Interlobular vein
Renal sinus (space)
Interlobular artery
Renal pelvis
Renal capsule
Minor calyx
Renal column
Ureter
Medullary ray
Renal pyramid

Plate 8 Blood supply of kidneys. (From Seeley RR, Stephens TD, Tate P: Anatomy and Physiology, 2nd ed. St. Louis: Mosby, 1986.)

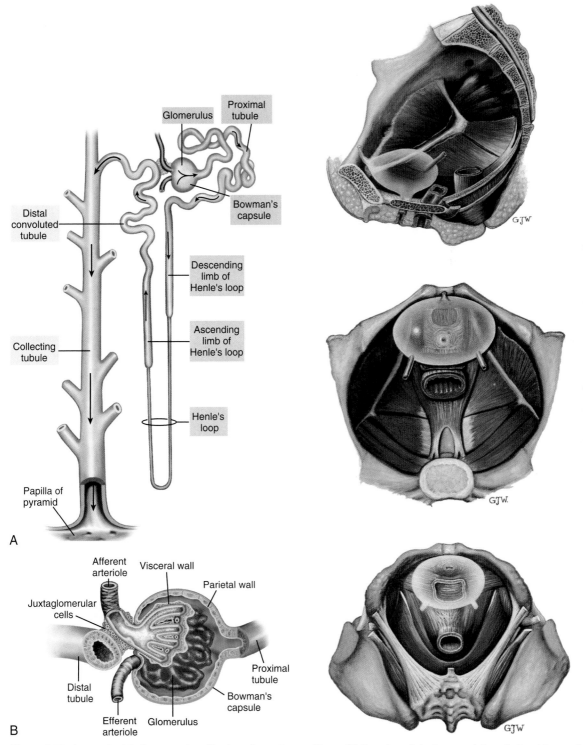

Plate 9 Nephron. **A,** Nephron and collecting duct. **B,** Glomerus. (From Thibodeau G, Patton K: Anatomy & Physiology, 6th ed. St. Louis: Mosby, 2007.)

Plate 10 Female pelvic floor and its relationship to the urinary bladder.

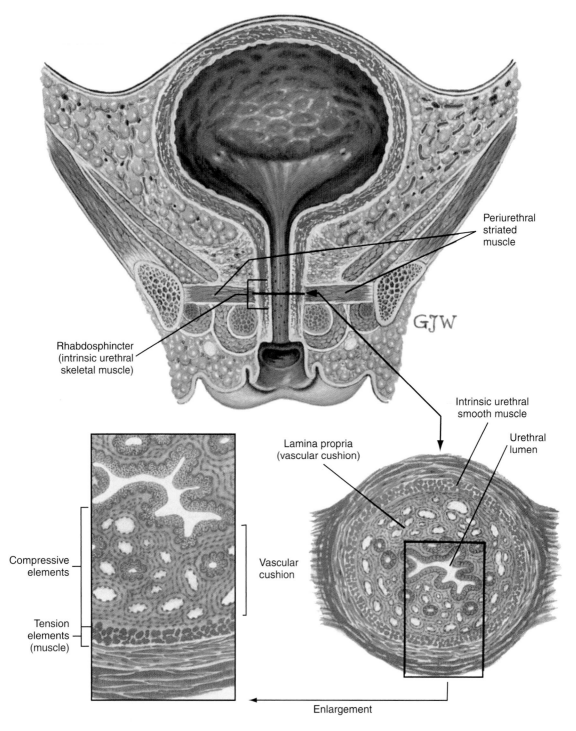

Plate 11 Urethral sphincter mechanism contains elements of compression and elements of tension.

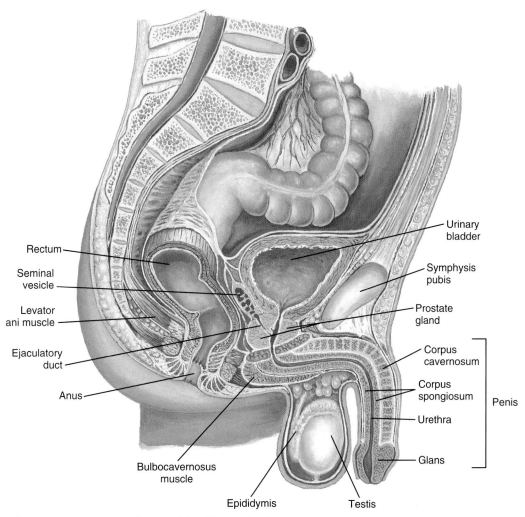

Rectum

Seminal
vesicle

Levator
ani muscle

Ejaculatory
duct

Anus

Bulbocavernosus
muscle

Epididymis

Testis

Urinary
bladder

Symphysis
pubis

Prostate
gland

Corpus
cavernosum

Corpus
spongiosum

Urethra

Glans

Penis

Plate 12 Cross-section of male pelvis with reproductive system. (From Seidel H, Ball J, Dains J, Benedict GW: Mosby's Guide to Physical Examination, 6th ed. St. Louis: Mosby, 2006.)

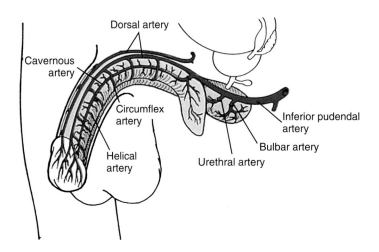

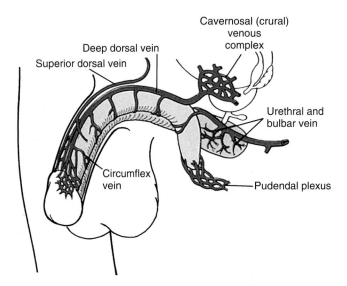

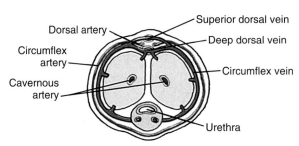

Plate 13 Vascular supply to penis.

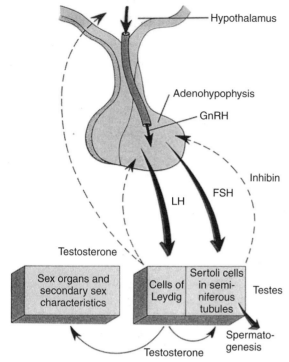

Fig. 2-19 The pituitary testicular axis regulates spermatogenesis and secondary sex characteristics of the male. (From Seeley RR, Stephens TD, Tate P: Anatomy and Physiology, 2nd edition. St Louis: Mosby, 1986.)

testosterone (T) and subsequent spermatogenesis. Within the testis, LH stimulates Leydig cells within the interstitium to produce T, and both FSH and LH stimulate Sertoli cells to create and support a microenvironment within the seminiferous tubule that supports and maintains spermatogenesis. Feedback loops that prevent excessive secretion of LHRH, FSH, and LH include increased serum levels of T and the presence of inhibin, which is produced in the testis.

The process of spermatogenesis is divided into three phases (Figure 2-19). During the first phase the stem cells (spermatogonia) enlarge and undergo *mitotic* divisions that lead to primary spermatocytes containing 92 chromosomes. A second phase is characterized by two consecutive *meiotic* divisions resulting in four spermatids containing the haploid number needed for fertilization of the ovum. A third phase, called spermiogenesis, consists of the transformation of the spermatid into the spermatozoon.

Specialized junctional complexes between the Sertoli cells create a barrier separating the developing spermatids from the bloodstream. This blood-testis barrier is formed at the onset of spermiogenesis; its purpose is not clear. However, it is postulated that the barrier may promote meiosis and protect the haploid sperm cells from exposure to the body's immune system, which may not recognize these unique cells. This barrier is significant from a clinical perspective because of its effect on pharmacotherapy aimed at the testis and because of the potential for infertility owing to an autoimmune response if it is violated.

Sperm maturation is divided into four phases and requires 72 days to complete. Phase 1 occurs when hyaluronidase, proteases, and other substances coalesce into an acrosomal granule that attaches to the nucleus and eventually forms the head of the mature, mobile spermatozoon. During phase 2 a cap forms around the acrosome, and the centrioles of the developing spermatid migrate to form the tail of the sperm. During the third phase, the spermatid assumes the characteristics of a mature sperm, including the formation of a mitochondrial sheath necessary for the forward motility of the sperm when injected into the female reproductive tract for the purpose of fertilization of an ovum. During phase 4, the tail is formed and excessive cytoplasm is shed with assistance from the Sertoli cells.

Accessory Organs of the Male Reproductive System

Sperm maturation occurs primarily in the epididymis,[53,54] a sausage-shaped organ located at the posterolateral surface of each testis (see Figures 2-18 and 2-19). The epididymis is approximately 5 cm long, and it is divided into three grossly visible regions: a head or globus major, a body (corpus), and a tail (globus minor). The internal architecture of the testis contains a single long tortuous canal; this tube contains no significant smooth muscle, but numerous cilia cause a slow forward movement of spermatozoa from the testis. At its tail, the ampulla of the epididymis opens into the more muscular vas deferens. The paired vasa deferentia connect the epididymis and the ejaculatory duct. The microscopic anatomy of the epididymis is characterized by an inner mucosa, smooth muscle tunic, and outer adventitia.

The blood supply of the epididymis and vas deferens is closely related. Both receive arterial blood from branches of the deferential artery, although the epididymis also may receive blood from the internal spermatic artery. Lymphatic channels of the epididymis empty into the external and hypogastric nodes, and those from the vas deferens empty into the internal and external iliac nodes.

Both the epididymis and vas deferens are responsible for sperm transport. Slow movement by cilia in the epididymal canal allows slow transport and maturation of spermatozoa from the testis. In contrast, the muscular tunic of the vas deferens acts under autonomic nervous system control to provide rapid movement of sperm during ejaculation.[55] Stimulation of adrenergic receptors causes contraction of smooth muscle within the walls of the vas deferens and transport of sperm toward the ejaculatory duct. However, other neurotransmitters (including acetylcholine, which may interact with norepinephrine to enhance the amplitude of smooth muscle contraction within the muscular tunic) also influence the process of ejaculation. Inhibition of ejaculation is modulated by a peptidergic neurotransmitter, neuropeptide Y (NPY), as well as endothelin, CGRP, and prostaglandins E_1 and E_2. Excitatory substances that influence contraction of smooth within the vas deferens include arginine vasopressin, bradykinin, and thromboxane.

The paired seminal vesicles lie between the posterior aspect of the bladder near its base and the rectum (see Figure 2-18).[56] Each organ is approximately 4 cm long, and they may be appreciated on digital rectal examination provided the examiner has relatively long fingers. The internal structure of the seminal vesicles contains a single coiled tube with irregularly placed diverticula that create its trabeculated appearance. The walls of the seminal vesicles comprise an inner mucosa, a muscular tunic, and a loose areolar tissue covered by dense connective tissue. Despite its name, the seminal vesicles do not serve as a storage compartment for sperm; this function is fulfilled by the epididymis. Instead, they have significant secretory functions postulated to contribute to semen production.

The ejaculatory ducts are found at the base of the prostate. They are formed by the terminal segments of the vas deferens and the seminal vesicles. Their walls are thin and include the inner mucosa, smooth muscle tunic and adventitia of the seminal vesicles, and vas deferens. Like the surrounding bladder neck, the smooth muscle bundles of the ejaculatory duct are rich with excitatory α-adrenergic receptors.

The prostate gland is a conical organ whose base lies just below the lissosphincter (bladder base).[56-58]

It tapers into an apex just superior to the membranous urethra. The proximal urethra travels through the prostate near its anterior surface. The prostate does not contain true lobes even though they are frequently described as such in clinical references. Instead, its internal architecture is best conceptualized as zones containing glandular elements and the fibromuscular stroma (Figure 2-20). The central zone of the prostate comprises about 25% of the glandular elements of the prostate. Its ducts contact the prostatic urethra at the superior end of the verumontanum. The embryonic origins of the central zone are distinct from the larger peripheral zone, which may account for its resistance to prostate cancer when compared with the glands of the peripheral zone. The peripheral zone comprises the largest portion of the prostate, accounting for approximately 70% of its glandular elements. The transition zone comprises a small group of ducts prone to more branching and acinar proliferation compared with the glandular elements of the central or peripheral zones. They comprise less than 5% of the glandular elements of the prostate in a young man, but they are the origin of the benign prostatic hyperplasia (BPH) common among elderly men.

The anterior fibromuscular stroma is a layer of connective tissue and smooth muscle that covers the entire anterior surface of the prostate and surrounds the bladder neck. The preprostatic tissue surrounds the anterior urethra to the level of the verumontanum. It is significant because it acts as a sphincter during ejaculation, preventing retrograde movement of semen into the bladder.

In the adult male, the prostate contains 30 to 50 lobules that combine into 15 to 30 secretory ducts that open into the proximal urethra. The epithelium of the prostate contains three metabolically active cell types.[56] Secretory epithelial cells manufacture the prostate-specific antigen, acid phosphatase, and other enzymes important to human semen. The role of basal cells within the prostate glands is less clear. They are probably involved in active transport needed to produce the high concentrations of specific elements within human semen. Neuroendocrine cells within the glandular epithelium regulate cellular activity through secretion of hormonal substances. Our understanding of the hormonal interactions that regulate prostatic growth and function is incomplete. The conversion of T to dihydrotestosterone (DHT) in

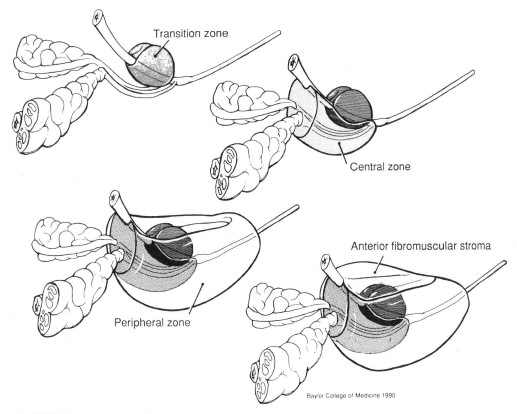

Transition zone

Central zone

Anterior fibromuscular stroma

Peripheral zone

Baylor College of Medicine 1990

Fig. 2-20 Zonal anatomy of prostate. (From Walsh PC, Retik AB, Vaughan ED, Wein AJ (eds): Campbell's Urology, 8th edition. Philadelphia: Saunders, 2002.)

the presence of the enzyme 5α-reductase is important to the development of BPH and administration of 5α-reductase inhibitors such as finasteride and dutasteride reduce prostatic size. Proloactin influences cell proliferation in multiple organs, including the prostate; age-related changes in prolactin are also hypothesized to contribute to BPH.[56a] The hormone oxytocin has been shown to regulate both prostatic cellular growth and smooth muscle tone; its levels have also been shown to be altered in men with BPH, suggesting that it also may play a role in this age-related condition.[56b] The smooth muscle of the fibromuscular component of the prostate contains abundant α-1$_A$ receptors; they contract during ejaculation, adding needed nutrients and other substances to seminal contents.[59] Stimulation of these receptors increases smooth muscle tone and urethral resistance. The primary function of the prostate gland is to manufacture and release specific substances that form the semen needed for sperm cells to fertilize a mature ovum.

The process of ejaculation begins with powerful contractions of the smooth muscle of the vas deferens that move mature sperm cells toward the ejaculatory ducts. As this occurs, muscular contractions of smooth muscle within the prostate and seminal vesicles mix the sperm with zinc, spermine, fructose, prostaglandins, immunoglobulins, proteases, esterases, and phosphatases. The semen protects the mature sperm cells against pathogens within the urethra or vagina, provides nutritional support as the sperm attempt to penetrate the ovum, and buffers the sperm from the more acidic environment of the female reproductive tract.

SUMMARY

The urinary system filters the blood to remove harmful toxins and maintain the internal homeostasis essential for life. After the kidneys manufacture urine, it is transported to the lower urinary tract by way of the renal pelves and ureters. Once it enters the lower urinary tract, it is stored until a combination of physiologic, psychological, and cultural factors prompts the individual to urinate. From a biologic perspective, the male reproductive system has two primary functions: generation of an erection sufficient for vaginal penetration and ejaculation of sperm-rich semen capable of fertilizing the mature ovum.

REFERENCES

1. Anderson JK, Kabalin JN, Cadeddu JA: Surgical anatomy of the retroperitoneum, adrenals, kidneys and ureters. In Wein AJ, Kavoussi LR, Novick AC, Partin AW, Peters CA (eds): Campbell-Walsh Urology, 9th edition. Philadelphia: Saunders, 2007; pp 3-37.
2. McDougal WS: The kidney. In Gillenwater JY, Grayhack JT, Howards SS, Mitchell ME: Adult & Pediatric Urology, 4th edition. Philadelphia: Lippincott, Williams & Wilkins, 2002; pp 563-87.
3. Rosol TJ, Yarrington JT, Latendresse J, Capen CC: Adrenal gland: structure, function, and mechanisms of toxicity. Toxicologic Pathology, 2001; 29:41-48.
4. Valtin H, Schafer JA: Renal Function, Mechanisms Preserving Fluid and Solute Balance in Health, 3rd edition. Boston: Little-Brown, 1995.
5. Vander AJ: Renal Physiology, 5th edition. New York: McGraw-Hill, 1995.
6. Noland LR: Renal system. In Thompson JT, MacFarland GK, Hirsch JE, Tucker SM: Clinical Nursing, 5th edition. St Louis: Mosby, 1997; pp 857-916.
7. Tisher CG, Madsen KM: Anatomy of the kidney. In Brenner BM (ed): The Kidney, 6th edition. Philadelphia: Saunders, 2000; pp 1-67.
8. Guyton AC: Medical Physiology, 11th edition. Philadelphia: Elsevier/Saunders, 2006.
9. Marunka Y: Hormonal and osmotic regulation of NaCl transport in renal distal nephron epithelium. Japanese Journal of Physiology, 1997; 47:499-511.
10. Giebisch G, Klein-Robbenhaar G: Recent studies on the characterization of loop diuretics. Journal of Cardiovascular Pharmacology, 1993; 22(supp. 3):S1-S10.
11. Schafer JA: Experimental validation of the countercurrent model of urinary concentration. American Journal of Physiology—Renal Physiology, 2004; 287(5):F861-3.
12. Nejsum LN: The renal plumbing system: aquaporin water channels. Cellular and Molecular Life Sciences, 2005; 62:1692-1706.
13. Wilcox CS: Diuretics. In Brenner BM (ed): The Kidney, 6th edition. Philadelphia: Saunders, 2000; pp 2219-52.
14. Giebisch G, Malnic G, Berliner RW: Control of renal potassium excretion. In Brenner BM (ed): The Kidney, 6th edition. Philadelphia: Saunders, 2000; pp 417-54.
15. Aviv A, Hollenberg NK, Weder A: Urinary potassium excretion and sodium sensitivity in blacks. Hypertension, 2004; 43(4):707-13.
16. Suki WN, Lederer ED, Rouse D: Renal transport of calcium, magnesium and phosphate. In Brenner BM (ed): The Kidney, 6th edition. Philadelphia: Saunders, 2000; pp 520-76.
17. Hayashi M: Physiology and pathophysiology of acid-base homeostasis in the kidney. Internal Medicine, 1998; 37:221-5.
18. Ludat K, Paulitschke M, Riedel E, Hampl H: Complete correction of renal anemia by recombinant human erythropoietin. Clinical Nephrology, 2000; 53(suppl):S42-9.
18a. Besarab A, Salifu MO, Lunde NM, Bansal V, Fishbane S, Dougherty FC: Beyer UBa16285 Study Investigators. Efficacy and tolerability of intravenous continuous erythropoietin receptor activator: a 19-week, phase II, multicenter, randomized, open-label, dose-finding study with a 12-month extension phase in patients with chronic renal disease. Clinical Therapeutics, 2007; 29(4):626-39.
19. Brown NJ: Aldosterone and end-organ damage. Current Opinion in Nephrology and Hypertension, 2005; 14(3):235-41.
20. Feldman D: Vitamin D, parathyroid hormone, and calcium: a complex regulatory network. American Journal of Medicine, 1999; 107:637-9.
21. Gray ML, Brown KC: Genitourinary system. In Thompson JT, MacFarland GK, Hirsch JE, Tucker SM (eds): Clinical Nursing, 5th edition. St Louis: Mosby, 2002; pp 917-99.
22. Weiss RM: Physiology and pharmacology of the renal pelvis and ureter. In Wein AJ, Kavoussi LR, Novick AC, Partin AW, Peters CA, (eds): Campbell-Walsh Urology, 9th edition. Philadelphia: Saunders, 2007; pp 1891-1921.
23. Shafik A, Shafik I, El Sibai O, Shafik AA: Changes in the urine composition during its passage through the ureter: a concept of urothelial function. Urological Research, 2005; 33(6):426-8.
23a. Lang RJ, Zoltkowski BZ, Hammer JM, Meeker WF, Wendit I: Electrical characterization of interstitial cells of Cajal-like cells and smooth muscle cells isolated from the mouse ureteropelvic junction. Journal of Urology, 2007; 177(4):1573-80.
23b. Jankovic SM, Jankovic SV, Stojadinovic D, Jakovljevic M, Milovanovic D: Effect of exogenous glutamate and N-methyl-D-aspartic acid on spontaneous activity of isolated human ureter. International Journal of Urology, 2007; 14(9):833-7.
24. Van Arendonk KJ, Madsen MT, Austin JC, Hawtrey CE, Graham MM, Cooper CS: Nuclear cystometrogram-determined bladder pressure at onset of vesicoureteral reflux predicts spontaneous resolution. Urology, 2007; 69(4):767-70.
25. Dixon J, Gosling J: Structure and innervation in the human. In Torrens M, Morrison JFB (eds): The Physiology of the Lower Urinary Tract. London: Springer-Verlag, 1987; pp 3-22.
26. Elbadawi A: Functional anatomy of the organs of micturition. Urologic Clinics of North America, 1996; 23:177-210.
27. Kumar V, Cross RL, Chess-Williams R, Chapple CR: Recent advances in basic science for overactive bladder. Current Opinion in Urology, 2005; 15(4):222-6.
28. Ashton-Miller JA, Howard D, DeLancey JO: The functional anatomy of the female pelvic floor and stress continence control system. Scandinavian Journal of Urology and Nephrology, (207):1-7 discussion 106-25.
29. Sampselle CA, Delancey JOL: Anatomy of female continence. Journal of Wound, Ostomy and Continence Nursing, 1998; 25:63-74.
30. Myers RP, Cahill DR, Devine RM, King BF: Anatomy of radical prostatectomy as defined by magnetic resonance imaging. Journal of Urology, 1998; 159:2148-58.
31. Mikuma N, Tamagawa M, Morita K, Tsukamoto T: Magnetic resonance imaging of the male pelvic floor: the anatomical configuration and dynamic movement in healthy men. Neurourology and Urodynamics, 1998; 17:591-7.
32. DeGroat WC: Innervation of the lower urinary tract: an overview. In 20th Annual Meeting of the Society for Urodynamics & Female Urology. Dallas, May 2001.
33. Gray M: Physiology of voiding. In Doughty DB (ed): Urinary and Fecal Incontinence: Nursing Management. St Louis: Mosby, 2000; pp 1-28.
34. Yoshimura N, Chancellor MB: Physiology and pharmacology of the bladder and urethra. In Wein AJ, Kavoussi LR, Novick AC, Partin AW, Peters CA (eds): Campbell-Walsh Urology, 9th edition. Philadelphia: Saunders, 2007; pp 1922-72.
35. Kavia RB, Dasgupta R, Fowler CJ: Functional imaging and the central control of the bladder. Journal of Comparative Neurology, 2005; 493(1):27-32.
36. Athwal BS, Berkley KJ, Hussain I, Brennan A, Craggs M, Sakakibara R, Frackowiak RS, Fowler CJ: Brain responses to changes in bladder volume and urge to void in healthy men. Brain, 2001; 124(pt 2):369-77.
37. Nour S, Svarer C, Kristensen JK, Paulson OB, Law I: Cerebral activation during micturition in normal men. Brain, 2000; 123(pt 4):781-9.

38. Hegde SS, Eglen RM: Muscarinic receptor subtypes modulating smooth muscle contractility in the urinary bladder. Life Sciences, 1999; 64:419-28.

39. Barrington FJ: The relationship of the hind brain to micturition. Brain, 1921; 44:23-53.

40. Staskin DR, Zimmern PE, Hadley HR, Raz S: Pathophysiology of stress incontinence. Clinics in Obstetrics and Gynecology, 1985; 12:357-88.

41. Zinner NR, Sterling AM, Ritter R: Role of inner urethral softness in urinary incontinence. Urology, 1980; 16:115-7.

42. Elbadawi A, Matthews R, Light JK, Wheeler TM: Immuno-histochemical and ultrastructural study of rhabdosphincter component of the prostatic capsule. Journal of Urology, 1997; 158:1819-38.

43. Sumino Y, Sato F, Kumamoto T, Mimata H: Striated muscle fiber compositions of human male urethral rhabdosphincter and levator ani. Journal of Urology, 2006; 175(4):1417-21.

44. Mostwin JL, Burnett AL: Anatomic aspects of urinary incontinence. In O'Donnell PD (ed): Urinary Incontinence. St Louis: Mosby, 1997; pp 25-32.

45. Aboseif SR, Tanagho EA: Anatomy of the penis. In Hellstrom WJG (ed): The Handbook of Sexual Dysfunction. San Francisco: American Society of Andrology, 1999; pp 2-6.

46. Moscovici J, Galinier P, Hammoudi S, Lefebvre D, Juricic M, Vaysse P: Contribution to the study of the venous vasculature of the penis. Surgical and Radiologic Anatomy, 1999; 21:193-9.

47. Lue TF: Physiology of penile erection and pathophysiology of erectile dysfunction and priapism. In Wein AJ, Kavoussi LR, Novick AC, Partin AW, Peters CA (eds): Campbell-Walsh Urology, 9th edition. Philadelphia: Saunders, 2007; pp 718-49.

48. Burnett AL: Neurophysiology of erectile function and dysfunction. In Hellstrom WJG (ed): The Handbook of Sexual Dysfunction. San Francisco: American Society of Andrology, 1999; pp 12-17.

49. Argiolas A, Melis MR: Central control of penile erection: role of the paraventricular nucleus of the hypothalamus. Progress in Neurobiology, 2005; 76(1):1-21.

49a. Miyagawa Y, Tsujimura A, Fujita K, Matsuoka Y, Takahashi T, Takao T, Takada S, Matsumiya K, Osaki Y, Takasawa M, Oku N, Hatazawa J, Kaneko S, Okuyama A: Differential brain processing of audiovisual sexual stimuli in men: comparative positron emission tomography study of the initiation and maintenance of penile erection during sexual arousal. Neuroimage, 2007; 36(3):830-42.

50. Andersson KE: Pharmacology of erectile function and dysfunction. Urologic Clinics of North America, 2001; 28:233-47.

51. Veldhuis JD, Iranmanesh A, Mulligan T, Pincus SM: Disruption of the young-adult synchrony between luteinizing hormone release and oscillations in follicle-stimulating hormone, prolactin, and nocturnal penile tumescence (NPT) in healthy older men. Journal of Clinical Endocrinology and Metabolism, 1999; 84:3498-3505.

52. Brooks JD: Anatomy of the lower urinary tract and male genitalia. In Walsh PC, Retik AB, Wein AJ, Vaughan ED (eds): Campbell's Urology. Philadelphia: Saunders, 1998; pp 89-128.

53. Schelegel PN, Hardy MP, Goldstein M: Male reproductive physiology. In Wein AJ, Kavoussi LR, Novick AC, Partin AW, Peters CA, (eds): Campbell-Walsh Urology, 9th edition. Philadelphia: Saunders, 2007; pp 577-608.

54. Lipschultz LI, Howards SS: Infertility in the Male. St Louis: Mosby, 1991.

55. Steers WD: Physiology of the vas deferens. World Journal of Urology, 1994; 12:281-5.

56. Veltri R, Rodriguez R: Molecular biology, endocrinology and physiology of the prostate and seminal vesicles. In Wein AJ, Kavoussi LR, Novick AC, Partin AW, Peters CA (eds): Campbell-Walsh Urology, 9th edition. Philadelphia: Saunders, 2007; pp 2677-2726.

56a. Crepin A. Bidaux G. Vanden-Abeele F. Dewailly E. Goffin V. Prevarskaya N. Slomianny C: Prolactin stimulates prostate cell proliferation by increasing endoplasmic reticulum content due to SERCA 2b over-expression. Biochemical Journal, 2007; 401(1): 49-55.

56b. Nicholson HD. Whittington K: Oxytocin and the human prostate in health and disease. International Review of Cytology, 2007; 263:253-86.

57. Grayhack JT, McVary KT, Kozlowski JM: Benign prostatic hyperplasia. In Gillenwater JY, Grayhack JT, Howards SS, Duckett JW (eds): Adult and Pediatric Urology, 4th edition. St Louis: Mosby, 2002; pp 1401-70.

58. Naz R: Prostate: basic and clinical aspects. Boca Raton, Fla: CRC Press, 1997.

59. Shafik A, Shafik AA, El Sibai O, Shafik IA: Contractile activity of the prostate at ejaculation: an electrophysiologic study. Urology, 2006; 67(4):793-6.

3

Signs and Symptoms in the Urologic Patient: Basic Principles of Screening and Assessment

Because assessment is an essential component of the nursing care for any patient with a urologic disorder, it is far too complex to integrate into a single chapter. Instead, essential components of assessment, including focused history, physical assessment, and diagnostic testing, are integrated throughout this textbook. This chapter will focus on common presenting signs and symptoms and techniques for physical examination of the urologic and reproductive system.

COMMON UROLOGIC SIGNS AND SYMPTOMS

A symptom is defined as subjective evidence of a disorder as perceived by the patient, whereas a sign is defined as objective evidence of a disorder.[1] For the purposes of this chapter, signs and symptoms will be defined based on their relationships to potential underlying urologic disorders. Nevertheless, it is essential to remember that the presenting sign or symptom (the principal complaint that drives a patient to seek care) represents the most worrisome or frightening manifestation as interpreted by the patient or care provider. Its meaning and significance from a *clinical* perspective can only be accurately assessed when the nurse determines the context in which the symptom occurs. Although the presence of other signs and symptoms may seem less significant to the patient, they may prove more revealing than the primary complaint when determining the nature of the underlying condition.

The first major segment of this chapter reviews common urologic signs and symptoms from the perspective of an initial or follow-up contact with a urologic nurse. Clinical Highlights for Advanced and Expert Practice: Telephone Consultation and the Urologic Nurse focuses on principles of successful telephone consultation (sometimes referred to as telephone triage) because it is an increasingly important means for initiating and maintaining communication with patients and their families in order to enable them to self-manage urologic problems while avoiding excessive and costly clinic visits or formal consultations.[2]

CONSTITUTIONAL SYMPTOMS

Constitutional symptoms indicate systemic effects of a disease. For the patient with a urologic disorder, constitutional symptoms usually indicate severely compromised renal function, a urologic tumor that has reached an advanced stage (i.e., metastasis to one or more distant organs), or a systemic infection.

Constitutional symptoms related to renal failure include fatigue and weakness, inability to concentrate, irritability, shortness of breath, exertional dyspnea, and cramping or restlessness of the legs. A rising creatinine may lead to nausea, hiccups, a loss of appetite, and weight loss. Advanced-stage urologic tumors produce many of the same symptoms, including fatigue and weakness, as well as nausea, a lack of appetite, and weight loss. These manifestations are often accompanied by bone pain or spontaneous (pathologic) fractures, and lower back pain if the tumor metastasizes to the vertebral bodies. Fever, hematuria, abdominal mass, flank pain, and lower urinary tract symptoms may accompany both conditions. These are discussed separately.

When constitutional symptoms are reported as an initial complaint by a patient or a care provider, the nurse should recommend a prompt and thorough evaluation by the patient's primary care provider when urologic symptoms are not present or by a urologist when they are associated with indications of a urologic source, such as hematuria, urinary system pain, or lower urinary tract symptoms. A report of constitutional symptoms in a patient undergoing treatment for a known urologic disorder may indicate progression of a malignancy or a deterioration of renal function, indicating the need for further evaluation.

Clinical Highlights for Advanced and Expert Practice: Telephone Consultation and the Urologic Nurse[2]

Telephone consultation is becoming an increasingly important tool for urologic practice. Effective communication on the telephone is aided by adhering to several simple principles that maximize the nurse's ability to gain essential information from the caller while offering rational and accurate advice and counseling to the patient or care provider.

Introduction

The nurse should introduce herself by name and title and clearly ascertain with whom she is speaking and his or her relation to the patient if this person is a care provider. Ensuring the caller's identity is particularly important to ensure the patient's privacy when providing support and counseling to a care provider. If the caller is a care provider, it may be advisable to ask to speak to the patient directly to obtain permission to reveal personal medical information. A caring and nonjudgmental approach, punctuated by clear questions about the patient's symptoms, helps to establish rapport and alleviate anxieties sometimes generated when speaking to someone other than "my doctor." The key to a successful call is gently enabling the patient or care provider to focus on the problem at hand while avoiding excessive extraneous conversation that impinges on the time of all parties involved.

Assessment of Signs and Symptoms

Unless the urologic nurse and patient have access to telemedicine technology, the telephone conversation is audible only, which limits the nurse's ability to assess for visual, gustatory, or other clues intuitively used in a face-to-face encounter. Remaining alert for verbal and nonverbal expressions, such as breathing patterns, sighs, and other clues, may reveal the patient or care provider's emotional state, anxiety level, and perceptions of his or her care to date. Background noises and conversations also may provide valuable clues about the patient's home environment. For example, sounds of children playing or construction may interfere with rest and recuperation, or interruptions by a family member in the background may provide clues to conflict in the home setting that may exert an influence on the patient's perceived symptoms. If a call comes from a care provider, the nurse may ask to speak directly with the patient to gain more direct information about her or his symptoms, emotional status, and mental acuity. Solicitation of presenting and related signs or symptoms articulated by a patient or care provider is critical to assessment by telephone, and this chapter provides a detailed discussion of the most common presenting signs and symptoms encountered in routine urologic practice.

Advice, Education, and Counseling

Several tools are invaluable when offering counseling, education, or advice by telephone consultation. These include the patient's medical record; a resource book containing key procedures, protocols, and practice guidelines for that practice; and access to consultation with the urologist, nurse practitioner, or another urologic professional. In addition, protocols for telephone consultation may be developed for a urologic practice, and these can be incorporated into standardized documentation forms that both provide a record of the call and assist the nurse to organize the complex information obtained from a telephone consultation into a rational and knowledge-based plan of action.

Documentation

Similar to a face-to-face counseling session, it is critical to document all telephone consultations. We recommend use of a standardized document form whenever feasible and particularly when the interaction involves secondary consultation with a urologist or other clinician.

Fever

Fever is a constitutional symptom whose presence raises an immediate suspicion of underlying infection. When presented with a report of a fever by telephone or verbally, it is important to determine who measured the patient's temperature and when the measurement was taken. A *high-grade fever* is usually defined as one that is 101° F (38.3° C) or higher, and a *low-grade fever* is above normal for that patient but beneath 101° F. The most common cause of a fever in a urologic setting is an acute urinary tract infection, typically (but not always) involving the upper urinary tracts (see Chapter 14 for a detailed discussion of febrile urinary tract infections in children). Other causes of high-grade fevers include acute bacterial prostatitis in men, acute epididymitis, or a complication of a procedure requiring urinary tract instrumentation. Additional symptoms related to a systemic infection include flank pain, nausea, vomiting, and chills. If a systemic infection is not promptly treated, the patient may progress to septic shock with cool, clammy skin; edema; and delirium.

Low-grade fever may be seen in patients with renal colic caused by urinary extravasation from the renal pelvis or a calyx. Although high-grade fevers are more commonly associated with an acute systemic infection than low-grade fevers, it is important to remember that neonates and frail elders may only develop a low-grade fever despite the presence of pyelonephritis or urosepsis.

Counseling the patient with a low- or high-grade fever begins with an assessment of its underlying cause. Patients or care providers are counseled that immediate evaluation and intervention are indicated for patients with high-grade fevers, and prompt evaluation is justified for most patients with a new complaint of a low-grade fever. Patients with a persistent fever may require additional evaluation, particularly when the fever persists despite an adequate appropriate antimicrobial therapy course of 3 to 5 days. For example, a patient diagnosed with pyelonephritis who calls the urologic nurse complaining of persistent fever despite 10 to 14 days of appropriate antimicrobial therapy should undergo evaluation for possible perirenal abscess.

Hematuria

Hematuria is usually classified as gross or microscopic. *Gross hematuria* is visible to the naked eye and may be reported by a patient as a presenting symptom, whereas *microscopic hematuria* can only be detected on urinalysis. The phrase *gross painless hematuria* refers to the presence of bloody urine in the absence of dysuria, and it raises an immediate suspicion of a urologic malignancy, such as bladder cancer. Although the painless hematuria seen in patients with urologic malignancies implies the absence of dysuria, it is frequently associated with lower urinary tract symptoms including day and nighttime voiding frequency, urgency, or urge urinary incontinence.

When hematuria is reported, the urologic nurse should inquire about the specific color of the urine, the timing of hematuria within the context of micturition, and its duration. Fresh blood in the urine will create a pink or reddish color, depending on the volume of blood in relation to urinary volume. Old blood is more likely to produce a dark red or brownish color, which may be an expected finding following certain urologic procedures.

Questions about the timing of hematuria may yield clues to the location of the associated urologic lesion.[3] Hematuria that occurs at the beginning of micturition is called *initial hematuria* and is associated with urethral disease, whereas hematuria that occurs during the end of voiding is called *terminal hematuria* and is associated with disorders of the bladder neck or prostatic urethra. Bloody urine that persists throughout micturition is called *total hematuria*, and it may be associated with a tumor, lesion, or disease of the kidney, ureter, or bladder. Blood from the urethra also may stain the underclothing or pajamas in the absence of hematuria during micturition. It is usually associated with a disorder affecting the anterior urethra.

The duration of hematuria may also provide clues to the underlying disorder. Many patients are alarmed by an initial episode of hematuria, but others may not perceive its clinical significance and may experience multiple episodes of hematuria before electing to seek care. Persistent hematuria is unusual as a presenting symptom, but it is common following urologic surgery or during an acute urinary tract infection.

An initial report of grossly visible hematuria justifies additional urologic evaluation. More than 100 medical disorders are associated with hematuria.[4] Patients reporting hematuria may be counseled that a large variety of conditions can produce hematuria. Nevertheless, a retrospective review of 1000 patients presenting with gross hematuria revealed that 22% had an associated urologic malignancy, illustrating the necessity for excluding this condition before considering other causes.[5] Table 3-1 outlines common nonmalignant causes of hematuria and associated clinical manifestations. Although acute urinary tract infection is known to be a common cause of hematuria in women and young adult men, additional evaluation is indicated to ensure that the hematuria abates following resolution of the infection and the patient is counseled that a recurring episode of hematuria should be promptly reported to the patient's primary care provider or urologist.

A report of persistent hematuria after a urologic procedure may or may not indicate a clinically relevant complication. Pink-tinged or light red urine is common following many open, laparoscopic, or

TABLE 3-1 Common Nonmalignant Causes of Hematuria

DISORDER	ASSOCIATED SIGNS AND SYMPTOMS
Acute urinary tract infection	Dysuria, urinary frequency, suprapubic pain
Urinary tract anomaly	Obstruction of the urinary system, such as at the UPJ
Urinary calculi	Renal colic
Acute glomerulonephritis	Oliguria, hypertension, constitutional symptoms
Benign prostatic hyperplasia	Lower urinary tract symptoms
Blood dyscrasias including sickle cell anemia	Bleeding disorder, easy bruising, joint pain, and erectile dysfunction

UPJ, Ureteropelvic junction.

endoscopic procedures and may indicate a very small amount of blood in a comparatively large volume of urine. It often persists for a period of days to several weeks depending on the type of procedure and is expected to gradually diminish as postoperative healing progresses. In contrast, passage of bright red urine or the presence of clots indicates a larger volume of blood in the urine that may be associated with significant blood loss from the urinary system. Many patients will contact the urologic nurse when a small amount of hematuria occurs 10 to 14 days after a urologic procedure, often accompanied by the passage of several small, dark-colored clots. Patients reporting these manifestations can be reassured that these signs are usually caused by the sloughing of scabs, indicating healing of the underlying mucosa, and require no further intervention unless accompanied by the passage of bright red clots or a recurrence of bright red urine, indicating significant blood loss.

The urologic nurse also may be asked to counsel patients found to have microscopic hematuria. Microscopic hematuria is less likely to be associated with urologic malignancies than gross hematuria and more likely to be associated with an underlying renal disorder as compared with a urologic disorder.[2] Nevertheless, approximately 13% of patients with persistent asymptomatic microscopic hematuria will be found to have an underlying urologic cancer.[6] Patients reporting this condition should be advised to undergo additional evaluation by a physician.

Abdominal Mass

Adults rarely complain of an abdominal mass, but the urologic nurse sometimes interacts with a parent who notices an abdominal mass when bathing or dressing a younger child or infant. Among infants, most abdominal masses arise from the urinary system and are typically attributable to benign conditions, such as hydronephrosis. However, a new mass in a school-aged child raises suspicion for a malignant condition, such as Wilms, tumor.[7] Patients or parents reporting an abdominal mass should be counseled to consult a physician for further evaluation.

Pain

Because of its subjective nature and multiple etiologies, it is essential that the urologic nurse employ a systematic approach to the evaluation of pain. Patients reporting pain should be asked to describe it by location, nature (type or character), duration, intensity, and known alleviating or aggravating factors. In addition, patients should be asked if they are experiencing any *referred pain*, defined as discomfort that is projected to an area distant from its primary source. Greater knowledge of these characteristics will assist the urologic nurse to identify possible causes of the pain and provide a more rational basis for recommending management strategies.

Flank Pain and Renal Colic. For patients, the flank usually refers to the back below the ribs to the upper portion of the pelvic bone. From a urologic perspective, flank pain is usually associated with a disorder of the underlying kidney or renal pelvis, particularly when it is unilateral. A continuous, dull ache that is localized within the flank is usually associated with chronic obstruction or infection. The pain varies from mild to severe in its intensity and is exacerbated if external pressure is placed on the costovertebral angle. Patients with flank pain associated with an infection will report signs and symptoms of pyelonephritis including fever, nausea, and dysuria and may also report constitutional symptoms related to urosepsis as discussed earlier. Patients with flank pain associated with chronic obstruction may note that the intensity of their discomfort is exacerbated by drinking a large volume of fluid. Rarely, they may also report constitutional symptoms indicating renal insufficiency.

Acute obstruction of a renal pelvis or ureter leads to a characteristic type of pain called *renal colic*.[3] Patients experiencing renal colic typically localize their discomfort to the flank (costovertebral angle) and outer aspect of the abdomen if an obstructing stone is located in the renal pelvis or proximal ureter. Discomfort from obstructing stones in the mid ureter is localized in the inguinal canal, and discomfort from stones entrapped in the lower ureter is localized in the suprapubic area. Renal colic has an acute onset and often awakens the patient from sleep. The pain waxes and wanes in response to peristaltic waves that persist for several minutes as intraluminal pressure rises and distends the ureteral or pelvic lumen. Periods of intense pain often occur, persisting for 20 to 30 minutes, followed by periods of less intense discomfort. The intensity of colicky pain varies from moderate to extremely severe, and patients exhibit restlessness as they seek in vain to find a position to alleviate their discomfort. Renal colic may cause referred pain transmitted to the inguinal canal or groin (i.e., testis, scrotum, or tip of penis in men; round ligament or labia in women).

After differentiating renal colic from the more continuous and dull ache of flank pain, the patient is queried about hematuria, fever, and the presence of lower urinary tract symptoms including a new onset of dysuria and urinary frequency. Patients with a new onset of renal colic require prompt evaluation and management. Patients with flank pain or renal colic and signs and symptoms of infection, such as a fever, also require rapid evaluation and intervention to prevent an infection from progressing to urosepsis.

Lower Urinary Tract and Pelvic Pain. Although a urinary tract infection is the most common cause of lower urinary tract or pelvic pain, it is essential to remember that multiple other factors also must be considered before concluding that a male patient experiencing suprapubic or pelvic pain has prostatitis or a female patient has acute cystitis. As noted earlier, a systematic approach to pain assessment will assist the urologic nurse in identifying possible underlying causes of pelvic pain and move beyond the traditional but limited view of pelvic pain as almost exclusively associated with urinary tract infection or prostatic inflammation.

Dysuria is the symptom of pain or discomfort associated with urination.[8] It is usually characterized as burning and reaches a peak in intensity sometime during urination, but many patients report a persistent burning or cramping pain in the urethra and suprapubic area that persists several minutes following micturition. It is typically associated with infection of the lower urinary tract, but it also may be seen with acute prostatic inflammation, urologic tumors, trauma, atrophic urogenital changes in women, urethral stricture, or interstitial cystitis. When querying a woman with dysuria, it is important to carefully determine the location of the pain; burning that is localized to the external genitalia may indicate the passage of urine over inflamed labia, while internal burning is more likely to suggest cystitis or urethritis. Questions about the onset and duration of the pain are also suggestive of possible etiologies. The pain associated with an acute urinary tract infection usually includes dysuria and suprapubic pain in the older child or young adult associated with lower urinary tract symptoms including voiding frequency and urgency. Suprapubic pain is exacerbated by bladder filling and postponing urination and relieved by urination. It also may be exacerbated by consuming caffeine or other bladder irritants. Cystitis may exacerbate urinary incontinence, but we have found that it does not commonly cause incontinence in the previously continent, community-dwelling young adult. In contrast, acute cystitis may exacerbate or even cause incontinence in the adult with a paralyzing spinal disorder, in younger children, or in frail elders.

A report of chronic pain that does not respond rapidly to antimicrobial treatment raises a suspicion of interstitial cystitis.[9] Similar to acute cystitis, interstitial cystitis is frequently associated with dysuria and suprapubic pain that is transiently relieved by micturition and exacerbated by consumption of a wide variety of substances capable of irritating the bladder mucosa. In contrast to acute cystitis, the pain of interstitial cystitis has a cyclic pattern with periods of acute exacerbation frequently associated with physical activities, sexual intercourse, or emotional distress that persist for a period of weeks to months or even years despite multiple attempts to treat with antimicrobials. The intensity of pain associated with interstitial cystitis varies widely, and it may be very intense in certain patients and milder in others.

Chronic pelvic pain in men has traditionally been attributed to prostatic inflammation, but more recent research has challenged this hypothesis.[10] Chronic male pelvic pain syndrome is associated with suprapubic or perineal pain. Lower urinary tract symptoms may include urgency or dysuria, often combined with hesitancy or difficulty initiating the urinary stream and feelings of incomplete bladder emptying. Postponing urination may or may not alleviate the pain of prostatitis, and ejaculation is reported to alleviate pain in some men but to exacerbate perineal pain in others. Queries about pelvic pain in men should exclude the presence of constitutional symptoms, such as fever, that indicate the presence of acute bacterial prostatitis.

Although not a medical emergency, chronic pelvic pain indicates the need for a thorough evaluation by a urologist or other clinician with expertise and interest in diagnosing and managing these challenging disorders. Patients are often distressed, anxious, and frustrated by previous attempts to seek care for persistent pain, and they may express these multiple emotions as distrust or even anger toward any health care provider. A patient and supportive attitude, combined with knowledge-based answers and advice about possible underlying conditions, helps to reassure the patient that her or his complaint is being taken seriously and that effective treatments are available.

LOWER URINARY TRACT SYMPTOMS

Lower urinary tract symptoms (LUTS) is a broad term meant to describe a variety of individual symptoms.[11] They are divided into three main categories: storage, voiding, and postmicturition. LUTS are closely associated with a variety of disorders affecting the lower (and often the upper) urinary tract. Specific LUTS tend to be associated with a variety of underlying conditions, and their presence may not readily distinguish one contributing condition from another.

Storage Symptoms

Daytime voiding frequency refers to the number of times a person urinates while awake. It can be expressed as the total number of urinations per day or the typical lag time between urinations. Patients who urinate more than eight times per day or more often than every 2 hours are defined as having *increased daytime frequency*.[11] Nighttime voiding frequency, more commonly referred to as *nocturia*, is defined as the number of times sleep is interrupted by the desire to urinate. Three or more episodes of nocturia per night are considered excessive nocturia.

Urgency (sometimes referred to as bothersome urgency) must be carefully distinguished from the physiologic desire to urinate. A physiologic desire to urinate is perceived as a growing awareness of the need to urinate that corresponds with vesicle filling and that is subsequently relieved by urination. It can be postponed for a matter of minutes to hours depending on intravesical volume, and it is completely relieved by urination. Urgency is defined as a strong and immediate desire to urinate that is not easily deferred. It interrupts activities of daily living and may lead to urge urinary incontinence if the person is unable to rapidly act on the desire. Based on media campaigns, many patients now refer to this symptom as "gotta go, gotta go, gotta go right now."

Urinary incontinence (UI) is an uncontrolled loss of urine, sometimes referred to by patients as a "bladder control problem," "dripping," or "leaking." When querying patients about urine loss, it is important to remember that many patients may deny a diagnosis of UI because of perceptions that this diagnosis implies a "total loss of control" requiring an adult containment brief, rather than any leakage. In addition, we recommend asking patients whether they require pads or absorbent products and why. Surprisingly, we have observed that many patients will deny urine loss or UI if their symptom is adequately contained within such a device.

A positive response to queries about urine loss should prompt the nurse to differentiate a sudden onset of leakage from established UI and to ask additional questions concerning the type of UI. Because of its typically insidious onset, UI is often considered to be "not bothersome" by patients or to be irrelevant (provided it can be hidden using absorbent products or preventive voiding behaviors). Nevertheless, it is important to counsel patients concerning the nature of UI, its diagnosis, and the presence of effective treatments. Refer to Chapters 6 and 15 for more detailed discussion of the assessment of UI in children and adults.

Voiding Symptoms

Patients may report a variety of voiding symptoms.[11] A slow stream is defined as a perceived reduction in urine flow compared with previous performance or compared with others. The severity of a slowed stream varies considerably, from a dribble or trickle to alteration in force perceptible only to the patient. A reduction in the force of the urinary stream occurring near the end of micturition is called a *terminal dribble*. An *interrupted or intermittent stream* starts and stops; patients often describe the need to strain to restart or maintain an intermittent stream. *Hesitancy* is defined as a delay in the onset of the start of the urinary stream, despite a desire to urinate. Two underlying disorders, poor detrusor contraction strength and bladder outlet obstruction, frequently produce voiding LUTS. Urodynamic evaluation may be indicated to further define the underlying cause of voiding LUTS and to guide treatment.

Postmicturition Symptoms

Two postmicturition symptoms are most likely to prompt patients to seek care. *Feelings of incomplete bladder emptying* are defined as a perception that residual urine remains in the bladder despite micturition; they may or may not indicate an elevated postvoid residual volume. A *postvoid dribble* is defined as the involuntary passage of a small volume of urine after voiding. Men often report a postvoid dribble after placing the penis back in the underclothing, and women may experience the symptom as they arise and leave the toilet, or when urine loss occurs as they wipe the perineal area immediately after urination.

DIFFICULTY URINATING

It is not unusual for the urologic nurse to be contacted by a patient experiencing significant difficulty or a complete inability to urinate. The two principal causes of the inability to urinate are urinary retention and oliguria or anuria. Urinary retention is most common in a urologic practice setting. The two forms of urinary retention are acute and chronic.[12] Acute urinary retention is defined as a sudden inability to urinate despite adequate (or quite large) intravesical volume. Patients are usually acutely aware of the problem and frequently complain of a growing desire to urinate, waxing suprapubic pressure and discomfort, and dribbling or complete absence of a urinary stream despite multiple attempts to void. A care provider may report acute urinary retention in a patient who is experiencing increasing agitation, restlessness, and confusion. Chronic urinary retention is characterized by incomplete bladder emptying despite persistent micturition. Many patients are unaware of incomplete bladder emptying, but others may experience feelings of incomplete bladder emptying, a diminished force behind their urinary stream, interrupted voiding, hesitancy, or postvoid dribbling. Patients with oliguria or anuria have underlying renal insufficiency and will be experiencing the constitutional symptoms discussed earlier.

The patient experiencing acute urinary retention can be given instructions on simple techniques to prompt voiding. Instruction includes consuming a bladder stimulant (i.e., irritant), such as a cup of brewed coffee or hot tea, warming up by taking a warm shower or bath, and permission to urinate while in the shower stall or tub. If urination has not occurred in more than 8 hours or if the patient remains unable to void despite adequate efforts at home, he or she is advised to seek care immediately, through either the urology service or local emergency department. Patients with chronic urinary retention are advised of the risk for acute urinary retention and counseled to seek care from a urologist. Those with evidence of renal insufficiency are also advised to seek care immediately.

SCROTAL SWELLING OR PAIN

Acute scrotal swelling in a child or young adult should be managed as a medical emergency. It usually occurs in children or adolescents after trauma or as a result of testicular torsion or acute epididymitis. Swelling in a young adult male after a viral illness, such as mumps, may indicate orchitis. Elderly patients are more likely to experience scrotal swelling and pain in response to acute epididymitis, but they may be caused by cellulitis or necrotizing fasciitis in rare cases. Patients or parents reporting acute scrotal swelling and pain are instructed to seek immediate care from a urologist or emergency department.

SEXUAL DYSFUNCTION IN THE MALE

A number of conditions may cause men to seek care from a urologic clinician, but the most common is erectile dysfunction (ED). ED is defined as the inability to achieve or sustain an erection sufficient for sexual activity. In contrast to a persistent cultural myth, a penile erection is not simply a mechanical event and all men experience occasional inability to achieve an erection despite the desire to engage in sexual activity. Clinically relevant ED is defined as a failure rate of approximately 50%.[13] Other complaints may include low sexual desire (libido), which is typically associated with hypogonadism, often in combination with ED.

Even less is known about ejaculation disorders, although sparse epidemiologic evidence suggests that these disorders are more common than previously suspected.[14] *Premature ejaculation* is variably defined as ejaculation occurring in 1 to 3 minutes following penetration or within 8 to 15 thrusts. Its cause is unknown, but ongoing research may expand treatment options and awareness of the condition among both patients and providers. *Retrograde ejaculation* is defined as absence of seminal emission despite subjective experience of ejaculation. It is caused by an autonomic nervous system dysfunction or iatrogenic disorder following retroperitoneal lymph node dissection surgery for testicular cancer.

Similar to UI, sexual dysfunction is shrouded in myth and tradition, and it typically provokes anxiety for both the male and his sexual partner. Adopting a knowledge-based and tolerant attitude is essential when counseling men and their partners presenting with sexual dysfunction. Because of advances in treatment options for ED, many cases can be evaluated and treated in the primary care setting, although complex cases or those refractory to initial treatment should be treated by a urologist. The evaluation and management of a loss of libido may be undertaken by a urologist or endocrinologist. In addition, it is important to counsel elderly men who may seek advice concerning "male menopause" or andropause to seek care from a qualified urologist and to avoid "specialty clinics" that purport to administer hormone replacement therapies without adequate evaluation and counseling about intended effects and potential adverse side effects.

PHYSICAL EXAMINATION

Because of its sensitive nature, the historical interview and physical examination are completed in an environment that ensures patient confidentiality and privacy. The urologic nurse can assist the anxious patient to relax and instill confidence in the professional by doing the following: avoiding bulky desks and tables

between the interviewer and the patient; maintaining eye contact; being professionally dressed and groomed; and projecting an attentive, warm, and cordial manner. Figure 3-1 illustrates equipment that may be needed for a focused physical examination. Additional equipment will be required if the patient is undergoing an integrated history and physical examination in preparation for a urologic surgical procedure (see Chapter 11).

GENERAL ASSESSMENT

A focused physical examination of the genitourinary system typically includes the abdomen and external genitalia. Before beginning the examination, the nurse should ensure proper privacy. Materials are collected beforehand, to avoid entering and leaving the room during the examination, and a chaperone is arranged for when indicated. In general, the presence of a chaperone is recommended for any examination that involves the genitalia. Supervision is considered mandatory when examining a person of the opposite gender or an individual with mental health or cognitive disorders that may alter his or her ability to recall the events of the evaluation reliably.

The patient is typically asked to urinate before the examination begins. This allows the patient to provide a urine specimen, and the opportunity may be used to measure a postvoid residual volume when indicated. The urologic nurse can also observe the person's gait and dexterity as the patient walks to

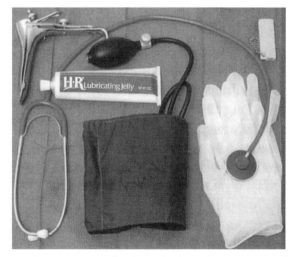

Fig. 3-1 Equipment for focused physical examination of the urinary system.

the washroom and handles a specimen cup. It is helpful to note the individual's mobility, dexterity, and cognition, including the use of assistive devices, such as a walker, cane, or wheelchair, and the person's ability to transfer onto a chair or examining table. If indicated, the nurse may wish to observe the patient's ability to remove clothing, specifically the ability to manipulate zippers or buttons. An evaluation of the patient's cognitive status begins at this time and continues throughout the history and physical examination.

The patient is also assessed for constitutional symptoms and general health. Vital signs are taken, including blood pressure, which should be obtained in supine and sitting or standing positions when indicated. Elevated blood pressure may be renovascular in origin, indicating a defect in a single kidney or primary vascular abnormalities. Skin integrity may be altered, with a proneness to bruises and slowed wound healing. Chronic anemia may be noted as pallor accompanied by general weakness and low tolerance of physical exertion. Electrolyte imbalance also may occur, causing fatigue, nausea, vomiting, and impaired cognition in severe cases. Peripheral edema may be noted, and certain individuals may experience shortness of breath or other signs of congestive heart failure. The hair may appear thin and brittle as a result of protein wasting; weight loss and muscle wasting may be detectable. The presence of any fever is noted, and subsequent evaluation is completed to determine its source.

Assessment of the Abdomen

General Approach. The patient is approached slowly and deliberately when preparing to examine the abdomen, and the clinician carefully explains each component of the evaluation. Placing the person in a comfortable position, using pillows as indicated, and asking the patient to breathe slowly through the mouth will promote relaxation of the abdominal muscles and enable optimal deep palpation of abdominal structures.

Inspection. The abdomen is inspected from a seated position at the patient's right side. The clinician particularly observes the contour of the abdomen and skin. The skin may be pale or tanned and may contain a fine venous network noticeable to the naked eye. Jaundice, discrete lesions, or generalized redness may indicate several specific disorders,

including infection. The presence, size, and location of scars are noted. Trauma or surgical procedures may affect the urinary system and adjacent structures. Abdominal scars also alert the nurse to the potential for adhesions, which may cause abdominal discomfort and may be perceived by the patient as pelvic, bladder, or renal pain.

The abdomen is also inspected for contour and symmetry. The normal abdomen may appear flat in normal persons, rounded with ample adipose tissue in obese individuals, or concave in thin adults. A visible mass of the upper abdominal quadrants may indicate the presence of a renal tumor or obstruction with severe hydronephrosis in children, although it is difficult to visualize even markedly enlarged kidneys in the adult. A centrally located protrusion in the suprapubic area may be visible in an adult or child, and it may indicate a distended bladder.

Auscultation. After the inspection, the abdomen is auscultated *before* light and deep palpation, because these maneuvers alter normal peristalsis. A warmed stethoscope is placed gently on the skin of the abdomen, and the clinician listens for bowel sounds, noting their presence, frequency, and character (Figure 3-2). Normal peristalsis is noted as clicks and gurgles that occur without any distinguishable pattern. As few as 5 or as many as 35 peristaltic sounds may be heard per minute. Evaluating the presence of bowel sounds is particularly significant after urologic surgery requiring manipulation or reconstruction of the bowel.

Percussion. Percussion is included in examination of the genitourinary system whenever incomplete

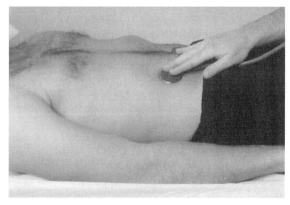

Fig. 3-2 Auscultation of the abdomen.

bladder emptying is suspected (Figure 3-3). Percussion of the suprapubic area follows general percussion of all abdominal quadrants to evaluate tympany versus dullness for that individual. Tympany is

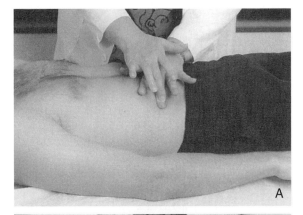

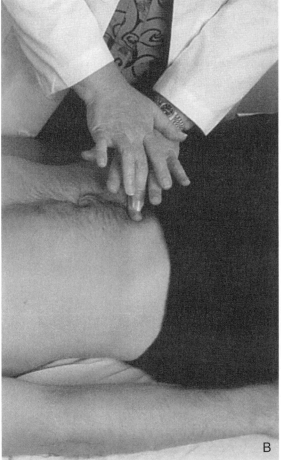

Fig. 3-3 A, Percussion of the lower abdomen. **B,** Percussion of the suprapubic area provides clues to intravesical volume.

noted over lower quadrants, where hollow bowel predominates, and dullness is noted over the liver. If the bladder has less than 150 ml of fluid it usually remains below the symphysis pubis and percussion will reveal tympany in the suprapubic area. In contrast, dullness in the suprapubic area will be heard when a large volume of urine is present in the bladder. In the obese patient, percussing the abdomen for bladder volume is not reliable. If a postvoid residual urine is suspected, a portable ultrasound or in-and-out catheterization is required for accuracy.

Palpation. The nurse should stand at the patient's side and begin light palpation with warm hands while giving a thorough explanation (Figure 3-4). Efforts should be taken to ensure that the patient is placed in a relatively comfortable position before beginning palpation. Light palpation is used to detect areas of tenderness and muscular resistance. A significant mass or urinary system infection that causes tenderness may produce resistance on light palpation. A pelvic mass or distended bladder also may be noted as resistance on light palpation over the lower quadrants of the abdomen and suprapubic area.

Deep palpation is used to delineate the abdominal organs and to detect subtle masses. The nurse uses the palmar surface of the fingers to press deeply but gently into the abdominal wall (Figure 3-5). The liver, spleen, loops of bowel, and borders of abdominal muscles also may be palpated using this technique. Slight tenderness over the cecum, sigmoid colon, and aorta may be noted in normal individuals. Any mass that causes muscle guarding is evaluated for size, shape, consistency, and magnitude of tenderness provoked by palpation.

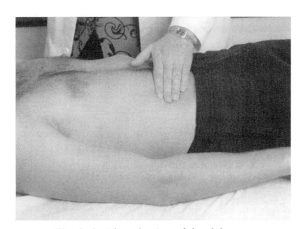

Fig. 3-4 Light palpation of the abdomen.

The kidneys are assessed for tenderness and masses, as are adjacent organs, including the liver, spleen, and gallbladder. To evaluate the kidneys, ask the patient to assume a sitting position. Place the palm of your right hand over the left costovertebral angle (Figure 3-6).

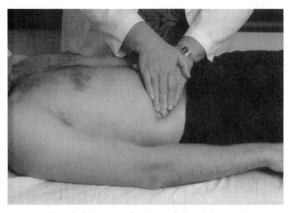

Fig. 3-5 Deep palpation of the abdomen.

Strike your hand lightly with the fist of the left hand. The patient should perceive this light blow as a dull thud rather than as sharp tenderness or pain. The maneuver is repeated over the right costovertebral angle. Testing for costovertebral tenderness is useful for detecting flank pain in patients with acute or chronic pyelonephritis, particularly when symptoms of flank pain are not clearly delineated through the history. However, this maneuver can be quite painful and is not typically indicated or advised in patients with renal colic and high fevers accompanied by unambiguous signs and symptoms of pyelonephritis.

Palpation of the kidneys is realistic in younger children, but it can only be accomplished in very thin adults. The patient is asked to assume a supine position. The nurse reaches her left hand to the patient's left flank in order to palpate the left kidney. It may help to ask the patient to inhale deeply, which will elevate the left flank. An alternate approach is to capture the kidney by asking the

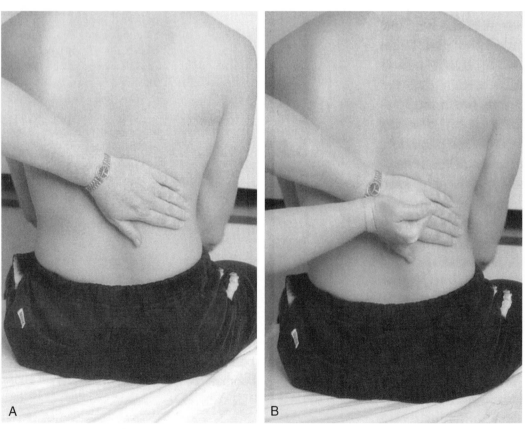

Fig. 3-6 Assessment of costovertebral angle tenderness. **A,** The open palm of one hand placed over the costovertebral angle. **B,** The fist of the second hand is used to gently strike the open palm.

patient to inhale and then exhale deeply during deep palpation. The nurse stands on the patient's left side and places the left hand over the flank and the right hand over the costal margin. The patient is asked to inhale deeply and exhale slowly. The descending kidney may be felt between the fingers. The right kidney may be more easily palpated than the left. The nurse stands on the patient's left side and places the left hand under the right flank (Figure 3-7). The left hand is placed under the right costal margin, and the patient is asked to inhale deeply and exhale slowly; the kidney may be palpable as it slips between the fingers (Figure 3-8). Deep palpation is required to locate the kidney, and the nurse should be reassured that these maneuvers are not feasible in most adult patients.

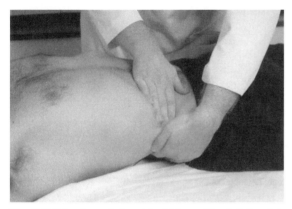

Fig. 3-7 Palpation of the right kidney. The left hand is placed under the patient's right flank.

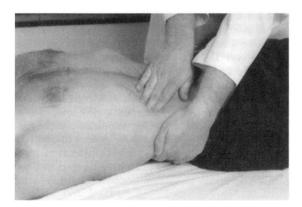

Fig. 3-8 Alternative technique for palpating the right kidney. The patient is asked to inhale deeply and exhale slowly, and the kidney may be palpable as it slips between the fingers.

Assessment of Male Genitalia

General Approach. Men may be quite anxious when the genitalia are examined. Therefore the patient is approached using a gentle and deliberate manner. It is important to avoid changing facial expressions if unexpected findings are discovered on evaluation and to remain alert to the possibility that the male patient may experience dizziness if examination provokes intense anxiety.

Inspection. The distribution of the hair on the genitalia is inspected initially, and younger patients may be asked if they routinely shave hair in this area. Scrotal hair typically is coarser than scalp hair and assumes a triangular distribution, with the apex pointing toward the scrotum. The scrotum is lightly covered with hair, and the penis is relatively hair free. The perineal skin is carefully inspected for signs of incontinence-associated dermatitis and secondary infection, such as candidiasis. Care is taken to inspect all skinfolds for evidence of moisture-related skin damage, often beginning with the folds between the scrotum and upper thigh.

The penis and scrotum are inspected next (Figure 3-9). The skin of the penis may be more pigmented than adjacent abdominal integument. The foreskin should be inspected for rashes or lesions, paying close attention to the presence of premalignant lesions or evidence of possible penile cancer. The foreskin is then retracted in the uncircumcised male and the glans penis carefully inspected. Inability to retract the foreskin is called phimosis and may indicate additional evaluation and treatment when seen in an adult male or older child although it is normal during infancy. The glans penis and corona are also inspected for rashes or lesions. In the uncircumcised man the glans is relatively moist and pink and may contain smegma, a whitish substance created by secretions from local sebaceous glands. Inspection of the glans penis in the circumcised male will reveal dryer skin than the uncircumcised male and than the surrounding skin and absence of smegma, but the glans should remain free from rashes or lesions. The urethral meatus is examined next (Figure 3-10). It should be ovoid and located on the ventral surface of the glans several millimeters from the tip. The glans penis should be gently pressed between the thumb and forefinger to expose and inspect the mucosa of the fossa navicularis (terminal portion of the urethra). The mucosa should readily separate, exposing pink, moist tissue. Discharge,

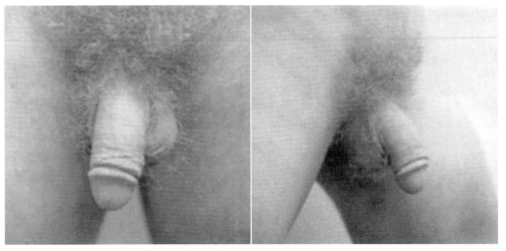

Fig. 3-9 Inspection of the penis and scrotum.

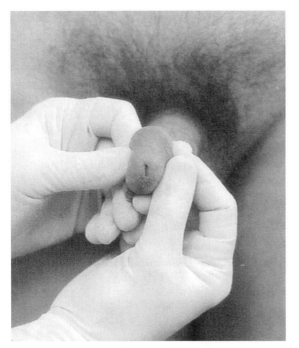

Fig. 3-10 Inspection of the urethral meatus in a circumcised male.

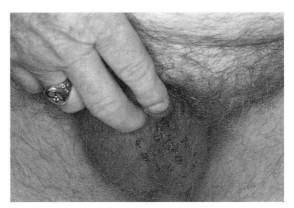

Fig. 3-11 Angiokeratoma of the scrotal skin. (From Walsh P, Retik AB, Vaughan ED, Wein AJ [eds]: Campbell's Urology, 8th edition. Philadelphia: Saunders, 2002.)

indicating urethritis, should be absent. Scarring or inability to expose distal mucosa may indicate stenosis and coexisting voiding dysfunction.

The scrotal skin is characterized by wrinkles (rugae), allowing retraction of the testes toward the body and divided by a central raphe creating the two hemiscrotums, which contain the paired testes. The scrotal skin may be slightly reddened in fair-skinned individuals, but redness indicates inflammation in darker-skinned males. As men age, the scrotum is more likely to contain one or more angiokeratomas, which are small, papular, purplish lesions caused by vascular malformations in the scrotal integument (Figure 3-11); they rarely require treatment. Sebaceous cysts also may be seen; these cutaneous cysts have a whitish appearance and a central pore from which a whitish, keratin-rich substance can be expressed (Figure 3-12). They require treatment only if they produce bothersome symptoms.

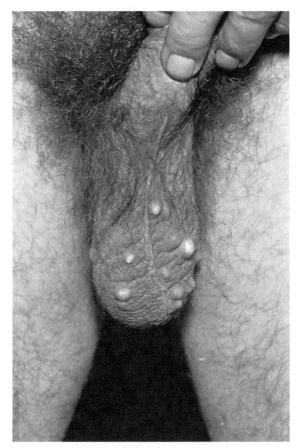

Fig. 3-12 Sebaceous cysts of the scrotum. (From Walsh P, Retik AB, Vaughan ED, Wein AJ [eds]: Campbell's Urology, 8th edition. Philadelphia: Saunders, 2002.)

A light source (a strong pen light or endoscopic light sourse) can be held behind the scrotum in a darkened room to transilluminate its contents. The testes should appear as darker organs within the scrotum, but other dark areas are abnormal and indicate inflammation, herniation of a bowel loop, or a tumor. Alternatively, a hydrocele or spermatocele will transilluminate as illustrated in Figure 3-13. Finally, the anal area is inspected; the perianal mucosa tends to be pinkish red, but adjacent skin should be free from lesions or rashes.

Palpation. The penile shaft is palpated for evidence of masses or tenderness. In addition to apparent masses, discrete hardened nodules, indicating Peyronie's disease, may be noted. A careful explanation precedes scrotal palpation. Warm hands and a slow, deliberate approach are necessary when palpating the scrotum. The nurse begins by identifying the presence of a testis

in each hemiscrotum (Figure 3-14). The testis should feel oval with a C-shaped tube, the epididymis, at its dorsal aspect. The testis should not be tender on light palpation but should be sensitive to pressure. Orchitis or epididymoorchitis produces exquisite tenderness on palpation because of the swelling and redness of the affected hemiscrotum. Testicular tenderness with elevation of a testis (i.e., "high-riding testicle") may indicate torsion. The inflammation associated with orchitis or epididymoorchitis is transiently relieved in some men by gentle elevation of the testis (Prehn's sign), but pain in the torsive testicle remains unaffected by elevation. Testicular tumors produce a distinct nodule with sensations of scrotal fullness or pressure. Testicular examination provides an excellent opportunity to teach the patient how to perform monthly testicular self-examination.

The scrotum is also examined for the presence of a hernia (Figure 3-15). The patient assumes a standing position, and he is asked to bear down while the nurse observes the area of the inguinal canal for evidence of a bulging hernia. The gloved examining finger is then gently inserted into the inguinal canal, using the loose skin of the scrotum dorsal to the testis. Again, the patient is asked to cough or perform Valsalva's maneuver, and the nurse feels for the sudden appearance of the hernia against the examining finger.

The rectal examination includes palpation of the prostate and an assessment of rectal vault contents and pelvic floor muscle strength (Figure 3-16). The patient is asked to lie on his side with the legs flexed at the knees or to stand up and lean over the examining table. The procedure is explained, and the patient is warned that insertion of the finger is expected to cause a sensation of pressure and vague discomfort. Alternatively, the patient may be asked to lean over an examining table with the arms folded in front of the abdomen, or he may be asked to separate the buttocks. We have found that placing the patient in a supine position with his legs placed comfortably in stirrups provides an ideal position for a digital rectal examination, particularly if the examiner's hands are comparatively small. Regardless of which position is selected, the patient is asked to bear down slightly to relax the anal sphincter as the well-lubricated and gloved examining finger is gently inserted. The nurse should slowly rotate the examining finger toward the individual's bladder to palpate the prostate for size, consistency, symmetry, and contour.

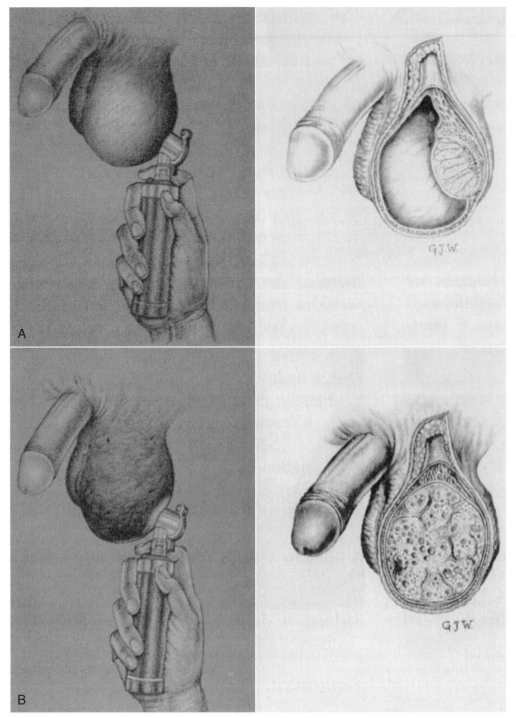

Fig. 3-13 Transillumination of scrotal contents. **A,** A hydrocele or spermatocele is not a solid mass and will reflect light. **B,** Solid masses, such as a testicular tumor, block light and do not transilluminate.

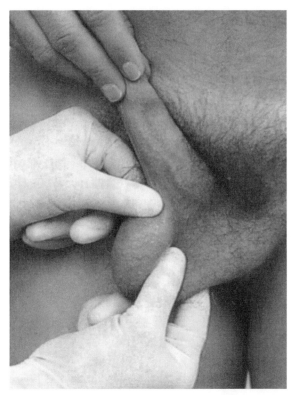

Fig. 3-14 Palpation of scrotal contents.

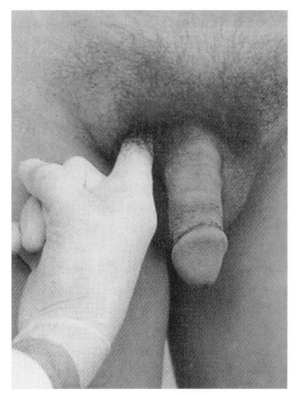

Fig. 3-15 Assessment for inguinal hernia.

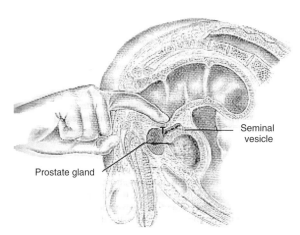

Fig. 3-16 Digital rectal palpation includes palpation of the prostate gland and assessment of pelvic floor muscle strength.

The prostate is approximately 4 cm in diameter and protrudes about 1 cm into the rectal vault. The palpable "lobes" should be symmetric and have a firm, smooth consistency. Symmetric enlargement of the prostatic lobes with loss of the central sulcus indicates benign prostatic hypertrophy, whereas asymmetric enlargement of one lobe, one or more hardened nodules, or induration raises a suspicion of prostatic cancer. Inflammation of the prostate (prostatitis) is associated with symmetric enlargement and a boggy character on palpation. Chronic male pelvic pain syndrome usually reveals a normal-sized prostate, but hypertonicity of the anal sphincter and increased discomfort occur as the examiner inserts the finger into the anal sphincter. Palpation of the prostate may cause emission of fluid into the urethra. Secretions obtained during digital examination may be examined under a light microscope or cultured if the patient is undergoing evaluation for prostatitis.

After palpating the prostate, the patient is asked to tighten the anal muscle around the examiner's finger to assess pelvic floor muscle tone. Low-tone pelvic floor muscle dysfunction is characterized by poor or lax circumferential tone and a brief, almost imperceptible contraction of the sphincter around the examiner's finger. High-tone pelvic floor muscle dysfunction is characterized by increased resting tone, discomfort when a finger is inserted, and weak or absent ability to contract the anal sphincter around the examiner's finger owing to excessive resting tone. The examination is completed by eliciting the bulbocavernosus reflex. The glans penis is gently compressed while the examining finger remains in the rectum. In the normal individual, the anal sphincter will contract, or "wink." Absence of the bulbocavernosus reflex also may indicate neurologic abnormality.

Assessment of Female Genitalia

General Approach. The patient is assisted to lie in a dorsal lithotomy position, and the legs are placed in stirrups or propped comfortably on the examining table. The female patient is typically anxious when the genitourinary system is examined and may recall specific, uncomfortable experiences caused by pelvic examination. This understandable anxiety can be relieved by ensuring privacy through adequate draping, preventing people from entering or leaving the room during the examination and by providing careful explanations before any maneuvers. The examiner should also maintain eye contact with the patient before examination whenever possible. Approaching the patient slowly and deliberately and enabling her to breathe slowly and deeply during anxiety-provoking maneuvers will diminish anxiety and discomfort associated with examination of the genitalia and vaginal vault.

Inspection and Palpation. The perineum and external genitalia are initially inspected, observing for hair distribution and skin integrity (Figure 3-17). Typically the pubic hair is coarser than scalp hair. Inspect the skin for redness, rashes, or lesions, paying careful attention to inspecting all skinfolds, particularly in the obese patient. The skin should be inspected for evidence of redness and erosion, paying careful attention to note maculopapular central and satellite lesions associated with cutaneous candidiasis. Women who wear adult containment briefs or absorbent products and who have significant volume urinary leakage are at high risk for incontinence-associated dermatitis as a result of chronic exposure of the skin to urine.

The vaginal mucosa and labia of postmenopausal or older women are inspected for evidence of atrophic urogenital changes. The labia majora are examined for size and appearance. Atrophic labia may be shriveled and partially or entirely fused with the pelvic skin. The labia majora should be gently separated, using the gloved fingers to inspect the labia minora; the

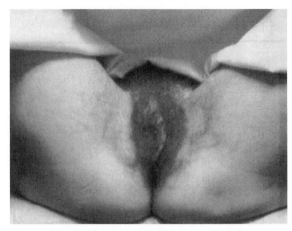

Fig. 3-17 Inspection of female genitalia.

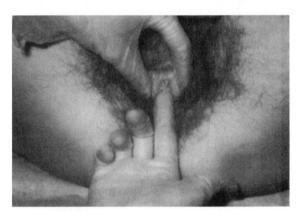

Fig. 3-18 Examination of the female urethra.

skin should be free from redness or lesions. The introitus and vaginal mucosa are inspected. The mucosa should be moist and nontender to gentle palpation, and rugae should be clearly visible. An atrophic vaginal vault will demonstrate thinning or disappearance of rugae and a dried and tender mucosa that may bleed if the vaginal vault is stretched.

The urethral meatus is carefully inspected (Figure 3-18). It should appear as a rosette or ovoid slit. It should lie within the midline and may be slightly within the vagina. The strength of the circumvaginal (pelvic floor) muscles is assessed by asking the woman to squeeze one or two of the examiner's fingers. Normal pelvic floor muscle strength will be appreciated as circumferential pressure against the finger, which will be pulled slightly toward the cervix. A vigorous contraction should offer mild resistance if the examiner's fingers are gently wiggled.

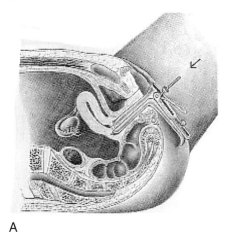

A

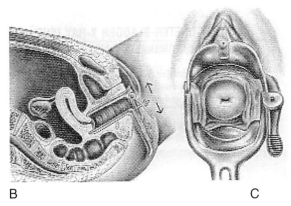

B   C

Fig. 3-19 Pelvic examination in a female using a speculum.
A, Insertion of the speculum. **B,** Gentle seperation of the blades.
C, Visualization of the cervix.

Vaginal wall support may be evaluated using the fingers or during a speculum examination (Figure 3-19). If the fingers are used, one or two gloved fingers are rotated to the posterior vaginal wall and the patient is asked to perform Valsalva's maneuver and/or cough. Descent of the anterior vaginal walls raises a strong suspicion of hypermobility of the bladder base and a corresponding cystocele. This maneuver also provides an opportunity to observe for urine loss. The presence of urine loss with physical exertion and in the absence of a strong urge to urinate is a sign of stress urinary incontinence. Following this maneuver, the examiner should rotate the fingers to support the anterior vaginal wall and the patient is again asked to perform Valsalva's maneuver or cough. Prolapse of the posterior vaginal wall provides strong evidence of a rectocele.

Speculum Examination. Examination with a speculum may or may not be included in the assessment of the female patient with a urologic complaint (see Figure 3-19). If a speculum is used, it should be warmed and adequately lubricated. The patient is advised just before the speculum is inserted and the inner aspect of the patient's thigh may be touched with the back of the gloved hand to help distract the patient and render insertion less uncomfortable. A water-soluble lubricant may be used unless cytologic specimens need to be obtained during the examination. The examiner should locate the cervix and inspect it for color, position, size, and shape of the os. A normal cervix is pink and moist; pregnancy may cause a more bluish appearance and anemia a paler color. The cervix should be located in the midline; its position correlates with the position of the uterus. Anterior orientation of the cervix indicates a retroverted uterus, whereas posterior orientation indicates an anteverted uterine position. Deviation to the left or right may indicate a mass, adhesions, or pregnancy. Any cervical discharge should be noted. Normal cervical discharge is odorless and murky or clear, and it varies in consistency from viscous to clear and thin. Discharge from bacterial or fungal infection is malodorous and yellow, gray, or green. Following inspection, the speculum is gently removed while carefully inspecting the vaginal mucosa for evidence of discharge, inflammation, and atrophic changes.

A single blade of the speculum may then be inserted to assess for vaginal wall prolapse. The speculum is initially oriented toward the woman's rectum, and she is asked to cough or perform Valsalva's maneuver while the nurse observes for evidence of anterior vaginal wall prolapse, indicating probable bladder base hypermobility and cystocele. Next, the blade is oriented toward the anterior vaginal wall, and the woman is asked to cough or bear down, again observing for prolapse of the posterior wall, indicating probable rectocele. As noted previously, the urethra should be observed for leakage, which provides the sign of stress urinary incontinence. As the speculum is withdrawn, the cervix is inspected for evidence of forward migration, indicating uterine prolapse.

The clinician then explains to the woman that a bimanual examination will follow inspection with the speculum. The glove is removed from one hand, and the index and middle finger of the gloved examining hand are lubricated. The full length of these fingers is gently inserted into the vaginal vault, allowing adequate time for the patient to relax her circumvaginal muscles to the fullest extent feasible. The vaginal wall is palpated for evidence of nodules, cysts, or masses. The cervix is located with the palmar aspect of the examiner's gloved fingers, and it is gently palpated circumferentially for size, length, and shape. The cervix is then grasped gently between the examiner's gloved fingers and gently moved from side to side. A normal cervix moves 1 to 2 cm without causing discomfort. A tender, fixed cervix may indicate pelvic inflammatory disease or an ectopic pregnancy. The tip of the finger may be inserted into the os of the cervix to assess its patency; it should admit approximately 0.5 cm of a fingertip.

The uterus is palpated for position, size, shape, and masses. The normal nongravid uterus is pear shaped and 5 to 8 cm long. Enlargement may indicate pregnancy in a young adult woman or a mass in postmenopausal women or those who are not pregnant. The ovaries are palpated if possible. They should feel firm, smooth, and ovoid and measure $3 \times 2 \times 1$ cm. A normal ovary is tender on examination, although exquisite pain is not expected. Nodules and enlargement are abnormal.

Bimanual palpation of the bladder can be painful and is often performed by the urologist during a procedure requiring anesthesia. It is typically used to assess local invasion in patients with bladder cancer.[15]

A clean pair of gloves is donned, and a digital rectal examination is completed to evaluate anal sphincter tone and the presence of the bulbocavernosus reflex. Gently tapping the clitoris should elicit the bulbocavernosus reflex. Poor anal sphincter tone, absence of the bulbocavernosus reflex, and diminished sensations may indicate neurologic disease contributing to voiding dysfunction or urinary retention.

SUMMARY

Urologic evaluation typically occurs in the context of a referral, either from a primary care provider or a specialist from a related field, such as general surgery or neurosurgery. Regardless of the context of the first contact with the patient with a urologic complaint, knowledge of common presenting signs and symptoms, combined with a rational approach to their evaluation, is essential to accurately diagnose and treat the underlying urologic disorder.

REFERENCES

1. Mosby's Medical, Nursing, and Allied Health Dictionary, 6th edition. St Louis: Mosby, 2002.
2. Charles-Jones H, May C, Latimer J, Roland M: Telephone triage by nurses in primary care: what is it for and what are the consequences likely to be? Journal of Health Services Research and Policy, 2003; 8(3):154-9.
3. Nadler RB, Bushman W, Wyker AW: Standard diagnostic considerations. In Gillenwater JY, Grayhack JT, Howards SS, Mitchell ME (eds):Adult and Pediatric Urology, 4th edition. Philadelphia: Lippincott, Williams & Wilkins, 2002; pp 47-64.
4. Resnick MI, Caldamone AA, Spirnak JP: Decision Making in Urology, 2nd edition. St Louis: Mosby, 1990.
5. Lee LW, Davis E: Gross urinary hemorrhage: a symptom, not a disease. Journal of the American Medical Association, 1953; 153(9):2-4.
6. Carson CC 3rd, Segura JW, Greene LF: Clinical importance of microhematuria. Journal of the American Medical Association, 1979; 241(2):149-50.
7. Young G, Toretsky JA, Campbell AB, Eskenazi AE: Recognition of common childhood malignancies. American Family Physician, 2000; 61(7):2144-54.
8. Bremnor JD, Sadovsky R: Evaluation of dysuria in adults. American Family Physician, 2002; 65(8):1589-96.
9. Gray M, Hufstuttler S, Albo M: Interstitial cystitis: a guide to recognition, evaluation and management for the nurse practitioner. Journal of Wound Ostomy and Continence Nursing, 2002; 29:93-102.
10. Krieger JN, Nyberg L Jr, Nickel JC: NIH consensus definition and classification of prostatitis. Journal of the American Medical Association, 1999; 282:236-7.
11. Abrams P, Cardozo L, Fall M, Griffiths G, Rosier P, Ulmsten U: The standardization of terminology of lower urinary tract function: report from the Standardization Sub-Committee of the International Continence Society. Neurourology and Urodynamics, 2002; 21:167-78.
12. Gray M: Urinary retention: management in the acute care setting. Part 1. American Journal of Nursing, 2000; 100(7):40-8.
13. Lewis JH, Rosen R, Goldstein I, Consensus Panel on Health Care Clinician Management of Erectile Dysfunction: Erectile dysfunction. American Journal of Nursing, 2003; 103(10):48-58.
14. Jannini EA, Lenzi A: Ejaculatory disorders: epidemiology and current approaches to definition, classification and subtyping. World Journal of Urology, 2005; 23(2):68-75.
15. Gerber GS, Brendler CB: Evaluation of the urologic patient. In Wein AJ, Kavoussi CR, Novick AC, Partin AW, Peters CA: Campbell-Walsh Urology, 9th edition. Philadelphia: Saunders, 2007; pp 81-110.

4 *Diagnostic Procedures*

From the development of the cystoscope, imaging procedures have historically played a central role in urologic practice. Imaging techniques continue to evolve at a rapid pace, and urologic clinicians routinely use radiographic, tomographic, ultrasonic, magnetic resonance, and pressure monitoring techniques to evaluate anatomic and functional aspects of the upper and lower urinary tract. This chapter will review diagnostic studies commonly used in urologic practice, focusing on associated nursing management.

RADIOGRAPHIC STUDIES

Although magnetic resonance and ultrasonography have gained in popularity, radiographic imaging continues to play a central role in urinary tract evaluation. Because the kidneys are able to concentrate and excrete certain materials into the urinary tract, contrast materials may be injected intravenously to highlight urinary tract morphology and assess renal concentrating function. Alternatively, contrast materials may be injected into the renal pelvis, ureter, bladder, or urethra to assess relevant anatomy and urine transport and filling function.

KIDNEY, URETER, AND BLADDER X-RAY (PLAIN ABDOMINAL FILM)

A plain abdominal x-ray is an anteroposterior (oriented from front to back) film of the kidneys, ureters, and bony pelvis, obtained without contrast material (Figure 4-1). A single film is obtained in the supine position showing the spine, ribs, bony pelvis, gas in the intestinal tract, and shadows of various organs, including the kidneys and psoas muscles. The kidney, ureter, and bladder film (KUB) is completed to detect the presence and estimate the size of larger radiopaque urinary calculi[1] (Figure 4-2, A). It is also used to detect abnormalities in bowel gas patterns that may indicate the presence of a large abdominal, pelvic, or renal mass; fecal impaction; or paralytic ileus. The renal shadows are usually visible on KUB, allowing rough determination

of renal size, location, and proximity to suspected calculi. Evaluation of anatomic defects of the bony spinal column and sacrum may indicate neuropathic bladder dysfunction caused by dysraphism of the lower spine (see Figure 4-2, B). Defects of the lower ribs and bony pelvis also may be detected.

Indications

Urinary calculi
Preliminary x-ray for intravenous pyelogram/urogram (IVP/IVU)
Preliminary x-ray for voiding cystourethrogram, cystogram, or videourodynamic testing

Contraindication

Pregnancy in the first trimester

Nursing Management

Preparation for a KUB varies according to its purpose. Bowel preparation ("bowel prep") may be required when a KUB is obtained before an IVP, but none is required when a KUB is taken as a single view or as a preliminary film before a cystogram, voiding cystourethrogram, or videourodynamics. The patient is advised that a KUB is a painless procedure but may not detect every urinary stone, particularly if the calculi are small, obscured by bowel gas, or radiolucent.

INTRAVENOUS PYELOGRAM/UROGRAM WITH NEPHROTOMOGRAMS

An IVP/IVU is a series of contrast-enhanced x-rays providing detailed information about the shape, position, structure, and excretory function of the kidneys, ureters, and bladder[2] (Figure 4-3). It is particularly useful for identification of urinary calculi, tumors, or anatomic defects. An ionic contrast solution, such as sodium diatrizoate (Hypaque) or methylglucamine iothalamate (Conray), is injected through the antecubital vein. Alternatively, a nonionic preparation, such as diatrizoate meglumine (Isovue) or iohexol (Omnipaque), may

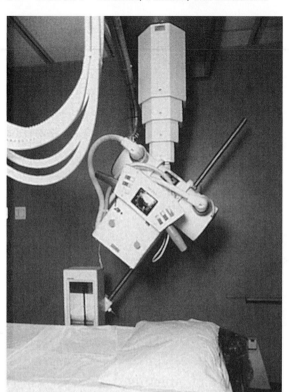

Fig. 4-1 Kidney, ureter, and bladder (KUB) equipment.

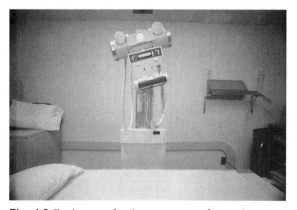

Fig. 4-3 Equipment for intravenous pyelogram/urogram with tomography.

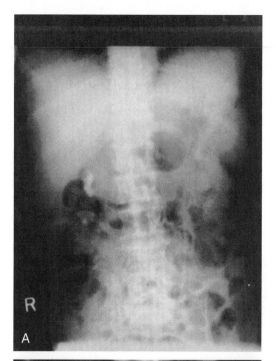

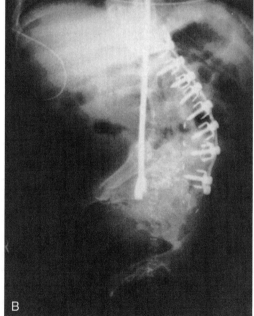

Fig. 4-2 A, Kidney, ureter, and bladder (KUB) image of urinary stone. **B,** KUB image demonstrating spina bifida plus rods with neuropathic bladder dysfunction.

be used for patients who are hypersensitive to ionic solutions or at risk for contrast-associated nephrotoxicity (see Clinical Highlights for Advanced and Expert Practice: Contrast-Induced Nephrotoxicity and Contrast-Induced Allergic-Like Reactions, p. 66).[3-8] A series of x-ray films is taken to obtain information about the transport of urine from the renal pelvis to the bladder (Figure 4-4). Mechanical compression of the abdomen may enhance the quality of certain views. X-rays of the partly filled bladder provide a limited cystogram. The patient's ability to empty the bladder may be assessed through a postvoid x-ray. The IVP/IVU requires approximately 45 to 60 minutes to complete, and results can be interpreted immediately when necessary.

Nephrotomograms are used to enhance the IVP. They image a single plane of the kidney instead of the multiplane view obtained during routine radiography. Tomography is particularly useful in the evaluation of urinary calculi or renal tumors.

Indications

Urinary calculi
Urinary system mass
Hematuria
Obstruction of the urinary system, particularly the
    upper tracts (i.e., renal, pelvic, or ureteral)
Urinary system anomaly

Contraindications

Hypersensitivity to contrast media
Hypersensitivity to iodine-based cleansing solutions
Hypersensitivity to seafood

Nursing Management

Screen the patient for hypersensitivity to intravenous (IV) contrast (see Clinical Highlights for Advanced and Expert Practice: Contrast-Induced Allergic-Like Reactions, pp. 67–68). Assess the patient for dehydration and for factors increasing the risk of nephrotoxicity, including mild renal insufficiency (creatinine above 1.3 to 1.5 mg/dl) and associated conditions (e.g., diabetes mellitus, cardiovascular disease, or multiple myeloma). Explain the procedure and the purpose of the test. Consult with the physician or nurse practitioner concerning proper bowel preparation, which is typically required for optimal visualization of the kidneys and ureters. Bowel preparation is influenced by the patient's age, health, patterns of bowel

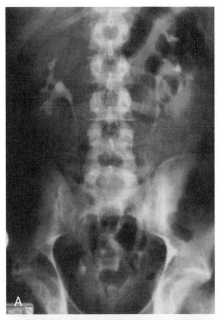

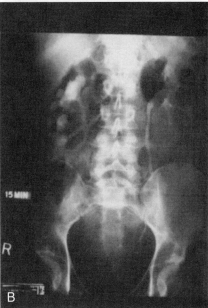

Fig. 4-4 A, Normal intravenous pyelogram (IVP) image. **B,** Hydronephrosis of right kidney.

elimination, and hydration status. It may include catharsis and a brief period of food and fluid restriction.

Catharsis is achieved by administration of castor oil or bisacodyl tablets (Dulcolax). A bisacodyl suppository may also be required the morning of the test to stimulate further bowel evacuation. Patients with chronic constipation may require a more vigorous

Clinical Highlights for Advanced and Expert Practice: Contrast-Induced Nephrotoxicity[3,4]

Background

Nephrotoxicity may occur with any radiographic study involving the injection of a contrast material. In most cases, the adverse reaction is limited to an asymptomatic and transient rise in serum creatinine that persists for 3 to 5 days. However, if the patient undergoes a surgical procedure or additional testing requiring further injection of contrast, the risk for a more severe and long-lasting adverse response rises. Severe contrast-induced nephrotoxicity is characterized by oliguria and an elevated serum creatinine that peaks 2 to 4 days following contrast injections and persists for 5 to 10 days.

Risk Factors

The primary risk factor for contrast-induced nephrotoxicity is preexisting renal insufficiency. This risk is in proportion to the creatinine when contrast is injected; it is also affected by the route of delivery (arterial injection carries a higher risk than does venous) and the type of contrast material used (ionic materials carry a higher risk than do nonionic products). For example, the risk of nephrotoxicity following venous injection of contrast in a patient with a creatinine less than 1.3 to 1.5 mg/dl is less than 1%. Contrast injection in patients with mild renal insufficiency (generally defined as creatinine of 1.5 to 2 mg/dl) is associated with a risk of 9% to 40%, and the chance of nephrotoxicity in a patient with severe renal insufficiency (creatinine above 2 mg/dl) is 50% to 90%.

- Additional risk factors include diabetes mellitus, cardiovascular disease, and multiple myeloma. However, they have been shown to present a significant risk *only* when associated with renal insufficiency. Dehydration also acts as a risk factor when associated with renal insufficiency, but it is reversible.
- The choice of contrast material and route of injection also affect the risk of nephrotoxicity. The overall risk of nephrotoxicity (including patients at all levels of predisposing risk) associated with venous injection of contrast is 2% to 5%, whereas the incidence with arterial injection is 7% to 8%. Ionic contrast materials and those with higher osmolarity also increase the risk of transient renal toxicity.
- Metformin (Glucophage) can exacerbate contrast-induced nephrotoxicity. It should be discontinued immediately before and for 48 hours following contrast injection, and it may be held until a follow-up serum creatinine is obtained if the risk of nephropathy is significant.

Evaluation

- Serum creatinine: acute elevation from baseline peaks 2 to 4 days after contrast injection; persists for 3 to 5 days in mild cases, 5 to 10 days in severe cases
- Radiographic appearance
- Bilateral persistence of contrast on nephrotomogram up to 24 hours after injection
- Concentration of calyceal system and parenchyma will increase over time rather than diminish with excretion of contrast
- Contrast may be excreted by alternate route, leading to visualization of biliary system, gallbladder, or bowel

Nursing Management

- When the creatinine is 1.3 to 1.5 mg/dl or less:
  - No special preparation
- When the creatinine is 1.6 to 2 mg/dl:
  - Ensure adequate hydration
  - Consult with urologist and radiologist concerning use of low-osmolar or nonionic contrast material
  - Consider alternate imaging study (e.g., computed tomography [CT] or ultrasound)
- When the creatinine is 2 mg/dl or higher:
  - Consult with urologist and radiologist about alternative imaging study
  - Injection may be considered in life-threatening situations or when patient is on dialysis

Clinical Highlights for Advanced and Expert Practice: Contrast-Induced Allergic-Like Reactions[3,5-8]

- -

Background

Injections of contrast materials lead to adverse reactions in some patients. These reactions range from transient and mild bothersome symptoms, such as a perception of warmth or flushing and nausea, to severe, life-threatening anaphylactoid reactions and death in rare cases. Mild reactions occur in approximately 3% of all cases when contrast media are injected into the vascular system. Anaphylactoid reactions occur in approximately 1% to 2% of patients receiving an IV injection of an ionic, high-osmolar material such as that often used with IV pyelography. Deaths are rare, occurring in 0.002% to 0.009% of patients.

Adverse responses to contrast media are typically described as "allergic," implying that they arise from an immunologic response similar to that seen in classic severe allergies to drugs, foods, or environmental sources. Associations between adverse materials and allergy to seafood or atopy support this hypothesis, but contrary evidence also exists that must be considered. For example, anaphylactoid responses to contrast materials frequently occur during initial exposure, they are dose dependent, and they do not always recur with subsequent administration. In addition, efforts to create an antiserum to contrast materials have not been successful, further confirming a weak rather than strong immunogenic element to these responses. Instead, considerable evidence exists that reactions to contrast media may represent activation of basophils and mast cells by an immunoglobulin E (IgE)–*independent* mechanism. Finally, some patients who initially tolerate intravascular injection of contrast materials experience "delayed" adverse reactions. These responses typically occur 1 to 48 hours after injection, but they may occur as long as 7 days after injection. They are characterized by mild to moderate urticaria, although more severe responses and erythema multiforme may occur in rare cases. The pathophysiology of these responses is even less well understood; it is usually postulated to represent a belated immunogenic response, possibly mediated by a T-cell mechanism rather than the IgE pathway observed in classic allergic reactions.

Because of these persistent and unanswered questions about the pathophysiology of adverse reactions to contrast materials, this Clinical Highlight for Advanced and Expert Practice has been purposely labeled "*allergic-like*" reactions to contrast materials. The choice of wording is highlighted because it is more than semantic; instead, it reflects some of the subtle but clinically relevant differences nurses face when seeking to prevent, recognize, and manage contrast-induced allergic-like reaction.

Risk Factors

- Previous allergic reaction to injection of contrast media
- Allergy to seafood
- Atopy
- Renal insufficiency (leads to prolonged exposure and delayed excretion of contrast media)
- Ionic and high osmolar contrast media (associated with a higher overall risk of allergic-like responses, but the risk of severe, anaphylactoid reactions and mortality rates are similar)

Evaluation

- Responses may occur as isolated events or progress from mild symptoms to severe anaphylactoid response
- Nausea (may lead to vomiting), perception of heat or flushing
- Urticaria or hives
- Mild, nonprogressive urticaria: often associated with itching, few lesions typical or limited to one area of body
- Extensive urticaria involving chest and abdomen, back, one or more extremities; often progressive and associated with other symptoms
- Wheezing: may occur as isolated finding but often associated with urticaria
- Bronchospasm
- Laryngeal edema: shortness of breath, hoarseness of voice, patient agitated and may complain of tightness or swelling in throat
- Hypotension
- Normal or slow pulse generally indicates vasovagal reaction
- Hypotension and rapid pulse indicate allergic-type response
- Anaphylactoid reaction: widespread urticaria, hypotension, hypotension, bronchospasm, laryngoedema, angioedema

Continued

Clinical Highlights for Advanced and Expert Practice: Contrast-Induced Allergic-Like Reactions[3,5-8]—Cont'd

Nursing Management

Premedicate high-risk patients when directed by the radiologist or urologist; alternatives include the following:

- Dexamethasone (Decadron), 4 mg every 6 hours for 18 to 24 hours before contrast injection
- Prednisone, 50 mg, 13, 7, and 1 hour before injection
- Methylprednisolone, 32 mg, 12 and 2 hours before injection
- Diphenhydramine, 50 mg by mouth (PO) as adjunctive therapy (diphenhydramine is *not* effective as monotherapy)

Arrange for use of nonionic contrast media in high-risk patients (reduces overall risk fivefold)

Prepare for contrast reaction before occurrence; ensure readiness of crash cart, and assemble medication box for contrast reactions, including the following:

- Diphenhydramine, 250-mg vials and one or two alternative medications (e.g., cimetidine, ranitidine)
- β_2-agonist inhalers: terbutaline, albuterol, and metaproterenol
- Atropine
- Corticosteroids
- Nitroglycerin
- Furosemide (Lasix)
- Normal saline

Observe for

- Nausea, vomiting, sensation of heat or flushing

Observe patient for signs and symptoms of allergic-type response

Mild, nonprogressive urticaria

- Counsel patient that isolated nausea, vomiting, or perception of heat does not indicate allergic reaction to contrast
- Check vital signs, including blood pressure, pulse, and respirations
- Auscultate for wheezing or evidence of bronchospasm
- Observe until urticaria clears or diminishes

Extensive or progressive urticaria

- Check vital signs, including blood pressure, pulse, and respirations
- Auscultate for wheezing or evidence of bronchospasm
- Diphenhydramine, 50 mg intramuscularly (IM) unless bronchospasm present (contraindicated with bronchospasm; may lead to hypotension)
- If antihistamine fails to control urticaria: epinephrine, 1 mg = 1 ml of 1:1000 (NB carefully check concentration; IV epinephrine used only when IM does not control symptoms

Wheezing

- Oxygen, 10 L/min
- β_2-agonist inhaler: two or three premeasured puffs or doses
- Norepinephrine, 1:1000 0/1 mg (0.1 ml) IM if β_2-agonist inhalers are not effective; IV epinephrine used if patient is hypotensive

Laryngeal edema

- Oxygen, 10 L/min
- IV epinephrine: 1:10,000 solution, administered as 1-ml slow IV push (over a period of 3 to 5 minutes)
- *Avoid* β_2-agonist inhalers; they exacerbate rather than alleviate laryngeal edema
- If patient does not promptly respond, initiate code

Anaphylactoid reaction (therapies are given concurrently)

- IV epinephrine: 1:10,000 solution, administered as 1-ml slow IV push (over a period of 3 to 5 minutes); repeat every 5 to 10 minutes to maximum dose of 1 mg
- Normal saline or Ringer's lactate through IV access
- Oxygen, 10 L/min
- Diphenhydramine, 25 to 50 mg IV
- Hydrocortisone, 1 g IV
- Initiate code

preparation. Children do not typically undergo a bowel preparation, unless constipation is a particular problem.

Fluid and food restriction may be recommended to optimize visualization of the urinary system anatomy. Adults may be asked to remain NPO (nothing by mouth) for approximately 4 hours before the examination, but children are rarely restricted.

During the test the patient is carefully monitored for signs of allergic reaction to contrast material, including respiratory difficulty, diaphoresis, numbness, and palpitations (see Clinical Highlights for Advanced and Expert Practice: Contrast-Induced Allergic-Like Reactions). Some patients experience nausea, flushing, and an unpleasant metallic or salty taste in the mouth, but these do not indicate hypersensitivity to contrast materials.

The patient is also carefully monitored for allergic reactions and contrast nephropathy immediately following the procedure. Hypersensitivity reactions vary in severity from transient nausea, urticaria, and itching to respiratory failure and death. An antihistamine such as diphenhydramine, corticosteroids, and an emergency cart are kept readily available. Ensure adequate fluid intake following the procedure, and measure urine output, which should be at least 30 ml/hr, to assess for contrast-induced nephropathy. Advise the patient who is unable to consume or retain fluids because of nausea and vomiting to promptly consult a physician in order to minimize the risk of contrast nephropathy.

RETROGRADE PYELOGRAM

A retrograde pyelogram (RPG) is a series of x-rays that provide detailed anatomic views of the ureter, ureteropelvic junction, renal pelvis, and calyces. The procedure is performed under endoscopic visualization of the ureterovesical junction. A ureteral catheter (Figure 4-5) is placed into the lower segment of the ureter, and contrast material is *gently* injected or infused by means of gravity into the upper urinary tract. Retrograde pyelography may be technically difficult when the patient has significant prostate enlargement, an ectopic ureter, or prior ureteral reimplantation.

Indications

Visualization of the ureter and renal pelvis when the kidney is unable to concentrate and excrete contrast material on IV urography

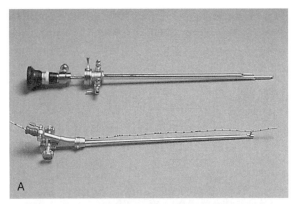

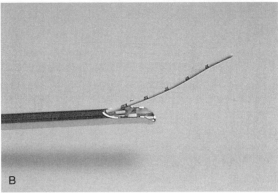

Fig. 4-5 Rigid cystoscope with McCarthy bridge for retrograde pyelogram (RPG). **A,** Bridge. **B,** Placement of ureteral catheter.

Alternative for visualization of ureter and renal pelvis in the patient hypersensitive to iodine-bound contrast materials *(Some risk of hypersensitivity remains.)*
Urinary calculi
Anatomic defect or mass
Obstruction
Placement of ureteral stent for drainage or manipulation of a stone

Contraindications

Hypersensitivity to contrast media
Hypersensitivity to iodine-bound cleansing solutions or shellfish

Nursing Management

Bowel preparation is not required before RPG, but the patient is prepared for cystoscopy and insertion of ureteral stents. Although the risk of allergic-like reaction is low, patients must nevertheless be monitored for hypersensitivity to infusion of contrast media. Postprocedure complications are uncommon and include perforation of the ureter or renal pelvis, infection, and acute renal failure caused by edema and ureteral obstruction. The patient is advised to call his or her physician if signs and symptoms of infection or ureteral perforation, such as persistent or escalating flank pain, dysuria, chills, and fever, occur. The patient is also alerted that injection of contrast material may cause transient flank pain.

CYSTOGRAM AND VOIDING CYSTOURETHROGRAM

A cystogram or voiding cystourethrogram (VCUG) requires catheterization and instillation of contrast material into the bladder. A cystogram is a series of x-rays of the bladder obtained during filling; the VCUG combines images of the cystogram with x-rays of the bladder and urethra during micturition (Figure 4-6).

Indications

Recurring urinary tract infection (particularly in children)
Pyelonephritis (febrile urinary tract infection)
Vesicoureteral reflux
Congenital anomaly of the lower urinary tract
Trauma of the lower urinary tract or pelvis (e.g., rupture of urethra or bladder, straddle injury, or pelvic fracture)
Suspected fistulae (i.e., vesicovaginal, vesicocutaneous, urethrovaginal, or urethrocutaneous)
Preoperative evaluation of patients undergoing renal, pancreatic, or combined transplant
Postoperative evaluation of suspected anastomotic leak

Contraindications

Hypersensitivity to intravesical contrast media
Hypersensitivity to iodine-based cleansing solutions, such as povidone-iodine (Betadine)
Current urinary tract infection

Nursing Management

The patient is advised that a cystogram or VCUG will require catheterization. A urinalysis or urine culture may be performed to exclude clinically relevant urinary tract infection. The patient is advised that

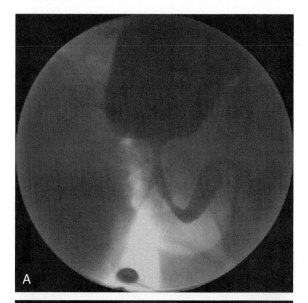

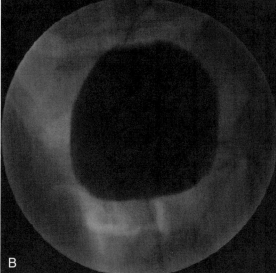

Fig. 4-6 A, Normal cystogram in a male. **B,** Voiding cystourethrogram demonstrating obstruction of the prostatic urethra.

the procedure may produce transient urethral and bladder discomfort that can be relieved by fluid intake and by a warm bath or shower. The patient is advised to increase the volume of fluids consumed for the first 4 to 6 hours following a VCUG in order to dilute and flush remaining contrast materials from the urinary tract. The patient is also taught the signs and symptoms of a urinary tract infection (i.e., dysuria, suprapubic or lower back pain, frequency, and hematuria) and instructed to contact the physician should symptoms occur.

RADIOGRAPHIC IMAGING OF URINARY DIVERSIONS (LOOPOGRAM AND POUCHOGRAM)

Contrast media may be infused into continent or incontinent urinary diversions in order to assess their anatomy, test the integrity of anastomotic sites, and assess their functional ability to store urine or serve as a conduit for its rapid expulsion from a reconstructed urinary tract. A KUB is usually performed before an imaging study of the pouch, particularly if there is a risk of stones such as seen with long-term continent urinary diversions.

Imaging an incontinent ileal conduit is done by inserting a relatively large catheter (18F to 24F) into the abdominal stoma and infusing contrast media under gravity. The stoma may be transiently obstructed by partially filling the retention balloon of the catheter. The architecture of the conduit is assessed, and the upper urinary tracts are imaged since the ureters are implanted in a refluxing manner. Drainage of the conduit can be assessed by removing any fluid from the retention balloon and removing the catheter from the stoma. Retention of contrast within the conduit or absence of ureteral reflux is significant because it indicates possible obstruction of the abdominal stoma or ureteroileal junction, respectively.

Imaging a continent urinary diversion requires infusion of contrast media into the reservoir of the urinary diversion by way of a catheter placed into the abdominal stoma. A low-volume image is usually obtained to ensure anatomic integrity and identify filling defects. The reservoir is then filled to capacity, and anastomotic integrity is again assessed. Vesicoureteral reflux is not necessarily expected when imaging a continent urinary diversion because the ureters may be implanted in a nonrefluxing manner or other techniques may be used to reduce the likelihood of reflux.

Urodynamic testing may be combined with upper tract imaging studies, particularly if urinary leakage occurs in a continent urinary diversion.

Indications

Baseline evaluation for subsequent comparison (usually obtained within first 6 to 12 weeks of construction)
Recurring pouchitis (i.e., infection of urine within a continent urinary diversion)
Febrile urinary tract infections
Incontinence of a continent urinary diversion
Suspected obstruction of the stoma or ureteroenteric anastomosis
Calculi

Contraindications

Current urinary tract infection (consult with physician concerning need for suppressive antibiotics)
Allergic-like reaction to contrast materials (consult radiologist or urologist concerning need for nonionic contrast media, premedication, or alternative imaging procedure)

Nursing Management

Obtain a urine specimen *directly* from the conduit or urinary reservoir as directed in order to identify and eliminate urinary tract infection. Review laboratory results in consultation with the physician or nurse practitioner to ensure accurate differentiation of asymptomatic bacteriuria, present in most continent and nearly all incontinent diversions, from clinically relevant infection. Consult with the radiology department, and arrange for the patient to self-catheterize during the continent urinary diversion imaging whenever feasible. This reduces patient anxiety and the risk of trauma to the stoma if radiologic personnel do not have extensive experience with continent urinary diversions. Inform the patient with an incontinent urinary diversion to bring an extra pouch since removal of the existing pouch is necessary so contrast media can be infused into the ileal conduit. Following the procedure, the patient is monitored for bleeding or infection. Light pink discharge, indicating bleeding of only a small volume of blood, may occur, but passage of bright red urine or clots is abnormal and requires prompt assessment and intervention. Infection of an incontinent urinary diversion is associated with an increased mucus production, a change in urinary odor, flank or abdominal discomfort, malaise, and fever. Infection of a continent urinary diversion also causes an increase in mucus production, a change in urine odor, acute incontinence in a previously continent diversion, or fever. Patients are advised that symptomatic infection of a continent or incontinent diversion requires prompt assessment and treatment, particularly when associated with a fever.

RETROGRADE URETHROGRAM

A retrograde urethrogram (RUG) is a series of x-ray images obtained during instillation of contrast media into the male urethra. The fluid is instilled in one of three ways. A catheter-tipped syringe may be placed in the meatus and advanced until it is blocked (Figure 4-7). Alternatively, an 8F to 10F Foley catheter is placed in the fossa navicularis, and its retention balloon is inflated with approximately 1 to 2 ml of fluid until the urethral meatus is blocked. Finally, a Brodney clamp can be placed; this device is specially designed to allow injection of contrast media while distancing the clinician's hand in order to minimize radiation exposure during the procedure. Oblique x-rays of the urethra are obtained during and after instillation of approximately 15 to 30 ml of contrast material.

Indications

Urethral stricture
Urethral fistula
Trauma
Urethral diverticulum
Urethral tumor

Contraindications

Hypersensitivity to intravesical contrast media
Hypersensitivity to iodine-based cleansing solutions

Nursing Management

The patient is advised that the RUG will require placement of a catheter or catheter-tipped syringe just beyond the urethral meatus. Children, in particular, should be reassured that the syringe will not be attached to a needle. Whenever possible a urinary tract infection should be treated before an RUG. Management following the procedure focuses on alleviating dysuria and urethral burning that are typically transient. Advise the patient to drink fluids and to take a warm bath or shower to reduce discomfort. A urinary analgesic, such as phenazopyridine, may be prescribed for persons with moderately severe to severe urethral sensitivity. The patient is also taught signs and symptoms of urinary tract infection and advised to contact his or her physician should symptoms occur.

COMPUTED TOMOGRAPHY

A computed tomography (CT) scan provides computer-generated axial images of the abdominal contents, including the kidneys, ureters, bladder, and major renal vessels, and male genitalia, including the pelvic lymph nodes (Figures 4-8 and 4-9).[9] CT images of the pelvis are useful for detecting and evaluating urinary system tumors and enlarged lymph nodes caused by metastatic invasion or pelvic abscess or distortion caused by a

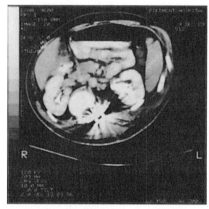

Fig. 4-8 Normal abdominal computed tomography (CT) scan demonstrating kidneys.

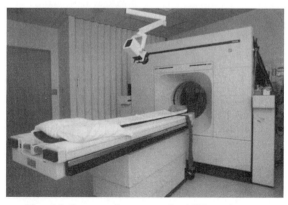

Fig. 4-9 Computed tomography (CT) equipment.

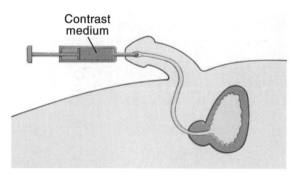

Contrast medium

Fig. 4-7 One technique for retrograde urethrography.

primary pelvic mass. CT also provides an estimate of tissue densities expressed as Hounsfield units. Normal parenchyma measures 80 to 100 Hounsfield units. Fluid-filled cysts have a lower density, whereas solid tumors have a density similar to normal parenchyma. Evaluation may be enhanced by administration of oral and/or IV contrast media.

The unenhanced CT scan has largely replaced other imaging modalities in the evaluation of acute flank pain in the emergency department setting. This technique has gained popularity because it provides an accurate method of diagnosing obstructing urinary stones, as well as images of the upper urinary tracts that help the physician determine the need for immediate treatment, urgent intervention, or delayed treatment.[10]

Newer techniques of CT imaging include multi-detector helical CT (sometimes called spiral CT), which uses a computer to generate three-dimensional images of the urinary system. These images are useful in the evaluation of abdominal masses and in tumor staging. This technique allows rapid imaging and is particularly useful when evaluating urinary calculi in an urgent care setting, such as the hospital-based emergency department.

The patient is placed in a supine position while a belt mechanism slowly moves the body while obtaining 10-mm axial views. A single longitudinal view is obtained to outline the location of subsequent cuts.

Indications

Acute flank pain
Urinary system anomalies
Abdominal trauma
Renal vein thrombosis
Renal artery stenosis
Chronic pyelonephritis
Acquired immunodeficiency syndrome (AIDS)–related
    nephropathy
Complex renal cysts
Evaluation of abdominal masses
Enlargement of abdominal lymph nodes
Tumor staging
Suspected non-Hodgkin's lymphoma
Urinary calculi

Contraindications

Hypersensitivity to contrast media
Morbid obesity (above 300 lb [136 kg])

Nursing Management

Advise patients that they will be placed on a pallet that will move through a tunnel-like imaging chamber. Regular CT scans require up to 60 minutes, but a spiral CT may be completed in 5 minutes or less. Remaining still is critical to an accurate study, and children or patients with severe claustrophobia may require sedation. The patient may be asked to hold respirations repeatedly for several seconds for optimal results. Hypersensitivity reactions may occur when contrast materials are ingested or injected.

MAGNETIC RESONANCE IMAGING

Magnetic resonance imaging (MRI) uses radio waves to alter the magnetic fields produced by the body rather than roentgen rays (x-rays) to produce images of the internal environment. MRI can produce images from any perspective, including cross-sectional, sagittal, transaxial, or coronal, without requiring the patient to move with respect to the imaging chamber (Figure 4-10). It is not useful in detecting urinary calculi.

Newer MRI techniques include open chamber imaging units capable of generating dynamic images

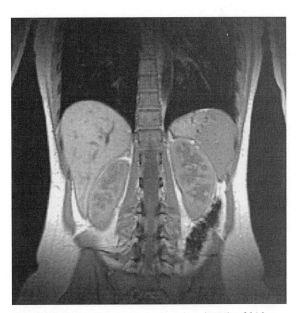

Fig. 4-10 Magnetic resonance imaging (MRI) of kidneys, coronal view. Note the bowel loop, psoas muscle, and liver causing the right kidney to lie lower than the left. (From Pollack HM, McClennan BL: *Clinical Urography*, 5th edition. Philadelphia: Saunders, 2000.)

useful in the characterization of pelvic organ prolapse.[11] MR urography requires IV injection of gadolinium (a contrast material that is not nephrotoxic).[12] Images are obtained as the contrast medium is concentrated and excreted by the kidneys. A diuretic (furosemide) is then injected to ensure adequate washout of the contrast and optimal imaging of the upper and lower urinary tracts. MR urography is particularly useful in the evaluation of dilated urinary tracts with poorly functioning kidneys.

Indications

Abdominal or pelvic mass
Staging renal and adrenal tumors
Congenital anomalies
Renal vein thrombosis
Renal artery stenosis
Renal vessels following transplant
Staging prostate and bladder cancer
Characterizing pelvic organ prolapse

Contraindications

Electric, magnetic, or mechanically activated implants, such as neurostimulators, cochlear implants, hearing aids, or pacemakers
Metal joint prostheses
Intracranial aneurysm clips
Intraorbital metal fragments or shrapnel

Nursing Management

The patient is asked to remove jewelry, watches, glasses, hairpins, and any other metal objects. IV poles, wheelchairs, and stretchers must be removed from the MRI chamber. Although most surgical clips are safe, patients must be carefully screened for cerebral clips used for aneurysm repairs, since some are ferromagnetic. Pacemakers and other implants contain metals. Preparation includes carefully explaining that scanning requires the patient to lie completely still on a narrow table with a cylindric scanner surrounding him or her while images are taken (Figure 4-11). Once in the machine, the patient cannot move out. This realization and the act of being placed in the machine can cause a disturbing sense of helplessness and claustrophobia. The patient should be advised that the MRI machine will make a repeated and loud knocking noise, which occurs when the coils change pulse direction. Mild sedation may be required to assist the patient to relax and

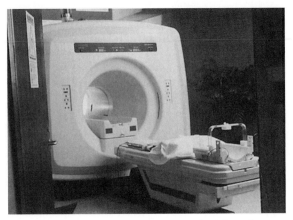

Fig. 4-11 Magnetic resonance imaging (MRI) equipment.

remain still throughout the examination. Reassure the patient that a technologist will remain in verbal communication throughout the procedure, but the technologist will not be in the room with him or her. Playing music also may relieve anxiety. The entire procedure may require up to 90 minutes. Consult the physician about sedating a patient who cannot cooperate or follow directions (i.e., children or adults with a history of claustrophobia).

ENDOSCOPY

Endoscopy is the visualization of hollow viscera within the body by means of light-enhanced telescopic or fiberoptic imaging. Endoscopy of the urinary system allows direct visualization of the renal pelvis and calices, ureters, and lower urinary tract. Rigid endoscopy requires insertion of a metal sheath followed by introduction of telescopes attached to a powerful light source for visual inspection (Figure 4-12). Flexible endoscopy uses fiberoptic technology for visualization through a relatively slender one-piece system. Both flexible and rigid endoscopic instruments provide working ports for obtaining biopsy specimens, ureteral catheterization, or other procedures requiring direct visualization of the urinary system. Three of the endoscopic procedures common to urology are cystoscopy, ureteroscopy, and percutaneous nephroscopy.

Cystoscopy (Cystourethroscopy). Cystoscopy is the most common endoscopic procedure in urology. The urethra, bladder urothelium, trigone, and ureterovesical junctions are visualized from a retrograde perspective. Rigid cystoscopy requires

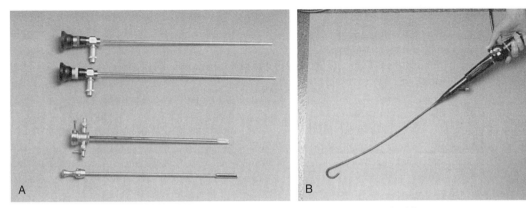

Fig. 4-12 Endoscopy equipment. **A,** Rigid cystoscope. **B,** Flexible cystoscope.

introduction of a 19F to 21F metal sheath followed by insertion of a telescope allowing direct visualization. The bladder neck and urethra are visualized during withdrawal of the sheath. Flexible cystoscopy uses a softer, 14F to 16F sheath that contains a fiberoptic system attached to a powerful light source. Fiberoptic instruments also allow visualization from an antegrade perspective by reorienting the scope on itself. It is more comfortable compared with the rigid cystoscope and is preferred in the office setting. Rigid cystoscopy is required in the evacuation of clots, when inserting a cone-tipped ureteral stent for ureteral imaging, and for transurethral resection procedures.

Ureteroscopy (Ureteropyeloscopy). Ureteroscopes are commonly available in 6.5F and 8.5F and combine a fiberoptic telescope encased in a metal sheath. Although this instrument allows flexibility and durability for visualizing the ureter and renal pelvis, it only provides a stippled visual field and a limited working port. Patients undergoing ureteroscopy are initially evaluated by cystourethroscopy in order to identify the ureteral orifice. The ureter may be dilated before insertion of the ureteroscope, or a specially designed guidewire and dilator may be inserted under ureteroscopic visualization. A rigid ureteroscope can be passed all the way into the renal pelvis, allowing visualization of the entire upper urinary tract. Following ureteroscopy most urologists will place a double pigtail ureteral catheter or ureteral stent.

Percutaneous Nephroscopy. Nephroscopy allows visualization of the renal pelvis and calices from an antegrade perspective. Fluoroscopic or ultrasonic guidance is used to gain access to the renal pelvis.

The tract is then dilated by sequential passage of dilators or inflation of a high-pressure balloon. A nephroscope is then inserted that has an offset lens and is specially designed for visualization and manipulation of renal calculi. A nephrostomy tube is placed when the procedure is completed to avoid the risk of obstruction.

Indications

Cystoscopy
Hematuria
Lower urinary tract filling defects or masses
Recurrent urinary tract infection
Foreign body
Stricture disease
Tumor surveillance
Suspected fistula
Bladder outlet obstruction of unknown etiology

Ureteroscopy
Obstruction
Filling defect or mass of upper urinary tract
Gross hematuria
Ureteral calculi
Ureteral stricture
Evaluation of foreign body
Surveillance following treatment of ureteropelvic tumor

Percutaneous Nephroscopy
Filling defect or mass of the renal pelvis or calices
Calculi
Incision of ureteropelvic junction (UPJ) obstruction

Contraindication
Urinary tract infection

Nursing Management

Cystourethroscopy. Advise the patient that cystourethroscopy requires urethral instrumentation. After ensuring adequate privacy, the patient is usually placed in a lithotomy position, and the perineum is draped and prepared with an antiseptic cleanser. Regional or systemic anesthesia is occasionally indicated, but the urethra is typically anesthetized with a 2% lidocaine lubricating gel. The lubricant should be injected into the urethra 3 to 5 minutes *before* insertion of the cystoscope. In men the urethra is occluded with a penile clamp to maximize local anesthesia, and a cotton ball or gauze is used to obstruct the urethral meatus in women. During the procedure, the patient is monitored for excessive pain and bladder overdistention. Following the procedure, the patient is counseled that urethral discomfort and hematuria may persist for 1 to 2 days. Consumption of fluids and a warm bath or shower usually relieve this discomfort. A urinary analgesic such as phenazopyridine (Pyridium) also may be prescribed following cystourethroscopy, particularly if inspection is completed with a larger rigid system or combined with invasive procedures, such as biopsy. After routine cystourethroscopy the urine may be pink tinged. Reassure the patient that even small amounts of blood can discolor a significant volume of urine. Patients undergoing biopsy procedures should also be counseled that they are likely to pass small, dark-colored flecks of blood (scabs) 7 to 10 days following the procedure. Alternatively, lysis of red blood cells within the urine may lighten the color of these clots to a grayish white color resembling sloughed tissue. Nevertheless, the passage of bright red blood or clots at any time following cystourethroscopy is abnormal and justifies prompt notification of the physician.

Because of the small but significant risk of urinary tract infection, patients must be taught to recognize the symptoms of cystitis and proper management. Infection may affect only the lower urinary tract, producing dysuria, suprapubic and lower back pain, hematuria, and voiding frequency. Rarely, infection may enter the systemic circulation through minute tears in the urinary mucosa, causing fever, chills, rapid pulse, and tachypnea. This medical emergency must be rapidly managed with fluid replacement and IV antibiotics to avoid septic shock characterized by hypothermia, diminishing blood pressure, and death.

Ureteropyeloscopy. Inform the patient that endoscopic examination of the ureter or renal pelvis requires cystoscopy followed by dilation of the ureter before or during visualization. This procedure typically requires regional or general anesthesia with its associated precautions. Bleeding may cause pink-tinged urine, but passage of bright red blood or clots is abnormal and should be promptly reported to the physician. Bothersome symptoms, including voiding frequency, urgency, dysuria, flank pain, and urge incontinence, may occur as a result of the ureteral stent. However, postprocedural urinary tract infection also may occur, producing similar symptoms coexisting with fever and chills requiring prompt assessment and management as described under Endoscopy.

Percutaneous Nephroscopy. General anesthesia is required for percutaneous nephroscopy, and patients should be advised of the care associated with anesthesia. Patients who are hypersensitive to contrast media are premedicated with corticosteroids. During the procedure, the patient should be monitored for extravasation of irrigation fluid, which can rapidly fill the intrapleural or intraperitoneal spaces. In order to avoid this complication, the nurse should measure both the volume of fluid infused and the volume drained by means of suction. Should extravasation occur, the procedure is terminated and a nephrostomy tube is placed until the renal pelvic perforation heals (usually in 2 to 3 days).

Bleeding is not unusual during percutaneous nephroscopy, particularly when a large stone or tumor is removed or an endopyelotomy is performed. In these cases, the patient may be expected to bleed 1 to 2 units. If rapid venous bleeding is encountered, the procedure may be temporarily halted and a nephrostomy tube placed and clamped to provide intrarenal tamponade. Venous bleeding is expected to resolve within 30 minutes, and the resulting clot is expected to lyse within 24 hours. Arterial bleeding is a more serious complication; patients undergoing endopyelotomy are at particular risk. A nephrostomy is used to provide tamponade, but an arteriogram is usually required and the transected vessel requires embolization if the bleeding persists.

Since percutaneous nephroscopy involves the renal pelvis, the risk of pyelonephritis and systemic infection is significant and requires prompt and aggressive management (see Endoscopy). Late bleeding may occur when the nephrostomy tube is removed. Bleeding is usually self-limited, but it may cause distention of the renal pelvis and severe renal colic. In some cases, bleeding is attributable to an arteriovenous (A-V) fissure. Symptoms of an A-V fissure include gross hematuria and obstruction requiring arteriography and selective embolization.

URODYNAMICS AND VIDEOURODYNAMICS (OF THE LOWER URINARY TRACT)

Urodynamics is a set of tests that measure lower urinary tract function (i.e., bladder filling and storage and bladder evacuation). A typical urodynamic evaluation includes uroflowmetry, a filling cystometrogram (CMG), sphincter electromyography (EMG), and a voiding pressure flow study. When these tests are performed together, this combined procedure is often referred to as multichannel urodynamics (Figure 4-13). Videourodynamics refers to the combination of multichannel urodynamic measurements with anatomic imaging of the lower urinary tract. Fluoroscopy is most commonly used, but ultrasound may be used in selected cases (Figure 4-14). Interpretation of these studies provides a detailed characterization of bladder filling, storage, and micturition (Table 4-1, p. 80).

Uroflowmetry. A urinary flow study (uroflow or flow rate) is a graphic representation of urethral flow. The patient is asked to arrive for testing with a comfortably full bladder and to urinate into a funnel incorporated into a machine that measures flow as milliliters per second (ml/sec). Uroflowmeters rely on one of several technologies to produce a flow rate, such as a transducer that measures the weight of the urine as it collects in a beaker. Alternatively, a spinning disk, capacitance, or air displacement meter may be used to measure flow. Uroflowmetry can be completed as a screening study to detect abnormal flow patterns. It is also obtained immediately before multichannel testing to provide a baseline flow pattern for comparison with results obtained during the voiding pressure flow study.

Cystometrogram. The CMG is a graphic representation of pressure as a function of bladder volume. The patient is asked to urinate in order to empty the bladder, or a uroflow study is performed. A specially designed urodynamic catheter is commonly inserted. These catheters are typically small (5F to 10F) and

contain two or three lumina capable of bladder infusion and measurement of intravesical and urethral pressures. Alternatively, cystometric pressures may be measured by a microtip, fiberoptic sensor, or air-charged catheter. The catheter is used to fill the bladder and simultaneously measure intravesical and/or urethral pressure. A postvoid residual urine volume is obtained and compared with the residual volume obtained immediately following the voiding pressure flow study. A tube with a small balloon is frequently placed into the rectum; it is used to measure abdominal pressures. Cystometry also may be performed using a two-catheter technique. In this case, a small, straight catheter (8F to 12F) is inserted and used to instill fluid into the bladder alongside a much smaller catheter (4F to 5F) used to measure intravesical pressure. Single-lumen catheters are used in selected cases where a small multilumen catheter cannot be inserted, but this technique is generally discouraged because of artifacts caused by turbulence when the bladder is filled and pressures are measured through a catheter with a single lumen.

The catheter or catheters and the rectal tube are connected to pressure transducers, and the bladder is filled with sterile water, saline, or contrast media until the patient perceives fullness or is unable to inhibit a detrusor contraction, indicating urge urinary incontinence. Provocative maneuvers are completed during the filling CMG in an attempt to reproduce bothersome lower urinary tract symptoms. For example, if stress urinary incontinence is suspected, filling is interrupted between 150 and 200 ml and the patient is asked to perform several slow Valsalva's maneuvers while the clinician assesses for urine loss. Similarly, the patient is filled to the point where a very strong urge to urinate is perceived. This provocative maneuver is often followed by a request that the patient refrain from toileting for a period of time despite the presence of this strong urge. These provocative maneuvers are completed in an attempt to reproduce urge urinary incontinence associated with an overactive bladder.

Voiding Pressure Flow Study. A filling CMG is typically followed by a voiding pressure flow study. The patient is assisted onto a voiding chair attached to a uroflowmeter, provided maximum privacy, and asked to urinate. If a two-catheter technique is used, the larger catheter used to fill the bladder is removed; otherwise, the patient is asked to urinate around any

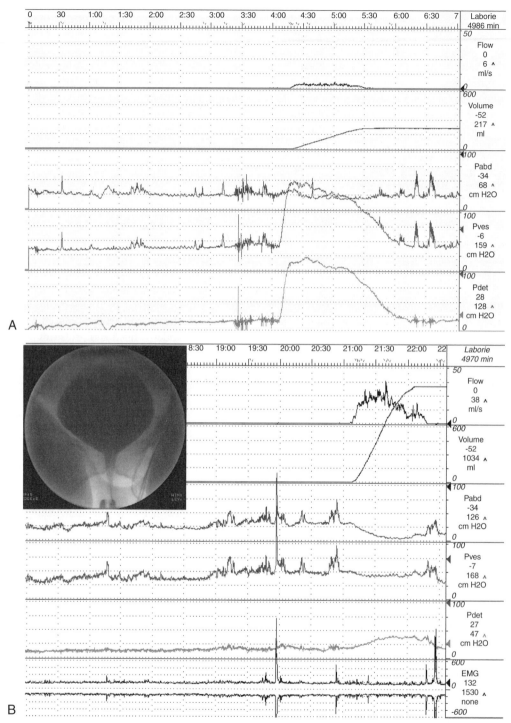

Fig. 4-13 A, Multichannel urodynamics. **B,** Videourodynamic tracing combines a fluoroscopic image with pressure, flow, and sphincter electromyogram (EMG) tracings.

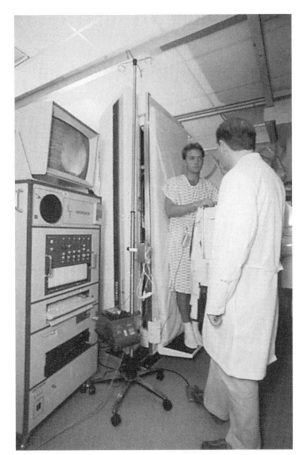

Fig. 4-14 Fluoroscopic equipment is typically used for videourodynamic testing.

catheters in the urethra. Urinary flow, intravesical, and abdominal pressures are measured simultaneously. In videourodynamics, fluoroscopic images are also obtained during the voiding pressure flow study, allowing visualization of the bladder outlet and urethra.

Sphincter Electromyography. The sphincter EMG is a graphic representation of the electrical activity produced by neuromuscular units within skeletal muscles. During urodynamic testing, an EMG is used to assess gross motor movements of the pelvic floor muscles (including the rhabdosphincter muscle, periurethral striated muscle, and levator ani). Typically, EMG patches or percutaneous electrode wires are inserted for the purpose of measuring gross muscle movements (kinesiology). In certain settings, however, needle electrodes may be inserted to assess both kinesiology and individual action

potentials, allowing diagnosis of pelvic floor muscle denervation. Sphincter EMG is measured during both filling cystometry and the voiding pressure flow study.

Urethral Pressure Study. A urethral pressure study is a graphic representation of urethral pressures; several techniques have been used to quantify urethral pressure and its relationship to sphincter competence during bladder filling and urethral resistance during micturition. The Brown-Wickham urethral pressure profile (UPP) is completed by filling the bladder to a moderate volume (approximately 200 ml) or to fullness and slowly pulling a catheter through the urethra. Pressure rises as the catheter passes through the urethral sphincter mechanism. This pressure is subtracted from intravesical pressure to derive the maximum urethral closure pressure. In addition, the UPP can be used to estimate the functional length of the sphincter mechanism. A cough UPP is designed to measure sphincter competence in patients with stress urinary incontinence. Urethral and intravesical pressures are measured simultaneously, and a computer-based recording device calculates and displays differential pressure. This differential pressure is calculated by subtracting intravesical from urethral pressure. The procedure is similar to the Brown-Wickham UPP except that the patient is asked to cough as the catheter is slowly withdrawn. If intravesical pressure exceeds the magnitude of pressure transmitted to the urethral sphincter mechanism, the differential pressure channel records a negative spike indicating stress urinary incontinence. In contrast, a positive deflection indicates preservation of sphincter closure and maintenance of continence. A micturition urethral pressure profile (MUPP) may be completed in male patients when the location of an obstructive lesion is not easily identified.

A triple-lumen catheter capable of measuring intravesical and urethral pressures is selected for the MUPP; the urethral pressure port or transducer is further distinguished by the presence of a small radiopaque marker. The test is completed by slowly pulling a catheter through the urethra while the patient urinates. Both urethral and intravesical pressures are recorded, and fluoroscopic images are taken to identify the precise point where urethral pressures are being recorded. During normal micturition, urethral pressure is approximately equal to intravesical

TABLE 4-1 Quick Reference to the Interpretation of Multichannel Urodynamics

FILLING CYSTOMETROGRAM	NORMAL RANGE	CLINICAL SIGNIFICANCE
Capacity	300-600 ml for adults (Age + 2) × 30 for children	Large capacity: chronic overdistention, sensory or motor denervation Small capacity: low bladder wall compliance, detrusor overactivity, irritation or inflammation of the bladder wall
Compliance	>20 ml/cm H_2O	High compliance: no clinical relevance as an isolated finding Low compliance: values < 10 ml/cm H_2O indicate high risk of upper urinary tract distress (febrile UTI, hydronephrosis, reflux, renal insufficiency)
Competence of the sphincter	Infinity (abdominal LPP, above measurable range)	Any measurable abdominal LPP indicates diagnosis of stress urinary incontinence Abdominal LPP < 90 cm H_2O indicates intrinsic sphincter deficiency
Sensations of bladder filling	First sensation at 90-200 ml Strong urge at 250-450 ml Fullness at 300-690 ml	See Capacity
Detrusor response	Absence of overactive detrusor contractions; contractions must cause leakage or compromise capacity to be defined as unstable	Overactive detrusor contractions associated with urge or reflex urinary incontinence
Voiding pressure study	Qualitative	ICS or Schäfer nomograms
Normal voiding pressure: male	Normal flow pattern, maximum flow > 12 ml/sec Pdet, max: 30-60 cm H_2O Quiet EMG	*A-G nomogram:* URA: <20 WF$_{max}$: ≥10 (7 lowest acceptable) *Schafer nomogram:* linPURR obstruction grade: 0-1 Contractility: normal or higher
Normal voiding pressure: female	Normal or explosive flow pattern Qmax: >15 ml/sec Pdet, max: <30 cm H_2O Quiet EMG	*A-G nomogram:* URA: ≤15 WF$_{max}$: ≥1 *Schafer nomogram:* linPURR obstruction grade: 0-II Contractility: normal or higher
Obstruction	Prolonged or intermittent flow pattern High voiding pressure Pdet, max: >60 cm H_2O EMG quiet or dyssynergic	*A-G nomogram:* URA: >20 in men or 20 in women WF$_{max}$: ≥10 unless detrusor decompensated with obstruction *Schafer nomogram:* linPURR obstruction grade: III-VI Contractility: normal or higher
Deficient detrusor contraction strength	Prolonged or intermittent flow pattern Low voiding pressure	*A-G nomogram:* URA: varies WF$_{max}$: usually ≤6 *Schäfer nomogram:* linPURR obstruction grade: varies Contractility: "weak +" or lower

EMG, Electromyogram; *ICS,* International Continence Society; *LPP,* leak point pressure; *URA,* urethral resistance algorithm; *UTI,* urinary tract infection.

pressure when pressures are measured between the bladder neck and the membranous urethra. In the patient with obstruction, a precipitous drop in urethral pressure occurs just distal to an obstructive lesion. Correlation of this pressure drop with the location of the radiopaque marker allows a precise diagnosis of the obstructive lesion.

Indications

Multichannel Urodynamics

Urinary incontinence that does not respond to empiric treatment

Urinary incontinence that cannot be adequately characterized by a focused history and physical examination

Urinary retention (differentiation of obstruction from deficient detrusor contractility)

Neuropathic bladder dysfunction

Videourodynamics

Urinary incontinence complicated by pelvic organ prolapse

Voiding dysfunction associated with upper urinary tract distress (e.g., ureterohydronephrosis, vesicoureteral reflux, febrile urinary tract infections, or renal insufficiency)

Voiding dysfunction associated with a congenital or acquired defect of the lower urinary tract (e.g., fistula, ectopia, or surgical reconstruction)

Urinary retention (e.g., differentiation of deficient detrusor contraction strength from obstruction and localization of any obstructive lesion)

Contraindications

Acute urinary tract infection

Acute overdistention of bladder (urodynamics typically deferred until bladder has been allowed to "rest" by indwelling catheter drainage or intermittent catheterization for 2 to 4 weeks)

Nursing Management

Encourage normal fluid intake, and ask the patient undergoing uroflowmetry to refrain from micturition for approximately 2 to 4 hours before the test. Counsel the patient undergoing uroflowmetry alone that the procedure is noninvasive but it is important to arrive with a comfortably full bladder in order to achieve optimal results. Patients may be counseled against attempting to overfill the bladder and to alert staff if they feel a very strong urge to urinate on arrival at the clinic so the uroflowmetry study can be completed before consultation with the urologist.

Advise the patient undergoing multichannel urodynamics that the procedure will require urethral catheterization, but reassure the person that a small catheter will be inserted and remain in place only for the duration of the examination. Assisting the patient in learning techniques of pelvic floor muscle relaxation will minimize discomfort associated with catheter insertion. Counsel the patient that a tube will also be placed in the rectum or posterior vaginal vault. Reassure the patient that a rectal tube is not expected to provoke a bowel movement and that placement is not associated with significant discomfort.

Consult with the urodynamic service concerning techniques for EMG measurement. Patch electrodes are placed in the perianal area and cause no discomfort. Needle or percutaneous wire electrodes cause transient discomfort when placed in the periurethral area. After the catheter and rectal tubes are connected to pressure transducers, inform the patient that the bladder will be filled with sterile water, saline, or contrast media until fullness is perceived or the individual is unable to inhibit a detrusor contraction and leakage occurs. Reassure the person that urine loss is an anticipated event during urodynamic testing and its presence assists the clinician in determining the cause of bothersome lower urinary tract symptoms.

Advise the patient that there is a small risk of urinary tract infection following urodynamic testing and that some increase in urinary urgency or suprapubic discomfort may occur. Consumption of fluids and a sitz bath will relieve transient urgency or discomfort. Consult with the physician concerning the need for prophylactic antibiotic therapy in patients with a history of recurring urinary tract infections.

URODYNAMICS OF THE UPPER URINARY TRACT: WHITAKER TEST

Urodynamics of the upper urinary tract are designed to measure urine transport from the renal pelvis to the ureterovesical junction. The Whitaker test is the most commonly performed urodynamic test of the upper urinary tracts. A large-bore needle or nephrostomy tube is placed in the renal pelvis by an interventional radiologist or urologist, and a catheter is placed in the bladder. Saline or contrast material is infused through the needle or nephrostomy tube at a rate of 10 ml/min. Renal pelvic pressure is measured through the needle or nephrostomy tube, and intravesical pressure is measured through the catheter. The goal of the test is to measure ureteral resistance in order to determine the magnitude and location of a ureteral obstruction. Measurement of upper urinary tract resistance is expressed as the differential renal pelvic pressure. Calculation is a two-step process. First, intravesical pressure is subtracted from renal pelvic pressure measured during ureteral perfusion. Second, the perfusion pressure of the needle or nephrostomy tube is subtracted to determine the differential renal pressure. The second step is necessary because perfusion of fluid through a single-lumen tube creates a turbulence artifact that must be eliminated. This pressure is determined by perfusing the tube or needle onto a towel placed parallel to the pressure transducer. Differential pressures that are less than 14 cm H_2O indicate no obstruction; values of 14 to 20 cm H_2O indicate mild (sometimes called equivocal) obstruction. Values of 21 cm H_2O to 34 cm H_2O indicate moderately severe obstruction, and differential pressures of 35 cm H_2O or higher indicate severe obstruction.[13] Although differential pressures can be calculated using saline, simultaneous fluoroscopy is strongly recommended since it allows localization of the level of obstruction.

Indications

Suspected ureteral obstruction not diagnosed by radionuclide study

Distal ureteral obstruction, particularly in the presence of massive dilation of the upper urinary tract or tracts

Contraindications

Urinary tract infection (pyelonephritis)

Hypersensitivity to contrast media

Nursing Management

Advise the patient of the purpose of the examination, and prepare for placement of a nephrostomy tube or spinal needle into the renal pelvis if necessary. Consult with the physician concerning the location of the examination, use of anesthesia, and plans for the tube following completion of the test. Spinal needles are removed after a Whitaker test, but a nephrostomy tube may remain in place in order to ensure

drainage of an obstructed kidney. Reassure the patient that infusion of contrast materials during the Whitaker test will be suspended if renal colic is provoked. Should this event occur, pain would be promptly relieved by draining contrast materials from the upper urinary tract. Renal colic following a Whitaker test is uncommon, and the patient is advised to consult the urologist should it occur. There is a small risk of pyelonephritis following a Whitaker test, and the patient should be taught to recognize these manifestations and instructed to promptly consult the urologist or nurse practitioner should they occur. The urologist may be consulted before the test concerning the need for prophylactic antibiotics, particularly for patients who have a history of febrile urinary tract infections.

RADIONUCLIDE IMAGING (NUCLEAR SCAN OR RADIONUCLIDE SCAN)

Nuclear imaging studies, unlike radiographic images, rely on injection or infusion of a radionuclide tracer substance that binds to renal tubular cells or is excreted by glomerular filtration (Figure 4-15).[14] Radionuclide scans of the kidneys allow assessment of the renal parenchyma, differential kidney function (expressed as each kidney's contribution to total renal function), and evaluation of excretory and transport function of the upper urinary tracts. Infusion of a radionuclide into the lower urinary tract (nuclear cystogram) provides an alternative means of obtaining a cystogram or voiding cystourethrogram in patients who are hypersensitive to intravesical instillation of contrast media.

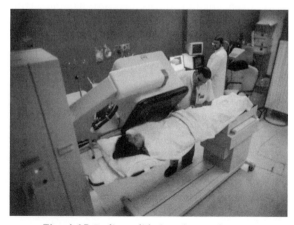

Fig. 4-15 Radionuclide imaging equipment.

Technetium 99m Diethylenetriamine Penta-acetic Acid. Diethylenetriamine pentaacetic acid (DTPA) is excreted from the kidneys by glomerular filtration. The radionuclide is injected as an IV bolus, and sequential computer images are obtained to evaluate renal and upper urinary tract function. A 30-second image assesses renal cortical blood flow and subsequent images are obtained at 1, 5, 10, 15, and 20 minutes. These images assess excretory and transport functions of the kidneys and upper urinary tracts. Furosemide (Lasix) may be administered during a DTPA scan; it is usually given between 15 and 20 minutes after initial injection. Injection is followed by rapid serial images evaluating radionuclide washout from each kidney (Figure 4-16, A). Computer analysis of a DTPA scan allows calculation of the glomerular filtration rate, effective renal blood flow, and differential renal function. In addition, an X-Y plot comparing time in seconds and the concentration of nuclear tracer substances in the kidney is obtained to assess obstruction of the upper urinary tracts. In the normal kidney, injection causes a precipitous decline in radionuclides in the kidney, indicating rapid washout under the influence of the diuretic. In an obstructed kidney, however, the time required to wash out radionuclide from the kidneys is prolonged, creating a plateau or a rise in the curve (see Figure 4-16, B). The time required to wash out radionuclide materials from the kidney can also be quantified as the $T_{1/2}$ (length of time required to eliminate 50% of the nuclear tracer from the kidney following administration of a diuretic). A $T_{1/2}$ of 10 minutes or less is normal in the patient with good renal function, values of 10 to 20 minutes are interpreted as equivocal, and values greater than 20 minutes indicate obstruction. When interpreting $T_{1/2}$ values, it is important to remem-ber that results are predicated on the assumption that renal function is normal (i.e., the kidney is capable of excreting the radionuclide from the parenchyma).

The DTPA scan provides a more thorough assessment of renal function than does the IVP/IVU. However, it provides less anatomic detail and is not as useful in the evaluation of urinary system masses or calculi. Significant dilation of the renal pelvis or ureter or distal ureteral obstruction may obscure results of the DTPA washout study. In this case a Whitaker test should be obtained to quantify the magnitude of obstruction and to identify the location of the blockage.

Technetium 99m Dimercaptosuccinic Acid. Dimercaptosuccinic acid (DMSA) is bound to the basement membrane of the proximal tubule of the nephron. A bolus of the DMSA radionuclide is injected

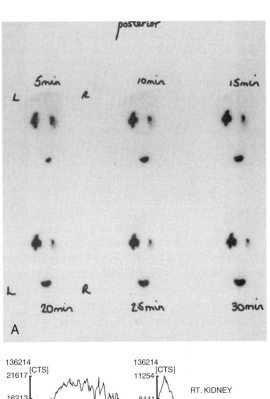

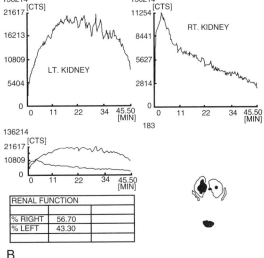

Fig. 4-16 A, Diethylenetriamine pentaacetic acid (DTPA) scan showing left ureteropelvic junction obstruction and hydronephrosis. **B,** X-Y plot showing radionuclide wash-out in right versus left kidney. The right kidney washes out rapidly after furosemide is administered, but the curve rises in the left kidney, demonstrating obstruction.

intravenously, and computer-generated images of the renal parenchyma are obtained. Because DMSA binds to the tubule of the nephron, it provides excellent images of the volume of functioning renal parenchyma. These images allow assessment of differential renal function and identification of renal scars (Figure 4-17). Because the DMSA scan is bound to the renal tubules, it does not allow assessment of upper urinary tract obstruction.

Technetium 99m Glucoheptonate. Glucoheptonate (GHA) is similar to DMSA in both its chemical structure and clinical application.

Iodine-131 Orthoiodohippurate. Orthoiodohippurate (OIH, hippurate, or Hippuran) is excreted in the urine by means of glomerular filtration (20%) and by tubular excretion (80%). Its clinical utility is limited because it exposes the patient to higher doses of radiation (particularly gamma energy) when compared with other radionuclides, such as DTPA.

Technetium 99m Mercaptoacetyltriglycine. Mercaptoacetyltriglycine (MAG$_3$) allows assessment of the renal parenchyma comparable to the DMSA radionuclide and evaluation of renal washout comparable to the DTPA scan. It is also preferred over DTPA or hippurate scans in patients with chronic renal failure.

Technetium 99m Pertechnetate. In urology, technetium 99m pertechnetate is used to differentiate torsion from epididymitis in the acutely painful scrotum. The patient is given an oral dose of potassium perchlorate or potassium iodide 30 minutes before injection of the radionuclide in order to block thyroid uptake. The penis is taped to the abdominal wall, and the affected hemiscrotum is supported on a sling that is slightly higher than the thigh in order to maximize the accuracy of imaging. An IV bolus of pertechnetate is injected, and multiple images are obtained immediately following injection and at 5 and 10 minutes. It is also used in an intravesical preparation for nuclear cystography.

Technetium 99m–Labeled Phosphate and Phosphonate. Several radionuclides have been developed that gradually collect in metabolically active bones. For example, technetium 99m methylene diphosphonate is injected by means of an IV bolus 3 hours before images are obtained. After 3 hours, approximately 60% of the radionuclide has been excreted through the urine. The remaining nuclear tracer will be concentrated in the kidneys and metabolically active areas of the bone. Metastatic tumors in patients with advanced-stage prostate cancer will show up as areas of increased uptake (sometimes called hot spots), reflecting their abnormally accelerated metabolism.

NUCLEAR CYSTOGRAPHY

Unlike the radionuclides mentioned previously, a nuclear cystogram is performed by intravesical infusion rather than IV injection. Technetium 99m pertechnetate is mixed with 250 to 500 ml of sterile saline and infused into the bladder by means of gravity. The images obtained are useful in the diagnosis and grading of vesicoureteral reflux. Nevertheless, the nuclear cystogram lacks the anatomic detail of a radiographic cystogram or VCUG.

Indications

Diethylenetriamine Pentaacetic Acid
Obstruction
Differential renal function
Glomerular filtration rate

Dimercaptosuccinic Acid and Glucoheptonate
Assessment of renal parenchyma and scars
Differential renal function

Hippurate
Individual and total effective renal plasma flow
Obstruction

Mercaptoacetyltriglycine
Assessment of renal parenchyma
Differential renal function

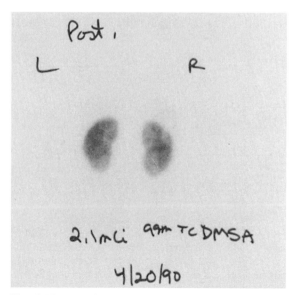

Fig. 4-17 Normal dimercaptosuccinic acid (DMSA) scan.

Glomerular filtration rate

Obstruction

Pertechnetate

Differentiation of epididymitis from testicular torsion (IV bolus)

Vesicoureteral reflux (intravesical infusion)

Technetium 99m–Labeled Phosphonate and Phosphate

Identification of bony metastasis in advanced-stage prostate cancer

Contraindications

None

Nursing Management

Instruct the patient that bowel preparation is not required for a radionuclide study. If the radionuclide is introduced intravenously the injection site is observed for signs of irritation from the tracer substance. While injection of radionuclide substance yields only very minimal radiation, pregnant women are advised to refrain from holding a child for 24 hours after the test. Consult the radiology department for policies pertaining to disposal of diapers or incontinent containment devices immediately following radionuclide testing.

Preparation for nuclear cystography is similar to that described for a radiographic cystogram or VCUG.

ANGIOGRAPHY OF THE URINARY SYSTEM

Kidneys. Contrast-enhanced renal angiography produces a set of radiographic images that provide a detailed evaluation of the kidney's arterial supply.[18] The procedure is usually performed in an interventional radiology suite. Access to the vascular system is obtained by catheterizing the femoral artery. A radiopaque catheter is threaded from the femoral artery to the abdominal aorta and into the renal artery. Contrast is injected into the artery, and rapid sequence films are obtained to characterize the arterial supply of the kidney. Patients who are hypersensitive to contrast media may be premedicated (see Clinical Highlights for Advanced and Expert Practice: Contrast-Induced Nephrotoxicity and Clinical Highlights for Advanced and Expert Practice: Contrast-Induced Allergic-Like Reactions). Technical advances in renal angiography allow more quantitative measurement of several aspects of renal artery stenosis, including differential pressure measurements, which

can be used to diagnose arterial obstruction, and measurement of renin levels in the renal veins.[19]

Alternatively, carbon dioxide or a gadolinium-based contrast may be substituted for an iodine-bound contrast medium, particularly if the patient has preexisting renal insufficiency. Digital subtraction angiography is a technique that uses a computer to trace the movement of contrast throughout the renal vascular system that is similar to the images produced by real-time fluoroscopy. It is particularly useful in the evaluation of renal artery stenosis because of its ability to quantify vessel diameter (Figure 4-18).

Other imaging studies may be used to image the renal vasculature. Nevertheless, contrast-enhanced renal angiography remains the gold standard for the diagnosis of renal artery stenosis when renovascular hypertension is suspected.[20]

Adrenal. Although the CT scan is typically used to image adrenal disease, angiography is sometimes useful for patients with small but hormonally active tumors, such as an aldosteronoma. Arteriography may be useful for larger tumors including pheochromocytomas or carcinomas. Vascular access is obtained from the femoral vein or artery. The adrenal system is difficult to access and must be differentiated from the larger hepatic veins by initial instillation of a small volume of contrast (about 1 ml). Venography is typically accompanied by differential hormonal analysis to aid in the diagnosis of

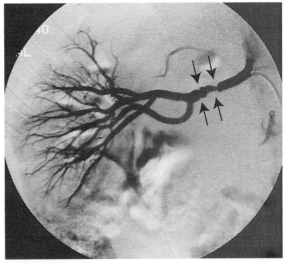

Fig. 4-18 Digital subtracted angiogram demonstrating renal artery stenosis. (From Pollack HM, McClennan BL: *Clinical Urography*, 5th edition. Philadelphia: Saunders, 2000.)

small but functionally relevant tumors. Arteriography is accompanied by aortography in order to identify extra-adrenal masses and to localize the three principal arteries that typically supply the gland. Arteriography is then used to characterize larger tumors and their blood supply.

Penis. Penile angiography (dynamic infusion cavernosography) may be undertaken in the evaluation of vasculogenic erectile dysfunction or priapism.[21] It is usually combined with dynamic measurement of intracavernosal pressure measurements (dynamic infusion cavernosometry). A small IV needle is inserted to achieve vascular access to the cavernosa, and a vasodilating agent (prostaglandin E_1) is injected to provoke an erection. Radiographic images are then combined with intracavernosal pressure measurements to determine the etiology of vasculogenic impotence. Alternatively, these studies can be used in cases of high-flow priapism that fail to respond to empiric treatment with α-adrenergic agonists. With the rise of effective oral agents for the management of erectile dysfunction and limited long-term success in surgical correction of vascular disorders, penile angiography is now performed only in highly selected cases.

Gonadal Angiography. Venography is useful in the evaluation of selected cases of varicoceles associated with male factor infertility or cryptorchid testes.[22] The right femoral or right internal jugular vein is used to gain access to the gonadal venous system.

Indications

Renal Angiography
Renal mass
Renal artery stenosis
Renovascular hypertension
Renal transplant
Adrenal Gland
Small, hormonally sensitive masses (venography)
Carcinoma or pheochromocytoma staging (arteriography)
Penis
Vasculogenic erectile dysfunction
Priapism
Testicular
Varicocele

Contraindication
Hypersensitivity to iodine-bound contrast media

Nursing Management

Ensure that appropriate premedication has been administered to all patients with a history of hypersensitivity to iodinated contrast materials (see Clinical Highlights for Advanced and Expert Practice: Contrast-Induced Allergic-Like Reactions). Advise the patient of the differences between iodine-bound and alternative contrast materials when indicated. Preparation for angiography may include administration of an opioid analgesic or anxiolytic medication. Advise the patient that injection of contrast will produce only transient discomfort.

Following the procedure, assess the puncture site to ensure that adequate pressure has been applied to the dressing to prevent bleeding. Assess pedal pulses and capillary refill of the toes to ensure adequate perfusion. Counsel the patient that 4 to 8 hours of strict bedrest are critical to prevent disruption of the pressure dressing and significant bleeding from the vascular access site.

ULTRASONOGRAPHY OF THE URINARY TRACT

Ultrasound uses short pulse bursts of ultrasonic pulses to image the urinary system, thus avoiding exposure to x-rays.[15] Pulses are emitted from a probe directly into the tissues, and the resulting echoes from these pulses are used to generate images (Figure 4-19). Within the genitourinary system, pulse frequencies of 1 to 10 MHz are used to image the kidneys, bladder, prostate, testes, and bladder.

Ultrasonic imaging may be combined with Doppler methods to assess blood flow. The Doppler shift is created by differences in a sound wave reflected from

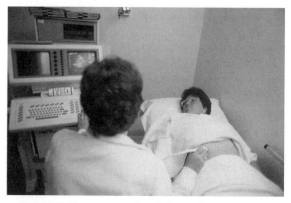

Fig. 4-19 Ultrasonography of the genitourinary tract.

a moving target. This shift can be used to detect whether movement is toward or away from the ultrasound probe and to detect the speed of the moving object. When applied to blood flow, the movement of erythrocytes creates a Doppler shift that can be used to evaluate both the volume and velocity of flow in specific vessels. This information has multiple clinical uses, including those discussed below.

Adrenals. The adrenal glands can be visualized using ultrasound. The patient is assisted into a supine or lateral decubitus position (oblique 45 to 90 degrees). Both glands are difficult to visualize in the obese patient, and the left gland may be difficult to image in any patient with gas in the stomach or colon. Ultrasound of the adrenal glands is used to identify masses or evaluate adrenal hemorrhage.

Kidneys and Ureters. Ultrasonic probes using 2.5 to 5 MHz can be placed over the abdomen or flank in order to generate images of the kidneys (Figure 4-20). The resulting images are used to assess the volume and architecture of the renal parenchyma and pelvicalyceal collecting system. Solid and cystic masses, calculi, and hydronephrosis can be readily detected by ultrasound. Ultrasound is also used in the evaluation of acute or chronic pyelonephritis, perinephric abscess, renal transplant rejection, acute tubular necrosis, and congenital defects of the upper urinary tract. The renal pelvis is well visualized by ultrasound, but the ureter is difficult to image unless it is massively dilated.

Bladder. The suprapubic area is preferred when imaging the bladder, although transvaginal, transrectal, or transurethral approaches also may be used for ultrasonography. A 3.5- to 5-MHz probe is used to generate transverse and sagittal images of the bladder wall and its contents. Images of the bladder wall may reveal thickening (indicating voiding dysfunction or obstruction), diverticula, masses, or congenital defects, such as a patent urachal remnant. Examination of the bladder base may reveal ureteroceles or pathologic opening of the bladder neck indicating severe stress urinary incontinence. The contents of the bladder vesicle should be completely anechoic; calculi or debris in the bladder is readily differentiated from surrounding urine during an ultrasound. Imaging of the posterior aspects of the bladder may reveal enlarged ureters.

Special ultrasonic instruments can also be used to measure bladder volume (Figure 4-21). These instruments are used to measure postvoiding residual volumes without resorting to urethral catheterization.

Penis and Urethra. Duplex ultrasonography is a highly specialized technique used to assess erectile function. A high-frequency probe is placed over the ventral aspect of the penis, and the diameter of each cavernosal artery is measured. The patient is then given an intracavernosal injection of a vasodilating agent, such as papaverine, phentolamine, or prostaglandin E_1. Blood flow velocities are measured in both cavernosal arteries at 5, 10, 15, and 20 minutes. Ultrasonic techniques also may be used to assess priapism, Peyronie's plaques, penile tumors, or trauma.

Five-megahertz probes can be placed on the dorsal aspect of the penis to image urethral strictures in males.[16] Although retrograde or antegrade urethrography remains the gold standard for imaging urethral narrowing, ultrasonography offers a noninvasive alternative to the RUG or VCUG.

Scrotum and Testes. Higher-frequency ultrasonic probes (5 to 10 MHz) can also be used to image scrotal contents, including the testis and epididymis. Scrotal ultrasonography is used to assess testicular masses, such as spermatoceles or solid tumors, as well as scrotal masses involving one or both testes, such as a hydrocele. Doppler-enhanced ultrasound provides a noninvasive and rapid method of differentiating hyperemia associated with epididymitis from testicular ischemia associated with torsion. It is also combined with imaging of the inguinal canals and lower abdomen when searching for undescended testes. Scrotal ultrasound is sometimes used in the evaluation of male factor infertility. Testicular size and the character of the parenchyma

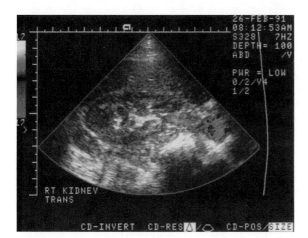

Fig. 4-20 Ultrasound of the kidney. (From Brundage D: Renal Disorders. St Louis: Mosby, 1992.)

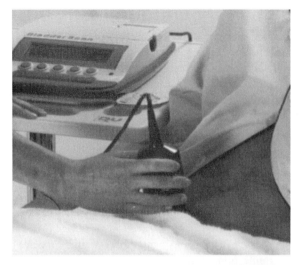

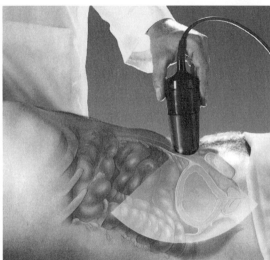

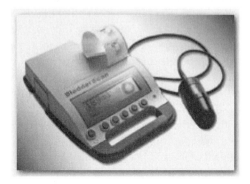

Fig. 4-21 Ultrasonic residual of the bladder provides a noninavasive alternative to catheterization.

can be assessed. Imaging of the epididymis may provide clues to the cause of infertility, including obstruction or absence of one or both epididymides.

Prostate. A 5- to 7-MHz transrectal probe is used to image the prostate. Imaging reveals prostatic calculi, and hypoechoic areas raise a suspicion of prostate cancer (Figure 4-22). However, because of the poor sensitivity of transrectal ultrasonography alone, imaging should be combined with prostate biopsy. A prostate biopsy specimen is obtained using a specially designed needle instrument that is attached to the transrectal probe. Real-time ultrasonic images are used to obtain biopsy specimens of both suspicious and normal-appearing areas of the prostate, or multiple (up to 27) biopsy specimens are obtained in an attempt to sample the entire gland.

After prostate cancer has been definitively diagnosed, transrectal ultrasonography is used to map the prostate and guide placement of irradiated seeds during brachytherapy.

Indications

Kidneys and Adrenals
Adrenal mass
Adrenal hemorrhage
Renal mass
Hydronephrosis
Transplant (rejection or obstruction)
Renovascular disorders

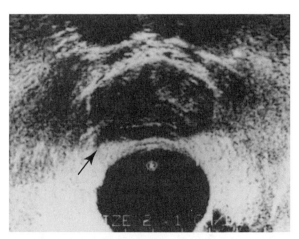

Fig. 4-22 Prostate ultrasound image showing invasive adenocarcinoma; a prostate biopsy will be obtained for pathologic analysis and tumor grading. (From Gillenwater JY: Adult and Pediatric Urology, 2nd edition. St Louis: Mosby, 1991.)

Bladder
Bladder wall defects (i.e., masses, diverticula, or ureteroceles)
Calculi or debris
Postvoiding urinary residual volume
Penis and Urethra
Masses
Trauma
Urethral stricture
Vasculogenic erectile dysfunction
Scrotum and Testes
Scrotal or testicular mass
Hydrocele
Hernia
Trauma
Undescended testis
Infertility (i.e., testicular parenchyma, volumes, varicocele, or epididymal defects or absence)
Prostate
Diagnosis of prostate cancer (i.e., suspicious digital rectal exam [DRE], abnormal serum prostate-specific antigen [PSA], or fractionated PSA or PSA velocity)
Guidance for prostate biopsies
Mapping for brachytherapy

Contraindications
None

Nursing Management
The nursing management of patients undergoing ultrasound imaging is profoundly affected by the purpose of the study and the organs to be imaged. Renal and bladder ultrasonography does not require bowel preparation and is painless. Advise the patient that a probe will be placed on the abdomen, suprapubic area, and flank in order to obtain images and that gentle pressure may be applied to achieve optimal results. A gel that feels and looks like K-Y jelly is placed on the skin and is wiped away as soon as the images are obtained. The time required for examination varies from 5 to 15 minutes.

Ultrasonic imaging for the evaluation of a urethral stricture, penile mass, or trauma requires placement of a probe on the dorsal aspect of the penis. In contrast, duplex ultrasonography requires placement of a probe on the ventral aspect as well as injection of a vasodilating agent. Since these agents sometimes provoke priapism, an antidote (i.e., ephedrine or pseudoephedrine) should be immediately available. Patients undergoing duplex ultrasonography are advised that the procedure will require 30 to 45 minutes to complete.

Scrotal ultrasound requires placement of a probe underneath the scrotum; the procedure is not painful and typically requires only 10 to 15 minutes to complete. Prostatic ultrasonography and biopsy are more invasive than other ultrasonic techniques and require more extensive preparation.[17] A careful explanation of the procedure should include use of a transrectal probe. Advise the patient that the probe will produce sensations of pressure or fullness in the rectal area that is relieved as soon as the probe is removed. Counsel the man that obtaining a biopsy produces a sudden noise as the specimen is obtained and a brief sensation of discomfort. This transient discomfort may be localized to the rectal area or referred to the penis. Some patients may experience a vasovagal response during the procedure. All anticoagulant medications, including prescribed agents such as warfarin, over-the-counter drugs such as aspirins, or dietary supplements such as high-dose vitamin E, must be discontinued, usually for 7 days before and 1 day following prostate ultrasound with biopsy. The bowel may be prepared with an enema or stimulant, and antimicrobial therapy is typically administered on the day of the procedure.

Following prostate ultrasound and biopsy the patient is taught to monitor the stool for the presence of excessive bleeding or passage of bright red clots. Patients are advised to inform the nurse or physician if excessive blood in the urine is noted that does not readily clear with increased fluid intake, particularly if blood clots occur that interfere with urination. Body temperature is measured twice daily for 48 hours after the procedure, and the patient is counseled to report fevers greater than 100° F (37.7° C). Anticipated responses to prostate biopsy include blood-streaked stools for 24 to 48 hours after the procedure, as well as passage of one or two small blood clots. Blood may be seen in the ejaculate for up to 6 weeks, and the rectal area may ache for 1 to 2 days.

BIOPSY PROCEDURES
Biopsy of the genitourinary system involves obtaining a small sample of tissue for pathologic analysis. The procedures required to obtain a useable biopsy specimen vary according to its location.

Renal Calyx, Pelvis, or Ureter. A biopsy specimen from the pelvicalyceal system is usually obtained during ureteroscopic examination. A number 3 or 5 cup forceps is introduced through the working channel of a flexible or rigid ureteroscope. The forceps instrument is advanced carefully with its jaws oriented parallel to the ureteral wall. The suspicious lesion is then grasped with the jaws, and gentle traction is applied until a specimen is obtained. The biopsy specimen that is obtained will be quite small, and the endourologist will take special care ensuring that it is not lost as the forceps is removed from the endoscope. Because of the small volume of discrete cup biopsy specimens from the upper urinary tracts, the pelvicalyceal system or ureter may be washed with saline and the fluid sent for cytology. In many cases, cold cup biopsy will be followed by tumor fulguration or laser ablation.

Bladder and Urethra. Bladder or urethral biopsy specimens are obtained during cystoscopic examination. When a malignant lesion is suspected, sterile water is typically used for irrigation, because its cytolytic properties are postulated to minimize the risk of reimplantation of viable cancer cells elsewhere in the lower urinary tract. The biopsy specimen is obtained at the time of tumor resection, fulguration, or laser ablation. If lesions are fulgurated, biopsy tissue is obtained from a small lesion using a cold cup technique. A grasping forceps is inserted through a working port of a rigid cystoscope, and the entire lesion is removed using gentle traction. A separate specimen may be submitted so the depth of the tumor can be assessed, a critical analysis when staging bladder or urethral tumors. Random biopsy specimens of healthy-appearing tissue are also obtained, clearly labeled, and submitted separately from the initial biopsy specimen.

Prostate. Refer to Prostate under Ultrasonography of the Urinary Tract.

Testicular. A biopsy specimen of the testis may be obtained as part of an evaluation of male factor infertility.[17] It is generally indicated in men with azoospermia and may fulfill both diagnostic and therapeutic roles, given advancements in sperm retrieval techniques including intracytoplasmic sperm injection (ICSI). Several techniques are used to obtain a testicular biopsy specimen. Open biopsy specimens can be obtained with the patient under general, spinal, or local anesthesia. When obtaining an open biopsy specimen, the urologist takes care to obtain an adequate biopsy specimen while avoiding damage to the epididymis or testicular blood supply. Percutaneous testicular biopsy is performed using a 16- to 18-gauge biopsy gun designed for obtaining prostate tissue specimens. Since this procedure is blind, a small risk of damage to the epididymis or blood supply exists. Percutaneous testicular aspiration is performed with a 23-gauge needle. The procedure carries less risk than the standard percutaneous approach, and it is less painful. In addition, it allows three or four aspirations so adequate material can be obtained for ICSI if sperm cannot be obtained from the epididymis. A biopsy specimen also may be obtained in the male undergoing evaluation for hypogonadotropic hypogonadism. Pathologic analysis is used to determine the presence of seminiferous tubules and germ cells. Testicular cancer tissue analysis is usually obtained during radical orchiectomy.

Indications

Urinary Tract (Pelvicalyceal System, Ureter, Bladder, and Urethra)

Mass

Hematuria (i.e., gross hematuria or persistent hematuria of unclear etiology)

Testicular

Male factor infertility with azoospermia

ICSI

Hypogonadotropic hypogonadism

Contraindications

If the nurse identifies potential contraindications, such as infection in the biopsy area or anticoagulant therapy, the physician must be notified because postbiopsy treatment may need to be adjusted.

Nursing Management

Patients undergoing biopsy of the upper or lower urinary tracts usually require general anesthesia. In addition to preparing the patient for anesthesia, a prophylactic antimicrobial may be administered.

Since biopsy specimens, especially those obtained from the upper urinary tracts, are very small, the resulting specimen should be treated with great care. A calyceal, renal pelvic, or ureteral biopsy specimen should be immediately placed in a fixative solution, and special notation of the minute specimen size should be included with documentation attached to the biopsy specimen. The specimen should be promptly forwarded to the laboratory for pathologic analysis in order to ensure optimal quality of the specimen needed to provide the patient with accurate results. Upper urinary tract cytology samples also must be handled with care, including accurate labeling of the specimen, notation of the area of the washing (e.g., right ureter or left renal pelvis), and prompt transport to the laboratory for analysis (usually within 1 hour of specimen collection).

Following biopsy, the patient is advised that a stent or catheter may be left in place, particularly if cold cup biopsy is performed with tumor fulguration, resection, or laser ablation since this increases the risk for clots and obstruction. Bleeding is controlled initially during the endoscopic procedure, but some pink or red-tinged urine may be anticipated following the procedure. However, passage of bright red clots indicates significant bleeding that requires prompt intervention. Advise the patient that small flecks of darker red "scabs" are typically passed from 7 to 10 days following the procedure as the underlying urothelium heals. This may be accompanied by pink-tinged urine, but bright red urine or clots should not be seen at this time.

The patient undergoing testicular biopsy also may require preparation for general or spinal anesthesia. Following the procedure, advise the patient that a hematoma may occur. Pain or pressure may accompany a hematoma and can be relieved by scrotal elevation and analgesics. Although scrotal hematomas are typically self-limiting, they occasionally require incision and drainage. Prophylactic antimicrobial therapy is rarely necessary.

SUMMARY

Advances in our technical abilities to assess the anatomy and function of the urinary system have greatly increased the time nurses spend on preparing patients for diagnostic procedures and monitoring patients' responses during testing. Enabling them to interpret results. It is increasingly essential that urologic nurses remain knowledgeable of the various tests, engage in clinical research in order to determine patients' responses to specific procedures, and enable our patients to interpret the meaning of results when they seek care for urologic disorders.

REFERENCES

1. Kampa RJ, Ghani KR, Wahed S, Patel U, Anson KM: Size matters: a survey of how urinary-tract stones are measured in the UK. Journal of Endourology, 2005; 19(7):856-60.
2. Fredenberg RM, Harris RD: Excretory urography in the adult. In Pollack HM, McClennan BL (eds): Clinical Urography, 5th edition. Philadelphia: Saunders, 2000; pp 147-256.
3. Older RA: Contrast media: basics, reactions and management: an interactive program, Baltimore: Urologic Multimedia, 2000.
4. Tublin ME, Murphy ME, Tessler FN: Current concepts in contrast media–induced nephropathy. American Journal of Roentgenology, 1998; 171:933-9.
5. Hosoya T, Yamaguchi K, Akutsu T, Mitsuhashi Y, Kondo S, Sugia Y, Adachi M: Delayed adverse reactions to iodinated contrast media and their risk factors. Radiation Medicine, 2000; 18:39-45.
6. Meth MJ, Maibach HI: Current understanding of contrast media reactions and implications for clinical management. Drug Safety, 1996; 29(2):133-41.
7. Laroche D, Namour F, Lefrancois C, Aimone-Gastin I, Romano A, Sainte-Laudy J, Laxenaire MC, Gueant JL: Anaphylactoid and anaphylactic reactions to iodinated contrast material. Allergy, 1999; 58:13-6.
8. Adkinson SC: Pathophysiology of contrast media anaphylactoid reactions: new perspectives on an old problem. Allergy, 1998; 53:1111-3.
9. Brink JA, Siegel CL: Computed tomography of the upper urinary tract. In Pollack HM, McClennan BL (eds): Clinical Urography, 5th edition. Philadelphia: Saunders, 2000; pp 473-503.
10. Hoppe H, Studer R, Kessler TM, Vock P, Studer UE, Thoeny HC: Alternate or additional findings on stone disease on unenhanced computerized tomography for acute flank pain can impact management. Journal of Urology, 2006; 175(5):1725-30.
11. Wefer AE, Wefer J, Frericks B, Truss MC, Galanski M: Advances in uroradiological imaging. BJU International, 2002; 89:477-87.
12. Garcia-Valtuille R, Garcia-Valtuille AI, Abascal F, Cerezal L, Arguello MC: Magnetic resonance urography: a pictorial overview. British Journal of Radiology, 2006; 79(943):614-26.
13. Weiss RM: Physiology and pharmacology of the renal pelvis and ureter. In Walsh PC, Retik AB, Wein AJ, Vaughan ED (eds): Campbell's Urology. Philadelphia: Saunders, 1998; pp 839-69.
14. Fine EJ, Blaufox MD, Rossleigh MA: Urological applications of radionuclides. In Pollack HM, McClennan BL (eds): Clinical Urography, 5th edition. Philadelphia: Saunders, 2000; pp 621-60.
15. Scoutt LM, Burns P, Brown JL, Hammers L, Rosenfield AT: Ultrasonography of the urinary tract. In Pollack HM, McClennan BL (eds): Clinical Urography, 5th edition. Philadelphia: Saunders, 2000; pp 388-472.
16. Morey AF, McAninch JW: Sonographic staging of anterior urethral strictures. Journal of Urology, 2000; 153:1070-75.
17. Gray M: A prostate cancer primer. Urologic Nursing, 2002; 22:151-72.
18. Dickey KW, Glickman MG, Bookstein JJ: Angiography of the genitourinary tract: techniques and applications. In Pollack HM, McClennan BL (eds): Clinical Urography, 5th edition. Philadelphia: Saunders, 2000; pp 555-601.
19. Garcia-Donaire JA, Alcazar JM: Ischemic nephropathy: detection and therapeutic intervention. Kidney International—Supplement, 2005;(99):S131-6.
20. Bloch MJ, Basile J: Clinical insights into the diagnosis and management of renovascular disease: an evidence-based review. Minerva Medica, 2004; 95(5):357-73.
21. Ford PL: Dynamic infusion cavernosometry and cavernosography. Urologic Nursing, 2000; 20:239-240, 243-245, 253.
22. Sigman M, Jarow JP: Male infertility. In Wein AJ, Kavoussi LR, Novick AC, Partin AW, Peter CA (eds): Campbell-Walsh Urology, 9th edition. Philadelphia: Saunders, 1998; pp 1287-1330.

CHAPTER

5   *Urinary Tract Infections*

....

OVERVIEW OF URINARY TRACT INFECTIONS

....

Epidemiology

In his now classic article, Kass wrote that urinary tract infections (UTIs) are "amongst the most frequently encountered, most frequently undiagnosed, and most difficult to manage of all infections."[1] Each year UTIs continue to account for losses in work time, morbidity, and medical costs.[2] The annual incidence of UTI in a community-based population in Canada is 1.75 episodes per 1000 persons.[2a] As many as 14% of community-dwelling women experience dysuria and urinary frequency,[3] with the prevalence increasing with age. For those living in long-term care settings the prevalence may be as high as 50%.[4] It is estimated that 7 million office visits per year are due to UTIs at an annual cost to the healthcare system of over $1 billion.[5]

Pathogenesis

A UTI occurs when a bacterial, fungal, or parasitic pathogen overwhelms the patient's (host's) defenses, resulting in inflammation of one or more components of the urinary tract. The pathogenesis of a UTI is complex and not well understood. Currently the interaction of biofilms,[6] the role of type 1 fimbriae in the colonization of the urethra and bladder,[7,8] and the role of bladder surface mucin[9] are all being investigated.

Biofilms in the Pathogenesis of a Urinary Tract Infection. Bacteria exist in two physical states: planktonic, free-floating, individual cells and sessile, adherent cells, attached to surfaces, which form biofilms and function as a sophisticated microcolony often impenetrable to macrophages and antibiotics. Biofilms are believed to have three layers: a linking film that attaches, a base film of compact microorganisms, and a surface film on which the planktonic organisms attach and then spread. It is in the planktonic state that bacteria are susceptible to antibiotic therapy, and it is only the free-floating planktonic organisms that are cultured in a urine specimen. The treatment challenge in complicated UTI is that the organisms are established and are not only free floating but also in the biofilm stage. Those organisms in the biofilms may be notably different from the free-floating ones, and such differences are proposed as a major reason for antibiotic failure in complicated or chronic UTI.[10]

Type 1 Fimbriae in the Pathogenesis of a Urinary Tract Infection. Strains of *Escherichia coli* may invade bladder epithelial cells and become intracellular. Attachment of *E. coli* through adhesive type 1 fimbriae contributes to the virulence of organisms; interactions between the proteins and bladder luminal surface of the epithelial cells lead to colonization of the bladder and invasion of the epithelial cells. Protected in the bladder tissue, the organisms are immune to antibiotic treatment[11] and may be a source for recurrent infections.

Bladder Surface in the Pathogenesis of a Urinary Tract Infection. Lining the luminal surface of the bladder is a transitional layer of epithelium (urothelium) about three or four cell layers deep[11] that is separated from the smooth muscular and serous layers by a thin basement membrane and lamina propria. In the healthy bladder the low urine pH and osmolarity as well as salts, urea, and organic acids in the urine inhibit bacterial survival. Moreover, antiadherence factors, including Tamm-Horsfall protein, low molecular weight sugars, secretory immunoglobulin A (IgA), and uromucoid, all inhibit bacterial attachment (Figure 5-1).[11]

The Agent and the Host

Infections depend on the contact between an infectious agent and a susceptible host. In the urinary tract, such factors include diminished host defenses in the urethra, urine, and bladder (internal environment), virulence features of infectious bacteria (agent), and the use of instruments such as urinary catheters or cystoscopes

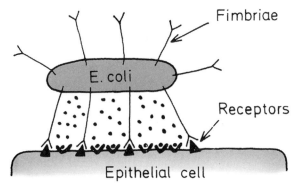

Fimbriae

E. coli

Receptors

Epithelial cell

Fig. 5-1 Bacterial adherence. (From Wein AJ, Kavoussi LR, Novick AC, Partin AW, Peters CA: Campbell-Walsh Urology, 9th edition. Philadelphia: Saunders, 2007.)

(external environment). Risk factors for UTIs in women include sexual activity, use of a diaphragm and/or spermicide, cystocele, anatomic or structural factors such as uterine prolapse, or estrogen deficiency,[12] whereas in young men, UTIs are rare.[13] Genetic factors such as blood group secretor status, recent antibiotic exposure, functional status, receptive anal intercourse, or human immunodeficiency virus (HIV) infection may also play a role.[14] In the older adult, UTI rates are similar in both men and women, and risk factors may include estrogen deficiency, diabetes, neurologic diseases, prostatism, dementia, and urinary and/or fecal incontinence.[4]

Urinary Pathogens

The majority of UTIs are caused by either coliforms or enterococci. Coliforms are generally gram-negative enteric (commensal to the intestinal tract) rods (bacilli). They include the Enterobacter family members of E. coli, species of Klebsiella, Enterobacter, and Citrobacter that ferment lactose,[15] and other family fermentative members, such as Serratia and Providencia species. E. coli is a member of the bacteria family Enterobacteriaceae, a commensal intestinal inhabitant that usually resides in humans without problem. In the urinary tract, E. coli is a rapid reproducer and the primary cause of 80% to 90% of uncomplicated UTIs.[16] Staphylococcus saprophyticus accounts for 10% to 20%, and other members of the family Enterobacteriaceae (e.g., Klebsiella, Proteus, and Enterobacter) account for approximately 5%. However, in complicated UTIs, E. coli is only responsible fosr about 20%, whereas Enterobacteriaceae, Pseudomonas, Acinetobacter, and gram-positive

organisms such as Staphylococcus aureus play a more significant role.[13,17] Anaerobic bacteria, such as Bacteroides melaninogenicus, and aerobic bacteria, such as lactobacilli, Staphylococcus epidermidis, Corynebacteriaceae, and α-hemolytic Streptococcus species, are also cultured in the urethra and are occasionally pathogenic, usually in compromised patients. Enterococci, α-hemolytic Streptococcus species, Candida albicans, lactobacilli, and Bacteroides species are commonly found in the anterior urethra of women but are rarely pathogenic.[18]

Enterococci constitute a subgroup of gram-positive Streptococcus group D species. This subgroup includes Enterococcus faecalis and Enterococcus faecium (previously known as Streptococcus faecalis and Streptococcus faecium). Of the two, Enterococcus faecalis is more commonly involved in UTIs. Both species are developing significant resistance to antibiotics. Enterococci commonly cause UTIs in hospitalized patients.[19]

Nosocomial Urinary Tract Infections

Nosocomial (hospital-acquired) UTIs are caused by a variety of pathogens; the most common species are E. coli or Enterococcus.[20] Patients with spinal cord injury are susceptible to Pseudomonas species colonization, especially if wearing external urinary catheters or using intermittent catheterization, and they may begin to colonize in as little as 2 days after hospital admission.[21,22] Of major concern is the increasing resistance to antibiotics of many bacterial strains.[23,24] The common infectious organisms in intensive care areas are E. coli, Pseudomonas species, S. epidermidis, S. aureus, coagulase-negative staphylococci, and Enterococcus species.[25] Under normal circumstances, many of these bacteria are commensal (symbiotic) with humans and the environment.[15] S. epidermidis, for example, is commonly found in the environment and on the skin and usually does not cause disease in healthy individuals. Infections emerge because commensal bacteria become opportunistic pathogens, taking advantage of diminished host defenses. S. epidermidis demonstrates this capacity in intensive care units since it frequently causes bacteremias associated with intravascular devices.[13]

Routes of Infection

The three routes of bacterial invasion into the bladder are ascension through the urethra, the hematogenous route, and the lymphatic channels. The most common is the ascending urethral pathway. Bacteria often migrate into the bladder but do not necessarily cause infection (e.g., with intercourse). The determinants of bacterial cystitis depend on the virulence and inoculum size of invasive bacteria and the adequacy of the host defense mechanisms. Data concerning the number of bacteria needed to produce a bladder infection are based solely on animal studies, which show that an extremely large inoculum (more than 1 million) is needed to produce cystitis in the noncompromised host. Fortunately, the number of bacteria that normally enter the bladder through the urethra is considerably smaller (fewer than 100).

Women are particularly susceptible to colonization of the urethra and to bacterial cystitis because of the relatively short, straight urethra; the close relationship between the vagina and urethra; and the normal flora of the genital area. Urethral colonization arises from the vaginal introitus and vestibule rather than from the rectum, as is commonly assumed. Longitudinal studies show that cultures of the vaginal vestibule and distal urethral mucosa are more predictive of recurrent bacterial cystitis than analysis of rectal flora.[26]

Natural Defenses of the Urinary Tract

The natural host defense mechanisms of the male and female urethra and bladder provide protection against bacterial colonization and infection in the healthy person.[27] The healthy bladder empties completely and is a sterile system. Protection is offered by properties in the urethra, a high-pressure zone at the sphincter, bactericidal properties of the bladder, and the urine. Any condition that alters complete emptying or contaminates the system favors colonization by microorganisms.[25]

The Urethra. The female urethra is approximately 3 to 4 cm in length. It is protected by periurethral mucus-secreting glands that surround the distal two thirds. Mucus traps bacteria attempting to ascend the urethra and may delay or prevent organisms from reaching the fourth centimeter of the urethra that is contiguous with the bladder.[9] Women who experience chronic UTIs seem to have an increased adherence of bacteria to urethral and vaginal mucosa and are less likely to have the protective effect of a secretor blood group antigen.[13] In the male the urethra extends approximately 20 cm through the prostate gland, fibrous sheath, and

penis and serves both the urinary and reproductive tracts. The prostatic urethra passes through the prostate gland, which produces an antibacterial substance and can synthesize IgA locally.[28] The long cavernous urethra receives secretions from the bulbourethral reproductive glands near its proximal end.

Colonization. The number and location of urethral microorganisms vary among individuals. Gram-negative and gram-positive bacteria in gradually decreasing numbers have been identified in two classic studies as far as the fifth and sixth urethral segments in the male urethra.[29] In the majority of females with a UTI, organisms have been identified along the entire urethra but particularly in the first centimeter.[30] Of note is that women without a UTI may be colonized in the first centimeter but are rarely colonized in the second, third, and fourth centimeters.[31] UTIs in young males are rare unless they have undergone urinary instrumentation or have functional or anatomic abnormalities of the genitourinary tract.[13,32]

High-pressure zone. The distal striated sphincters in the male (within the membranous urethra) and in the female (approximately 1.5 cm from the meatus) create high-pressure zones that are still accepted as relative barriers to bacterial ascent from the distal urethra to the bladder.[33,34] An association between the urethral high-pressure zone and distribution of colonized microbes within the urethra is believed to exist. The urethral high-pressure zone may partially determine, as a relative barrier, whether colonized microbes ascend from the meatus or periurethral area to the bladder. During urethral catheterization, for example, the catheter passes through the distal urethra and penetrates the natural barrier, carrying microbes that may be inoculated into the bladder.

The bladder. Early research providing the foundation of understanding UTI illustrated that bladder overdistention may disrupt tissue integrity by decreasing blood supply to the bladder wall.[35] This renders the bladder susceptible to bacteria by way of the hematogenous route. Natural bladder defenses mean that under normal circumstances, bacteria in contact with the bladder wall are rapidly killed. Small numbers of bacteria are killed more effectively than large numbers, and some bacterial strains are more susceptible (e.g., *Proteus mirabilis*) than others (e.g., *Staphylococcus aureus*).[36] In an animal model, it has been shown that while organisms are multiplying in urine (e.g., *E. coli*), the bladder wall continues to exert a bactericidal effect on organisms attached to the bladder surface.[37] It is believed that women with recurrent UTIs have an increased adherence of bacteria to urothelial cells by fimbrial adhesins compared with women who do not experience UTI. Moreover, blood group phenotypes in women with recurrent UTIs may differ in the proportion of protective secretor blood group antigens that affect the ability of the urothelium to resist bacterial adherence.[25]

Urine. Urine is generally bacteriostatic for small inocula (fewer than 10^2 organisms/ml) under optimal conditions (e.g., low pH).[38] Properties of urine, such as pH, osmolality, glucose and amino acid content, organic acids, and urea, can promote or inhibit the growth of bacteria.[28] The frequency of bladder emptying, high urinary flow, and the amount of residual urine have been suggested to contribute to the presence or absence of bacteria in the urine,[39] but further research is still needed to confirm these statements.

Urine flow and voiding flush unattached or weakly adherent microbes out of the bladder vesicle.[40] Multiplication of bacteria in the urine occurs in four phases: lag phase, logarithmic phase, maximum stationary phase, and phase of decline identified in a classic study by Asscher, Sussman, and Weiser.[41] The lag phase is a high-energy phase in which the bacteria adapt to the new environment rather than increasing in cell mass or in number. The logarithmic phase begins once bacteria have adapted and accounts for growth at a constant energetic rate until the condition of the urine changes enough to inhibit growth (e.g., reduced nutrients, increased toxic waste). The time it takes viable *E. coli*, for example, to double in number (generation time) can be as short as 12.5 minutes[42] whereas for other organisms the generation time may be hours (e.g., *Mycobacterium tuberculosis*). Eventually the maximum stationary phase may be reached while at the same time resources in the urine decline. Because of lack of nutrients and buildup of toxic waste, the phase of decline sets in and bacteria begin to die.[40]

Alterations in Host Defense Mechanisms

Abnormalities such as obstruction to urine flow, vesicoureteral reflux, underlying disease such as urinary calculi, and pregnancy will all alter the natural defense mechanisms and increase the risk of UTI.

Obstruction. Any obstruction to urine flow, such as prostatism, bladder tumor, urethral strictures, cystocele, constipation, vaginal sling procedure, pessary, or neurologic conditions causing poor detrusor contractility, will result in residual urine. High colony counts and invasion of the urothelial cells of the bladder will ensue.[43] In addition, obstruction causes physiologic changes in the detrusor itself, further resulting in reduced ability to cope with bacterial invasion.

Vesicoureteral Reflux. Vesicoureteral reflux compromises the defense mechanisms by allowing colonized or infected urine to move from the lower to the upper tract and possibly into the renal parenchyma.

Urinary Calculi. Urinary calculi are often obstructive to urinary outflow and serve as a nidus for infection during antibiotic therapy. In addition, any disease or circumstance that interferes with the body's immune system decreases the efficiency of the bladder wall to react against bacteriuria.

Bacteriuria in Pregnancy. Asymptomatic bacteriuria in pregnancy is nearly double that of nonpregnant women. Although asymptomatic bacteriuria is not a health issue in nonpregnant women, pregnant women whose bacteriuria progresses to pyelonephritis have an increased risk of preterm delivery.[44] Pregnant women with bacteriuria are at a significantly increased risk (20% to 40%) for developing pyelonephritis, and this risk is dramatically reduced by treating the bladder infection. Risk factors for bacteriuria are catheterization during pregnancy, diabetes, sickle cell anemia, low socioeconomic status, multiple births, or UTIs as a child. Bacteriuria during pregnancy is also a risk factor for UTI after delivery. Treatment of UTI in pregnancy should be with penicillins or cephalosporins. Quinolones and trimethoprim-sulfa are both contraindicated in pregnancy.

Changes in the urinary tract unique to pregnancy increase a woman's likelihood for having recurring UTIs or experiencing a first UTI. The primary urologic change is the "physiologic hydroureter of pregnancy," which is the reversible dilation of the ureters and renal pelvis. This dilation often begins as early as the seventh week of gestation and progresses until delivery. The right ureter is affected more often than the left, and ureteral peristalsis is significantly slowed after the second month of gestation, so that intraureteral volume may be as great as 25 times normal.[44]

Clinical Manifestations of Acute Cystitis/ Uncomplicated Urinary Tract Infection

Symptomatic differentiation of lower urinary tract (bladder) infection from upper tract symptoms is relatively straightforward in an otherwise healthy adult. Typical symptoms are listed in Box 5-1.

History and urinalysis should separate cystitis from vaginitis, urethritis, or sexually transmitted infections (STIs). Women with vaginitis will complain of discomfort with voiding but not urgency, frequency, dysuria, or hematuria; vaginal discharge may be present, and the vaginal vault will be red and inflamed. Differential diagnosis may be herpes simplex virus, chlamydia, trichomoniasis, *Candida*, bacterial vaginosis, or gonorrhea. Table 5-1 describes the STIs that cause symptoms similar to a UTI, particularly dysuria and suprapubic discomfort.[45] In STIs the urinalysis may show pyuria but will not culture positive for organisms. Urethritis is characterized by dysuria with or without frequency and urgency; symptoms are uncomfortable but not excessively painful and gradual in onset; urethral discharge may be present and in the male is characteristic of urethritis. Differential diagnosis includes gonorrhea, chlamydia, herpes simplex virus, or *Trichomonas*.

Urethral injury or irritation can occur from sexual intercourse, chemical irritants such as vaginal perfumes or soaps, or allergies. Urethral discharge and pyuria are absent.

Unresolved or Recurrent Urinary Tract Infections

Unresolved bacteriuria during therapy may arise from several causes: bacterial resistance to antimicrobial treatment; development of a secondary strain as the primary organism is eliminated; bacteriuria caused by two different organisms with mutually exclusive susceptibilities; renal insufficiency (azotemia) causing inadequate concentrations of antibiotic in the urinary tract, although the correct agent has been chosen; staghorn calculus large enough to support a critical mass of bacteria too great for antibiotics to resolve; and papillary necrosis from analgesic abuse.[43]

Recurrent Urinary Tract Infections

Recurrent UTIs are due to either bacterial persistence or reinfection. Symptoms may recur 5 to 10 days after therapy, resulting in a positive urine culture. Bacterial persistence is from the same organism; reinfections occur at varying intervals and are usually caused by different species. Differentiating between persistent and recurrent infections is important to management. Persistent infections may occur in men with chronic bacterial prostatitis who have a persistent focus for ascending urethral infection from the prostatic ductal system or in patients with struvite stones in the urinary tract; in persistent infections the infectious agent can be identified and treated or removed. Box 5-2 on p. 100 lists the causes of bacterial persistence. Women with reinfection rarely have a urologic abnormality and require long-term suppressive antibiotics; reinfection in men is rare and should be investigated by endoscopy.

Sexual intercourse is associated with an increased incidence of recurrent UTIs, and some women specifically correlate intercourse and recurrence. Compared with the general population, nuns have a 0.4% to 1.6% incidence of UTI and married women have a higher incidence than single women. Intercourse predisposes susceptible women because of transference of bacteria into the bladder and/or related minor urethral injury that may result in infection.[46]

RENAL INFECTIONS (UPPER URINARY TRACT INFECTIONS)

Acute Uncomplicated Pyelonephritis (Bacterial Nephritis)

Patients with upper tract infections may experience concurrent lower tract symptoms. Classic symptoms of uncomplicated pyelonephritis are rapid onset of temperature, chills, malaise, and lower back or unilateral or bilateral flank pain. However, not all patients with these symptoms have renal infections,

---

BOX 5-1 Typical Upper and Lower Urinary Tract Symptoms

Lower Urinary Tract Symptoms (Localized Symptoms)
Dysuria (often described like voiding needles or razor blades)
Suprapubic pain/aching
Frequency
Hematuria

Upper Urinary Tract Symptoms (Systemic Symptoms)
Temperature > 102.2° F (39° C)
Flank pain, lower back pain
Lethargy, malaise, fatigue
Chills, sweats
Hematuria

TABLE 5-1 Urologic Symptoms Associated with Sexually Transmitted Infections

PATHOGEN	MODES OF TRANSMISSION	SYMPTOMS	DIAGNOSIS	TREATMENT
Bacterial Infections				
Gonorrhea (*Neisseria gonorrhoeae*)	Transmitted by vaginal, oral, or anal sexual activity or from mother to newborn during delivery	Symptoms usually appear 2-10 days after infection *Women:* yellow-bloody discharge, dysuria, frequency, pain and swelling of the labia, irregular menstrual bleeding (80% of women are asymptomatic) *Men:* whitish penile discharge (early stage); yellowish, thick penile discharge (late stage); dysuria, frequency	Clinical inspection, culture of sample discharge	Cefixime, azithromycin, doxycycline
Syphilis (*Treponema pallidum*)	Transmitted by vaginal, oral, or anal sexual activity or by touching an infectious chancre	In primary stage, a hard, round, painless chancre or sore appears at site of infection within 2-4 wk; may progress through secondary, latent, and tertiary stages, if left untreated; rashes usually covering the body—especially on the palms of the hands and the soles of the feet	Primary-stage syphilis diagnosed by clinical examination and by examination of fluid from a chancre; secondary-stage syphilis diagnosed by a blood test (i.e., the VDRL)	Penicillin; or doxycycline, tetracycline, or erythromycin for nonpregnant, penicillin-allergic patients
Chlamydia and NGU (*Chlamydia trachomatis* and NGU in men may also be caused by *Ureaplasma urealyticum* and other pathogens)	Transmitted by vaginal, oral, or anal sexual activity; to the eye by touching one's eyes after touching the genitalia of an infected partner; or to newborns passing through the birth canal of an infected mother	Usually occur 1-3 wk after infection *Women:* frequency, dysuria, lower abdominal pain and inflammation, vaginal discharge or bleeding, painful intercourse, bleeding with intercourse (75% of women symptom free)	The Abbott Testpack analyzes a cervical smear in women; in men an extract of fluid from the penis is analyzed	Doxycycline, cefixime, or azithromycin

Continued

TABLE 5-1 Urologic Symptoms Associated with Sexually Transmitted Infections—cont'd

PATHOGEN	MODES OF TRANSMISSION	SYMPTOMS	DIAGNOSIS	TREATMENT
		Men: symptoms similar to but milder than those of gonorrhea—burning or painful urination, slight penile discharge, sore throat may indicate infection from oral-genital contact (25% of men asymptomatic)		Oral metronidazole
Vaginitis				
Bacterial vaginosis (*Gardnerella vaginalis* and others)	Can arise from overgrowth of organisms in vagina, allergic reactions, etc.; also transmitted by sexual contact	*Women:* thin, foul-smelling, white/gray vaginal discharge; genitalia irritated and slight dysuria; vaginal itching and burning caused by the discharge *Men:* inflammation of penile foreskin and glans, urethritis, and cystitis May be asymptomatic in both genders	Culture and examination of bacterium	
Candidiasis (yeast infection) (*Candida albicans*)	Overgrowth of fungus in vagina; may also be transmitted by sexual contact or by sharing a washcloth with an infected person	*Women:* vulval itching; white, cheesy, foul-smelling discharge; soreness or swelling of vaginal and vulval tissues, dysuria *Men:* itching and burning on urination or a reddening of the penis, cheesy material under foreskin of penis	Diagnosis usually made on basis of symptoms	Vaginal suppositories, creams, or tablets containing miconazole, clotrimazole, or tioconazole
Trichomoniasis (*Trichomonas vaginalis:* a protozoan)	Almost always transmitted sexually	Symptoms appear 4-20 days after exposure *Women:* foamy, yellowish, odorous vaginal discharge; itching or burning sensations in vulva, painful intercourse, frequency; many women asymptomatic	Microscopic examination of a smear of vaginal secretions or of culture of the sample (latter method preferred)	Metronidazole

Viral Infections

	Transmission	Symptoms	Diagnosis	Treatment
Genital herpes (herpes simplex virus type 2)	Almost always by means of vaginal, oral, or anal sexual activity; most contagious during active outbreaks of infection	*Men:* usually asymptomatic but mild urethritis possible When a person becomes infected for the first time symptoms usually appear within 2-10 days Appearance of painful, reddish bumps around the genitalia, thighs, or buttocks; in women, may also be in the vagina or on the cervix; bumps become blisters or sores that fill with pus and break, shedding viral particles; symptoms: burning urination, fever, aches and pains, swollen glands; in women, vaginal discharge	Clinical inspection of sores; culture and examination of fluid drawn from the base of a genital sore	Acyclovir may provide relief and prompt healing but is not a cure; people with herpes often benefit from counseling and group support
Genital (venereal) warts (human papilloma virus [HPV])	Transmission by sexual and other forms of contact, such as with infected towels or clothing	Symptoms usually develop within 3 mo of contact with an infected individual Appearance of painless warts, often resembling cauliflowers, on the penis, foreskin, scrotum, or internal urethra in men; on the vulva, labia, wall of the vagina, or cervix in women; may occur around the anus and the rectum of both genders	Clinical inspection	Methods include cryotherapy (freezing), podophyllin, burning, surgical removal

NGU, Nongonococcal urethritis; *VDRL,* Venereal Disease Research Laboratory.

BOX 5-2 Etiology of Bacterial Persistence

Infection from a renal calculus
Chronic bacterial prostatitis
Infected calyceal diverticulum
Infected nonrefluxing stump following nephrectomy
Atrophic infected kidney
Medullary sponge kidney
Infected urachal cyst
Infected necrotic papilla from papillary necrosis

and some patients with renal infections do not exhibit such typical symptoms. Appropriate radiologic and laboratory studies are required to establish a diagnosis (Figures 5-2 and 5-3). Of note is that the absence of pyuria does not rule out pyelonephritis because the ureter draining the infected kidney may be obstructed.

Symptoms may be managed by oral antibiotics; at-risk patients requiring more aggressive therapy with aminoglycosides include pregnant women, immunocompromised patients, or acutely ill patients.

Acute Focal or Multifocal Bacterial Nephritis

Acute focal or multifocal bacterial nephritis is an uncommon, severe form of acute renal infection affecting one or more lobes of the kidney. Leukocytosis and gram-negative UTI are found clinically, and half of the patients are bacteremic. Radiologic examination shows a poorly marginated mass suggestive of renal abscess or tumor. Treatment includes hydration and intravenous antibiotics for 7 days, followed by oral antibiotics for another 7 days (Figure 5-4).

Infected Hydronephrosis and Pyonephrosis

Pyonephrosis refers to infected hydronephrosis associated with destruction of the renal parenchyma and total or near total loss of renal function. The patient presents clinically with high fever, chills, and flank pain. Excretory urography shows poorly functioning hydronephrotic kidneys. Treatment involves appropriate antibiotic therapy; however, immediate drainage of the kidney is mandatory. Patients with pyonephrosis are particularly susceptible to perinephric abscess formation. Clinical presentation is similar to pyelonephritis, with laboratory tests showing leukocytosis, elevated levels of serum creatinine, and pyuria. Treatment for perinephric abscess involves intravenous antibiotic therapy followed by surgical drainage (Figure 5-5).

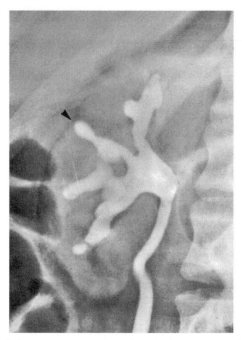

Fig. 5-2 Excretory urogram (IVU) demonstrates focal, coarse scarring in the right kidney of an 18-year-old girl with a history of many recurrent fevers between 2 months and 2 years of age. A cystogram when the patient was 2 years old established an atrophic left kidney with marked reflux up to the left kidney and slight reflux up to the right kidney. IVU at the age of 6 years established severe atrophy of the left kidney. She had no infections between the ages of 6 and 15 years. Several reinfections occurred at the age of 15 years, and they ceased with prophylactic therapy. Her blood pressure has remained normal, and her serum creatinine level was 0.9 mg/dL at the age of 18 years. At 21 years of age she stopped antimicrobial prophylaxis for 18 months without infections or introital colonization with Enterobacteriaceae. Note that all calyces are blunted and that one extends to the capsule (*arrowhead*) because of atrophy of the overlying cortex. (From Wein AJ, Kavoussi LR, Novick AC, Partin AW, Peters CA: Campbell-Walsh Urology, 9th edition. Philadelphia: Saunders, 2007.)

Renal Abscess

Gram-negative organisms are implicated in renal abscess, the collection of purulent material in the renal parenchyma (Figure 5-6). Symptoms include fever, chills, flank pain, and general malaise often accompanied by lower urinary tract symptoms. The patient presents with leukocytosis and positive blood cultures. In advanced cases, radiologic findings may demonstrate generalized renal enlargement. Computed tomography (CT) and ultrasonography are the diagnostic procedures

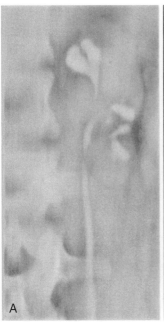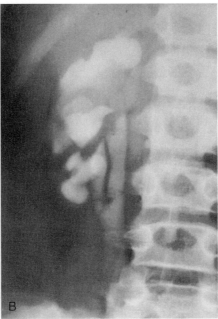

Fig. 5-3 A, IVU of the left kidney. The severe pyelonephritic atrophy, undoubtedly caused by febrile urinary infections during early infancy with reflux into different segments of the kidney, produced irregular cortical scarring. Note how all the calyces extend to the capsule with irregular, intervening areas of cortex. **B,** Pyelonephritic atrophy, suggestive of postobstructive atrophy, in a 20-year-old woman with spina bifida, neurogenic bladder, and many episodes of fever and bacteriuria in early childhood. Observe the uniform, regular atrophy of the renal cortex that suggests reflux of bacteria simultaneously into virtually all nephrons. This type of pyelonephritic atrophy is uncommon compared with that shown in **A** and is characteristic of obstruction with superimposed infection. (From Wein AJ, Kavoussi LR, Novick AC, Partin AW, Peters CA: Campbell-Walsh Uro-logy, 9th edition. Philadelphia: Saunders, 2007.)

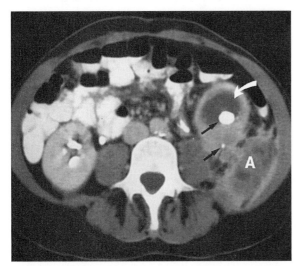

Fig. 5-4 Xanthogranulomatous pyelonephritis. Enhanced CT scan shows collecting system and parenchymal calculi (*straight arrows*) with lower pole pyonephrosis (*curved arrow*) and an irregular, predominantly low-density perinephric abscess (A) extending into the soft tissues of the flank. (From Wein AJ, Kavoussi LR, Novick AC, Partin AW, Peters CA: Campbell-Walsh Urology, 9th edition. Philadelphia: Saunders, 2007.)

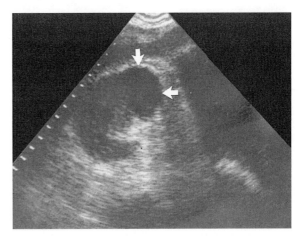

Fig. 5-5 Acute renal abscess. Transverse ultrasonographic scan of the right kidney demonstrates a poorly marginated rounded focal hypoechoic mass (*arrows*) in the anterior portion of the kidney. (From Wein AJ, Kavoussi LR, Novick AC, Partin AW, Peters CA: Campbell-Walsh Urology, 9th edition. Philadelphia: Saunders, 2007.)

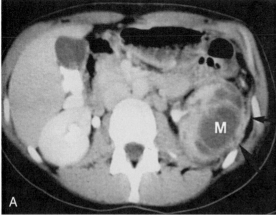

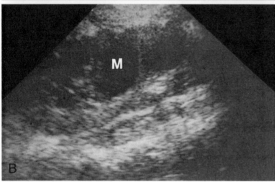

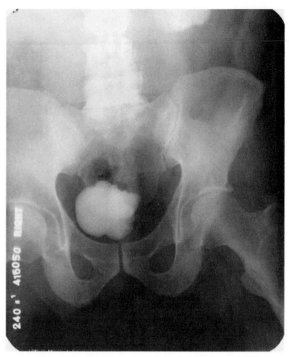

Fig. 5-6 Chronic renal abscess. **A,** Enhanced CT scan shows an irregular septated low-density mass (M) extensively involving the left kidney. Note thickening of perinephric fascia (*arrowheads*) and extensive compression of the renal collecting system. Findings are typical of renal abscess. **B,** Ultrasound longitudinal scan demonstrates a septated hypoechoic mass (M) occupying much of the renal parenchymal volume. (From Wein AJ, Kavoussi LR, Novick AC, Partin AW, Peters CA: Campbell-Walsh Urology, 9th edition. Philadelphia: Saunders, 2007.)

Fig. 5-7 The cystogram portion of an intravenous pyelogram in a patient with left renal tuberculosis. Note the contracted left side of the bladder that is secondary to fibrosis from the tuberculosis. (From Wein AJ, Kavoussi LR, Novick AC, Partin AW, Peters CA: Campbell-Walsh Urology, 9th edition. Philadelphia: Saunders, 2007.)

of choice because they provide excellent delineation of tissue. Management involves the use of intravenous antibiotic therapy and careful observation. If there is no improvement within 48 hours, aspiration and drainage should be done.[43]

Renal Tuberculosis/Infectious Granulomatous Nephritis

The kidneys are the most common site for extrapulmonary tuberculosis. Renal tuberculosis is primarily a disease of young to middle-aged adults (Figure 5-7). Because it progresses slowly, there is no classic clinical presentation. Symptoms can include dull, vague flank discomfort; gross hematuria; and ureteral colic

caused by passage of clots or calculi. Urinalysis is abnormal in the majority of patients, indicating a sterile pyuria accompanied by hematuria and proteinuria. Positive urine cultures for *M. tuberculosis* are usual. The majority of patients will have abnormal excretory urograms.

Renal tuberculosis should be considered when chronic or recurrent cystitis does not respond to treatment, sterile pyuria is noted on urine culture, or gross hematuria is present. Treatment includes a strict medical regimen with a combination of drugs given over a 6-month course.[43]

Tubercular Cystitis

Tuberculosis of the bladder results from the implantation of the tubercle bacilli into the wall, causing an uneven mix of inflamed areas interspersed with normal mucosal segments. The cystoscopic picture of the bladder may resemble interstitial cystitis or candidal infection with patches of inflamed tissue and reddened ureteral orifices. The anterior urethra is not affected by the infection, but the posterior urethra and prostate are heavily involved in men, representing progression from prostate to bladder. The trigone is relatively spared from inflammatory changes, but the dome of the bladder is extensively affected, resulting in a marked loss in capacity.

The primary symptoms of tubercular cystitis are marked frequency and urgency. Bladder volume rapidly decreases and may result in irreversible changes in advanced stages of the infection.[26] Urodynamic assessment in advanced cases may reveal poor bladder wall compliance and a functional capacity of 60 ml of urine or less.

Emphysematous Pyelonephritis or Cystitis

Emphysematous pyelonephritis is a necrotizing renal infection characterized by gas in the renal parenchyma and should be considered a complication of severe pyelonephritis.[47] The condition usually occurs in diabetic patients. Many patients have obstructed urinary tracts and significant renal function impairment as well as diabetes. The causative organism is generally *E. coli*, which produces carbon dioxide by the fermentation of sugar. The condition generally affects women more than men. The usual clinical presentation involves acute, severe pyelonephritis that does not respond to antibiotic treatment, as well as flank pain, fever, and vomiting. The diagnosis is made by radiographic confirmation of gas shadows over the affected kidney and positive urine cultures for *E. coli*. Treatment involves fluid resuscitation along with intravenous broad-spectrum antibiotic administration. Emphysematous pyelonephritis is a surgical emergency, because many patients are septic. Nephrectomy is recommended for patients who do not respond to medical therapy in a few days.

Cystitis emphysematosa is a rare form of bladder inflammation resulting from infection by gas-forming urinary bacteria or (more commonly) vesicoenteric fistula. The condition may also be observed after urologic instrumentation or urodynamic testing using carbon dioxide. Pneumaturia is associated with this form of cystitis.[43]

Bacteriuria in Elders. The prevalence of bacteriuria increases with age for both men and women, especially for those in institutions.[48,49] The reasons for increased prevalence are not well studied, but comorbid conditions, such as diabetes, neurologic diseases, obstruction, and impaired mobility, may

all play a role.[50] Bacteriuria in elders is often persistent, recurrent, and long lasting. Whereas in the younger person the presence or absence of pyuria can be used to differentiate infection from colonization of the urinary tract, in the elderly person, where virtually all subjects in institutions have pyuria, a positive urine dip is unlikely to be a meaningful concept.[27] Moreover, the relationship between symptoms and UTI is often vague and nonspecific when compared with a younger population.[51] Symptoms might include, but are not restricted to, fever, a general decline in status, or alterations in genitourinary function, such as incontinence. Despite the high prevalence of bacteriuria in elders, the majority of bacteriuric subjects are asymptomatic. Treatment of asymptomatic bacteriuria is not recommended because of the frequent recurrence of bacteriuria after conclusion of treatment, adverse drug effects, and increased drug resistance.[52] Treatment of symptomatic infections follows the same principles as for younger populations although the difficulty of identifying a symptomatic infection may be more challenging and antibiotic treatment should follow a 7- to 10-day course rather than the shorter 3-day course that is standard therapy in younger women.

Funguria

The most common fungal infection of the bladder is candidiasis. *Candida albicans* is endemic to the human body and can often be found in the pharynx, stomach, intestinal tract, and vaginal vault (particularly in pregnant or diabetic women). Risk factors for candidiasis include the presence of an indwelling catheter, antimicrobial therapy, diabetes mellitus, hospitalization, and immunosuppression. Patients with obstructive prostatic enlargement or who are pregnant are also at risk.

Normal bacterial flora and polymorphonuclear leukocytes in the mucosa of the urethra and bladder have marked anticandidal effects that usually inhibit fungal growth. In addition, prostatic fluid in men is fungicidal, which helps explain the relatively low incidence of candidal cystitis in men compared with women. Cell-mediated immunity and other white blood cells (WBCs) also help prevent candidiasis. Administration of antibiotics is thought to stimulate the production of *C. albicans* by altering the pH of gastrointestinal mucosa, suppressing normal bacterial flora that compete with the fungus for food, and inhibiting polymorphonuclear phagocytosis that helps the body guard against overgrowth.

The symptoms are similar to those of bacterial cystitis and include urgency, marked frequency, dysuria, suprapubic pain, and nocturia. Pyelonephritis-like symptoms will be present with renal fungal infections. Pneumaturia (the expression of gas or air through the urethra during or after micturition) may be noted.

Parasitic Cystitis

Although schistosomiasis is rare in the United States, it is relatively common elsewhere in the world. The ova of the parasite enter the bloodstream by penetrating the skin. The veins of the bladder are a popular breeding site for the parasites. The eggs are then extruded into the vesicle for further spread of the parasitic organisms. The healing of the affected areas of the bladder causes thickening and contraction of the bladder wall. Damage of the ureterovesical junction often occurs, resulting in vesicoureteral reflux. Contracted bands mark the bladder and may extend into the lower ureter. Urinary stasis and ova in the urine contribute to urinary calculi.[43]

Chemotherapy- and Radiation-Induced Cystitis

Chemotherapy- or radiation-induced cystitis is characterized by inflammatory changes in the bladder wall in the absence of infection. The symptoms are similar to those of infectious cystitis and include urgency, frequency, and suprapubic pain. Detrusor instability and urge incontinence may occur.

Although the bladder is relatively resistant to radiation, therapeutic doses greater than 6000 to 7000 rad over a 6- to 7-week period may result in cystitis. Chemotherapy-induced cystitis may arise from systemic cyclophosphamide or intravesical antineoplastic drugs, such as mitomycin. The diagnosis is made when symptoms of cystitis are reported with a normal culture and positive history of exposure to radiation or a chemotherapeutic agent.[53]

Inflammatory lesions of the bladder cause intense, irritative symptoms, including dysuria, frequency, and urgency. Lesions may represent a complication of chronic bacterial infection or outlet obstruction. Inflammatory lesions often resemble malignant tumors, and certain lesions are considered premalignant. Table 5-2 summarizes three of the most common types of lesions.

Catheter-Associated Urinary Tract Infections

Catheter-associated UTI is defined as presence of a symptomatic infection in a person with an indwelling urinary catheter. Bacteriuria occurs in as few as 2 days after catheterization, depending on insertion technique, state of the patient's health, and gender (women usually develop bacteriuria more quickly than men). Bacteria are introduced into the bladder in several ways: through the urethra with catheterization, through the drainage bag, and on the catheter itself. The catheter acts as a nidus for organisms adhering to the catheter surface.[54] Prevention of catheter-associated UTI requires meticulous insertion technique during catheterization, maintenance of a closed

TABLE 5-2 Inflammatory Lesions of the Bladder

LESION	GROSS APPEARANCE	MALIGNANT POTENTIAL
Infectious cystitis	Reddened and inflamed bladder neck and trigone	Unlikely
Cystitis cystica	1-cm cysts in bladder base, may extend into upper urinary tract	May resemble tumor
Cystitis glandularis	Generalized inflammation of bladder wall, bladder neck, and trigone	May represent premalignant lesion or coexist with cancer
Eosinophilic cystitis	Polypoid lesions with generalized bladder wall inflammation	Not considered premalignant
Tubercular cystitis	Alternating areas of inflamed and normal bladder mucosa	
Catheterized patient		Potential for epithelial changes and squamous cell carcinoma

drainage system, and removal of the catheter as quickly as possible.[54a] Inoculation of catheters with silver alloy shows positive benefits in some studies but not in others,[55] and the use of antibiotic-soaked filters in catheter drainage bags shows limited benefit.[56] Prevention of catheter-associated UTI is especially important in the acute setting where the prevalence of indwelling catheterization is comparatively high (33% to 35%),[55a] especially with the advent of prospective payment changes by the US Centers for Medicare and Medicaid Services beginning in 2008.[55b] These changes provide explicit economic incentives that shift the emphasis from treatment of catheter-associated UTIs acquired in hospital to prevention.

After 30 days of catheterization, nearly all patients will have bacteriuria, but most remain symptom free. For this reason, neither routine cultures nor prophylactic antibiotics are recommended. Irrigations with saline, acetic acid solutions, and antibacterial solutions have not proved effective for the prevention of catheter-associated UTI, nor have meatal antibiotic ointments, antibiotic-impregnated catheters, or antibiotic prophylaxis.[54a] Care of the long-term indwelling catheter is based on comfort and quality of life for the patient and prevention of symptomatic catheter-associated UTI rather than attempts to resolve asymptomatic bacteriuria. Box 5-3 outlines general recommendations for reducing catheter-associated complications.

DIAGNOSIS OF URINARY TRACT INFECTION

Despite concerns about antibiotic overuse[57] and the difficulty in distinguishing a UTI from other common conditions affecting young women, such as vaginitis (e.g., *Chlamydia trachomatis*, *Neisseria gonorrhoeae*, herpes simplex virus), the treatment of a UTI is not always based on diagnostic tests.[58]

Kass[59] introduced the concept that bacterial counts of a single microorganism in excess of 10^5 colony-forming units (CFUs)/ml of urine had a 95% correlation with clinically determined cases of pyelonephritis, a concept that remains accepted today. Kass' research established catheter or midstream urine cultures as the gold standard of UTI diagnosis. However, this diagnostic method is expensive and time consuming, and the sensitivity of urine culture to detect significant UTI using this stringent cutoff value of 10^5 CFUs/ml has been often questioned for both adults[60] and children.[61] In young symptomatic women bacterial counts of 10^2 CFUs/ml may reflect a significant growth in the presence of symptoms[33]

BOX 5-3 Management of Problems Associated with Indwelling Catheters

- Try a hydrophilic catheter (Lubricious) or 100% silicone. The hydrophilic catheter has the advantage of less biofilm adherence than on other surfaces, including silicone; the silicone catheter has the advantage of a wider lumen that may allow better drainage of the mucous secretions.
- Bladder irrigation with saline (1 tsp table salt to 500 ml boiled tap water) or weak solution of acetic acid (1:10) is rarely effective in prolonging catheter life. However, for some patients, it is helpful. Patients or family members can be taught to do bladder irrigations.
- An alternative to bladder irrigation is weekly catheter change. If the catheter is changed weekly, then a less expensive product may be appropriate (rather than hydrophilic or silicone catheters).
- Maintain catheter size no larger than 16F with a 10-ml balloon. Increasing the size of the catheter or balloon will only cause major damage to the bladder neck, eventually rendering the patient incontinent even with a catheter in place.
- Keep the catheter well supported so that there is no tugging or drag on the bladder neck.
- Some wheelchair-bound patients will benefit from a suprapubic catheter. This is only possible, however, if the bladder neck is intact and the patient is continent when the urethral catheter is removed. If the patient is not continent, then, despite a suprapubic catheter, perineal maceration from leaking urine will occur. The condition of the bladder neck can be evaluated at cystoscopy.
- Patients who continue to have leakage or blocking of the catheter should be evaluated with a cystoscopy. Bladder calculi, formed from calcium oxalate crystals, are common in patients with long-term indwelling catheters and cause bladder spasms, increased mucus production, and blocking of the catheter.
- Once the bladder is assessed by cystoscopy and deemed to be healthy, the use of anticholinergics (e.g., oxybutynin) may help with bypassing (i.e., detrusor instability). Unfortunately the side effects of constipation may limit their use.

although typical practice relies on higher counts in part because of changes in laboratory procedures. Urine culture is also insensitive to *C. trachomatis* infection. The overall prevalence of *Chlamydia* in asymptomatic young women was 9.2% in a recent study.[62]

A validated alternative method assisting in the diagnosis of uncomplicated UTI is the demonstration of significant pyuria, usually defined as 10 or more leukocytes per microliter (10^+ WBCs/μl) in freshly voided urine. Pyuria is present in almost all symptomatic UTIs, including *C. trachomatis*, and its absence should strongly suggest another diagnosis, such as tuberculosis.[33] Pyuria is accurately determined by direct microscopy of unspun, undiluted urine, or an approximation of pyuria is derived using a rapid urinalysis assay for the presence of leukocyte esterase. This enzyme is found in primary neutrophil granules and reacts with a reagent impregnated into the dipstick pad to give a color change. Rapid urinalysis assays are cost effective (approximately $1.00 per test), easy to use, efficacious, and safe.[63] The sensitivity and specificity of leukocyte esterase urinalysis assays compared with direct microscopy have been previously reported as 89.4% and 90.4%, respectively.[64]

The nitrite test using rapid urine dip has been used to screen for significant gram-negative organisms. Although the positive predictive value of the test is good (i.e., if the test is positive the person has a high likelihood of having a gram-negative infection), the negative predictive value is low. *E coli* and *Proteus* reduce nitrates to nitrites, and if a urine specimen containing these organisms is obtained from urine that has been in the bladder at least 4 hours, a nitrite urine dip will be positive. However, if the urine has not been in the bladder for an adequate time or if the organisms are not *E. coli* or *Proteus*, then the nitrite test will be false negative. Thus nitrite should be a confirmation of gram-negative organisms, but its absence should not rule out a UTI in the presence of other symptoms. Table 5-3 lists common findings on urinalysis of a symptomatic patient and gives the indications for false-positive and false-negative readings.

Diagnosis of Funguria

Microscopic urinalysis will show budding fungi or pseudohyphae.[43] Pyuria does not correlate well with fungal infections. On cystoscopy, the mucosal lining of the bladder is marked by grayish white spots that result in mucosal bleeding if removed. The ureteral orifices may be affected so that cystoscopic findings may resemble tubercular infection of the bladder. In certain cases asymptomatic candidal colonization of the urine without inflammation of the bladder may be seen.

Collection of Urine. Midstream collection with careful perineal cleaning and labial separation has been the gold standard for urine collection in women. The validity of midstream collection has been challenged by at least two recent studies, both of which suggest that a clean voided sample without cleansing does not differ from a traditional midstream urinalysis.[65,66] Both can be prone to contamination from vaginal discharge but are usually accurate for detection of leukocytes and hemoglobin. Although the gold standard for urine collection has been catheterization, at least one study comparing voided midstream urine with urethral catheterization suggests that voided samples are as accurate as ones obtained by more invasive catheterization.[67]

Diagnostic Imaging. Imaging studies (see Chapter 4 for more details) are not used in routine evaluation of UTI since urinalysis and presenting symptoms are usually adequate for diagnosis. Patients with a UTI who are candidates for more invasive investigation include the following:

- Men who are otherwise healthy
- Patients with signs and symptoms of urinary obstruction
- Patients who fail to respond to antimicrobials or who have recurrent infections

Ultrasound, CT, and intravenous pyelogram may all be used. Ultrasound is rapid, noninvasive, and a good means of evaluating the renal collecting system, parenchyma, and surrounding retroperitoneum for infection. Ultrasound is particularly useful for identifying calculi, hydronephrosis, abscesses, and postvoid residual. CT scanning is used to identify an inflammatory process, tumors, and radiolucent calculi (see Chapter 4). Table 5-4 lists the diagnostic studies and possible findings in the investigation of UTI.

TREATMENT OF URINARY TRACT INFECTIONS

Antibiotic Therapy

In first (uncomplicated) UTI in premenopausal women, empiric treatment is indicated based on the results of the rapid urinalysis showing pyuria and

TABLE 5-3 Urinalysis

URINALYSIS NORMAL	ABNORMAL RESULTS	COMMON CAUSES OF FALSE-POSITIVE/FALSE-NEGATIVE RESULTS
Color: normally pale yellow because of pigment urochrome, sediment may be present	Hgb, urobilinogen	Colorless: overhydration Yellow: phenacetin, riboflavin (B vitamins) Green-blue: biliverdin, amitriptyline, triamterene Brown: aloe, fava beans, rhubarb, chloroquine, furazolidone, metronidazole, nitrofurantoin Brown/black: melanin, cascara, senna, methocarbamol, methyldopa, sorbitol
Turbidity: clear	Cloudy because of pyuria (WBCs); rare causes are chyluria, lipiduria, hyperoxaluria, hyperuricosuria	Cloudy: phosphaturia (after ingestion of high quantity of milk); vaginal discharge
SG: 1.001-1.035	Dehydration (SG < 1.008), overhydration (SG > 1.02); impaired renal function; diabetes insipidus; diabetes mellitus; inappropriate secretion of ADH	Overhydration/dehydration, diuretics; fever, sweating, vomiting; increased after iodinated contrast injection, patients taking dextran
pH range 5.5-6.5	>7.5 in patient with UTI suggests urea-splitting organism *Proteus*; metabolic acidosis or alkalosis; acidic urine in patients with uric acid and cystine stones; persistent pH < 5.5 used to diagnose RTA	
Hgb: negative or trace	Infection (bladder or renal), renal calculus, bladder tumor; IgA nephropathy; lupus erythematosus; papillary necrosis	False positive from ingestion of beets or blackberries, vitamin C, phenolphthalein (bowel evacuants), phenothiazines, rifampin, menstrual flow, heavy exercise; anticoagulants above therapeutic levels
Protein: negative	Renal impairment, multiple myeloma, fever, CHF	Concentrated urine; exercise; positional (e.g., prolonged standing)
Glucose: negative	Diabetes mellitus (always test for ketones if glucose positive)	Pregnancy, fasting; false positive in acidic urine with high SG
Ketones: negative	Diabetic ketoacidosis	Fasting; high-protein "fad" diets
Bilirubin: negative	Hepatic disease	Dehydration, phenazopyridine (pyridium), sulfasalazine, vitamin C
Leukocytes: negative	UTI if corresponds with symptoms	False positive: dehydration, reading the dipstick after the recommended time (usually 2 min); false negative: overhydration, glycosuria, ascorbic acid
Nitrates: negative	Gram-negative organisms convert nitrates to nitrites	False negative: dilute urine, <10^5 CFUs/ml; urine held in bladder less than 4 hr

ADH, Antidiuretic hormone; *CFUs,* colony-forming units; *CHF,* congestive heart failure; *Hgb,* hemoglobin; *IgA,* immunoglobulin A; *RTA,* renal tubular acidosis; *SG,* specific gravity; *UTI,* urinary tract infection; *WBCs,* white blood cells.

TABLE 5-4 Diagnostic Studies and Findings

DIAGNOSTIC TEST	FINDINGS
Urinalysis	See Table 5-3
Urine culture	>100,000 (10^5) colony-forming units (CFUs) per milliliter of agar indicates clinically significant infection; lesser colony counts significant when associated with symptomatic cystitis or in children
	Urine culture negative in parasitic, fungal, or chemotherapy- or radiation-induced therapy
Bladder wall biopsy	Infectious cystitis: consistent with acute inflammation
	Cystitis cystica: negative
	Cystitis glandularis: may demonstrate cancer
	Eosinophilic cystitis: extensive eosinophilic infiltration
	Chemotherapy- or radiation-induced cystitis: chronic inflammation of bladder mucosa
Voiding diary urodynamics	Reduced functional capacity, urinary frequency, nocturia
	Infectious cystitis, cystitis cystica, cystitis glandularis, eosinophilic cystitis: urodynamics contraindicated except in special cases
	Tubercular cystitis: small capacity with poor bladder wall compliance
	Chemotherapy- or radiation-induced cystitis: sensory urgency with low capacity; bladder wall compliance may be compromised; unstable detrusor may be noted
Voiding cystourethrogram	Cystitis emphysematosa: lucent filling defect produced by gas-producing bacteria

the typical symptom presentation of rapid onset of dysuria, suprapubic pain, and frequency.[68] For premenopausal women, current recommendations are a 3-day course of empiric treatment (rather than waiting for a urine culture) with a fluoroquinolone or ciprofloxacin because of the high likelihood of gram-negative coliforms, particularly *E. coli*, the 48-hour wait required for definitive diagnosis with culture and sensitivity, and the cost of urine culture. If the patient has a sulfa allergy, a fluoroquinolone or trimethoprim alone can be prescribed. Previously suggested single-dose therapy has not been as effective in eradicating the organism as the 3-day regimen.[69] In recurrent or complicated UTIs antibiotic therapy should be guided by individual culture and sensitivity reports. As well, bacteriuria in symptomatic men and older women has slower eradication rates so that therapy should be prescribed for 7 to 10 days. Figure 5-8 shows a treatment algorithm for UTIs.

Antibiotics have three routes of action in the bacterial cell wall: inhibition of nucleic acid synthesis, inhibition of cell wall synthesis and β-lactam production, or inhibition of protein synthesis. Box 5-4 provides details on the mechanism of action of the antibiotics used in urology.

Inhibition of Nucleic Acid Synthesis. Trimethoprim-sulfamethoxazole (TMP/SMX), nitrofurantoin, and quinolone antibiotics inhibit nucleic acid synthesis and are the preferred agents for the treatment of uncomplicated UTIs. The sulfonamides were among the first group of drugs used as antibiotics. They achieve high concentrations in the kidney through which they are eliminated. Before the combination of trimethoprim with sulfamethoxazole (TMP/SMX or co-trimoxazole), sulfamethoxazole alone was the most frequently prescribed antibiotic. Combined with phenazopyridine, which has analgesic properties, it was marketed as Azo-Gantanol. Adding the antimetabolite trimethoprim to sulfonamide (1:5) causes a synergistic effect inhibiting two steps in the folic acid pathway that is required for the synthesis of DNA by the bacterial organism. TMP/SMX is not effective against *Enterococcus* and *Pseudomonas* species.

Nitrofurantoin (microcrystalline) does not achieve high enough concentrations to be effective in upper tract or complicated UTI. It is a safe medication, with low acquired resistance, and is used effectively in prophylaxis. Nitrofurantoin (Macrobid, Macrodantin) is a macrocrystalline form that is absorbed more slowly than the microcrystalline form and causes less gastrointestinal distress.

Quinolone antibiotics are bactericidal. An early quinolone for UTI was nalidixic acid, but the narrow spectrum and side effects limited its use. Adding a fluorine atom to the quinolone molecule (*fluoroquinolone*) resulted in creation of the newer quinolones,

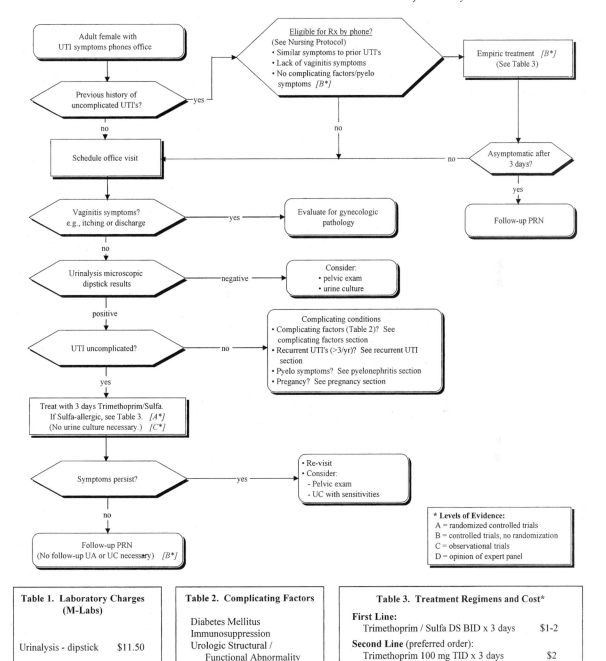

Fig. 5-8 Algorithm for treatment of UTI. (Reproduced with premission from University of Michigan Health System. Guidelines for Clinical Care: Urinary tract infection. Ann, Mich: Author, 1999.)

BOX 5-4 Mechanism of Action of the Antibiotics Used in Urology
. . . .

Inhibition of Nucleic Acid (Sulfonamides and Fluoroquinolones)

- Bacteriostatic
- Inhibit bacterial growth by preventing synthesis of folic acid, a B vitamin necessary for synthesis of purines and nucleic acid
- B vitamins consist of p-aminobenzoic acid (PABA), pteridine, and glutamic acid
- Sulfonamides compete with PABA for the enzyme that incorporates the PABA into the folic acid molecule
- Sulfonamides called *antimetabolites* because they block part of the biosynthetic pathway

Inhibition of Cell Wall Synthesis (β-Lactams: Penicillins and Cephalosporins)

- Bactericidal
- Prevent the cross-linking between linear peptidoglycan polymer chains that make up the cell wall
- Most staphylococci resistant to β-lactams because they produce enzymes (β-lactamases) that open the β-lactam ring

Inhibition of Protein Synthesis (Aminoglycosides, Tetracycline, Macrolides, and Chloramphenicol)

- Bactericidal
- Aminoglycosides are the most important drugs in this class for urology
- Bind to the 30S subunit on bacterial ribosome
- Inhibit binding of the aminocyl–transfer ribonucleic acid (tRNA), which is required to elongate the peptide chain
- Cause misreading of messenger ribonucleic acid (mRNA) so that nonfunctional proteins are synthesized
- Risk for nephrotoxicity and damage to cranial nerve VIII causing ototoxicity

which are highly effective against a broad range of gram-negative and gram-positive organisms.[70] The fluoroquinolones inhibit DNA gyrase, leading to "unwinding" of the DNA supercoils and causing cell death. Ciprofloxacin and norfloxacin are broad-spectrum fluoroquinolones with relatively low toxicity. The fluoroquinolones are highly effective against Enterobacteriaceae, *Pseudomonas aeruginosa, S. aureus,* and *S. saprophyticus.* Because most anaerobes are

resistant to all these medications, there is no alteration in vaginal or fecal flora and *Candida* infections are not a problem.

Inhibition of Cell Wall Synthesis and β-Lactam Production. β-Lactams are so called because of the β-lactam ring in their chemical structure.[71] They include penicillins, cephalosporins, and related compounds. They are effective against many gram-positive, gram-negative, and anaerobic organisms by interfering with the structural cross-linking of peptidoglycans in bacterial cell walls. Because many of these drugs are well absorbed after oral administration, they are clinically useful in the outpatient setting and are the recommended first choice in pregnant women. A concern about the use of β-lactams is bacterial resistance, particularly with ampicillin. One mechanism of resistance is the production of *β-lactamases,* enzymes that cleave the β-lactam ring.[72] Such activity is found in gram-positive organisms, gram-negative organisms, and anaerobes. Because of the potential for bacterial resistance, treatment of UTI with β-lactam antibiotics should be the second-line agents. β-Lactams also affect anaerobic organisms and predispose patients to *Candida* infection. Combining penicillins with β-lactamase inhibitors prevents the breakdown of penicillin. One example of this is ampicillin and clavulanate.

Inhibition of Protein Synthesis. Inhibitors of protein synthesis include aminoglycosides, tetracyclines, and macrolides. In the treatment of severe systemic UTI, aminoglycosides are the drug of choice. They act by inhibiting bacterial protein synthesis, binding at the subunit, and inhibiting binding of the aminoacyl RNA as well as causing misreading of mRNA so that nonfunctional proteins are synthesized.[71] Gentamycin is the most important aminoglycoside in urologic cases. It must be given intravenously and is important in the treatment of severe systemic infections caused by *P. aeruginosa.* Gentamycin has been associated with significant nephrotoxicity and ototoxicity and must be used cautiously and for a short term. Box 5-4 and Table 5-5 provide details of antibiotic usage in patients with a UTI.

Antifungals in the Management of Funguria. The first step in management of funguria is to remove potentially infectious sources, particularly indwelling catheters. Nutritional status should be assessed and optimized and any broad-spectrum

TABLE 5-5 Antibiotic Therapy for Bacterial Cystitis

TYPE OF THERAPY	ANTIBIOTIC AGENTS	NOTES
Short-term therapy (3-5 days) or 7-10 days in men or postmenopausal women	TMP/SMX, one double-strength tablet bid	First-line choice; effective for 3- to 5-day regimen; inexpensive but growing resistance means fluoroquinolone may be first-line therapy
	Fluoroquinolones (ciprofloxacin, norfloxacin)	Lower risk of bacterial resistance than TMP/SMX but more expensive
	Nitrofurantoin (Macrobid), 50-100 mg qid	
β-lactams more effective if taken for >5 days Suppressive therapy for recurrences (6-24 mo)	Ampicillin, 2 g in four divided doses Amoxicillin, 2 g in four divided doses TMP/SMX, one regular-strength tablet daily; may be alternated monthly with nitrofurantoin (Macrodantin), 50-100 mg/day, to reduce bacterial resistance	Second-line agents for UTI

bid, Twice daily; *qid,* four times daily; *TMP/SMX,* trimethoprim-sulfamethoxazole; *UTI,* urinary tract infection.

antibiotics stopped. Antibiotic treatment may be intravesical amphotericin B bladder irrigation or intravesical miconazole (50 g in 1 L of sterile water by way of a three-way catheter over a 24-hour period, or 200 ml of irrigant instilled and catheter clamped for 1 to 2 hours).[73] Oral antibiotics include flucytosine or fluconazole. Table 5-6 outlines doses and anticipated side effects of these antibiotics.

Pharmacokinetics: Distribution, Metabolism, and Elimination of the Antibiotics. The nucleic acid inhibitors, β-lactams, aminoglycosides, and antifungals are all metabolized in the liver and excreted in the urine. Apart from gentamycin, all are well absorbed from the gastrointestinal tract. All should be used with caution in elders or patients with decreased renal function, but particularly the fluoroquinolones and aminoglycosides. Box 5-5 on p. 116 outlines the physiologic changes that affect pharmacokinetics in elders.[70]

Alternative Treatments of Urinary Tract Infections

Alternatives to antibiotic therapy for uncomplicated UTI are attracting increasing interest. Cranberry juice or tablets are commonly believed to prevent or treat UTIs. The mechanism of action is not clear. Cranberries and blueberries contain high concentrations of quinic acid, which is aromatized to benzoic acid, activated by glycine, and changed to hippuric acid. It is believed that bacterial attachment by type 1 fimbriae of *E. coli, Proteus, Klebsiella, Enterobacter,* and *Pseudomonas* strains is inhibited by one or a combination of the following molecules: hippuric acid, fructose, ascorbic acid, or proanthocyanidins. In a study evaluating 150 community-dwelling sexually active women who had had at least two symptomatic UTIs in the past year, the subjects who were randomized to cranberry tablets or cranberry juice had significantly fewer symptomatic UTIs than the placebo control.[74] A systematic literature review[75] noted the following clinical points about the use of cranberry products: the incidence of UTIs in community-dwelling women may be reduced, there does not appear to be benefit in patients using intermittent catheterization, and no data are available on the products in long-term care.

Probiotics, such as *lactobacilli,* have been suggested for recurrent UTIs or vaginal infections. Clinical evidence for probiotics is scarce, but they are a promising area for further research.[76] Other strategies have been recommended but have no research to support them: namely, wearing cotton underwear, wiping front to back, avoiding bubble baths, and voiding immediately after intercourse. Women should be advised that some people find these strategies helpful and they may wish to try them.

Text continued on p. 116

TABLE 5-6 Antibiotics, Doses, and Indications

DRUG NAME (TRADE NAME)	DOSE/ROUTE	INDICATIONS, CONTRAINDICATIONS, ADVERSE EFFECTS, DRUG/DRUG INTERACTIONS	ONSET	PEAK	T½	DURATION	ABSORPTION
Nucleic Acid Inhibitors							
TMP/SMX: trimethoprim-sulfamethoxazole (Bactrim)	Tablet: 400 mg SMX/80 mg TMP; 800 mg SMX/160 TMP (DS) Adult: One tablet bid × 3-10 days; one DS bid × 3-10 days Pediatric: 4 mg/kg/day in divided doses every 12 hr	Indications: Escherichia coli, Klebsiella, Morganella morganii, Serratia, Staphylococcus Contraindications: Hypersensitivity to any sulfa drug or any component; porphyria; megaloblastic anemia caused by folate deficiency; severe renal insufficiency; hepatic dysfunction; pregnancy; infants younger than 2 mo because of wide distribution Adverse effects: Nausea/vomiting, anorexia, megaloblastic anemia, hallucinations, depression, seizures Drug/drug interactions: Cytochrome P-450 effect: CYP2C9 enzyme inhibitor Decreased effect: Decreased effect of cyclosporines and tricyclic anti-depressants; procaine and indomethacin may decrease effect of TMP/SMX Increased effect/toxicity: Sulfamethoxazole may cause an increased effect of sulfonylureas and oral anticoagulants; increases serum concentration of methotrexate, phenytoin, or cyclosporine	Rapid	Peak blood levels occur from 1-4 hr	10-11 hr Half-life prolonged in renal failure	12-24 hr	Oral absorption: 90%-100% Plasma protein binding: TMP: 44% SMX: 70%
Nitrofurantoin (Macrobid, Macrodantin)	Oral suspension: 25 mg/5 ml Capsule: 50 mg, 100 mg Adult: 50-100 mg/dose	Indications: Proteus mirabilis, group D streptococcus, Enterococcus faecalis Contraindications: Hypersensitivity to nitrofurantoin; renal impairment; pregnant patients at term and during labor and delivery	Not known	30 min	20-60 min	6-12 hr	Foods or agents delaying gastric emptying increase the bioavailability

| | every 6 hr × 5-10 days not to exceed 400 mg/24 hr
Pediatric: >1 mo: 5-7 mg/kg/day in divided doses every 6 hr | *Adverse effects:* Nausea, pulmonary allergic reaction, dizziness, hemolytic anemia
Drug/drug interactions: None reported
Decreased effect: Antacids decrease absorption of nitrofurantoin
Increased effect/toxicity: probenecid decreases renal excretion of nitrofurantoin | Rapid | 1-2 hr | |
| Fluoroquinolones (ciprofloxacin, norfloxacin) | *Adult:*
Oral: 400 mg bid for 3-10 days
IV: 200-400 mg every 12 hr for 7-10 days | *Indications: Escherichia coli, Klebsiella, Pseudomonas aeruginosa, Morganella morganii, Serratia:* choose over aminoglycosides in patients with reduced renal function
Contraindications: Hypersensitivity to fluoroquinolones; pregnancy; absorption can be reduced by aluminum- or magnesium-containing antacids, iron salts, zinc salts, and sucralfate
Adverse effects: Nausea, diarrhea, headache, insomnia, photosensitivity, CNS stimulation, dizziness, tendonitis/tendon rupture
Drug/drug interactions: Cytochrome P-450 effect: CYP1A2 and 3A3/4 enzyme inhibitor
Decreased effect: Decreased absorption with antacids containing aluminum, magnesium, and/or calcium
Increased effect/toxicity: Increased serum levels of caffeine, warfarin, cyclosporine, and theophylline; cimetidine and probenecid may increase norfloxacin serum levels | | Adults with normal renal function: 3-5 hr; prolonged in reduced renal function | 12 hr | Oral:
Ciprofloxacin: rapid from GI tract (~50%-85%)
Norfloxacin: rapid up to 40% |

Continued

TABLE 5-6 Antibiotics, Doses, and Indications—cont'd

Inhibition of Cell Wall and β-Lactam Production

DRUG NAME (TRADE NAME)	DOSE/ROUTE	INDICATIONS, CONTRAINDICATIONS, ADVERSE EFFECTS, DRUG/DRUG INTERACTIONS	ONSET	PEAK	T½	DURATION	ABSORPTION
Penicillins (ampicillin, amoxicillin, amoxicillin-clavulanate)	*Ampicillin:* *Adult:* Oral: 250-500 mg every 6 hr × 3 days IM: 500-1500 mg every 4-6 hr *Amoxicillin:* *Adult:* 250-500 mg every 8 hr × 3 days (nb: two 250-mg tablets are not equivalent to one 500-mg tablet since both 250-mg and 500-mg tablets contain the same amount of clavulanate)	*Indications: Proteus mirabilis, Serratia,* group D streptococcus, *Pseudomonas aeruginosa;* pregnant patients with UTI/bacteriuria *Contraindications:* Hypersensitivity to amoxicillin, clavulanic acid, penicillins, cephalosporins, and imipenem; caution when given to nursing mothers since this may lead to sensitization of the infant *Adverse effects:* GI upset, rash, Stevens-Johnson syndrome, pseudomembranous colitis *Drug/drug interactions:* Decreases the effectiveness of oral contraceptives and increases breakthrough bleeding; interacts with probenecid, causing decreased renal tubular secretions, resulting in increased blood levels and possible toxicity; false-positive clinitest	0.5-1.4 hr	1-2 hr	60-90 min	4-8 hr (varies among medications)	Oral: 50% Plasma protein binding: 20%
Cephalosporins (cefazolin, cefoperazone, cefotetan, cephalexin)	IM, IV *Adult:* 1-2 g every 8 hr (max: 12 g/day) *Pediatric:* >1 mo of age: 25-100 mg/kg/day divided every 6-7 hr	*Indications: Staphylococcus, Klebsiella,* first-generation gram-positives, second-generation gram-negative and gram-positive anaerobes, third-generation ceftazidime gram-negative *Pseudomonas,* fourth-generation wider gram-positive bactericidal range *Contraindications:* Contraindicated in anyone with allergies to cephalosporins	0.5-2.2 hr	0.5-1 hr	0.5-9 hr Depends on first, second, third, or fourth generation	6-24 hr	

Protein Synthesis Inhibitors

Drug	Dosage	Indications / Contraindications / Adverse effects / Drug interactions	Onset	Peak	Half-life	Duration	Absorption / Notes
		Adverse effects: Diarrhea, GI upset, rash, headache, dizziness Drug/drug interactions: Interacts with probenecid, causing increased blood levels and possible toxicity; increased serum levels of anticoagulants, interacts with ethanol by inhibiting the second stage of ethanol metabolism, causing a disulfiram-like reaction					
Aminoglycosides (gentamycin, tetramycin)	IM, IV Adult: 1.5 mg/kg/dose	Indications: Pseudomonas aeruginosa, urosepsis Contraindications: Hypersensitivity to gentamicin or other aminoglycosides; used with caution in patients with renal impairment or preexisting hearing impairment (consider fluoroquinolone); patients with myasthenia gravis Adverse effects: Nephrotoxicity and ototoxicity Drug/drug interactions: Patients receiving ototoxic drugs, nephrotoxic drugs, and neuromuscular blocking agents	Varies	0.5-2 hr	1.5-3 hr With end-stage renal disease: 36-70 hr	8-12 hr	Parenteral only; plasma protein binding: 10%
Tetracyclines	Adult: Oral: 250-500 mg/dose every 6 hr Pediatric: Oral: 30-50 mg/kg/day divided every 6 hr	Indications: Klebsiella, Staphylococcus Contraindications: Hypersensitivity to tetracyclines, pregnancy, children younger than 5 yr of age, contraindicated for patients taking terfenadine, astemizole, and cisapride Adverse effects: Dizziness, lightheadedness, unsteadiness, photosensitivity, nausea, diarrhea, discoloration of teeth in children Drug/drug interactions: Should not be administered with calcium supplements, iron supplements, magnesium-containing laxatives, and most antacids; decrease the plasma levels of barbiturates, carbamazepine, hydantoins, and digoxin	Varies	Oral: 2-4 hr	Short-acting agents: 8 hr Long-acting agents: 16-18 hr	Short-acting agents: 6-12 hr	Oral: 75% Long-acting agents have the highest absorption and are bound to protein to the greatest extent

bid, Twice daily; CNS, central nervous system; DS, double strength; GI, gastrointestinal; IM, intramuscular; IV, intravenous; UTI, urinary tract infection.

BOX 5-5 Physiologic Changes in Elders Affecting Pharmacokinetic Properties of Medications

Absorption

- Gastric hydrochloride (H) is less acidic because of a gradual reduction in the production of hydrochloric acid in the stomach.
- Gastric emptying is slowed because of a decline in tone and motor activity.
- Movement throughout the gastrointestinal (GI) tract is slower because of decreased muscle tone and motor activity.
- Blood flow to the GI tract is reduced by 40% to 50% because of decreased cardiac output and decreased blood flow.
- The absorptive surface area is decreased because the aging process blunts and flattens villi.

Distribution

- Total body water (TBW) in adults from 40 to 60 years of age is 55% (male) and 47% (female); for those over 60 years it is 52% (male) and 46% (female).
- Fat content is increased because of decreased lean mass.
- Protein (albumin) binding sites are reduced because of decreased production of proteins by aging liver and reduced intake.

Metabolism

- The levels of microsomal enzymes are decreased because the capacity of the aging liver to produce them is reduced.
- Liver blood flow is reduced by approximately 1.5% per year after the age of 25 years, decreasing hepatic metabolism.

Excretion

- Glomerular filtration rate is decreased by 40% to 50% primarily because of decreased blood flow.
- Number of intact nephrons is decreased.

SUMMARY

In conclusion, UTI is one of the most common urologic conditions, particularly in premenopausal women. Treatment should be based on past history, causative organism, and least expensive effective antibiotic. Complementary therapy such as cranberry juice or tablets may control symptoms in community-dwelling women.

REFERENCES

1. Kass EH: Bacteriuria and the diagnosis of infections of the urinary tract with observations on the use of methionine as a urinary antiseptic. Archives of Internal Medicine, 1957; 100:709-14.
2. Sheffield JS, Cunningham FG: Urinary tract infection in women. Obstetrics and Gynecology, 2005; 106:1085-92.
2a. Laupland KB, Ross T, Pitout JD, Church DL, Gregson DB: Community-onset urinary tract infections: a population-based assessment. Infection, 2007; 35(3):150-53.
3. Nicolle L, Anderson PA, Conly J, Mainprize TC, Meuser J, Nickel JC, Senikas VM, Zhanel GG: Uncomplicated urinary tract infection in women: current practice and the effect of antibiotic resistance on empiric treatment. Canadian Family Physician, 2006; 52:612-18.
4. Nicholle LE: Urinary tract infection in geriatric and institutionalized patients: urinary tract infections and sexually transmitted diseases. Current Opinion in Urology, 2002; 12:51-5.
5. University of Michigan Health System—Academic Institution: Guidelines for clinical care: urinary tract infection, 1999. Retrieved July 19, 2002 from http://cme.med.umich.edu/pdf/guideline/UTI.pdf.
6. Choong S, Whitfield H: Biofilms and their role in infections in urology. BJU International, 2000; 86:935-41.
7. Snyder JA, Lloyd AL, Lockatell CV, Johnson DE, Mobley HLT: Role of phase variation of type 1 fimbriae in a uropathogenic *Escherichia coli* cystitis isolate during urinary tract infection. Infection and Immunity, 2006; 74:1387-93.
8. Wullt B, Bergsten G, Connell H, Rollano P, Gebretsadik N, Hull R, Svanborg C: P fimbriae enhance the establishment of *Escherichia coli* in the human urinary tract. Molecular Microbiology, 2000; 38:456-64.
9. Shupp-Byrne DE, Sedor JF, Soroush M, McCue PA, Mulholland SG: Interaction of bladder glycoprotein GP51 with uropathogenic bacteria. Journal of Urology, 2001; 165:1342-6.
10. Costerton JW: Introduction to biofilm. International Journal of Antimicrobial Agents, 1999; 11:217-21.
11. Mulvey MA, Schilling JD, Martinez JJ, Hultgren SJ: Bad bugs and beleaguered bladders: interplay between uropathogenic *Escherichia coli* and innate host defenses. Proceedings of the National Academy of Sciences of the United States of America, 2000; 97:8829-35.
12. Raz R, Gennesin Y, Wasser J, Stoler Z, Rosenfeld S, Rottensterich E, Stamm WE: Recurrent urinary tract infections in postmenopausal women. Clinical Infectious Diseases, 2000; 30:152-6.
13. Goldman HB: Evaluation and management of recurrent urinary-tract infections. In Kursh ED, Ulchaker JC (eds): Office Urology: the Clinician's Guide. Totowa, NJ: Humana Press, 2001; pp 105-11.
14. Harrington RD, Hooton TM: Urinary tract infection risk factors and gender. Journal of Gender-Specific Medicine, 2000; 3:27-34.
15. Sharp SE: Commensal and pathogenic organisms of humans. In Murray PR, Baron EJ, Pfaller MA, Tenover FC, Yolken RH (eds): Manual of Clinical Microbiology, 7th edition. Washington, DC: ASM Press, 1999; pp 23-32.
16. Fadda G, Nicoletti G, Schito GG, Tempera G: Antimicrobial susceptibility patterns of contemporary pathogens from uncomplicated urinary tract infections isolated in a multicenter Italian survey: possible impact on guidelines. Journal of Chemotherapy, 2005; 17:251-7.
17. Wagenlehner FM, Naber KG: Current challenges in the treatment of complicated urinary tract infections and prostatitis. Clinical Microbiology and Infection, 2006; 12:67-80.
18. Schlager TA: Urinary tract infections in infants and children. Infectious Disease Clinics of North America, 2003; 17(2):353-65.
19. Liu H, Mullholland SG: Appropriate antibiotic treatment of genitourinary infections in hospitalized patients. American Journal of Medicine, 2005; 118:14S-20S.
20. Wagenlehner FM, Loibl E, Vogel H, Naber KG: Incidence of nosocomial urinary tract infections on a surgical intensive care unit and implications for management. International Journal of Antimicrobial Agents, 2006; 28(supp 1):586-590. [Epub July 7, 2006].

21. Girard R, Mazoyer MA, Plauchu MM, Rode G: High prevalence of nosocomial infections in rehabilitation units accounted for by urinary tract infections in patients with spinal cord injury. Journal of Hospital Infection, 2006; 62:473-9.

22. Saint S, Kaufman SR, Rogers MA, Baker PD, Ossenkop K, Lipsky BA: Condom versus indwelling urinary catheters: a randomized trial. Journal of the American Geriatrics Society, 2006; 54:1055-61.

23. Moreno E, Prats G, Sabate M, Perez T, Johnson JR, Andreu A: Quinolone, fluoroquinolone and trimethoprim/sulfamethoxazole resistance in relation to virulence determinants and phylogenetic background among uropathogenic *Escherichia coli*. Journal of Antimicrobial Chemotherapy, 2006; 57(2):204-11.

24. Paterson DL: Resistance in gram-negative bacteria: Enterobacteriaceae. American Journal of Medicine, 2006; 119:S20-8.

25. Lark RL, Chenoweth C, Saint S, Zemencuk JK, Lipsky BA, Plorde JJ: Four year prospective evaluation of nosocomial bacteremia: epidemiology, microbiology, and patient outcome. Diagnostic Microbiology and Infectious Disease, 2000; 38:131-40.

26. Moreno E, Andreu A, Perez T, Sabate M, Johnson JR, Prats G: Relationship between *Escherichia coli* strains causing urinary tract infection in women and the dominant faecal flora of the same hosts. Epidemiology and Infection, 2006; 26(Jan):1-9.

27. Franco AV: Recurrent urinary tract infections. Best Practice and Research. Clinical Obstetrics and Gynaecology, 2005; 19:861-73.

28. Hummers-Pradier E, Ohse AM, Koch M, Heizmann WR, Kochen MM: Urinary tract infection in men. International Journal of Clinical Pharmacology and Therapeutics, 2004; 42:360-6.

29. Helmholz HF: Determination of the bacterial content of the urethra: a new method, with results of a study of 82 men. Journal of Urology, 1950; 64:158-66.

30. Cox CE, Lacy SS, Hinman F: The urethra and its relationship to urinary tract infection. II. The urethral flora of the female with recurrent urinary tract infection. Journal of Urology, 1968; 99:632-8.

31. O'Neil AGB: The bacterial content of the female urethra: a new method of study. British Journal of Urology, 1981; 53:368-70.

32. Kwok WY, de Kwaadsteniet MC, Harmsen M, van Suijlekom-Smit LW, Schellevis FG, van der Wouden JC: Incidence rates and management of urinary tract infections among children in Dutch general practice: results from a nation-wide registration study. BMC Pediatrics, 2006; 6(Apr 4):10.

33. Mayo ME, Hinman F: Role of mid-urethral high pressure zone in spontaneous bacterial ascent. Journal of Urology, 1973; 109:268-72.

34. Tanagho EA, Miller ER: Functional considerations of urethral sphincteric dynamics. Journal of Urology, 1973; 109:273-78.

35. Lapides J: Mechanisms of urinary tract infection. Urology, 1979; 14:217-25.

36. Norden CW, Green GM, Kass EH: Antibacterial mechanisms of the urinary bladder. Journal of Clinical Investigation, 1968; 47: 2689-2700.

37. Hand WL, Smith JW, Sanford JP: The antibacterial effect of normal and infected urinary bladder. Journal of Laboratory and Clinical Medicine, 1971; 77:605-15.

38. Kaye D: Antibacterial activity of human urine. Journal of Clinical Investigation, 1968; 47:2374-90.

39. Esclarin De Ruz A, Garcia Leoni E, Herruzo Cabrera R: Epidemiology and risk factors for urinary tract infection in patients with spinal cord injury. Journal of Urology, 2000; 164(4):1285-9.

40. Sobel JD: Pathogenesis of urinary tract infection: role of host defenses. Infectious Disease Clinics of North America, 1997; 11:531-49.

41. Asscher AW, Sussman M, Weiser R: Bacterial growth in human urine. In O'Grady F, Brumfitt W (eds): Urinary Tract Infection. London: Oxford University Press, 1968; pp 3-13.

42. Roberts AP, Clayton SG, Bean HS: Urine factors affecting bacterial growth. In O'Grady F, Brumfitt W (eds): Urinary Tract Infection. London: Oxford University Press, 1968.

43. Schaeffer AJ, Schaeffer EM: Infections of the urinary tract. In Wein AJ, Kavoussi LR, Novick AC, Partin AW, Peters CA (eds): Campbell-Walsh Urology, 9th edition. Philadelphia: Saunders, 2007; pp 223-303.

44. Macejko AM, Schaeffer AJ: Asymptomatic bacteriuria and symptomatic urinary tract infections during pregnancy. Urologic Clinics of North America, 2007; 34(1):35-42.

45. Rathus SA, Nevid JS, Fichner-Rathus L, McKenzie SW: Essentials of human sexuality. Canadian edition. Toronto: Pearson Education Canada, 2002; pp 330-2.

46. Stamm WE: Urinary tract infections. Infectious Disease Clinics of North America, 2003; 17:xiii-xiv.

47. Nemati E, Basra R, Fernandes J, Levy JB: Emphysematous cystitis. Nephrology Dialysis Transplantation, 2005; 20:652-3.

48. Bonadio M, Costarelli S, Morelli G, Tartaglia T: The influence of diabetes mellitus on the spectrum of uropathogens and the antimicrobial resistance in elderly adult patients with urinary tract infection. BMC Infectious Diseases, 2006; 6:54.

49. Loeb M, Brazil K, Lohfeld L, McGeer A, Simor A, Stevenson K, Zoutman D, Smith S, Liu X, Walter SD: Effect of a multifaceted intervention on number of antimicrobial prescriptions for suspected urinary tract infections in residents of nursing homes: cluster randomized controlled trial. British Medical Journal, 2005; 331:669.

50. Horn SD, Buerhaus p, Bergstrom N, Smout RJ: RN staffing time and outcomes of long-stay nursing home residents: pressure ulcers and other adverse outcomes are less likely as RNs spend more time on direct patient care. American Journal of Nursing, 2005; 105:58-70.

51. Junathi-Mehta M, Drickamer MA, Towle V, Zhang Y, Tinetti ME, Quagliarello VJ: Nursing home practitioner survey of diagnostic criteria for urinary tract infections. Journal of the American Geriatrics Society, 2005; 53:1986.

52. Lin YT, Chen LK, Lin MH, Hwang SJ: Asymptomatic bacteriuria among the institutionalized elderly. Journal of the Chinese Medical Association, 2006; 69:213-7.

53. Rosenberg JE, Carroll PR, Small EJ: Update on chemotherapy for advanced bladder cancer. Journal of Urology, 2005; 174(1):14-20.

54. Kunin CM: Urinary-catheter-associated infections in the elderly. International Journal of Antimicrobial Agents, 2006; 28(supp. 1): S78-S81. [Epub July 10, 2006].

54a. Gray M: What nursing interventions reduce the risk of symptomatic urinary tract infection in the patient with an indwelling catheter?. Journal of Wound, Ostomy and Continence Nursing, 2004; 31(1):3-13.

55. Brosnahan J, Jull A, Tracy C: Types of urethral catheters for management of short-term voiding problems in hospitalized adults. Cochrane Database of Systematic Reviews, 2004; (1), Art No.: CD004012.

55a. Junkin J, Selekof JL: Prevalence of incontinence and associated skin injury in the acute care patient. Journal of Wound, Ostomy and Continence Nursing, 2007; 34(3):260-9.

55b. Hess CT, Rook LJ: Understanding recent regulatory guidelines for hospital-acquired urinary tract infections and pressure ulcers. Ostonomy and Wound Management, 2007; 53(12):34-41.

56. Reiche T, Lisby G, Jorgensen S, Christensen AB, Nordling J: A prospective, controlled, randomized study of the effect of a slow-release silver device on the frequency of urinary tract infection in newly catheterized patients. BJU International, 2000; 85(Jan):54-9.

57. Goettsch W, van Pelt W, Nagelkerke N, Hendrix MG, Buiting AG, Petit PL, Sabbe LJ, van Griethuysen AJ, de Neeling AJ: Increasing resistance to fluoroquinolones in *Escherichia coli* from urinary tract infections. Journal of Antimicrobial Chemotherapy, 2000; 46:223-8.

58. Ronald AR, Nicolle LE, Stamm E, Krieger J, Warren J, Schaeffer A, Naber KG, Hooton TM, Johnson J, Chambers S, Andriole V: Urinary tract infection in adults: research priorities and strategies. International Journal of Antimicrobial Agents, 2001; 17(4):343-8.

59. Kass EH: Bacteriuria and the diagnosis of infections of the urinary tract with observations on the use of methionine as a urinary antiseptic. Archives of Internal Medicine, 1957; 100:709-14.

60. Stamm WE, Wagner KF, Amsel R, Alexander ER, Turck M, Counts GW, Holmes K: Causes of the acute urethral syndrome in women. New England Journal of Medicine, 1980; 303:409-15.

61. Hoberman A, Wald ER, Reynolds EA, Penchansky L, Charron M: Pyuria and bacteriuria in urine specimens obtained by catheter from young children with fever. Journal of Pediatrics, 1994; 124:513-9.

62. Gaydos CA, Howell MR, Pare B, Clark KL, Ellis DA, Hendrix RM, Gaydos JC, McKee KT, Quinn TC: *Chlamydia trachomatis* infections in female military recruits. New England Journal of Medicine, 1998; 339:739-44.

63. Smyth M, Moore JE, Goldsmith CE: Urinary tract infections: role of the clinical microbiology laboratory. Urologic Nursing, 2006; 26(3):198-203.

64. Moore KN, Murray S, Malone-Lee J, Wagg A: Rapid urinalysis assays for the diagnosis of urinary tract infection. British Journal of Nursing, 2001; 10(15):995-1001.

65. Lifshitz E, Kramer L: Outpatient urine culture: does collection technique matter?. Archives of Internal Medicine, 2000; 160(Sep. 11):2537-40.

66. Prandoni D, Boone MH, Larson E, Blane CG, Fitzpatrick H: Assessment of urine collection technique for microbial culture. American Journal of Infection Control, 1996; 24(June):219-21.

67. Walter FG, Knopp RK: Urine sampling in ambulatory women: midstream clean-catch versus catheterization. Annals of Emergency Medicine, 1999; 18:166-72.

68. Gradwohl SE, Chenoweth CE, Fonde KR, Van Harrison R, Zoschnick LB: Urinary tract infection: guidelines for clinical care. University of Michigan Health System, 2005. Retrieved Aug 1, 2006 at http://cme.med.umich.edu.

69. Fourcroy JL, Berner B, Chiang Y-K, Cramer M, Shore N: Efficacy and safety of a novel once-daily extended-release ciprofloxacin tablet formulation for treatment of uncomplicated urinary tract infection in women. Antimicrobial Agents and Chemotherapy, 2005; 49:4137-43.

70. Mazzei T, Cassetta MI, Fallani S, Arrigucci S, Novelli A: Pharmacokinetic and pharmacodynamic aspects of antimicrobial agents for the treatment of uncomplicated urinary tract infections. International Journal of Antimicrobial Agents, 2006; 28(supp. 1):S35. [Epub July 7, 2006].

71. Neal MJ: Medical Pharmacology at a Glance, 4th edition. Oxford: Blackwell Science, 2002.

72. Bush K, Jacoby GA, Medeiros AA: A functional classification scheme for beta-lactamases and its correlation with molecular structure. Antimicrobial Agents and Chemotherapy, 1995; 39:1211-33.

73. Drew RH, Arthur RR, Perfect JR: Is it time to abandon the use of amphotericin B bladder irrigation?. Clinical Infectious Diseases, 2005; 40(10):1465-70.

74. Stothers L: A randomized trial to evaluate effectiveness and cost effectiveness of naturopathic cranberry products as prophylaxis against urinary tract infection in women. Canadian Journal of Urology, 2002; 9:1558-62.

75. Gray M: Are cranberry juice or cranberry products effective in the prevention or management of urinary tract infection?. Journal of Wound, Ostomy and Continence Nursing, 2002; 29:122-6.

76. Falagas ME, Betsi GI, Tokas T, Athanasiou S: Probiotics for prevention of recurrent urinary tract infections in women: a review of the evidence from microbiological and clinical studies. Drugs, 2006; 66:1253-61.

CHAPTER

6 *Urinary Incontinence*

OVERVIEW OF URINARY INCONTINENCE IN ADULTS

Urinary incontinence (UI) is a complex condition that does not always respond to a single intervention. This chapter reviews assessment and treatment of the adult patient with UI. Chapters 15 and 16 review UI in children, and surgical procedures used to manage UI are discussed in Chapter 11.

The International Continence Society defines UI as the complaint of any involuntary leakage of urine.[1] Another definition describes UI as urine loss of sufficient severity that it is perceived as a problem for the affected person, family, or care providers, and a third definition states that it is any uncontrolled loss of urine.[2,3]

Epidemiology

The wide range of definitions makes it difficult to compile or summarize prevalence and incidence data. The annual incidence in adult women is approximately 8% to 10%, and it has been estimated as 9% in elderly men.[3] Recent studies report UI from 5% in healthy Belgian women age 15 years and older[4] to 38% in North American women[5] to 54% in a sample of Taiwanese women.[6] Diabetes,[7,8] depression,[9,10] and gender are all significant risk factors. Estimates of prevalence in men vary from 3% to 11%, and the proportion of women to men experiencing UI varies from 2:1 to 7:1.[11] If UI is defined by clinical criteria (limited to those with sufficient severity to create a problem), it affects approximately 9% of the general population.[3]

Although we know that aging is *not* a cause of UI, older adults are at greater risk when compared with younger adults.[12,13] UI affects more than 50% of persons residing in long-term care facilities[14] and remains inadequately addressed in many settings.[15] In women the prevalence of any urine loss reaches an initial peak of approximately 30% around age 50 years. It then remains relatively stable until the seventh decade of life, when it rises to as much as 50% or higher among women who are homebound or residing in a long-term care facility.[16] In men, UI remains at a relatively constant level until the sixth decade of life and then also begins to rise proportionally with aging.[11]

Racial or ethnic differences probably influence the type of UI rather than its overall risk. For example, several studies indicate that white and Hispanic women may be at greater risk for incontinence and pelvic organ prolapse than African-American women, whereas African-American women may be at higher risk for urge incontinence associated with detrusor overactivity.[17-19]

Classification of Urinary Incontinence

UI can be subdivided into acute or transient versus established or chronic. Although multiple classification systems have been proposed, the most useful for assessment and initial management remains symptom based.

Acute/Transient Urinary Incontinence. UI may occur in a previously continent patient, or it may be exacerbated by a number of treatable acute or transient conditions (Table 6-1).[20-22]

Chronic (Established) Urinary Incontinence. Chronic UI is insidious in its onset and may exist for months or years before the person seeks assistance; it is subdivided according to its predominant symptom. The most common forms of established UI are stress, urge, and mixed. Less common forms of UI include reflex, functional, extraurethral, and postprostatectomy. Urinary retention, sometimes associated with overflow UI, will be discussed separately.

Stress Urinary Incontinence. Stress UI occurs when physical activity such as coughing, sneezing, lifting a heavy object, climbing stairs, running, or walking leads to increases in abdominal forces and transient incompetence of the urethral sphincter mechanism. Pure stress UI is characterized by urine loss in the absence of the urge to urinate. The sign of stress UI can be elicited during the physical assessment by asking the patient to perform Valsalva's maneuver or cough while standing over a pad or while holding a paper towel near the urethral meatus or during the pelvic examination.[23,24] The urodynamic diagnosis of stress UI is based on observation of urethral leakage in response to increases in abdominal and intravesical pressure and in the absence of a detrusor contraction.[1]

Stress UI is attributable to two factors: pelvic descent (pelvic organ prolapse) and intrinsic sphincter incompetence. Pelvic organ prolapse is caused by weakness of the pelvic floor muscles and disruption in the endopelvic fascia that allow the pelvic organs to descend or "fall" into the potential space of the vaginal vault (Figure 6-1).[25] Descent of the vaginal walls within the vault or beyond its introitus is seen with physical exertion or at rest, depending on the

TABLE 6-1 Causes of Acute or Transient Urinary Incontinence[20-22]

FACTOR	CLINICAL RELEVANCE
Delirium (transient state of mental confusion, anxiety, disorientation, hallucinations, delusions, or incoherent speech caused by an acute systemic illness, high fever, metabolic imbalance from organ failure, or toxicity from alcohol, drugs, poisons, or anesthesia)	Often associated with acute UI in elders; treatment of the underlying cause of the delirium may resolve UI or restore the person to premorbid continence status
Infection (UTI characterized by bacteriuria and pyuria)	Although multiple researchers have documented an association between UI and UTI, it remains unclear whether infection causes UI or primarily acts as a risk factor for UTIs; in addition, any relationship between UI and asymptomatic bacteriuria in elders remains unclear
Atrophic urethritis and vaginitis	Genitourinary atrophy is associated with multiple bothersome symptoms, including vaginal dryness and itching as well as urinary urgency; however, systemic hormone replacement therapy may slightly *increase* UI frequency, whereas the efficacy of local replacement therapy has not been adequately studied
Pharmaceuticals (multiple agents)	Multiple classes of drugs affect lower UTI and may contribute to UI; common classes include the following: Diuretics (increase urine production) α-Adrenergic agonists (diminish urethral resistance) Anticholinergics (diminished detrusor contractility in selected patients increases risk of urinary retention and overflow UI) Hypnotics and sedatives (reduce awareness of urge to urinate and ability to respond to cues to void)
Excess urine output (polyuria)	Diuresis increases risk of UI; possible causes include the following: Undiagnosed or poorly controlled diabetes mellitus High-volume fluid intake (may be adopted as a behavioral strategy to blunt appetite and lose weight) Diabetes insipidus (uncommon disorder sometimes seen with traumatic brain injury)
Restricted mobility	Interferes with patient's ability to complete act of micturition
Stool impaction (severe constipation)	Increases risk of UTI, UI, and urinary retention, particularly in elders or children

UI, Urinary incontinence; *UTI*, urinary tract infection.

severity of the prolapse. Descent of the bladder is called a cystocele, descent of the rectum is termed a rectocele, and herniation of the small bowel into the vagina is referred to as an enterocele. When the pelvic organs prolapse, stress UI may occur because of disruptions to the transmission of passive pressures to the proximal urethra or because of a compromised neuromuscular response to increased abdominal pressures within the urethra or periurethral muscles.[26] Table 6-2 outlines risk factors for pelvic organ prolapse and stress UI.

Intrinsic sphincter incompetence occurs when components of the urethral sphincter mechanism are damaged, compromising its ability to form a watertight seal when faced with increasing abdominal pressures. In women intrinsic sphincter

incompetence may coexist with pelvic organ prolapse or follow surgical repair of prolapse (Figure 6-2).[27] *Intrinsic sphincter deficiency* is the urodynamic diagnosis used to describe stress UI caused by intrinsic sphincter deficiency.[28] Intrinsic sphincter incompetence typically affects neuromuscular control of the smooth or striated muscle of the sphincter mechanism. Defects in sphincter compression associated with estrogen deficiency in women or urethral scarring may contribute to sphincter incompetence in both women and men, but they are rarely the sole cause of stress UI. Common causes of intrinsic sphincter incompetence are outlined in Table 6-3.

Urge Incontinence and the Overactive Bladder. The symptom of urge UI is defined as urine loss associated with a precipitous desire to

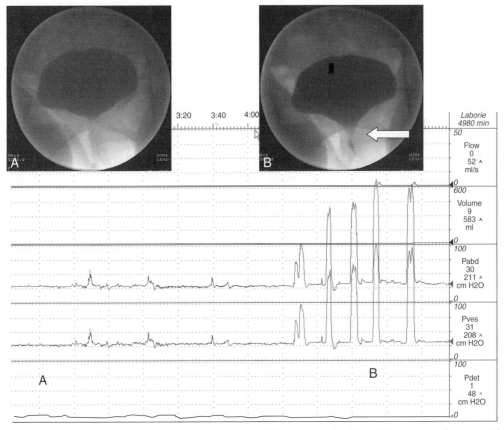

Fig. 6-1 Urodynamic diagnosis of stress urinary incontinence (UI) associated with pelvic organ prolapse. **A,** The *radiographic image* shows the bladder above the inferior margin of the symphysis pubis, and the corresponding *urodynamic tracing* demonstrates resting abdominal *(Pabd)* and intravesical *(Pves)* pressures. **B,** The *radiographic image* now shows descent of the bladder base below the inferior margin of the symphysis pubis with leakage of contrast from the urethra *(arrow).* The corresponding *urodynamic tracing* shows a sharp rise in abdominal and intravesical pressures with Valsalva's maneuver and urine loss registering on the "Flow" tracing.

TABLE 6-2 Risk Factors for Pelvic Organ Prolapse[27,75,118]

Constitutional factors	Age
	Family history (first-line relative with prolapse)
	Congenital anomalies (e.g., myelodysplasia, sacral agenesis, or imperforate anus)
Obstetric factors	Parity (risk rises proportionally with number of pregnancies)
	Vaginal delivery: risk increases when the following occur:
	Tearing
	Episiotomy
	Forceps use
	Breech presentation
	Delivery of a large-for-gestational-age infant
Gynecologic factors	Menopausal status
Obesity	Body mass index
	Android distribution of body fat increases risk
Surgery	Hysterectomy
Physical activity	Occupation-related factors (repetitive lifting)
	High-impact physical activity (e.g., paratrooping, long distance running, high-impact gymnastics or aerobics)
Chronic cough	Long-term smoking
	Chronic obstructive pulmonary disease
Chronic constipation	Although a relationship between constipation and pelvic organ prolapse clearly exists, the nature of this relationship remains unclear
Chronic steroid use	Chronic steroid use and differences in endogenous steroid metabolism may increase the risk of pelvic organ prolapse

urinate caused by an overactive detrusor contraction. The sign of urge UI is difficult to reproduce during physical examination, and it may or may not be readily reproduced by urodynamic testing.[24] The urodynamic diagnosis of detrusor overactivity is based on documentation of an overactive detrusor contraction in association with a strong desire to urinate.

Our understanding of urge UI continues to evolve, and it is now considered part of a larger symptom syndrome called the overactive bladder (OAB). OAB is defined as bothersome urgency, usually associated with daytime voiding frequency (more than every 2 hours) and nocturia (more than one episode per night for adults under 65 years of age and three or more episodes for adults aged 65 years or older) with or without urge UI and occurring in the absence of pathologic or metabolic conditions that might explain these symptoms.[1,29] Redefining urge UI as part of the OAB symptom syndrome changes its epidemiologic parameters, particularly since the majority of patients with OAB (67%) do not experience leakage.[30] Risk factors for OAB and urge UI include functional deficits such as impaired mobility or dexterity, cognitive difficulties, and female gender.

Table 6-4 describes conditions associated with overactive bladder and/or urge UI.

The prevalence of OAB was 11.8% in the adult population.[31] These results may appear lower than from previous studied due to the use of a more specific classification of OAB.[1] Women reported a slightly higher rate (12.8) than did men (10.8%). Before the age of 60, OAB is more common in women than in men, with women more likely to experience mixed UI with OAB. After the age of 60, equal numbers of men and women are likely to experience OAB with urge UI symptoms.[31]

Redefining urge UI within the context of OAB has also generated controversy.[32,33] Defined as a symptom syndrome, the diagnosis of OAB is based on history and physical examination rather than complex urodynamic testing. As a result, initial diagnosis and treatment are shifted from a specialist to a primary care setting and the apparent similarities between OAB with and without coexisting urge UI are bridged. Nevertheless, a diagnosis of OAB does not replace the need for detailed evaluation, often including urodynamic testing (Figure 6-3), for patients with complicating conditions or for those who prove refractory to

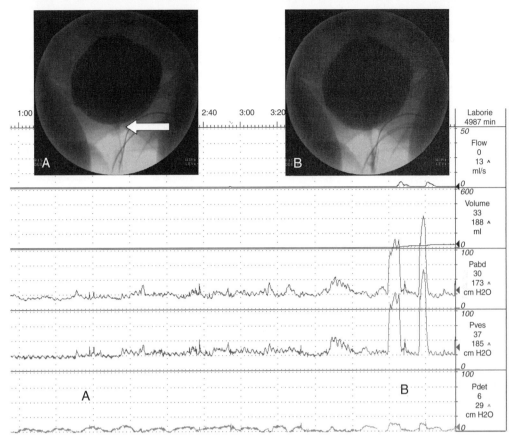

Fig. 6-2 Urodynamic diagnosis of stress urinary incontinence (UI) caused by urethral sphincter incompetence and occurring in the absence of pelvic organ prolapse. **A,** The *radiographic image* shows that the bladder base is above the inferior margin of the symphysis pubis at rest, but the bladder neck is slightly open *(arrow)*. The corresponding *urodynamic tracing* shows baseline abdominal *(Pabd)* and intravesical *(Pves)* pressure tracings. **B,** Leakage of contrast from the urethra occurs in the absence of bladder base descent. The corresponding urodynamic tracing demonstrates urine loss with only a moderate rise in abdominal pressures.

TABLE 6-3 Causes of Intrinsic Sphincter Incompetence[121,122]

Neuropathic Factors	Spinal cord injury affecting spinal segments S2 to S4
	Congenital defects affecting the lumbosacral spinal cord
	Myelodysplasia
	Sacral agenesis
	Imperforate anus
	Acquired disorders affecting the lumbosacral spine
	Postpolio syndrome
	Cauda equina syndrome
	Spinal stenosis
	Peripheral nerve disorders
	Pelvic bone fracture
	Polyneuropathies associated with diabetes mellitus, chronic alcoholism, etc.
Iatrogenic Causes	Urethral suspension procedures in women (particularly multiple surgeries)
	Y-V plasty of the urethra
	Bladder neck incision
	Radical prostatectomy
	Transurethral resection of the prostate

TABLE 6-4 Conditions Associated with Overactive Bladder

FACTOR	RELATIONSHIP TO OVERACTIVE BLADDER
Neurologic disorders (e.g., stroke, hydrocephalus, brain tumors, dementia, or parkinsonism)	Evidence in humans and animal models demonstrates that these disorders interfere with modulatory centers in brain, resulting in neurogenic detrusor overactivity.[122]
Obstruction (see Table 6-5)	Evidence in humans and animals shows a relationship between obstruction and overactive bladder; evidence in animals supports obstruction as a cause of detrusor overactivity, but evidence in humans is mixed.[123]
Stress UI	Clinical evidence reveals association among stress UI, overactive bladder, and urge UI in many women, but the nature of this relationship remains unclear.[124]
Inflammation (e.g., UTI, bladder stones, or tumors)	Clinical evidence links UTI, UI, and overactive bladder symptoms, but the nature of these relationships remains unknown.
Idiopathic	Many cases of overactive bladder and/or urge UI occur without apparent cause. Possible contributing factors include myogenic detrusor dysfunction,[125] depression, hypertension, and undetected neuropathy.[126]

UI, Urinary incontinence; *UTI*, urinary tract infection.

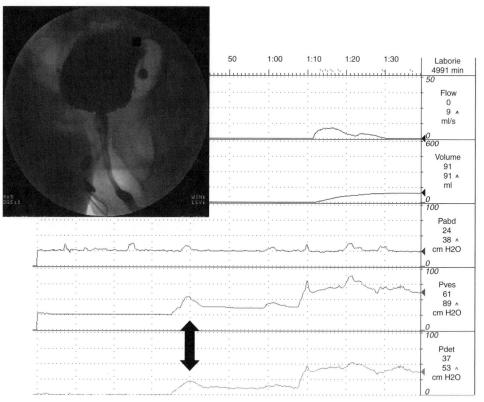

Fig. 6-3 Urodynamic diagnosis of urge urinary incontinence (UI) is based on demonstration of an overactive detrusor contraction that produces a precipitous desire to void and urinary leakage. The *radiographic image* demonstrates high-volume urine loss with relaxation of the urethral sphincter mechanism. The corresponding *urodynamic tracing* demonstrates simultaneous rises in intravesical *(Pves)* and detrusor *(Pdet)* pressure tracings and urinary leakage without any increase in abdominal *(Pabd)* pressures. A lower-pressure overactive detrusor contraction occurs before this event, causing bothersome urgency but no urinary leakage *(arrow)*.

conservative management, nor lessen the need for research into the underlying etiology and pathophysiology of detrusor overactivity and associated symptoms.

Mixed Urinary Incontinence. Mixed UI is a combination of urge and stress UI. The reported prevalence varies, but pooled estimates indicate that approximately 29% of women reporting urine loss experience mixed UI.[34] The pathophysiology of mixed UI is not known, but it is hypothesized that some relationship between sphincter incompetence and detrusor overactivity may exist. This relationship is supported by observations that 55% of women with stress UI symptoms also report bothersome urgency and episodes of urge UI, whereas 38% of women with detrusor overactivity documented on urodynamic evaluation are also found to have stress UI.[35]

Reflex Incontinence. Reflex UI is defined as leakage associated with detrusor overactivity but without precipitous urgency. It is caused by paralyzing disorders affecting spinal segments above the sacral micturition center (S2 to S4) but below the pontine micturition center. Examples include spinal cord injury, multiple sclerosis, spinovascular disease, spinal stenosis, spina bifida defects, or transverse myelitis.[24] Because these lesions occur below the pontine micturition center, detrusor overactivity often coexists with detrusor-sphincter (vesicosphincter) dyssynergia, defined as the loss of coordination between striated muscle of the sphincter mechanism and the detrusor. As a result, the detrusor and striated sphincter muscles contract simultaneously, creating a functional obstruction of the bladder outlet (Figure 6-4).

Autonomic dysreflexia (AD) also occurs in some patients with reflex UI. AD is defined as generalized firing of the sympathetic nervous system in response to a noxious stimulus, such as bladder or bowel distention. This neural discharge causes flushing, pupillary dilation, and a precipitous and potentially dangerous rise in blood

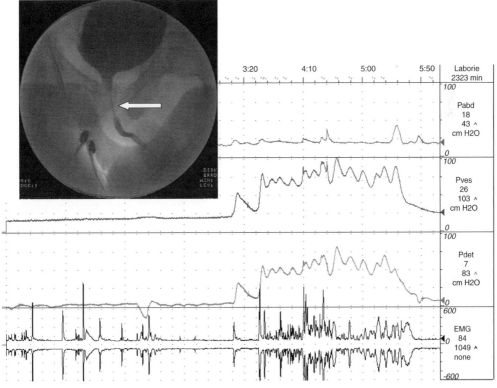

Fig. 6-4 Urodynamic diagnosis of reflex urinary incontinence (UI). The *radiographic image* demonstrates urine loss with narrowing of membranous urethra caused by dyssynergia of the striated muscle of the urethral sphincter mechanisms *(arrow)*. The corresponding *urodynamic tracing* demonstrates simultaneous rises in intravesical *(Pves)* and detrusor *(Pdet)* pressure tracings caused by an overactive detrusor contraction. Electromyogram *(EMG)* tracing shows activity indicating detrusor-striated sphincter dyssynergia.

pressure. Clinical manifestations include a pounding headache, tachycardia with palpitations, dilation of the pupils, and a feeling of anxiety or impending disaster. Bladder distention is the most common cause of AD, but other noxious stimuli, such as bowel distention, digital evacuation maneuvers, and infected pressure ulcers, are also factors.

Functional Incontinence. Functional UI is defined by NANDA International as urine loss caused by impaired functional status[3] and reflects impaired mobility and dexterity and cognitive deficits. Environmental barriers that block toilet access also adversely predispose people to functional UI. Although functional status is a critical concern for many people with UI, this condition is better conceived of as a complicating factor of existing incontinence, rather than an isolated cause.

Extraurethral Incontinence. Extraurethral UI occurs when urine bypasses the urethral sphincter mechanism. It is typically continuous and unaffected by physical exertion or the sensation to urinate. Extraurethral UI may be a continuous dribble superimposed on an otherwise normal urination pattern or may severely disrupt or replace any recognizable cycle of bladder filling and micturition.

Extraurethral leakage arises from one of three sources: reconstructive surgical procedures, urinary ectopia, or urinary fistula. Reconstructive surgical procedures, such as the Bricker ileal conduit or sigmoid conduit, deliberately bypass the bladder and create a conduit for continuous urine leakage from a stoma. Urinary ectopia is the result of a congenital

defect of the ureter, bladder, or urethra. An ectopic ureter may open into the vagina, causing dribbling UI that coexists with an otherwise normal voiding pattern (Figure 6-5). In rare cases an ectopic ureter terminates into the distal urethra. Ectopia of the bladder (exstrophy) is characterized by an externalized bladder wall and absence of a urethral sphincter mechanism (see Chapter 14).

A urinary fistula is defined as an epithelialized tract that creates an abnormal communication between two hollow organs or an organ and the skin. Fistulae are acquired defects and are labeled according to their origin and termination (Figure 6-6). *Vesicovaginal*

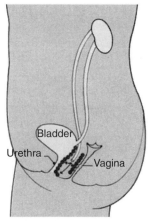

Fig. 6-5 Ureteral ectopia. Extraurethral urinary incontinence (UI) occurs when the ectopic ureter opens into the vagina or distal urethra, bypassing the urethral sphincter mechanism and causing dribbling urine loss superimposed on an otherwise normal urine elimination pattern.

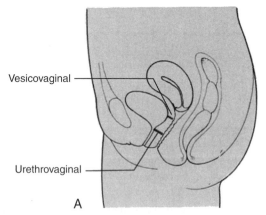

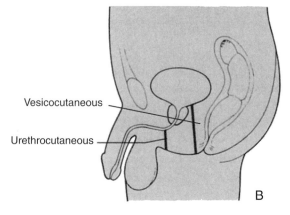

Fig. 6-6 Common fistulae. **A,** Female. **B,** Male. Extraurethral urinary incontinence (UI) occurs when a fistulous tract bypasses the urethral sphincter mechanism, allowing continuous urine loss. UI is often severe and may replace any identifiable voiding pattern.

fistula describes a communication between the bladder and the vaginal vault, and *urethrovaginal* fistula connects the urethra and vagina. Fistulae also may connect the bladder and urethra with the skin, such as a *urethrocutaneous* fistula or a *vesicocutaneous* fistula. Obstructed parturition is the most common cause of fistulae on a global basis,[36] but fistulae are typically iatrogenic, usually during hysterectomy, in industrialized countries.[37] Other causes include pelvic radiation, penetrating trauma, perineal wounds, and invasive malignancies. Fistulae also occur in the upper urinary tracts and following urinary diversion (see Clinical Highlights for Expert and Advanced Practice: Urinary Fistula and Vesicovaginal Fistula, pp. 128-129).

Urinary Incontinence after Radical Prostatectomy. Although postprostatectomy UI is not considered a separate type or form of chronic incontinence, its occurrence is of particular concern to the urologic nurse. The primary cause of UI following radical prostatectomy is damage to the sphincter mechanism, but additional factors, such as detrusor overactivity and low bladder wall compliance, also may occur.[38] The relative risk for UI after radical prostatectomy is affected by multiple factors, including presurgical lower urinary tract function, age, surgical approach, the ability to complete nerve- or bladder neck–sparing procedures during surgery, and postoperative radiation therapy.[38] Although more than 90% of men will experience urine loss immediately following catheter removal, the majority will achieve continence within 12 weeks postoperatively and less than 20% will have persistent UI requiring ongoing use of containment products (Figure 6-7).[39]

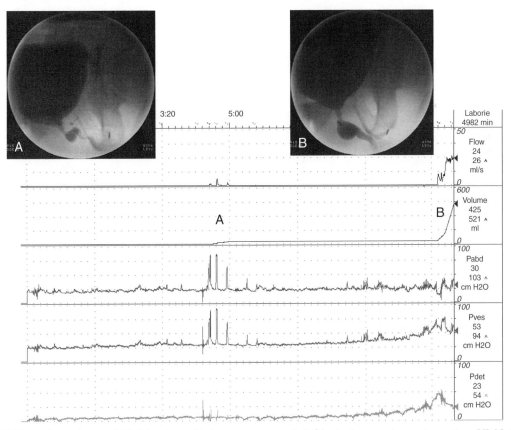

Fig. 6-7 Urinary incontinence (UI) following radical prostatectomy. **A,** Sphincter incompetence causes stress UI. Note urine loss from the urethra that corresponds with rises in abdominal *(Pabd)* and intravesical *(Pves)* pressures when patient performs Valsalva's maneuver. **B,** Overactive detrusor contraction causes urgency and urinary leakage. The corresponding *urodynamic tracing* demonstrates simultaneous rises in intravesical *(Pves)* and detrusor *(Pdet)* pressure tracings and urinary leakage caused by detrusor overactivity.

Clinical Highlights for Expert and Advanced Practice: Urinary Fistula and Vesicovaginal Fistula

Vesicovaginal Fistula

A vesicovaginal fistula causes significant morbidity, particularly when it occurs as a complication of obstructed and prolonged labor in developing countries.[36] In North America, Europe, and most of Asia vesicovaginal fistulae are more commonly associated with unintentional trauma during gynecologic procedures, such as a hysterectomy. A small number are caused by radiation, pelvic tumors, inflammation, or foreign bodies.[37,127] The continuous urine leakage places the patient at risk for skin breakdown, irritation of the vagina and vulva and perineum, as well as an unpleasant odor. Even when the fistula is repaired, the incidence of urinary incontinence remains as high as 26%.[128]

Clinical manifestations include continuous urine loss from the vagina after recent pelvic surgery. UI usually occurs between postoperative days 5 and 14. Patients with small fistulae may describe watery vaginal discharge superimposed on an otherwise normal voiding pattern or stress UI, particularly when urine has pooled in the vagina when the woman is supine and then leaks as she rises to a standing position. Larger fistulae produce severe, ongoing urine loss that replaces normal bladder filling and voiding patterns.

Urethrovaginal Fistula

A urethrovaginal fistula is less common. It is usually associated with a urethral diverticulectomy, anterior colporrhaphy, transurethral resection of bladder neck, or trauma. Clinical manifestations include continuous urine leakage when the fistula involves the bladder neck or proximal urethra. If it is located in the distal urethra, the fistula may be asymptomatic or the patient may complain of a "spraying" urine stream.[128]

Ureterovaginal/Ureterocutaneous Fistula

The ureters are susceptible to injury during vascular, gynecologic, urologic, and colorectal surgery. Total abdominal hysterectomy is the most common cause of ureterovaginal or ureterocutaneous fistula. Risk factors are endometriosis, obesity, pelvic inflammatory disease, and/or preoperative radiation.

Clinical manifestations include abdominal pain, flank tenderness, abdominal mass, or fever as urine collects. Urine drainage may occur days or weeks later and will be detected through copious incisional or vaginal drainage.[127]

Arterioureteral Fistula

Although very rare, a life-threatening fistula can form between the ureter and the iliac artery.[129] Ureteral injury related to stents used to relieve strictures or bypass calculi plus risk factors such as prior surgery or radiotherapy may cause injury to the vaso-vasorum, in turn causing leakage of blood, fibrosis, and adherence of the ureter to the arterial wall.

Clinical features are abdominal or flank pain, ureteric obstruction, and gross hematuria. An arterioureteral fistula should be suspected in patients with complicated pelvic surgery and massive hematuria, particularly if ureteral stents have been placed.

Rectourethral or Prostatic Fistula

Rectourethral fistula may be congenital or acquired. Congenital fistulae are rare and are usually associated with a high or intermediate imperforate anus.[130] Acquired rectourethral fistula is an uncommon side effect of radical prostatectomy, transurethral resection of the prostate, cryotherapy, or brachytherapy.[131,132] Direct trauma, particularly with pelvic fracture, and inflammatory processes such as prostatic abscess, urethral stricture, tuberculosis, and Crohn disease also may contribute.[133]

Clinical manifestations include pneumaturia or fecaluria with leakage of urine from the rectum during voiding, diarrhea, urinary tract infections, and epididymitis.

Vesicoenteric Fistula

Fistulae connecting the rectum, ilium, colon, or appendix may be caused by diverticulitis, malignancy, Crohn disease, therapeutic radiation, and trauma. Colovesical fistulae are most common.[130]

Clinical manifestations include recurring urinary tract infection and suprapubic pain. Urine and mucus may be passed through the rectum, or fecal material may be seen in the urine. Pneumaturia also may occur.

Rectovaginal Fistula

Rectovaginal fistulae are caused by obstructed labor and first-degree perineal tears, Crohn disease, diverticular disease, or surgical trauma. The primary clinical manifestation is fecal drainage through the vagina.

Clinical Highlights for Expert and Advanced Practice: Urinary Fistula and Vesicovaginal Fistula—cont'd

. . . .

Renal and Upper Urinary Tract Fistula

A variety of rare fistulae may form between the kidney and adjacent organs (e.g., bowel or lung). Trauma, percutaneous surgery, or inflammatory bowel disease is the most common cause. Obstruction or distal calculi have been associated with nephrocutaneous fistula.

Clinical manifestations include severe gastrointestinal symptoms, particularly nausea and vomiting, as well as recurrent symptomatic upper tract infections and flank pain. Urine drainage will be seen if the fistula is cutaneous.

Fistula of Urinary Diversion

Approximately 2% to 9% of the patients who undergo urinary diversion procedures develop a ureterointestinal fistula during the early postoperative period.[127] Later-forming ureterointestinal fistulae are usually related to necrosis at the anastomosis. Fistulae after urinary diversion are associated with a mortality rate as high as 50%.

Clinical manifestations include sepsis, bowel obstruction, elevated BUN, urine drainage through the incision, and increasing effluent from the conduit.

Assessment

Cystoscopy is often performed when a fistula is suspected, and vaginoscopy is done in selected cases. Endoscopy may reveal an orifice of the fistula, or it may reveal secondary evidence of communication, such as fecal material in an inflamed, edematous bladder. Smaller vesicovaginal fistulae are assessed by filling the bladder with a solution containing methylene blue and placing a tampon in the vagina. The solution is left in the bladder for a brief period of time, usually 15 to 30 minutes, and the tampon is assessed for evidence of blue staining, indicating communication between bladder and vaginal vault. Ureterovaginal fistulae are often associated with vesicovaginal fistulae. These must be excluded during diagnostic evaluation.[37] A barium enema, sigmoidoscopy, and colonoscopy may be performed when rectourethral fistula is suspected. They help define the extent of bowel disease and the presence of stenosis at the fistula site. Retrograde ureterography and CT scans are preferred when evaluating a fistula involving the upper urinary tracts. Diagnosis of fistula of urinary diversion is based on a loopogram or pouchogram, IVP, and presence of increased urea and creatinine in the drainage fluid.

Treatment

Approximately 10% of small vesicovaginal fistulae heal with an indwelling catheter left in place for 2 to 8 weeks. Fistulae that do not heal after 2 months of catheterization are unlikely to heal by this method.[37,128] Electrocoagulation of the mucosa may heal smaller vesicovaginal fistulae. Surgical repair is often postponed for 3 to 6 months to encourage spontaneous closure, to reduce inflammation and edema, and to allow time for treatment of underlying disease.

Patients who experience a fistula associated with extraurethral UI are given advice concerning appropriate urine containment devices until surgical repair is done. Small fistulae may be managed with a tampon, but larger defects typically require an incontinence containment brief or large absorptive pad. The patient is taught preventive perineal skin care, including regular cleansing with a skin-cleansing product, avoidance of excessive use of harsh soaps and friction, routine drying of the perineal skin, and judicious use of topical skin barrier products.

BUN, Blood urea nitrogen; *CT,* computed tomography; *IVP,* intravenous pyelogram; *UI,* urinary incontinence.

Urinary Retention and Overflow Urinary Incontinence. Urinary retention is defined as either the inability to fully empty the bladder of urine despite voiding or a complete inability to urinate.[40,41] It may be associated with overflow UI, defined as dribbling urine loss when bladder overdistention creates excessive pressure against the urethral sphincter mechanism. *Acute urinary retention* (AUR) is the complete inability to void and is a medical emergency requiring prompt intervention. People with AUR usually experience extreme discomfort, and their symptoms may be confused with an "acute abdomen." *Chronic urinary retention* is ongoing, incomplete bladder emptying despite micturition. Two conditions cause urinary retention: obstruction and/or deficient detrusor contraction strength. Obstruction is characterized by an anatomic lesion or structure that partially blocks urinary outflow (e.g., a urethral stricture, enlarged prostate, or vaginal sling procedure) or a functional blockage caused by paradoxic muscle contraction (e.g., detrusor-sphincter dyssynergia). Deficient detrusor contractility is characterized by a contraction that lacks amplitude (i.e., force) or duration (i.e., endurance) to effectively eliminate urine from the bladder.

Postvoid Dribble. Postvoid dribble is an annoying loss of urine several seconds to a few minutes after completion of voiding. In men it usually occurs when urine pools in the bulbar urethra at the termination of micturition. Bulbar urethral massage or pelvic floor muscle exercises are usually successful in alleviating the problem.[42] In women, however, postvoid dribbling may indicate a suburethral diverticulum requiring surgical management.[43]

Assessment

The evaluation of UI begins with a focused history and physical assessment. Laboratory evaluation begins with a urinalysis, followed by urine culture and sensitivity testing when indicated. More extensive testing, often including urodynamic evaluation, is indicated in select cases.

History. The history begins with the person's (or caregiver's) description of the problem and degree of bother, the duration of the UI, an appraisal of lower urinary tract symptoms, and review of treatments and their effectiveness. Appraisal of lower urinary tract habits includes daytime voiding frequency, nocturia, bothersome urgency, factors that provoke or prevent UI, character of voided stream, and perceptions of bladder emptying. Queries about daytime voiding frequency should be based on performance within a 2-hour time frame rather than estimates of total voids over 24 hours.[24] Diurnal voiding frequency is diagnosed when patients report voiding intervals of 2 hours or less while awake. Nocturia is assessed by asking about the number of times the person is awakened by the urge to urinate. Excessive nocturia is diagnosed if an adult who is less than 65 years of age reports two or more episodes per night or when an older adult reports three or more episodes per night. Urgency to urinate is a normal response to bladder filling; bothersome urgency occurs when the patient notes a strong urge to urinate that interferes with daily activities at lower bladder volumes. It is typically associated with daytime voiding frequency and excessive nocturia.

When assessing for UI, the nurse should ask about bladder control, urine loss, dripping before or after

voiding, or pad use in addition to questions about incontinence. Although the term *incontinence* is used by healthcare professionals to indicate any uncontrolled loss of urine, many individuals reserve the term for severe urine loss requiring the use of an adult containment brief. Activity-induced urine loss without frequency or nocturia suggests stress UI. A presumptive diagnosis of OAB should be based on a history of daytime voiding frequency, nocturia, and symptoms of urge UI (i.e., urine loss associated with a precipitous desire to urinate). Mixed UI is suspected when symptoms of activity-induced and urge-related urine loss are reported. Urine loss without sensory awareness may be reflex UI when it occurs in a patient with a paralyzing spinal disorder, or it may indicate overflow incontinence or extraurethral UI. The frequency, amount of leakage, and the type and number of pads worn provide a crude assessment of UI severity, although this perception is influenced by multiple subjective factors.

AUR is associated with abdominal discomfort, anxiety, and restlessness in a person who is unable to urinate. In contrast, no cluster of symptoms can be identified that accurately differentiate chronic urinary retention from other conditions affecting lower urinary tract function.[44] Some patients with chronic urinary retention report a poor force behind their urinary stream, intermittency, or perceptions of incomplete bladder emptying or even UI with increased abdominal pressure (Figure 6-8). Bothersome lower urinary symptoms associated with overactive bladder, such as diurnal frequency, nocturia, and bothersome urgency, occur in some; others have significant residual volumes but a complete absence of bothersome or even noticeable symptoms (Box 6-1).

A focused review of systems is completed to determine factors that may contribute to UI. Key systems in this review include the urinary, reproductive, neurologic, and gastrointestinal systems (Table 6-5). This review should include explicit questions about bowel and flatus incontinence, since people are unlikely to spontaneously volunteer such information unless directly asked.[45] Although these disorders are often considered separately, they frequently coexist and may reveal an underlying disorder of the pelvic floor muscles. For example, in one study, 24% of women respondents had *both* UI and fecal incontinence and those with fecal incontinence reported it as significantly more devastating than urinary incontinence.

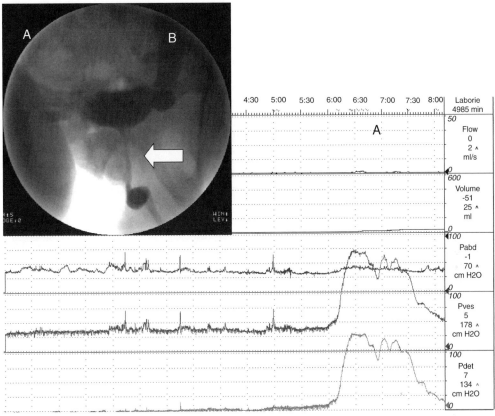

Fig. 6-8 Bladder outlet obstruction caused by benign prostatic hyperplasia. **A,** The *radiographic image* demonstrates narrowing of bladder neck and entire prostatic urethra and is associated with high-grade left vesicoureteral reflux. **B,** The *corresponding urodynamic tracing* shows high detrusor contraction pressure and prolonged, interrupted flow characteristic of obstruction.

BOX 6-1 Causes of Urinary Retention

Obstruction
- Bladder neck contracture
- Bladder neck dyssynergia
- Prostatic enlargement
  - Benign prostatic hyperplasia
  - Prostatitis (particularly acute)
  - Prostate cancer (advanced stage)
- Detrusor-sphincter dyssynergia
- Urethral stricture
- Pelvic organ prolapse (severe cases)

Deficient Detrusor Contraction Strength
- Spinal cord injury (i.e., lesions affecting spinal segments S2, S3, and S4)
- Cauda equina syndrome
- Peripheral polyneuropathies
  - Diabetes mellitus
  - Chronic alcoholism
  - Heavy metal poisoning

- Herpes zoster or simplex affecting sacral nerve roots
- Injury or extensive surgery causing denervation of pelvic plexus
  - Abdominoperineal (AP) resection
  - Pelvic exenteration
- Medication side effects
  - Anticholinergics
  - Antimuscarinics
  - Tricyclic antidepressants
  - Calcium channel blockers (particularly when combined with anticholinergic)
  - Opioid analgesics
  - Illegal drugs (e.g., hypnotics, cannabis)
- Impaction of stool

TABLE 6-5 Review of Systems: Implications of Positive Findings

FINDING	IMPLICATION FOR UI
Urinary tract infections Upper urinary tract problems Urinary tract calculi Renal insufficiency/failure	Urinary retention (febrile UTI; upper urinary tract problems; renal insufficiency, particularly associated with bladder outlet obstruction or low bladder wall compliance)
Urinary system tumor	Urge UI, indication for immediate referral
Disorders of the brain	Urge UI with detrusor hyperreflexia, also alter mobility or cognition and increase risk of functional UI
Disorders of the spinal cord	Reflex UI with detrusor-sphincter dyssynergia and urinary retention; paralyzing spinal disorders affect mobility, dexterity, and risk of functional UI
Disorders of the peripheral nerves	Urinary retention with diminished or absent sensations of bladder filling and deficient detrusor contraction strength, may reduce mobility and increase risk of functional UI Denervation also may cause intrinsic sphincter deficiency and stress UI
Disorders affecting multiple levels of the nervous system	Urge or reflex UI, urinary retention
Obstetric history	Multiple deliveries; deliveries requiring forceps assistance, central episiotomy; those complicated by breech presentation, central tearing increase risk of pelvic floor muscle denervation and stress UI
Gynecologic history	Vaginitis, endometriosis may contribute to irritative voiding symptoms and urge UI
Menstrual status	Atrophic vaginitis associated with atrophic urethritis causing irritative voiding symptoms and urge UI
Symptoms of pelvic organ prolapse	Pelvic organ prolapse associated with stress UI; urinary retention may occur when prolapse is severe
Prostatism problems	Prostate enlargement associated with bladder outlet obstruction and urinary retention Severe bladder outlet obstruction causes detrusor instability and urge UI Prostatitis causes irritative voiding symptoms and may produce detrusor instability and urge UI
Sexual dysfunction	Erectile dysfunction, ejaculatory dysfunction may be associated with disorders of spinal cord, peripheral nervous system causing urge UI, reflex UI
Scrotal disorders	Epididymitis may indicate reflux into male reproductive tract from detrusor-sphincter dyssynergia or reflex UI
Sexually transmitted diseases	Gonococcal or nongonococcal urethritis may cause secondary stricture with bladder outlet obstruction and urinary retention
Bowel elimination patterns/ fecal continence	Constipation, fecal incontinence may indicate neuropathic bladder dysfunction with urge or reflex UI, urinary retention
Metabolic disorders	Diabetes mellitus most common cause of peripheral polyneuropathies, associated with urgency, frequency, and urge UI in early stages and urinary retention in late stages
Hypertension	Hypertension may directly contribute to urinary urgency, medications used to treat hypertension contribute to transient UI (refer to current medications)
Disorders of special senses (i.e., vision and hearing)	Increased risk of functional UI
Cancer	May contribute to urinary retention or UI because of primary effect on urinary system or secondary effects on nervous system, gastrointestinal system, etc.
Surgical history	*Urologic procedures*

TABLE 6-5 Review of Systems: Implications of Positive Findings—cont'd

FINDING	IMPLICATION FOR UI
	Bladder suspension associated with risk of detrusor instability and urge UI or recurrent stress UI and intrinsic sphincter deficiency as well as urethral hypermobility, suspensions also associated with small risk of obstruction and urinary retention
	Transurethral procedures (TURP, TUIP, etc.) associated with small risk of sphincter damage and subsequent stress UI
	Gynecologic procedures
	Hysterectomy carries uncertain risk of subsequent stress UI
	Cystocele repair may increase risk of subsequent stress UI
	Neurologic procedures
	Risk of urge or reflex UI, urinary retention from preexisting condition and from surgical intervention
	Abdominal procedures (risk of urinary retention with extensive resection)
Current medications	Anticholinergics, antispasmodics, antidepressants, antipsychotics, sedative/hypnotics, narcotic analgesics associated with urinary retention or reduced ability to respond to toileting cues with subsequent transient UI
	α-Adrenergic agonists (decongestants) increase risk of urinary retention, particularly in men with prostatic enlargement
	β-Adrenergic agonists may increase risk of urinary retention, particularly when combined with agents listed above
	Calcium channel blockers increase risk of urinary retention, particularly when combined with agents listed above
	α-Adrenergic blockers (antagonists) increase risk of stress UI
	Diuretics increase risk of urinary frequency, urgency, and urge UI

Modified from Doughty DB: Urinary and Fecal Incontinence: Nursing Management. St Louis: Mosby, 2000.
TUIP, Transurethral incision of prostate; *TURP,* transurethral resection of prostate; *UI,* urinary incontinence; *UTI,* urinary tract infection.

Moreover, women with urinary incontinence were more likely to report fecal incontinence events than women continent of urine.[46] Although the relationship between constipation and UI is not completely understood, at least one study shows that older women with UI are more likely to have both constipation and fecal incontinence than are continent women.[47]

The initial history concludes with an assessment of the impact of UI on the person's life: his or her ability or willingness to socialize, to leave home for extended periods, to take holidays, or to attend church or temple. Financial impact should also be considered; UI containment products can be expensive, and people on fixed or limited incomes may not be able to afford the products they need or not know how to access services that can assist them.

Physical Examination. Physical assessment begins with an evaluation of the patient's dexterity, mobility, and cognition. The nurse should take note of any incontinence containment devices (e.g., pads or briefs, condom catheter, or penile clamp). The perineal skin and skinfolds are inspected for integrity, moisture, and dermatitis from urine or fecal incontinence. Inspection of the vaginal mucosa is helpful, and specific maneuvers may be attempted to reproduce UI, such as coughing or Valsalva's maneuver while lying or standing. A neurologic assessment focuses on sensory and motor function of the pelvic floor muscles and the perineal dermatomes. This includes the bulbocavernous reflex, ability to differentiate deep and light touch and sharp versus dull sensations, and two-point discrimination. A simple assessment of pelvic floor muscle tone is completed by asking the patient to squeeze (tighten) the circumvaginal muscles around the examiner's finger. Scales ranging from 0 to 3[48] or 0 to 5[49] provide a rough assessment of pelvic floor muscle strength (Table 6-6).

Laboratory Evaluation

Routine laboratory testing for the person with UI always includes urinalysis as well as a bladder log (sometimes called a voiding diary or frequency/volume chart).

TABLE 6-6 Assessment of Pelvic Floor Muscle Strength[48,49]

RATING	MOTION DEMONSTRATED
Oxford Scale	
0	No contraction
1	Flicker only
2	Weak contraction
3	Moderate contraction
4	Good contraction
5	Strong contraction
Brink Scale	
0	No contraction
1	Slight pressure around finger, duration < 1 sec
2	Moderate pressure around finger, duration 1-3 sec
3	Strong pressure persists > 3 sec

Measurements of postvoid residual volume, urodynamic testing, or imaging studies, such as a voiding cystourethrogram or renal/bladder ultrasound, are performed in selected patients.

Urinalysis. Urinalysis may be completed by means of a dipstick or microscopy. Urine culture and sensitivity testing are performed only when indicated. Table 6-7 reviews normal and clinically relevant urinalysis findings.

Bladder Log. The bladder log provides a record of urine elimination patterns for a period of 1 to 7 days. It is typically kept by the person or care provider. The simplest bladder log records only the frequency of urination and incontinence. More complex logs may include information about voided volume, the amount and type of fluid consumed, and the person's assessment of the reasons for urine loss (often recorded as related to activity or urgency). For the alert, motivated person, completion of a bladder log provides a

TABLE 6-7 Urinalysis: Normal and Significant Findings and Their Implications

NORMAL VALUE	SIGNIFICANCE OF ABNORMAL FINDING	FOLLOW-UP
Specific gravity: 1.003-1.029	*Low specific gravity:* excessive water intake, diabetes insipidus	*Low specific gravity:* obtain serum electrolytes; follow up evaluation by primary care physician or nephrologist
	High specific gravity: dehydration, diabetes mellitus with glucosuria	*High specific gravity:* bladder log including fluid intake, evaluation for diabetes mellitus if glucosuria present
Glucose: absent	*Positive glucose:* uncontrolled or undiagnosed diabetes mellitus	Refer to primary care physician for diagnostic evaluation or alteration in current management
Nitrites/leukocytes: absent	*Positive nitrites and negative leukocytes:* bacteriuria	Microscopic evaluation for presence of bacteria and WBCs; urine culture and sensitivity for bacteriuria and culture and sensitivity based on clinical judgment when bacteriuria present but pyuria (WBCs) absent
	Positive nitrites and leukocytes: bacteriuria and pyuria (urinary tract infection)	
Hemoglobin: negative	*Positive hemoglobin:* hematuria	Microscopic examination, urine culture and sensitivity if other signs of infection present (pyuria, bacteriuria); urine cytology and referral to urologist if hematuria present without coexisting infection
Protein: negative	*Positive with leukocytes or protein:* may indicate renal disease	Refer to physician or nephrologist unless UTI coexists

Modified from Doughty DB: Urinary and Fecal Incontinence: Nursing Management. St Louis: Mosby, 2000.
UTI, Urinary tract infection; *WBCs,* white blood cells.

valuable record of urine elimination patterns and a self-instruction tool that allows greater insights into bladder function and the behavioral antecedents of UI. Incomplete data entry is a potential problem, particularly when people are asked to measure fluid intake or voided volumes. In addition, individuals may record what they think the nurse wants to know, particularly when a bladder log is used to evaluate treatment outcome. These limitations are minimized by careful explanation of the purpose of the log, minimizing the time of data collection, careful review of data with the patient, and providing the patient with a clearly marked graduated receptacle to measure voided volume. Figure 6-9 provides examples of bladder logs.

	Sunday		Monday		Tuesday		Wednesday		Thursday		Friday		Saturday	
Time	Voided	Leaked	Voided	Leaked	Voided	Leaked	Voided	Leaked	Voided	Leaked	Voided	Leaked	Voided	Leaked

A

Time	Amount voided	Leakage	Amount of fluid consumed

B

Name _____ Date _____

Time toilet is offered	Leakage (yes or no)	Was patient aware of urge? (yes or no)	Did patient void? (yes or no)	Comments
0800				
1000				
1200				
1400				
1600				
1800				

(2000 and so forth)

C

Fig. 6-9 Examples of bladder logs (voiding diaries). **A,** Simple bladder log requires patient to indicate voiding and leakage episodes by a check mark or tick. **B,** A slightly more complex bladder log requires patient to record the volume voided and volume of fluid consumption. Patients may be asked to record the types of beverages consumed, which allows assessment of intake of beverages containing potential bladder irritants, such as caffeine. **C,** This bladder log is designed to assess the response of the patient undergoing a prompted voiding program. Continence status is assessed every 2 hours, and the caregiver records whether the patient's pad or brief was wet or dry and the patient's response to prompted toileting assistance. (From Doughty D: Urinary and Fecal Incontinence: Current Management Concepts, 3rd edition. St Louis: Mosby, 2006.)

Treatment

Effective treatment of UI depends on a collaborative approach among the nurse, physician, patient, and (in many cases) healthcare professionals such as physical or occupational therapists and lay caregivers. Successful UI management is rarely achieved by a single intervention but rather a combination of behavioral, pharmacologic, and/or surgical therapy. For example, a person with an overactive bladder and urge UI is more likely to respond to a bladder management program that includes changes in voiding frequency, fluid and dietary interventions, and pharmacotherapy as compared with pharmacotherapy or pelvic floor muscle rehabilitation in isolation.[50] Table 6-8 outlines treatment options based on UI type.

For the purposes of this discussion, treatment options will be divided into four key categories: containment devices, behavioral interventions, pharmacotherapy,

TABLE 6-8 Treatment Options for Chronic Urinary Incontinence

UI TYPE	TREATMENT OPTIONS
Stress UI	Behavioral*:
	Fluid and dietary counseling
	Pelvic floor muscle rehabilitation
	Habit training
	Weight loss and smoking cessation
	Urethral barrier devices (urethral insert)
	Pessary
	Pharmacologic†:
	Tricyclic antidepressants (imipramine)
	Serotonin-norepinephrine reuptake inhibitor (duloxetine)
	Surgical:
	Suburethral bulking agents (GAX collagen, silicone beads)
	Retropubic procedures (Burch colposuspension, Marshall-Marchetti-Krantz)
	Transvaginal needle procedures (Pereyra, Stamey, Raz, Gittes)
	Suburethral sling surgery (autologous fascia, cadaveric fascia, synthetic materials, tension-free vaginal tape, obturator tape)
	Artificial urinary sphincter
Overactive bladder	Behavioral:
	Pelvic floor muscle rehabilitation
	Bladder training
	Electrical stimulation (transvaginal, transrectal, transcutaneous)
	Pharmacologic:
	Antimuscarinics/anticholinergics (tolterodine, oxybutynin, trospium, darafenicin, solafenicin)
	Tricyclic antagonists (imipramine)
	Surgical (rare):
	Augmentation procedures (augmentation enterocystoplasty, autoaugmentation, gastrocystoplasty)
	Electrical stimulation (surgically implanted device)
	Urinary diversion
Mixed incontinence (OAB and stress UI)	Combination of interventions, initial therapy focuses on "predominant" (most bothersome or most severe) UI type
Postvoid dribble	Behavioral:
	Massage of bulbar urethra (men) or pelvic floor muscle exercises
	Surgical:
	Ablation of suburethral diverticulum (women)

TABLE 6-8 Treatment Options for Chronic Urinary Incontinence—cont'd

UI TYPE	TREATMENT OPTIONS

UI after radical prostatectomy	Behavioral:
	    Pelvic floor muscle rehabilitation
	    Urethral barrier device (penile clamp)
	    Incontinence products
	Pharmacologic:
	    Antimuscarinics/anticholinergics (tolterodine, oxybutynin, trospium, darafenicin, solafenicin)
	    Imipramine
	Surgical:
	    Suburethral sling surgery
	    Artificial urinary sphincter

Reflex incontinence	Behavioral:
	    Pelvic floor muscle rehabilitation (limited to persons with pseudodyssynergia and voiding dysfunction)
	    Scheduled voiding
	    Intermittent catheterization
	Pharmacologic:
	    Antimuscarinics/antispasmodics (usually combined with intermittent catheterization)
	    α-Adrenergic antagonists (doxazosin, terazosin, tamsulosin) (usually combined with condom catheter containment)
	Surgical:
	    Transurethral sphincterotomy (combined with condom catheter containment)
	    Transurethral injection of botulinum toxin
	    Augmentation procedures (augmentation enterocystoplasty, autoaugmentation, gastrocystoplasty)
	    Urinary diversion

Functional incontinence (environmental)	Behavioral:
	    Prompted toileting
	    Removal of environmental barriers to toileting
	    Interventions to maximize mobility and dexterity

Extraurethral incontinence	Pharmacologic:
	    Sclerosing therapy
	Surgical:
	    Repair of fistula
	    Reconstruction of ectopic urethra, bladder, or ureter

Urinary retention	Behavioral:
	    Scheduled toileting
	    Double voiding
	    Intermittent catheterization
	Pharmacologic:
	    α-Adrenergic antagonists (doxazosin, terazosin, tamsulosin)
	    Finasteride (limited to men with benign prostatic hyperplasia)
	    Urecholine
	Surgical:
	    Reconstruction or resection of surgical lesion

OAB, Overactive bladder; *UI,* urinary incontinence.
*Behavioral options include general advice concerning fluid, diet, smoking cessation, weight loss, bowel management, voiding frequency, and pelvic floor muscle exercises.
†Specific agents in this category are available in Europe but have not been approved by the U.S. Food and Drug Administration.

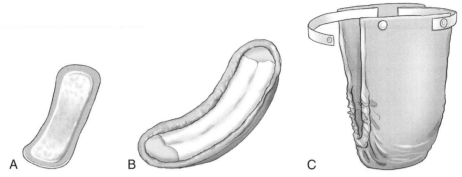

Fig. 6-10 Absorbent products designed specifically for containing urinary leakage. **A,** Minipads are inserted into underclothing. They are lightweight and easy to conceal; they are designed to absorb low-volume urine loss. **B,** Medium pads are also inserted into underclothing. They absorb larger volumes of urine loss, often up to 500 ml. They are attached to underclothing by an adhesive strip, or a mesh undergarment may be purchased to hold medium pads in place. **C,** Larger pads may be worn under regular underclothing. These pads are held in place by Velcro straps worn around the waist. They will absorb large volumes of urine (more than 500 ml).

and surgical options. Chapter 11 provides a detailed discussion of nursing management for patients with UI undergoing surgery.

Containment Devices. Absorbent products include a variety of devices designed to absorb urinary and/or fecal incontinence while protecting the perineal skin[51] (Figure 6-10). These products can be further subdivided into underpads that fit into the individual's underclothing, pad and pant systems, or incontinent briefs (sometimes called body-worns or adult diapers). Underpads incorporate fluff pulp (cellulose wood pulp) or superabsorbent material (synthetic particles made from cross-linked sodium polyacrylates) into disposable products, or they incorporate multiple layers of absorbent cotton-based cloth into a reusable product. Pad and pant systems incorporate an absorbent pad into specially designed disposable pads with a reusable brief or a reusable, washable device. Disposable briefs incorporate fluff pulp or superabsorbent material into a device that is designed to contain both urinary and fecal incontinence, whereas reusable products rely on layered cloth (Figure 6-11).

Counseling patients, families, or care providers about selection of containment devices must be individualized, but the main principles of selection are guided by a combination of clinical experience and limited research-based evidence. The use of home-based products, such as rags, paper towels, or toilet tissue, is discouraged since these products are ineffective for the containment of urine and offer no protection from odor or perineal skin irritation.

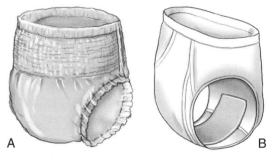

Fig. 6-11 Adult incontinence briefs are capable of absorbing large volume or continuous urine loss, and they are indicated when a patient experiences double (urinary and fecal) incontinence. **A,** Disposable incontinence brief. **B,** Reusable incontinence brief incorporates disposable pad into washable undergarment.

The use of feminine hygiene products is also discouraged. These products are designed to contain menstrual flow, not urine. Systematic reviews reveal no clinical differences between disposable versus reusable underpads,[51] and data are mixed on whether reusable or disposable products offer better perineal skin protection.[52] Disposable pads may be less expensive than reusable products and reduce the burden on weekly laundering as well as odor in the home. Interviews with incontinent women reveal that key criteria of containment products are the ability to reliably hold urine, to contain odor, to stay in place, to be discrete, and to be comfortable comfort when wet. At night, discreteness was replaced by the need to keep skin dry. Participants reported high levels of anxiety with perceived risk of poor pad performance or lack of discreteness.[51] When advising women of products, the choice should take into account personal needs at various times of the day and activities rather than one product that will meet all the individual's needs. Finally, containment products should be easily concealed under clothing, minimize noise when moving, and be easily donned, removed, or reapplied for toileting.

Condom catheters rely on a sheath that encases the penile shaft and a drainage port attached to a leg bag or bedside bag. A variety of products are available that incorporate a self-adhesive strip, separate adhesive strip, inflatable ring, or external strap holder to achieve a watertight seal. They are made of latex, silicone, or hydrocolloid adhesive wafer. Patients with allergies to latex or adhesive must be fitted with a silicone or hydrocolloid product that avoids the application of adhesive to the penile skin. Correct sizing of condom catheters based on penile circumferences and length is critical to proper functioning. The system should prevent leakage under most circumstances but must not be applied with sufficient force to cause ischemia to the penile skin. Patients or care providers are taught to routinely change the catheter and cleanse the underlying skin, usually every 24 hours. Condoms are associated with urinary tract infection (UTI), and the person will need instruction on signs or symptoms of UTI and what to do if symptoms occur.[53] Patients are also taught to routinely inspect the penile skin with every catheter change and to promptly contact their physician or nurse practitioner should pressure ulceration occur.

A condom catheter is reserved for men with moderate- to high-volume urine loss that cannot be managed by alternative means. It is preferable to an indwelling catheter because of comfort and avoidance of serious urologic complications associated with long-term indwelling catheter use.[54]

Barrier and Compressive Devices. Urethral barrier devices mechanically block urine loss from the urethra. They rely on a patch or suction cup that is placed at the urethral meatus or a soft tube that is inserted into the urethra to block urine outflow. Although these devices have been found to be effective,[55] cost and long-term patient acceptance have limited the use and availability of these products.

Penile compression devices (penile clamps) are typically used by men experiencing transient (and

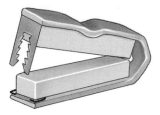

Fig. 6-12 Penile clamp devices may be worn to prevent moderate to severe urine loss following radical prostatectomy. Patients *must* have normal penile and bladder sensation, cognitive ability, manual dexterity, and adequate vision for skin checking.

often severe) UI immediately following radical prostatectomy (Figure 6-12). One study found that the traditional penile clamp was more effective and more comfortable than two other smaller products. Ultrasound revealed that the penile circulation was not impeded when the clamp was applied with adequate pressure to prevent leakage.[56] The authors emphasize that men who may benefit from a penile compression device meet the following criteria: have stress UI, a bladder capacity of at least 250 ml, normal penile and genital sensation and healthy skin, sufficient mental acuity to remember to release the device at regular intervals, and manual dexterity to be able to apply and remove the clamp. Relative contraindications include neurologic or vascular impairments that affect penile sensation or vascularity (e.g., multiple sclerosis, spinal cord injury, or diabetes). Since men can easily obtain the penile compression devices over the counter or on the Internet, urologic nurses should routinely include information about penile clamps to men with UI, including counseling that the device should be used only in close consultation with a healthcare provider.

Pessaries. Pessaries can play an important role in the management of women with prolapse and/or UI. They are often fitted for women with comorbid conditions who are not surgical candidates or for those with moderately severe to severe prolapse who do not wish to undergo surgery.[57] All pessaries are designed to restore the vaginal walls (including the bladder neck) to a more nearly normal relationship with respect to the rectum, pelvic bone, and adjacent structures (Figure 6-13). When properly sized and fitted, pessaries are effective and comfortable. Fitting requires considerable skill and expertise and should be undertaken by a healthcare professional with specialized training (e.g., advanced practice nurse,

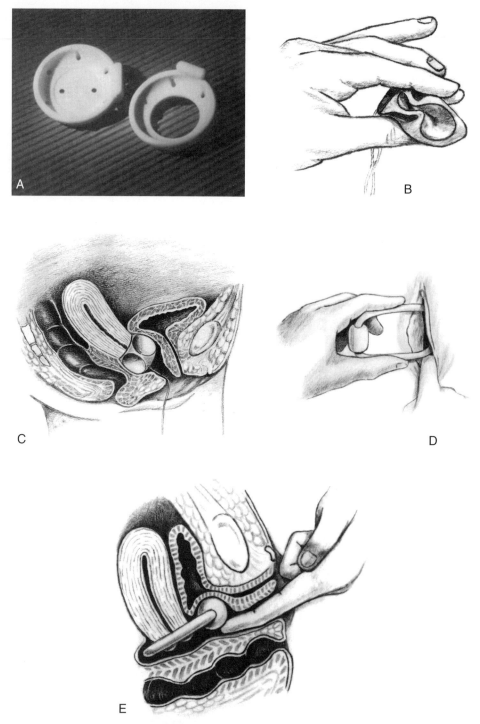

Fig. 6-13 A, Dish pessaries with and without support (available from Mentor Corporation, Santa Barbara, Calif), which can be used for stress incontinence. **B,** Cube pessary is compressed between the thumb and forefingers. If necessary the entering edge can be coated with suitable lubricant. **C,** Silicone cube in position. **D,** Ring incontinence pessary being inserted.. **E,** Ring incontinence pessary positioned. (**B** through **E,** *Courtesy of Milex Corporation,* Chicago, Ill).

urologist, gynecologist, or urogynecologist). Women using a pessary require local hormone replacement therapy (HRT) in order to prevent vaginal irritation, erosion, and discomfort (Table 6-9). For women with severe atrophic changes, local HRT may be undertaken over a period of several weeks in order to prepare the vaginal tissue for pessary insertion. Once in place, pessaries should be removed at least monthly, washed with soap and water, and replaced by the patient or care provider. Ideally, the woman should visit the advanced practice nurse or physician on a monthly basis for assessment of the vaginal vault although the frequency of follow-up visits will vary according to individual needs.[58] Provided the vaginal epithelium remains healthy and the woman is capable of removing and inserting the pessary independently, the time between visits can be extended to 3 to 6 months.[59] Complications of pessaries are unusual *provided* the patient is observed on a regular basis, is cognitively capable of being responsible for pessary care, and remains on localized HRT. However, without proper follow-up, the pessary may be forgotten, resulting in vaginal or urethral erosion, vaginosis, or urethrovaginal or rectovaginal fistula.

Behavioral Interventions. Behavioral interventions include a range of strategies that the patient can incorporate into daily routine to improve or relieve bothersome lower urinary tract symptoms. Common interventions are fluid and dietary adjustments, smoking cessation, weight loss, bowel management, adjustments of voiding frequency, and pelvic floor muscle rehabilitation.

Fluid adjustment. Many individuals with UI or overactive bladder reduce fluid intake in an attempt to reduce symptoms. Unfortunately, this strategy may paradoxically increase rather than diminish bothersome symptoms and increase the risk of constipation and UTI. A number of small studies and one systematic literature review have examined the relationship between fluid intake and UI, and they indicate that increasing noncaffeinated fluid intake increases voided volume and reduces UTI risk without increasing UI or voiding frequency.[60-62] In general, men and women are advised to consume 3.7 L and 2.7 L, respectively, of total fluids per day (approximately 30 ml per kilogram).[63] This intake may be increased with warm temperatures or exercise.

Whereas chronic fluid restriction paradoxically increases the frequency of UI episodes and fails to reduce voiding frequency, short-term restriction may be beneficial. For example, one study of the relationship among evening fluid intake, nocturia, and nighttime UI in elders with overactive bladder suggests that restriction of evening fluids may be beneficial.[64] Avoiding a large volume of fluid over a brief period of time and instead drinking smaller amounts throughout the day may help, particularly if confronted by a transient period of limited toilet access, such as during travel by car or airplane.

Bladder irritants. A number of substances have been described as "bladder irritants," primarily based on anecdotal association with bothersome lower urinary tract symptoms. Two potential irritants are caffeine and alcohol. Research in animals and humans demonstrates that caffeine activates intracellular calcium ions, stimulating the detrusor muscle and possibly precipitating urgency or urge incontinence.[65,66] Whereas some have identified caffeine as one factor,[61] others have been unable to identify a clear association between caffeine and UI in community-dwelling women or disabled people.[67,68] Of note, at least one randomized clinical study found a significant improvement in UI frequency among subjects who decreased caffeine intake to less than 100 mg/day.[69] Patients can be advised of this relationship and encouraged to reduce or eliminate caffeine from their diet as one component of a bladder management program.

Evidence is mixed concerning social consumption of alcohol and its relationship to the risk or severity of UI.[70] Alcohol acts as a diuretic through its effects on vasopressin (antidiuretic hormone) and in high doses depresses the central nervous system and diminishes the individual's awareness of cues to urinate. Single-photon emission computed tomography (SPECT) studies of the frontal cortex support an association between frontal lobe hypoactivity and advanced-stage alcoholism.[71] Other substances, such as aspartame, chocolate, carbonated drinks, and citrus juices, have been labeled bladder irritants. However, research to determine whether elimination would relieve bothersome lower urinary tract symptoms is inadequate.

Smoking cessation. Although no significant association between smoking and UI has been found in younger men, men aged 50 to 70 years who were smokers and former smokers have a significantly increased risk of lower urinary tract symptoms

Text continued on p. 146

TABLE 6-9 Medications Commonly Prescribed for the Treatment of Urinary Incontinence

CLASSIFICATION	GENERIC NAME	MECHANISM OF ACTION	DOSE	SIDE EFFECTS	CONTRAINDICATIONS
Drugs That Decrease Activity of Overactive Bladder (Urge UI)[16,137,144]					
Anticholinergics/ antimuscarinics	Oxybutynin	Antispasmodic and slight analgesic effect on smooth muscle; inhibits acetylcholine on smooth muscle	2.5-5 mg one to four times daily; oxybutynin XL available in 5 and 10 mg	Constipation, dry mucosa (mouth, vagina, eyes); in elders: confusion, decreased cognition (crosses blood-brain barrier); blurred vision; may result in urinary retention—at-risk patients should be monitored for residual urine	As per all anticholinergic medications: narrow-angle glaucoma; GI obstruction or atony; ulcerative colitis, myasthenia gravis; urinary retention or residual urine (can be used in conjunction with intermittent catheterization)
	Oxybutynin XL	All are metabolized primarily by liver		NB: gradual increase of oral dose increases tolerability, especially in elders; doses as low as 2.5 mg at bedtime are effective for some elderly patients NB: Warn patient that empty capsule from oxybutynin LA will be excreted in the feces	
	Transdermal oxybutynin patch	As above, transdermal route increases bioavailability and diminishes proportion metabolized by liver	3.9-mg patch applied to lower abdomen, buttocks, or hip every 3.5 days	As above, irritation of skin under patch occurs in some	
	Tolterodine Tolterodine LA	More selective on muscarinic (M3) receptors than oxybutynin, resulting in fewer anticholinergic side effects	1-2 mg twice daily; may take up to 8 wk to reach optimum benefit; LA, 4 mg	As above but less because of selectivity of M3 bladder receptors over salivary receptors	As above; adjust dosage if concurrent use of cytochrome P-450 3A4 inhibitors (fluoxetine increases concentration by 4.8 times)

Antimuscarinics				
Darifenacin hydrobromide	Highly selective M3 receptor antagonis[t]	7.5 mg daily; if after a minimum of 2 weeks symptoms persist, increase to 15 mg daily	As above; dry mouth and constipation most commonly reported	As above
Solifenacin succinate	Primarily M3 receptor antagonist, with antagonistic properties to M2 receptors as well	5 mg daily; if symptoms persist, may be increased to 10 mg daily if tolerated	As above; side effects specifically related to M3 blockade include dry mouth, constipation, and abnormal vision	As above; hepatic and/or renal impairment
Trospium chloride	Peripheral nonselective antimuscarinic activity; a quaternary amine compound, positively charged, water soluble and bulky that may be less likely to cross the blood brain barrier; NOT metabolized by cytochrome P450 system	20 mg twice daily	As above; most common are dry mouth, constipation, and headache; increased incidence of side effects in elderly (>75 years) NB: Should be taken 1 hour before meals on an empty stomach; as a water-soluble agent, absorption in the gut is decreased; taken with a high-fat meal results in reduced drug absorption	Excreted by renal tubular system; co-administration of drugs competing for active tubular secretion may increase serum concentration of trospium and increase concentrations of other common drugs, such as digoxin, metformin, and morphine
Trospium chloride extended release	Time and pH-dependent coating; not affected by antacids	60 mg daily	Decreased incidence of side effects with daily dose compared with twice daily trospium	Not metabolized by cytochrome P450 pathway therefore decreased likelihood of interactions with drugs using this pathway

Continued

TABLE 6-9 Medications Commonly Prescribed for the Treatment of Urinary Incontinence—cont'd

CLASSIFICATION	GENERIC NAME	MECHANISM OF ACTION	DOSE	SIDE EFFECTS	CONTRAINDICATIONS
	Fesoterodine	New antimuscarinic drug in development; acts functionally as a prodrug; rapid and extensive hydrolyzation by nonspecific esterases to 5-hydroxymethyl tolterodine; conversion is rapid and virtually com-plete; after oral dosing, only the metabolite, not parent compound, can be detected in patient plasma	4 mg and 8 mg daily	As above; decreased incidence of side effects reported in trials; dry mouth most common	As above; under investigation
Neuromuscular blocking agents	Botulinum A toxin (Botox)	Neurotoxin in trials for clinical use for OAB; appears to affect only presynaptic membrane of the neuromuscular junction; prevents calcium-dependent release of acetylcholine and produces a state of denervation; reversible as muscle inactivation persists until new fibrils grow from the nerve (3-9 months on average)	100-500 units per dose; dosage, number of injections, and injection rate remain under investigation	Under investigation; currently reported: muscle weakness, urinary retention, short duration of action (12–36 weeks)	Hypersensitivity to albumin, botulinum toxin, or any component of the formulation; infection at the proposed injection site; diseases of neuromuscular transmission; coagulopathy including therapeutic anticoagulation; uncooperative patient NB: Estimated that the cost of one intraoffice treatment session with intravesical anesthesia is about $1000 every 6 months

Tricyclic antidepressants	Imipramine, doxepin, desipramine, nortriptyline		25 mg at bedtime up to 25 mg three times daily	Anticholinergic side effects described above; α-adrenergic side effects and CNS side effects, including reduced short-term memory or confusion, especially in elderly patients	Decrease in nocturnal UI; side effects common

Drugs That Increase Urethral Sphincter Tone (Benign Prostatic Hyperplasia)

α-Adrenergic agent	Pseudoephedrine	Stimulates α-fibers at bladder neck and sphincter, causing increased tone	75 mg every 12 hr	Hypertension, insomnia, tremor, agitation, palpitations	Patients taking MAO inhibitors, those with hypertension, with narrow-angle glaucoma, and elders
Hormone replacement therapy	Premarin vaginal cream	Reduces irritation from atrophic vaginitis	Cream: 1-2 g at bedtime for 2 wk, then 2× per wk at bedtime	May cause sore breasts; spotting; must be applied intravaginally and not on the labia	Generally contraindicated in women with history of endometrial, ovarian, or breast cancer
	Slow-release estradiol ring	NB: Dose is too low to provide systemic benefits of estrogen therapy	Estradiol ring: change every 3 mo		

Drugs That Decrease Urethral Sphincter Tone (Benign Prostatic Hyperplasia)

α-Adrenergic blockers (agonists)	Terazosin, prazosin, doxazosin	Block α₁A-fibers at the bladder neck and sphincter, causing decreased tone and improving voiding in men with mild obstruction	Varies with medication; for all α-blockers start at a very low dose and gradually increase until therapeutic effect is achieved	Postural hypotension, syncope, fainting (especially with first dose)	Patients taking antihypertensive medications will need to have doses titrated
5-α reductase inhibitors	Finasteride	Inhibits the conversion of testosterone to dihydrotestosterone; this causes a reduction in prostate size and improves voiding symptoms from prostatic enlargement	5 mg/day	Medication taken on a long-term basis; when it is stopped the prostate will gradually increase in size again	Food may delay rate and extent of oral absorption; not indicated in patients with urinary obstruction unless they are being carefully monitored by a urologist

CNS, Central nervous system; GI, gastrointestinal; MAO, monoamine oxidase; PO, by mouth; UI, urinary incontinence.

compared with those who had never smoked.[72] In women cigarette smoking is a risk factor for both stress and urge incontinence[73,74] and increases the risk of UI in older women with chronic obstructive pulmonary disease and chronic respiratory symptoms.[75] These data add one more argument to the urgent need to assist all patients in reducing or stopping smoking.

Weight reduction. Obesity in women is a commonly cited risk factor in the development *and* recurrence of UI that is independent of obstetric history, surgery, smoking, and family history.[76] Obesity, defined as more than 120% of the ideal body weight for height and age, is significantly more prevalent both in women with genuine stress UI and in women with OAB than in the continent population.[77,78] The magnitude of weight loss required to significantly improve or relieve incontinence is not known. Women with profound weight loss after gastric bypass surgery report a significant improvement in stress UI, but more modest weight loss programs may not lead to noticeable improvements.[79] Although weight loss alone may not dramatically reduce UI severity or frequency, maintenance of an ideal body weight is known to produce multiple health benefits, including reduced risk of diabetes, heart disease, and UI.

Physical activity/exercise. An area that has attracted little research related to etiology of UI is physical activity associated with repeated or excessive increases in abdominal pressure. Approximately 31% to 33% of elite nulliparous female athletes and female soldiers report UI with strenuous physical activity.[80-82] How-ever, it should be noted that these women report UI *only* during specific, strenuous activities that may exceed physiologic thresholds of urethral resistance. It is not known whether repetitive exercise that places greater than normal physical stress on the pelvic floor support structures may, over time, lead to damage of the endopelvic fascia or pelvic floor muscles.

Although prevention of UI requires further study, focused pelvic floor muscle therapy may prevent or delay onset of incontinence in postmenopausal continent women.[83] Men aged 40 to 75 years who undertake moderate exercise (walk 2 to 3 hours each week) may have a 25% lower risk of benign prostatic hyperplasia, thus potentially reducing the risk for lower urinary tract symptoms or even obstruction.[84] Based on these observations and given the significant

health benefits associated with exercise, women should be encouraged to engage in routine aerobic exercise and strength training. Women who limit their activities or stop exercising because of UI should be encouraged to restart a regular exercise program as they undergo treatment. An important exception is the woman who has undergone recent urethral suspension surgery who should temporarily refrain from lifting a heavy object or repetitive exercises that stress the pelvic floor until the delicate anastomoses are allowed sufficient time to heal.

Bowel management. A growing body of evidence shows that UI, fecal incontinence, and pelvic organ prolapse are closely related conditions.[85-87] Although vaginal childbirth has been implicated as a major contributing event for UI and pelvic neuropathy, chronic constipation with repeated prolonged straining related to defecation also may contribute to progressive neuropathy and dysfunction.[88] Chronic constipation reduces urinary flow rate, increases voiding time and bladder capacity, and is associated with UI, incomplete bladder emptying, and UTI.[87,89]

Bladder training, scheduled toileting, and prompted toileting. Bladder training is a technique of gradually increasing the length of time between voidings by adherence to a set daytime schedule. Bladder training can improve continence for patients with pure urge, pure stress, and mixed UI symptoms.[90] The initial schedule is determined by the bladder log, and the ultimate goal of voiding frequency is negotiated with the patient. Typically a final goal of 2 to 3 hours is agreed on, and voiding intervals are gradually increased by increments of 15 to 30 minutes using techniques of urge suppression (e.g., pelvic floor muscle contractions, breathing/distraction, and relaxation) (Box 6-2). The program is based on three components: patient education, scheduled voiding, and positive reinforcement.[91,92] Determinants of success include good sensation of bladder fullness, adequate pelvic floor muscle tone (assessed by a pelvic examination), and motivation. Structured pelvic floor muscle therapy with or without biofeedback may improve the effectiveness of bladder training.

Scheduled toileting (timed toileting), usually every 2 to 3 hours, is an adjunct to pharmacotherapy. For example, although antimuscarinic agents are known to increase bladder capacity and diminish the frequency of urge UI episodes, they do not reduce the

BOX 6-2 Bladder Training Protocol (Urge Suppression)—Patient Handout

. . . .

1. Establish a voiding pattern: use a bladder log (fluid volume chart) to record frequency of voiding and fluid intake over 3- to 7-day period.
2. Determine goal for voiding frequency. This negotiation is affected by baseline voiding frequency, an understanding of your goals, and knowledge of the normal range of voiding frequency (every 2 to 4 hours). If frequency is more than every 60 minutes, the initial goal is usually set for voiding every hour. If it is less than every 60 minutes, then start with a 30-minute interval. After 2 to 7 days without urine leakage, increase the time between voids by 15 to 30 minutes. Continue this process until the voiding frequency goal is met.
3. Teach urge suppression along with pelvic floor muscle exercises and distraction techniques to help dissipate the urge to void. Teach the patient to control the urge, take a deep breath, and relax. Stand still or sit down and contract the pelvic floor muscles four or six times. Count backwards from 100. Concentrate on having the urge decrease. Wait until it passes, and then resume activities. If it is longer than 2 hours since they last used the toilet, advise to proceed slowly to the toilet to empty the bladder. Rushing to the toilet will make the symptoms of urgency much worse.
4. Record progress by bladder diary. A daily or weekly bladder log helps to track progress.
5. Follow up regularly. Bladder retraining requires work and commitment. Support and encouragement are important for success. Successful bladder retraining can take several weeks. *See your healthcare professional regularly.*

time between the onset of an overactive contraction and subsequent urine loss nor do they prevent *all* overactive contractions.[93] Scheduled toileting theoretically prevents bladder filling to a volume that triggers an overactive contraction or excessive urine loss with activity. Current research on the effectiveness of scheduled voiding is only modest, and further exploration of the topic is warranted.[94]

Prompted toileting (also called habit training) is scheduled toileting assistance provided by a caregiver and is used for patients with cognitive impairments.[95] A bladder log assesses response to prompted toileting (see Figure 6-9, C). A care provider prompts the person about whether he or she needs to empty the bladder and checks clothing, underpads, or incontinence briefs to assess continence on a prescribed basis, usually every 2 to 3 hours. The caregiver praises the person who is dry and assists the person to toilet. Successful toileting is praised, and the person is informed of the next scheduled toileting prompt. Predictors of success with a prompted voiding program include moderate to mild cognitive impairment, initial success during a 2- to 3-day trial period, and appropriate response to prompts to toilet. In structured settings, results may be improved when a physical exercise program is combined with the prompted voiding routine.[96] Reduction of incontinence episodes and improved skin health are benefits of prompted toileting, but the procedure is labor intensive and nurses must be sensitive to caregiver burden when recommending prompted voiding.[90]

Pelvic floor muscle rehabilitation. Pelvic floor muscle rehabilitation (PFMR) is a mainstay of behavioral therapy for UI and is shown to be effective for patients with stress,[97-98] urge,[99] or mixed UI[100] and following labor and delivery.[101] In women, PFMR combines three principal elements: biofeedback, muscle training, and neuromuscular reeducation. In men, after radical prostatectomy, it remains unclear whether preoperative and/or postoperative PFMR improves achievement of continence. However, the strategy is relatively noninvasive and men may benefit from the support provided by the nurse or physical therapist. A pelvic floor muscle contraction is thought to prevent UI by raising the urethra toward the symphysis pubis, preventing urethral descent, and improving structural support of the pelvic organs.[100] Clinical Highlights for Expert and Advanced Practice: Pelvic Floor Muscle Rehabilitation reviews techniques and principles of PFMR. The benefits of PFMR have been shown to last in patients for as long as 5 years.[102] It should be noted that biofeedback equipment is an adjunct to PFMR. Manual teaching without equipment is clinically effective.

Other behavioral interventions for urinary retention. AUR is a medical emergency that must be resolved by catheterization. However, some interventions may relieve retention, avoiding the need for catheterization. A cup of hot tea or coffee may stimulate micturition. The patient should attempt urination in complete privacy, with her or his feet placed solidly on the floor to maximize pelvic floor relaxation. A warm sitz bath or shower may allow

Clinical Highlights for Expert and Advanced Practice: Pelvic Floor Muscle Rehabilitation[23,135-138]

Pelvic floor muscle rehabilitation (PFMR) is a clinician-directed program of biofeedback, muscle training, and/or neuromuscular reeducation that enhances pelvic floor muscle awareness, improves muscle strength and function, and provides the patient with strategies to use the muscles to improve continence or alleviate retention.

Biofeedback

Biofeedback is any visual, auditory, or tactile intervention that provides cues to previously hidden muscle function. It is a critical element of PFMR necessary for the patient to identify, isolate, contract, and relax the pelvic floor muscles. Identification of the pelvic floor muscles occurs when the patient correctly contracts and relaxes the pelvic floor muscles when desired. Isolation occurs when the patient is able to contract these muscles without simultaneous contraction of the abdominal, thigh, or hip muscles. The significance of biofeedback to PFMR was documented by Bump and coworkers,[135] who demonstrated that when given verbal or written instruction alone, less than half of a group of community-dwelling women were able to effectively contract the pelvic floor muscles and 25% used a technique likely to promote rather than alleviate urine loss.

The following strategies may be used to provide biofeedback as one component of a PFMR program:

- Urine stream interruption: The patient is taught to interrupt the urine stream during micturition. Because this is sometimes confused as a muscle-training or strengthening maneuver, patients must be taught to attempt this maneuver no more than once daily or every other day. Urine stream interruption in women is enhanced by asking them to void backwards, squatting over the toilet rather than seated. This enhances visual feedback from the interrupted stream.
- Digital examination of the vaginal vault or rectum: Placement of the finger in the vaginal vault or rectum, followed by asking the patient to contract the anal or circumvaginal muscles, provides auditory (verbal) and tactile feedback as the patient contracts these muscles against the fixed finger. Gently moving the fingers may enhance tactile feedback. It also provides assessment of pelvic floor muscle strength (see Table 6-6).
- Verbal instruction: Patients may be asked to sequentially contract and relax muscle with verbal cues such as "tap your fingers," "make a fist," or "wink your eye," interspersed with the directive "wink your anus."
- Computer-assisted biofeedback: EMG or pressure can be used to provide biofeedback. An intravaginal probe is preferred for women, and an intrarectal probe is typically used in men. Alternatively, patch electrodes can be used when a vaginal or rectal probe is not desirable or feasible. Feedback is primarily visual information displayed on a computer monitor, but audible (i.e., clinician direction and verbal confirmation of muscle identification and isolation) and tactile feedback is also provided during this interactive process (Figure 6-14). The patient is instructed to squeeze the pelvic floor muscles as if interrupting the urinary stream or tightening (winking) the anus. Verbal instruction is enhanced by placement of the probe and additional instruction to contract the muscle around the probe as if grasping the device and pulling it toward the posterior vagina or rectum. The ultimate result of this instruction is then evaluated by the clinician and instantly displayed to the patient by means of verbal and/or audible feedback generated by electronic equipment.
- Electrical stimulation may assist the patient to identify the pelvic floor muscles. Stimulation may be applied for a period of 3 to 4 seconds followed by a relaxation period of 6 to 8 seconds. A brief series of stimulation/relaxation maneuvers (rest-duty cycles) is administered, and the patient is instructed to carefully attend to the sensations associated with these stimulated pelvic floor muscle contractions. This session is immediately followed by a traditional biofeedback session emphasizing identification, contraction, and relaxation of the pelvic floor muscles.

Muscle Training

Once the patient has been taught to identify, isolate, contract, and relax the pelvic floor muscles, an exercise program is begun to improve pelvic floor muscle function, including maximal strength and endurance. The following maneuvers may be taught:

- Separate maximal strength and endurance exercises are occasionally taught. Maximal strength is enhanced through short maximal contractions (2 to 4 seconds) followed by a brief relaxation period, and endurance can be enhanced through submaximal contraction held for longer periods (6 to 12 seconds) followed by an equal-length rest period.
- Alternatively, a single exercise, with 5 to 10 seconds of submaximal to maximal muscle contraction followed by a rest period of at least equal length, enhances both maximal strength and endurance.

Clinical Highlights for Expert and Advanced Practice: Pelvic Floor Muscle Rehabilitation[23,135-138]—cont'd

• •

- A graded exercise program is used to gradually increase the functional ability and strength of the pelvic floor muscles. The patient is started on fewer repetitions (as few as three to five) and gradually increased to a maximum number of 20 or not more than 50 repetitions each day.

- Patients are taught to exercise on a daily basis in order to allow adequate muscle recovery and to encourage muscle hypertrophy. Patients may be taught to divide the regimen into two sessions each day, but attempts to train the muscles to the point of exhaustion multiple times per day are discouraged since this strategy does not allow adequate time for rest, recovery, and hypertrophy.

- Teach the patient to integrate exercise into the daily routine and to devote a dedicated period for exercise. Exercise during the morning may be encouraged, since pelvic floor muscle performance may be optimal during this period, but regular, daily exercise is emphasized as most important. Exercising while stopped at a traffic light or when performing another task requiring concentration is *discouraged* since it detracts from the patient's appreciation of the proprioceptive sensations associated with pelvic floor muscle contraction and relaxation and it reduces the efficiency of these exercises.

- The time required for improvement and the number of clinician sessions needed to improve continence vary according to the diagnosis, the intrinsic strength of the pelvic floor muscles, and the patient's ability to comply with home exercises. Intense training usually requires 12 to 24 weeks and two to six clinician-directed sessions.

Neuromuscular Reeducation

Neuromuscular coordination teaches the patient to contract and relax pelvic floor muscles in a manner that promotes continence. Strategies of neuromuscular reeducation designed to improve specific UI types include the following:

- Contraction of the pelvic floor muscles immediately before coughing, climbing stairs, or lifting a heavy object in order to prevent stress UI

- Urge suppression to prevent urge UI: When the patient perceives a strong urge to urinate, she or he is advised to deliberately stop and contract the pelvic floor muscles rapidly and maximally for a period of 2 to 3 seconds, followed by a brief period of relaxation (2 to 6 seconds) until the urge to urinate subsides. The patient is then counseled to move to the toilet at a normal pace and urinate. General relaxation methods can be taught to enhance urge suppression (see Box 6-2).

EMG, Electromyography; *UI*, urinary incontinence.

---

adequate relaxation to stimulate voiding while still in the tub or shower stall. Voiding might be stimulated by gently rubbing trigger points within the perineal area, listening to running water, or running warm water over the perineal area. If these strategies do not resolve retention, if the person remains unable to urinate despite 2 to 4 hours of effort, or when urinary retention causes significant discomfort and distention, immediate care in the clinic or local hospital emergency department is required.

Chronic urinary retention (incomplete bladder emptying) may be managed by scheduled toileting, particularly in patients with sensory impairments caused by diabetes mellitus or neurologic disorders. The patient should be taught to urinate every 3 to 4 hours, even if the urge is not perceived. Initially, patients should be encouraged to allow adequate time and effort to urinate in order to "retrain" the bladder

to empty at smaller volumes. Double voiding may help. The patient is taught to urinate, remain seated on the toilet, and attempt a second urination after a brief rest period (approximately 5 minutes). Reading a book or magazine can encourage patience and relaxation while completing a double-voiding technique.

Catheterization. Catheterization is reserved for patients with urinary retention or UI complicated by retention. Intermittent catheterization (IC) can be performed by the patient, a significant other, lay caregiver, or healthcare professional. Experience with spinal cord–injured patients demonstrates that long-term IC is associated with fewer urologic complications than either indwelling or condom catheter containment.[103] Adherence to IC is as high as 71% to 92%, with a continence rate of 45%. Even among spinal cord–injured patients who report leakage

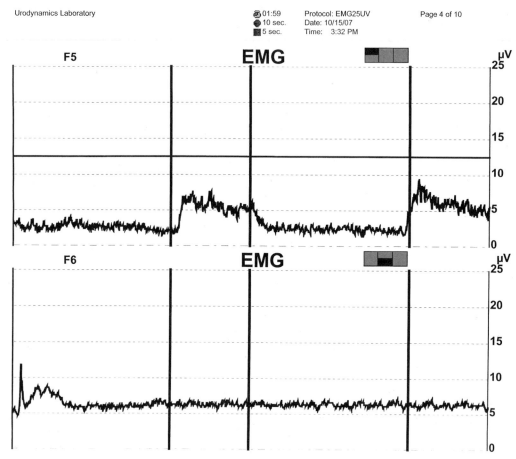

Fig. 6-14 Computer-assisted biofeedback provides immediate cues to pelvic floor and abdominal muscle activity. *EMG,* Electromyogram.

between catheterizations, the majority report urine loss as occurring every other day or less frequently.

In the community, patients are taught to insert the catheter using clean technique, following hand washing with soap and water or an antiseptic hand cleanser. The catheter is inserted until urine returns, and then the bladder is drained completely. The patient is taught to gently pinch or bend the catheter to prevent dribbling urine as the catheter is withdrawn. Following removal, the catheter is rinsed with cool water to remove mucus or other materials and then cleansed with soap and water and air-dried for additional uses. Sterile, single-use catheters are recommended for immunocompromised patients, pregnant women, or any individuals at high risk of systemic infection.[104] If patients wish to sterilize their catheters, microwaving is one alternative. The catheter is cleaned with soap and water and placed in a paper bag; the

catheter should be moist or nearly dry. An 8- to 10-oz glass of water is placed next to the bag to serve as a heat bath and to prevent catheters from melting. Catheters are microwaved on the high setting for 8 to 10 minutes and left to cool in the paper bag until ready to reuse. There is no strong evidence that sterilizing catheters or using a sterile, single-use polyvinyl chloride (PVC) or hydrophilic catheter reduces the incidence of UTI in community-dwelling people. Probably the most critical factor to bladder health is regular emptying with bladder volumes approximately 500 ml or less depending on urodynamic findings.

An indwelling catheter is considered a last resort in continence management. It is reserved for patients with urinary retention, with or without UI, or for persons with UI or retention in a palliative care setting when the demands of toileting cause significant burden. A transient indwelling catheter may be inserted when healing a high-stage pressure ulcer in the perineal area or if a patient is acutely ill and requires fluid output monitoring. Long-term use of an indwelling catheter is avoided because it carries an unacceptably high risk of urologic complications, including infection, calculi, pyelonephritis, and hydronephrosis. A urethral catheter also carries a significant risk of urinary leakage when left in place over a period of years and is associated with a high rate of patient dissatisfaction.[105] There is a 2% to 10% increased risk of bladder cancer in catheterized patients compared with the general population.[106] Although most bladder cancer in the general population is transitional cell carcinoma, squamous cell carcinomas are more common among people managed with a long-term indwelling catheter.[107]

Urethral catheterization is often used initially, but a suprapubic catheter offers potential advantages for some, avoiding the risk of urethral erosion and increasing patient comfort. A slight risk of bowel perforation with insertion of a suprapubic catheter is present. Infection rates and bladder stones are similar to those associated with urethral catheters.

In addition to deliberations about the catheterization site, the material of construction, catheter size, and drainage system should be carefully considered.[108] The ideal catheter is constructed of a material that minimizes mucosal irritation. Latex or silicone latex causes more urothelial inflammation than a silicone or hydrogel-coated catheter.[109] Bacteriuria remains an inevitable consequence of long-term catheterization. Bacteriuria is generally asymptomatic. Routine urine cultures are not indicated and should only be done using a new catheter when the patient is symptomatic. Measures such as urethral cleaning, prophylactic antibiotics, and routine changes are not effective prevention against UTI.

Catheter size and balloon size are also important considerations. A large catheter or improperly filled balloon causes discomfort and increases the risk of urethral erosion. Catheter size refers to the external diameter of the tube, usually quantified as a French size. Balloon size is quantified by the volume of fluid required to *fill* the balloon itself. Since dead space exists in the balloon port, a 5-ml balloon usually requires 10 ml to fill both the sphere and dead space. Improperly filled 30-ml balloons may increase irritation at the bladder neck and the risk of subsequent detrusor hyperreflexia. It is recommended that most adults use a 14F to 16F catheter with a 5-ml balloon

filled with 10 ml of fluid. The drainage system for the indwelling catheter must contain an antireflux valve preventing the backflow of urine from the bag to the bladder. The leg bag should hold at least 500 ml, and overnight bags should hold 2000 to 2500 ml. The patient and care providers are taught to clean the drainage bag using soap and water and then rinse with vinegar or dilute hypochlorite solution.

Pharmacologic Management. Drug therapy differs according to UI type. Table 6-9 provides an overview of the pharmacologic management of UI in adults.

α-Adrenergic agonists, such as pseudoephedrine, act peripherally to stimulate adrenergic receptors in the smooth muscle of the urethra and the rhabdosphincter. A meta-analysis of 15 randomized clinical trials revealed that adrenergic drugs can be effective for managing stress UI when compared with placebos, but insufficient evidence was found to definitively compare the magnitude of this effect with results achieved by PFMR or surgical repair.[110] These agents were previously available as over-the-counter agents, but are now restricted or unavailable because of tightened regulations. Side effects can be significant, including sleeplessness and restlessness, tachycardia, cardiac arrhythmias, and increased blood pressure.

Imipramine is a tricyclic antidepressant that exerts peripheral α-adrenergic and anticholinergic effects. In one small clinical trial, imipramine reduced or resolved stress UI in 60% of women.[111] However, the beneficial effects must be carefully weighed against potential side effects, including dry mouth, drowsiness, tachycardia, increased blood pressure, and cognitive effects.

A new compound, duloxetine (Yentreve), has received approval for the treatment of stress UI in Europe but has not yet been approved for use in the United States.[112,113] Duloxetine is a balanced serotonin and norepinephrine reuptake inhibitor that acts at the level of Onuf's nucleus to increase rhabdosphincter tone and alleviate stress UI. This effect is removed during micturition because of the actions of glutamine (see Chapter 2). The most common side effect is nausea, a common adverse effect for other serotonin-norepinephrine and serotonin reuptake inhibitors. Combining duloxetine with PFMR shows that both therapies are likely equally effective.[114]

Pharmacologic agents to manage OAB dysfunction with and without coexisting urge UI include several closely related types of drugs: anticholinergics, antimuscarinics, and anticholinergic/musculotropic agents.[115] Currently 5 different medications in 8 formulations and 14 doses are available.[116] In reviewing the data, all are similar in effectiveness; the differences lie in side effect profiles. These drugs increase bladder capacity and reduce the frequency of micturition, alleviate detrusor overactivity and bothersome urgency, and reduce the frequency of UI episodes. Assisting patients to understand and manage side effects of these agents is particularly important since their presence and severity profoundly influence long-term adherence to therapy. Common side effects include dry mouth, constipation, dry eyes, dry mucosa (including the vagina), and confusion in some elders. Side effects can be minimized by starting at the lowest possible dose and gradually increasing the dose to a point where an optimal balance between efficacy and side effects is achieved (Table 6-9) The most recent advance in treatment of OAB is the introduction of botulinum toxin-A (Botox). Botox inhibits the release of acetylcholine thus, in the case of the bladder, inhibiting unstable detrusor contractions. Success has been reported in people with idiopathic and neurogenic OAB, and the procedure may be a promising new alternative for individuals who are not successful with medication treatment. Side effects are urinary retention and bladder pain, and current issues are cost and durability of the treatment, ranging from 3 to 6 months at most.[144]

Although estrogen deficiency has been associated with bothersome lower urinary tract symptoms and UI in women, an epidemiologic study of 1525 women found that oral estrogen replacement therapy slightly exacerbated UI.[117,118] In contrast, topical administration of vaginal estrogen may relieve bothersome lower urinary tract symptoms associated with vaginal atrophy, such as urgency, dysuria, vaginal dryness and dyspareunia, or recurring UTI.[119] The decision to administer estrogen replacement therapy is based on multiple factors, and our understanding of the long-term effects of oral estrogen in combination with progestin, unopposed oral estrogen, and intravaginal or topical estrogens continues to evolve. Therefore HRT is prescribed only after close consultation with the patient's primary care provider, gynecologist, urologist, or other care provider.

Two types of drugs may be used for the treatment of urinary retention. Bethanechol chloride is a cholinergic agonist that is designed to increase detrusor contractility. It is administered orally as 25-mg capsules for a daily dosage of 50 to 100 mg. However, the few available clinical and urodynamic studies fail to demonstrate efficacy among most patients with poor detrusor contraction strength or acontractile detrusor function.[120] Side effects include flushing, nausea, vomiting, diarrhea, salivation, headache, and sweating.

α-adrenergic antagonists may be administered to reduce urethral resistance,[120] primarily in the management of benign prostatic hyperplasia (BPH), but may be prescribed to women and men with urinary retention because of bladder neck dyssynergia, prostatitis, vesicosphincter dyssynergia, or poor detrusor contraction strength. See Table 6-9 and Chapter 7 for detailed discussion.

Surgical Management. Surgery is reserved for selected patients with anatomic or functional deficits amenable to surgical reconstruction. Table 6-10 lists surgical options for patients with UI. Detailed nursing management related to individual surgical procedures is reviewed in Chapter 11.

SUMMARY

Recognition, assessment, and management of UI make up a significant portion of urologic nursing practice. Advances in treatment options mean that evaluation and treatment are increasingly initiated in the primary care setting. Nevertheless, many patients are not satisfied with simple interventions, and referral to a urologist or advanced practice nurse with specialized training and knowledge in continence management is indicated. Even within a specialty practice setting, routine evaluation begins with a focused history and physical examination, and more complex assessment is reserved for selected patients. Likewise, treatment begins with minimally invasive techniques, such as dietary and lifestyle modifications and PFMR, often combined with pharmacotherapy. However, even when more complex testing and surgical intervention are indicated, the urologic nurse continues to play a central role in managing the patient with UI.

TABLE 6-10 Surgical Management of Stress and Urge Urinary Incontinence in the Adult[134]

UI TYPE	PROCEDURE	BRIEF DESCRIPTION AND COMPLICATIONS
Stress UI	Retropubic procedures	Collection of surgical procedures designed to correct descent (hypermobility) of bladder base; the retropubic space is approached through a lower midline abdominal or Pfannenstiel incision. Compensatory support for the bladder base is achieved using the cartilage of the symphysis pubis (MMK), Cooper's ligament (Burch), or the arcus tendineus (paravaginal repair).
	Marshall-Marchetti-Krantz (MMK)	Postoperative complications
	Burch colposuspension	Transient postoperative urinary retention
	Paravaginal repair	De novo or persistent OAB dysfunction
		Exacerbation of posterior vaginal prolapse with enterocele
	Laparoscopic retropubic suspension	Uses laparoscopic approach to access retropubic space and provide compensatory support to bladder base and proximal urethra; potential advantages include avoidance of open incision and reduced hospital stay; potential disadvantages include prolonged surgical time and higher associated costs.
		Postoperative complications are similar to those for any retropubic suspension.
	Needle procedures	The bladder base is approached from a vaginal incision.
	Pereyra	The Pereyra uses a T-shaped vaginal incision and a needle stylet to fix absorbable sutures to periurethral tissue over the rectus fascia.
	Stamey	The Stamey modifies the Pereyra by (1) incorporating endoscopy to ensure sutures are placed at the bladder neck, (2) substituting nonabsorbable sutures with Dacron vaginal pledgets to buttress the periurethral tissue and reduce risk of sutures pulling through the tissue, and (3) using a blunt needle (Stamey needle) designed to provide greater technical ease when completing the procedure.
	Gittes	The Gittes uses two suprapubic stab incisions to pass two Stamey needles and sutures through the vaginal wall at the bladder neck. A Mayo needle is then used to take helical bites of tissue before the sutures are tied over the abdominal wall. Subsequent scarring is postulated to provide compensatory support for the bladder base.
	Raz needle suspension	The Raz procedure modified the Stamey by (1) incorporating a U-shaped incision, (2) entering the retropubic space through this vaginal approach, detaching periurethral tissue from the arcus tendineus, and (3) creating compensatory support by passing helical sutures through the vaginal and abdominal walls.
		Postoperative complications
		Transient urinary retention
		Persistent or de novo detrusor overactivity
		Pelvic pain or dyspareunia
		Exacerbation of pelvic organ prolapse

Continued

TABLE 6-10 Surgical Management of Stress and Urge Urinary Incontinence in the Adult[134]—cont'd

UI TYPE	PROCEDURE	BRIEF DESCRIPTION AND COMPLICATIONS
	Tension-free vaginal tape (TVT) procedure	A loose-weave polypropylene mesh tape is passed under the proximal third of the urethra to enhance compression. Tension against the urethra is avoided to prevent obstruction. Three small incisions are required for placement, including two 1-cm incisions in the abdominal wall and a 1.5-cm incision in the vagina.
	Bone-anchoring procedures	These procedures use approaches similar to vaginal suspensions described above, but anchors are placed in the pubic bones to prevent dislodgement of sutures from the vaginal wall, nerve entrapment and subsequent pain, and problems arising from mobility of the rectus fascia.
	Anterior colporrhaphy (Kelly plication)	Provides compensatory support when prolapse affects midline support resulting in a cystocele. A midline incision is made in the vagina to within 1 cm of the urethral meatus. Plication sutures are inserted to provide compensatory support for bladder base and proximal urethra.
	Suburethral sling procedures	Surgical techniques that enhance urethral compression by placing a sling (hammock) beneath the proximal third of the urethra, while avoiding any tension against the urethra. Access may be gained by abdominal or vaginal incision. A variety of materials have been used to create a sling including autologous fascia harvested from the fascia lata, abdominal wall, or vaginal wall; cadaveric fascia; or synthetic materials including Gore-Tex, Mersilene, or polypropylene.
	Suburethral injection	Synthetic materials are injected beneath the mucosa of the proximal urethra, avoiding the rhabdosphincter. Available synthetic materials include glutaraldehyde cross-linked (GAX) bovine collagen and nonresorbable pyrolytic carbon-coated zirconium beads (Durasphere). Autologous fat and blood have been investigated as potential alternatives to synthetic materials.
	Artificial urinary sphincter (AUS)	The device contains three principal components: (1) a silicone balloon reservoir, (2) a sleevelike cuff that wraps around the urethra creating compression, and (3) a pump mechanism with deactivation button connected by kink-resistant tubing. The AUS is placed in men through a midline perineal incision and in women through an abdominal or transvaginal incision. The urethral cuff is usually placed around the bulbar urethra in men, the reservoir in the lower abdomen, and the deactivation device in the scrotum. In women the urethral cuff is typically placed at the bladder neck, the balloon reservoir in the lower abdomen, and the pump within the labia majora. The device is initially left deactivated for 6 wk to allow healing. *Postoperative complications* Hematoma Infection (may require explantation and replacement) Tissue atrophy underneath the cuff Loss of bladder wall compliance, hydronephrosis, and upper urinary tract distress

TABLE 6-10 Surgical Management of Stress and Urge Urinary Incontinence in the Adult[134]—cont'd

UI TYPE	PROCEDURE	BRIEF DESCRIPTION AND COMPLICATIONS
Urge UI	Augmentation enterocystoplasty	An abdominal incision is used to bivalve the urinary bladder. An intestinal segment is isolated from the fecal stream, cut along its antimesenteric border, and folded in a U, S, or W configuration to create an approximately spherical structure when attached to the bivalved bladder. Following surgery, the bladder must be regularly drained by intermittent catheterization. *Postoperative complications* Excessive mucus production associated with blockage of catheter and incomplete bladder evacuation and increased risk for vesical calculi Disruption of anatomic integrity of augmented bladder Chronic diarrhea Metabolic acidosis Vitamin B_{12} deficiency (usually seen 1-2 yr postoperatively)
	Autoaugmentation	The bladder is approached through an abdominal incision or using laparoscopic techniques. The detrusor is incised in order to form a large diverticulum. Although this procedure clearly increases bladder wall compliance, it has been found to provide only modest improvement in bladder capacity. A potential advantage of the procedure is avoidance of metabolic acidosis, malabsorption, or stool elimination complications associated with augmentation enterocystoplasty. *Postoperative complications* Bladder wall scarring or contracture Recurrence of OAB symptoms over time
	Implantation of a neuromodulation device	The procedure is typically completed in two stages. Initially, percutaneous probes are placed into a sacral foramen and tested for potential efficacy (ablation of detrusor overactivity and OAB symptoms). If efficacy is achieved, a permanent four-lead device is implanted into the same sacral foramen and anchored to the periosteum of the sacral bone. The procedure requires general anesthesia, but paralytic anesthetic agents are avoided since they interfere with testing for placement when the device is implanted. A simpler, one-stage technique has been described and is now preferred by some surgeons. *Potential postoperative complications* Pain at the site of the generator or a lead site Lead migration with compromised efficacy Infection of the device

OAB, Overactive bladder; *UI,* urinary incontinence.

REFERENCES

1. Abrams P, Cardozo L, Fall M, Griffiths G, Rosier P, Ulmsten U, van Kerrebroeck P, Victor A, Wein A: The standardization of terminology of lower urinary tract function: report from the Standardization Sub-Committee of the International Continence Society. Neurourology and Urodynamics, 2002; 21:167-78.
2. Gray M: Gender, race and culture research in UI. American Journal of Nursing, 2003; 3(suppl):20-25.
3. Hunskaar S, Burgio K, Clark A, Lapitan MC, Nelson R, Sillén U, et al: Epidemiology of urinary (UI) and faecal (FI) incontinence, & pelvic organ prolapse (POP). In Abrams P, Cardozo L, Khoury S, Wein AJ (eds): Incontinence: 3rd International Consultation on Urinary Incontinence. Plymouth, UK: Plymbridge, 2005; pp 255-312.
4. Van Oyen H, Van Oyen P: Urinary incontinence in Belgium; prevalence, correlates and psychosocial consequences. Acta Clinica Belgica, 2002; 57:207-18.
5. Anger JT, Saigal CS, Litwin MS: The prevalence of urinary incontinence among community dwelling adult women: results from the National Health and Nutrition Examination Survey. Journal of Urology, 2006; 175:601-4.
6. Chen GD, Lin TL, Hu SW, Chen YC, Lin LY: Prevalence and correlation of urinary incontinence and overactive bladder in Taiwanese women. Neurourology and Urodynamics, 2003; 22:109-17.
7. Lewis CM, Schrader R, Many A, Mackay M, Rogers RG: Diabetes and urinary incontinence in 50- to 90-year old women: a cross-sectional population-based study. American Journal of Obstetrics and Gynecology, 2005; 193:2154-58.
8. Brown JS, Wing R, Barrett-Connor E, Nyberg LM, Kusek JW, Orchard TJ, Ma Y, Vittinghoff C, Kanaya AM: Lifestyle intervention is associated with lower prevalence of urinary incontinence: The Diabetes Prevention Program. Diabetes Care, 2006; 29:385-90.
9. Vigod SN, Stewart DE: Major depression in female urinary incontinence. Psychosomatics, 2006; 47:147-51.
10. Nygaard I, Turvey C, Burns TL, Crischilles E, Wallace R: Urinary incontinence and depression in middle-aged United States women. Obstetrics and Gynecology, 2003; 101:149-56.
11. Wilson PD, Berghmans B, Hagen S, Hay-Smith J, Moore K, Nygaard I: Adult conservative management. In Abrams P, Cardozo L, Khoury S, Wein AJ (eds): Incontinence: 3rd International Consultation on Urinary Incontinence. Plymouth, UK: Plymbridge, 2005; pp 855-964.
12. Pfisterer MH, Griffiths DJ, Schaefer W, Resnick NM: The effect of age on lower urinary tract function: a study in women. Journal of the American Geriatric Society, 2006; 54:405-12.
13. Dubeau CE: The aging lower urinary tract. Journal of Urology, 2006; 175:S11-15.
14. Anger JT, Saigal CS, Pace J, Rodriguez LV, Litwin MS: True prevalence of urinary incontinence among female nursing home residents. Urology, 2006; 67:281-87.
15. Wagg A, Mian S, Lowe D, Potter J, Pearson M: Continence Programme Working Party: National audit of continence care for older people: results of a pilot study. Journal of Evaluation in Clinical Practice, 2005; 11:525-32.
16. Hannestad YS, Rortveit G, Sandvik H, Hunskaar S: Epidemiology of incontinence in the County of Nord-Trondelag: a community-based epidemiological survey of female urinary incontinence: the Norwegian EPINCONT study. Journal of Clinical Epidemiology, 2000; 53:1150-7.
17. Thom DH, van den Eeden SK, Ragins AI, Wassel-Fyr C, Vittinghoff E, Subak LL, Brown JS: Differences in prevalence of urinary incontinence by race/ethnicity. Journal of Urology, 2006; 175:259-64.
18. Duong TH, Korn AP: A comparison of urinary incontinence among African American, Asian, Hispanic and white women. American Journal of Obstetrics and Gynecology, 2001; 184:1083-6.
19. Graham CA, Mallett VT: Race as a predictor of urinary incontinence and pelvic organ prolapse. American Journal of Obstetrics and Gynecology, 2001; 185:116-20.
20. Foxman B, Somsel P, Tallman P, Gillespie B, Raz R, Colodner R, Kandula D, Sobel JD: Urinary tract infection among women aged 40 to 65: behavioral and sexual risk factors. Journal of Clinical Epidemiology, 2001; 54:710-8.
21. Molander U, Arvidsson L, Milsom I, Sandberg T: A longitudinal cohort study of elderly women with urinary tract infections. Maturitas, 2000; 34:127-31.
22. Grady D, Brown JS, Vittinghoff E, Applegate W, Varner E, Snyder T: The HERS Research Group. Postmenopausal hormones and incontinence: the Heart and Estrogen/Progestin Replacement Study. Obstetrics and Gynecology, 2001; 97:116-20.
23. Miller JM, Ashton-Miller JA, Delancey JO: Quantification of cough-related urine loss using the paper towel test. Obstetrics and Gynecology, 1998; 91:705-9.
24. Gray ML, Moore KN: Assessment of patients with urinary incontinence. In Doughty DB (ed): Urinary and Fecal Incontinence: Current Management Concepts, 3rd edition. St Louis: Mosby, 2006; pp 341-412.
25. Shull BL: Pelvic organ prolapse: anterior, superior, and posterior vaginal segment defects. American Journal of Obstetrics and Gynecology, 1999; 181:6-11.
26. Ashton-Miller JA, Howard D, Delancey JO: The functional anatomy of the female pelvic floor and stress continence control system. Scandinavian Journal of Urology and Nephrology, 2001; supplement(207):1-7.
27. Olsen AL, Smith VJ, Bergstrom JO, Colling JC, Clark AL: Epidemiology of surgically managed pelvic organ prolapse and urinary incontinence. Obstetrics and Gynecology, 1997; 89:501-6.
28. Macura KJ, Genadry RR, Bluemke DA: MR imaging of the female urethra and supporting ligaments in assessment of urinary incontinence: spectrum of abnormalities. Radiographics, 2006; 26:1135-49.
29. Miller J, Hoffman E: The causes and consequences of overactive bladder. Journal of Women's Health, 2006; 15:251-60.
30. Stewart WF, Van Rooyen JB, Cundiff GW, Abrams P, Herzog AR, Corey R, Hunt TL, Wein AJ: Prevalence and burden of overactive bladder in the United States. World Journal of Urology, 2003; 20(6):327-36.
31. Irwin DE, Milsom I, Hunskaar S, Reilly K, Kopp Z, Herschorn S, Coyn K, Kelleher C, Hampel C, Artibani W, Abrams P: Population-based survey of urinary incontinence, overactive bladder, and other lower urinary tract symptoms in five countries: results of the EPIC study. European Urology, 2006; 50(6):1306-14.
32. Milsom I, Stewart W, Thuroff J: The prevalence of overactive bladder. American Journal of Managed Care, 2000; 6(11, suppl):S565-73.
33. Blaivas JG: Overactive bladder: symptom or syndrome?. BJU International, 2003; 92(6):521-2.
34. Chaikin DC, Blaivas JG: Voiding dysfunction: definitions. Current Opinion in Urology, 2001; 11(4):395-8.
35. Bump RC, Norton PA, Zinner NR, Yalcin I: Mixed urinary incontinence symptoms: urodynamic findings, incontinence severity and treatment response. Obstetrics and Gynecology, 2003; 102(1):76-83.
36. Flores-Carreras O, Cabrera JR, Galeano PA, Torres FE: Fistulas of the urinary tract in gynecologic and obstetric surgery. International Urogynecology Journal, 2001; 12:203-14.
37. Rovner ES: Urinary tract fistula. In Wein AJ, Kavoussi LR, Novick AC, Partin AW, Peters CA (eds): Campbell's Urology, 9th edition. Philadelphia: Saunders, 2007; pp 2322-60.
38. Hunter K, Moore KN, Glazener CM: Conservative management of post prostatectomy incontinence. Cochrane Database Systematic Reviews, 2007; 2:CD001843.
39. Jacobsen N, Moore KN, Estey E, Voaklander E: Open versus laparoscopic radical prostatectomy: a prospective comparison of postoperative urinary incontinence rates. Journal of Urology, 2007; 177:615-619.
40. Gray M: Urinary retention: management in the acute care setting. 1. 2000; 100(7):40-8.
41. Gray M: Urinary retention: management in the acute care setting. 2. American Journal of Nursing, 2000; 100(8):36-44.

42. Dorey G, Speakman M, Fenely R, Swinkels A, Dunn C, Ewings P: Pelvic floor muscle exercises for treating post-micturition dribble in men with erectile dysfunction: a randomized controlled trial. Urologic Nursing, 2004; 24:490-7,512.

43. Nezu FM, Vasavada SP: Evaluation and management of female urethral diverticulum. Techniques in Urology, 2001; 7:169-75.

44. Moore KN: Pathology and management of acute and chronic urinary retention. In Doughty DB (ed): Urinary and Fecal Incontinence: Current Management Concepts, 3rd edition. St Louis: Mosby, 2006; pp 225-53.

45. Norton C: Constipation in older patients: effects on quality of life. British Journal of Nursing, 2006; 15:188-92.

46. Meschia M, Buonaguidi A, Pifarotti P, Somigliana E, Spennacchio M, Amicarelli F: Prevalence of anal incontinence in women with symptoms of urinary incontinence and genital prolapse. Obstetrics and Gynecology, 2002; 100:719-23.

47. Roberts RO, Jacobsen SJ, Reilly WT, Pemberton JH, Lieber MM, Talley NJ: Prevalence of combined fecal and urinary incontinence: a community-based study. Journal of the American Geriatrics Society, 1999; 47:837-41.

48. Brink CA, Sampselle CM, Wells TJ, Diokno AC, Gillis GL: A digital test for pelvic muscle strength in older women with urinary incontinence. Nursing Research, 1989; 38:196-9.

49. Laycock J: Clinical evaluation of the pelvic floor. In Schussler B, Laycock J, Norton P, Stanton SL (eds): Pelvic Floor Reeducation, 1st edition. London: Springer-Verlag, 1994; pp 42-8.

50. Burgio KL, Locher JL, Goode PS: Combined behavioral and drug therapy for urge incontinence in older women. Journal of the American Geriatrics Society, 2000; 48:370-4.

51. Getliffe K, Fader M, Cottenden A, Jamieson K, Green N: Absorbent products for incontinence: 'treatment effects' and impact on quality of life. Journal of Clinical Nursing, 2007; 16(10):1936-45.

52. Dunn S, Kowanko I, Patterson J, Petty L: Systematic review of the effectiveness of urinary continence products. Journal of Wound, Ostomy and Continence Nursing, 2002; 29:129-42.

53. Saint S, Kaufman SR, Rogers MA, Baker PD, Ossenkop K, Lipsky BA: Condom versus indwelling urinary catheters: a randomized trial. Journal of the American Geriatrics Society, 2006; 54:1055-61.

54. Saint S, Lipsky BA, Baker PD, McDonald LL, Ossenkop K: Urinary catheters: what type do men and their nurses prefer?. Journal of the American Geriatrics Society, 1999; 47:1453-7.

55. Brubaker L, Harris T, Gleason D, Newman D, North B: The external urethral barrier for stress incontinence: a multicenter trial of safety and efficacy. Miniguard Investigators Group. Obstetrics and Gynecology, 1999; 93:932-7.

56. Moore KN, Schieman S, Ackerman T, Dzus HY, Metcalfe JB, Voaklander DC: Assessing comfort, safety, and patient satisfaction with three commonly used penile compression devices. Urology, 2004; 63:150-4.

57. Fernando RJ, Thakar R, Sultan AH, Shah SM, Jones PW: Effect of vaginal pessaries on symptoms associated with pelvic organ prolapse. Obstetrics and Gynecology, 2006; 108:93-9.

58. Hanson LA, Schultz JA, Flood CG, Cooley B, Tam F: Vaginal pessaries in managing women with pelvic floor prolapse and urinary incontinence: patient characteristics and factors contributing to success. International Urogynecology Journal, 2006; 17:155-9.

59. Wu V, Farrell SA, Baskett TF, Flowerdew G: A simplified protocol for pessary management. Obstetrics and Gynecology, 1997; 90:990-4.

60. Dowd TT, Campbell JM, Jones JA: Fluid intake and urinary incontinence in older community-dwelling women. Journal of Community Health Nursing, 1996; 13:179-86.

61. Tomlinson BU, Dougherty MC, Pendergast JF, Boyington AR, Coffman MA, Pickens SM: Dietary caffeine, fluid intake and urinary incontinence in older rural women. International Urogynecology Journal, 1999; 10:22-8.

62. Gray M: Does fluid intake influence the risk for urinary incontinence, urinary tract infection and bladder cancer?. Journal of Wound, Ostomy and Continence Nursing, 2003; 30:126-31.

63. Panel on Dietary Reference Intakes for Electrolytes and Water, Standing Committee on the Scientific Evaluation of Dietary Reference Intakes. In Dietary Reference Intakes for Water, Potassium, Sodium, Chloride, and Sulfate. Washington, D.C: The National Academies Press, 2004; p 73.

64. Griffiths DJ, McCracken PN, Harrison GM, Gormley EA: Relationship of fluid intake to voluntary micturition and urinary incontinence in geriatric patients. Neurourology and Urodynamics, 1993; 12:1-7.

65. Creighton SM, Stanton SL: Caffeine: does it affect your bladder?. British Journal of Urology, 1990; 66:613-4.

66. Gray M: Caffeine and urinary incontinence. Journal of Wound, Ostomy and Continence Nursing, 2001; 28:66-9.

67. Swithinbank L, Hashim H, Abrams P: The effect of fluid intake on urinary symptoms in women. Journal of Urology, 2005; 174:187-189.

68. Fried GW, Goetz G, Potts-Nulty S, Cioschi HM, Staas WE Jr: A behavioral approach to the treatment of urinary incontinence in a disabled population. Archives of Physical Medicine and Rehabilitation, 1995; 76:1120-4.

69. Bryant CM, Dowell CJ, Fairbrother G: Caffeine reduction education to improve urinary symptoms. British Journal of Nursing, 2002; 11:560-5.

70. Parazzini F, Colli E., Origgi G, Surace M, Bianchi M, Benzi G, Artibani W: Risk factors for urinary incontinence in women. European Urology, 2000; 37:637-43.

71. Denays R, Tondeur M, Noel P, Ham HR: Bilateral cerebral mediofrontal hypoactivity in Tc-99m HMPAO SPECT imaging. Clinical Nuclear Medicine, 1994; 19:873-6.

72. Koskimaki J, Hakama M, Huhtala H, Tammela TL: Association of smoking with lower urinary tract symptoms. Journal of Urology, 1998; 159:1580-2.

73. Danforth KN, Townsend MK, Lifford K, Curhan GC, Resnick NM, Grodstein F: Risk factors for urinary incontinence among middle-aged women. American Journal of Obstetrics and Gynecology, 2006; 194:339-45.

74. Hannestad Y, Rortveit G, Daltveit A, Hunskaar S: Are smoking and other lifestyle factors associated with female urinary incontinence? The Norwegian EPINCONT Study. BJOG: International Journal of Obstetrics and Gynecology, 2003; 110:247-54.

75. Diokno AC, Brock BM, Herzog AR, Bromberg J: Medical correlates of urinary incontinence in the elderly. Urology, 1990; 36:129-38.

76. Bouldin MJ, Ross LA, Sumrall CD, Loustalot FV, Low AK, Land KK: The effect of obesity surgery on obesity comorbidity. American Journal of the Medical Sciences, 2006; 331:183-93.

77. Richter HE, Burgio KL, Clements RH, Goode PS, Redden DT, Varner RE: Urinary and anal incontinence in morbidly obese women considering weight loss surgery. Obstetrics and Gynecology, 2005; 106:1272-7.

78. Kolbl H, Riss P: Obesity and stress urinary incontinence: significance of indices of relative weight. Urologia Internationalis, 1988; 43:7-10.

79. Bump RC, Sugerman HJ, Fantl JA, McClish DK: Obesity and lower urinary tract function in women: effect of surgically induced weight loss. American Journal of Obstetrics and Gynecology, 1992; 167:392-9.

80. Bø K, Stien R, Kulseng-Hanssen S, Kristofferson M: Clinical and urodynamic assessment of nulliparous young women with and without stress incontinence symptoms: a case control study. Obstetrics and Gynecology, 1994; 84:1028-32.

81. Caylet N, Fabbro-Peray P, Marès P, Dauzat M, Prat-Pradal D, Corcos J: Prevalence and occurrence of stress urinary incontinence in elite women athletes. Canadian Journal of Urology, 2006; 13:3174-9.

82. Davis G, Sherman R, Wong MF, McClure G, Perez R, Hibbert M: Urinary incontinence among female soldiers. Military Medicine, 1999; 164:182-7.

83. Diokno AC, Sampselle CM, Herzog AR, Raghunathan TE, Hines S, Messer KL, Karl C, Leite MC: Prevention of urinary incontinence by behavioral modification program: a randomized, controlled trial

among older women in the community. Journal of Urology, 2004; 171:1165-71.

84. Platz EA, Kawachi I, Rimm EB, Colditz GA, Stampfer MJ, Willett WC, Giovannucci E: Physical activity and benign prostatic hyperplasia. Archives of Internal Medicine, 1998; 158:2349-56.

85. Pannek J, Haupt G, Sommerfeld H-J, Schulze H, Senge T: Urodynamic and rectomanometric findings in urinary incontinence. Scandinavian Journal of Urology and Nephrology, 1996; 30:457-60.

86. Smith AR, Hosker GL, Warrell DW: The role of pudendal nerve damage in the aetiology of genuine stress incontinence in women. British Journal of Obstetrics and Gynaecology, 1989; 96:29-32.

87. Ng SC, Chen YC, Lin LY, Chen GD: Anorectal dysfunction in women with urinary incontinence or lower urinary tract symptoms. International Journal of Gynecology and Obstetrics, 2002; 77:139-45.

88. Lubowski DZ, Swash M, Nicholls RJ, Henry MM: Increase in pudendal nerve terminal motor latency with defaecation straining. British Journal of Surgery, 1988; 75:1095-7.

89. MacDonald A, Shearer M, Paterson PJ, Finlay IG: Relationship between outlet obstruction constipation and obstructed urinary flow. British Journal of Surgery, 1991; 78:693-5.

90. Ostaszkiewicz J, Johnston L, Roe B: Habit training for urinary incontinence in adults. Cochrane Database Systematic Review, 2004; 2:CD002801.

91. Elser DM, Wyman JF, McClish DK, Robinson D, Fantl JA, Bump RC: The effect of bladder training, pelvic floor muscle training, or combination training on urodynamic parameters in women with urinary incontinence. Continence Program for Women Research Group. Neurourology and Urodynamics, 1999; 18:427-36.

92. Wyman JF, Fantl JA: Bladder training in ambulatory care management of urinary incontinence. Urologic Nursing, 1991; 11:11-7.

93. Wein AJ: Pharmacological agents for the treatment of urinary incontinence due to overactive bladder. Expert Opinion on Investigational Drugs, 2001; 10:65-83.

94. Ostaszkiewicz J, Roe B, Johnston L: Effects of timed voiding for the management of urinary incontinence in adults: systematic review. Journal of Advanced Nursing, 2005; 52:420-31.

95. Pinkowski PS: Prompted voiding in the long-term care facility. Journal of Wound, Ostomy and Continence Nursing, 1996; 23:110-4.

96. Ouslander JG, Griffiths PC, McConnell E, Riolo L, Kutner M, Schnelle J: Functional incidental training: a randomized, controlled, crossover trial in Veterans Affairs nursing homes. Journal of the American Geriatrics Society, 2005; 53:1091-100.

97. Bø K, Talseth T, Holme I: Single blind randomized controlled trial of pelvic floor exercises, electrical stimulation, vaginal cones or no treatment in management of genuine stress incontinence in women. British Medical Journal, 1999; 318:487-93.

98. Wells TJ, Brink CA, Diokno AC, Wolfe R, Gillis CL: Pelvic muscle exercise for stress urinary incontinence in elderly women. Journal of the American Geriatrics Society, 1991; 38:785-91.

99. Burgio KL, Locher JL, Goode PS, Hardin JM, McDowell BJ, Dombrowski M, Candib D: Behavioral vs. drug treatment for urge urinary incontinence in older women: a randomized controlled trial. Journal of the American Medical Association, 1998; 280:1995-2000.

100. Hay-Smith EJ, Dumoulin C: Pelvic floor muscle training versus no treatment, or inactive control treatments, for urinary incontinence in women. Cochrane Database Systematic Review, 2006; 1(Jan 25):CD005654.

101. Chiarelli P, Cockburn J: Promoting urinary continence in women after delivery: randomised controlled trial. British Medical Journal, 2002; 324:1241-53.

102. Bø K: Adherence to pelvic floor muscle exercises and long-term effect on stress urinary incontinence: a five year follow up study. Scandinavian Journal of Medicine & Science in Sports, 1995; 1:36-9.

103. Ku JH, Choi WJ, Lee KY, Jung TY, Lee JK, Park WH, Shim HB: Complications of the upper urinary tract in patients with spinal

cord injury: a long-term follow-up study. Urological Research, 2005; 33:435-9.

104. Moore KN, Fader M, Getliffe K: Long-term bladder management by intermittent catheterisation in adults and children. Cochrane Database Systematic Reviews, 2007; 4.

105. Wilde MH, Cameron BL: Meanings and practical knowledge of people with long-term urinary catheters. Journal of Wound, Ostomy and Continence Nursing, 2003; 30:33-40.

106. Hess MJ, Zhan EH, Foo DK, Yalla SV: Bladder cancer in patients with spinal cord injury. Journal of Spinal Cord Medicine, 2003; 26:335-8.

107. West DA, Cummings JM, Longo WE, Virgo KS, Johnson FE, Parra RO: Role of chronic catheterization in the development of bladder cancer in patients with spinal cord injury. Urology, 1999; 53:292-7.

108. Cox AJ: Effect of a hydrogel coating on the surface topography of latex-based urinary catheters: an SEM study. Biomaterials, 1987; 8:500-2.

109. Talja M, Korpela A, Jarvi K: Comparison of urethral reaction to full silicone, hydrogen-coated and siliconised latex catheters. British Journal of Urology, 1990; 66:652-7.

110. Alhasso A, Glazener CMA, Pickard R, N'Dow J: Adrenergic drugs for urinary incontinence in adults. Cochrane Database Systematic Review, 2005; 3(July 20):CD001842.

111. Lin HH, Sheu BC, Lo MC, Huang SC: Comparison of treatment outcomes for imipramine for female genuine stress incontinence. British Journal of Obstetrics and Gynaecology, 1999; 106:1089-92.

112. Dmochowski RR, Miklos JR, Norton PA, Zinner NR, Yalcin I, Bump RC: Duloxetine Urinary Incontinence Study Group. Duloxetine versus placebo for the treatment of North American women with stress urinary incontinence. Journal of Urology, 2003; 170(4, pt 1):1259-63.

113. Norton PA, Zinner NR, Yalcin I, Bump RC: Duloxetine Urinary Incontinence Study Group. Duloxetine versus placebo in the treatment of stress urinary incontinence. American Journal of Obstetrics and Gynecology, 2002; 187(1):40-8.

114. Ghoniem GM, Van Leeuwen JS, Elser DM, Freeman RM, Zhao YD, Yalcin I, Bump RC: A randomized controlled trial of duloxetine alone, pelvic floor muscle training alone, combined treatment and no active treatment in women with stress urinary incontinence. Journal of Urology, 2005; 173:1647-53.

115. Hay-Smith J, Herbison P, Ellis G, Morris A: Which anticholinergic drug for overactive bladder symptoms in adults. Cochrane Database Systematic Review, 2005; 3(July 20):CD005429.

116. Taylor P: Pharmacologic management of overactive bladder. Journal of Wound, Ostomy and Continence Nursing, 2005; 32:S16-24.

117. Hendrix SL, Cochrane BB, Nygaard IE, Handa VL, Barnabei VM, Iglesia C, Aragaki A, Naughton MJ, Wallace RB, McNeeley SG: Effects of estrogen with and without progestin on urinary incontinence. Journal of the American Medical Association, 2005; 293:935-48.

118. Grady D, Brown JS, Vittinghoff E, Applegate W, Varner E, Snyder T: The HERS Research Group. Postmenopausal hormones and incontinence: the Heart and Estrogen/Progestin Replacement Study. Obstetrics and Gynecology, 2001; 97(1):116-20.

119. Cardozo L, Lose G, McClish D, Versi E, de Koning Gans H: A systematic review of estrogens for recurrent urinary tract infections: third report of the hormones and urogenital therapy (HUT) committee. International Urogynecology Journal, 2001; 12(1):15-20.

120. Wein AJ: Lower urinary tract dysfunction in neurologic injury and disease. In Wein AJ, Kavoussi LR, Novick AC, Partin AW, Peters CA (eds): Campbell's Urology, 9th edition. Philadelphia: Saunders, 2007; pp 931-1026 [Chapter 59].

121. Gray M, Rayome R, Moore KN: The urethral sphincter: an update. Urologic Nursing, 1995; 15(2):40-55.

122. de Groat WC: A neurologic basis for the overactive bladder. Urology, 1997; 50(6A, suppl):36-52.

123. Thomas AW, Abrams P: Lower urinary tract symptoms, benign prostatic obstruction and the overactive bladder. BJU International, 2000; 85(supp. 3):57-68.

124. Gunnarsson M, Mattiasson A: Female stress, urge, and mixed urinary incontinence are associated with a chronic and progressive pelvic floor/vaginal neuromuscular disorder: an investigation of 317 healthy and incontinent women using vaginal surface electromyography. Neurourology and Urodynamics, 1999; 18:613-21.

125. Brading AF: A myogenic basis for the overactive bladder. Urology, 1997; 50(6A, suppl):57-67.

126. Ahlberg J, Edlund C, Wikkelso C, Rosengren L: Fall M: Neurological signs are common in patients with urodynamically verified "idiopathic" bladder overactivity. Neurourology and Urodynamics, 2002; 21:65-70.

127. Romics I, Kelemen Z, Fazakas Z: The diagnosis and management of vesicovaginal fistulae. BJU International, 2002; 89:764-6.

128. Jonas D, Beecken WD: An easy method to localize the vesical opening of an enterovesical fistula. Journal of Urology, 2002; 167:1794-6.

129. Bergqvist D, Pärsson H, Sherif A: Arterio-ureteral fistula—a systematic review. European Journal of Vascular and Endovascular Surgery, 2001; 22:191-6.

130. Sharma AK, Kothari SK, Menon P, Sharma A: Congenital H-type rectourethral fistula. Pediatric Surgery International, 2002; 18:193-4.

131. Boushey RP, McLeod RS, Cohen Z: Surgical management of acquired rectourethral fistula, emphasizing the posterior approach. Canadian Journal of Surgery, 1998; 41:241-4.

132. Cherr GS, Hall C, Pineau BC, Waters GS: Rectourethral fistula and massive rectal bleeding from iodine-125 prostate brachytherapy: a case report. American Surgeon, 2001; 67:131-4.

133. Cools P, Vanderputte S, Van der Stighelen Y, Colemont L, Denis B: Rectourethral fistula due to Crohn's disease. Acta Urologica Belgica, 1996; 64:47-48.

134. Bump RC, Hurt WG, Fantl JA, Wyman JF: Assessment of Kegel pelvic muscle exercise performance after brief verbal instruction. American Journal of Obstetrics and Gynecology, 1991; 165:322-7.

135. Johnson VY: Effects of a submaximal exercise protocol to recondition the pelvic floor musculature. Nursing Research, 2001; 50:33-41.

136. Dougherty MC: Current status of research on pelvic muscle strengthening techniques. Journal of Wound, Ostomy, and Continence Nursing, 1998; 25:75-83.

137. Haab R, Corcos J, Siami P, Glavind K, Dwyer P, Steels M, Kawakami F, Lheritier K, Steers WD: Long-term treatment with darifenacin for overactive bladder: results of a 2-year, open-label extension study. BJU International, 2006; 98:1025-32.

138. Abrams P, Andersson KE: Muscarinic receptor antagonists for overactive bladder. BJU International, 2007; 100:987-1006.

139. Staskin D, Sand P, Zinner N, Dmochowski R: Once daily trospium chloride is effective and well tolerated for the treatment of overactive bladder: results from a multicenter phase III trial. Journal of Urology, 2007; 178:978-83.

140. Chapple C, Van Kerrebroeck P, Tubaro A, Haag-Molkenteller C, Forst HT, Massow U, Wang J, Brodsky M: Clinical efficacy, safety, and tolerability of once-daily fesoterodine in subjects with overactive bladder. European Urology, 2007; 52:1204-12.

141. Nitti VW, Dmochowski R, Sand PK, Forst HT, Haag-Molkenteller C, Massow U, Wang J, Brodsky M, Bavendam T: Efficacy, safety and tolerability of fesoterodine for overactive bladder syndrome. Journal of Urology, 2007; 178:2488-94.

142. Casanova N, McGuire E, Fenner DE: Botulinum toxin: a potential alternative to current treatment of neurogenic and idiopathic urinary incontinence due to detrusor overactivity. International Journal of Gynaecology and Obstetrics, 2006; 95:305-11.

143. Jeffery S, Fynes M, Lee F, Wang K, Williams L, Morley R: Efficacy and complications of intradetrusor injection with botulinum toxin A in patients with refractory idiopathic detrusor overactivity. BJU International, 2007; 100:1302-6.

144. Sahai A, Khan MS, Dasgupta P: Efficacy of botulinum toxin-A for treating idiopathic detrusor overactivity: results from a single center, randomized, double-blind, placebo controlled trial. Journal of Urology, 2007; 77:2231-36.

CHAPTER

7

Obstructive Uropathy

Urologic clinicians are often confronted by the question, Is this patient's urinary tract obstructed? Although the nature of the question implies that it can be answered by a simple "yes" or "no," obstruction is a physical and physiologic concept that must be measured using a scale of severity rather than as a dichotomous (yes/no) question. From a physical perspective, obstruction is defined as a phenomenon that prevents or blocks movement.[1] In the urinary system, obstruction is defined as a narrowed area somewhere within the urinary tract that increases resistance to urinary transport to a point that proximal pressure must be raised in order to maintain or reestablish flow.[2,3] Thus obstruction comprises three distinctive and interrelated concepts: increased resistance resulting from a structural or functional lesion, the abnormal rise in pressure needed to maintain some level of flow through the urinary system, and the physiologic consequences of this disruption to normal function.

An obstructive lesion can occur anywhere in the urinary tract, from nephron to distal urethra (Figure 7-1).[4,5] When faced with obstruction, the initial response of the urinary system is to increase contractile force (pressure) proximal to the level of the blockage. If the resistance caused by the obstruction is comparatively mild, this increase in pressure may be sufficient to restore normal flow. However, when faced with a more severe or complete narrowing within the tract, flow is greatly reduced or completely blocked, leading to urinary stasis and retrograde (backward) transmission of pressures to the proximal urinary tract. Obstruction of the upper urinary tract leads to a condition called hydronephrosis, defined as an enlargement of the renal pelvis and calices.[6] Obstruction of the ureter leads to ureteral dilation, usually accompanied by hydronephrosis, and is labeled ureterohydronephrosis. Obstruction of the lower urinary tract, usually referred to as bladder outlet obstruction, typically leads to enlargement of the vesicle, often

accompanied by trabeculation of the bladder wall, with or without grossly apparent dilation of the urethra proximal to the level of obstruction. Vesicoureteral reflux also may be noted, and urine may reflux into the prostatic ducts when obstruction occurs at the level of the membranous urethra.

DEFINITION

The term *obstructive uropathy* describes damage to the renal parenchyma resulting from complete or partial obstruction.[4] Strictly defined, obstructive uropathy is limited to abnormalities of the renal parenchyma, although this term is often applied to any pathologic change in the urinary tract resulting from an obstructive lesion or functional abnormality. From a clinical perspective, the latter (broader) definition is useful because it acknowledges that the urinary tract can be conceptualized as a continuous tube extending from the glomerulus, where blood is filtered in order to form urine, to the urethral meatus, where urine exits the body during micturition. The magnitude and character of obstructive uropathy are distinguished by the location, character, and severity of the obstruction and the presence of complicating conditions, such as infection.

The initial response to upper urinary tract obstruction is an increase in the force and frequency of peristaltic contractions.[7,8] If this process is unable to overcome an obstruction, the renal pelvis and ureter begin to dilate, the smooth muscle in the ureteral wall hypertrophies, and collagen is deposited (presumably in an attempt to regulate the magnitude of dilation). Because the urinary tract acts as a single tube, this process adversely affects all structures proximal to the obstruction, including the nephrons of the renal parenchyma. Retrograde transmission of pressure from the obstruction diminishes renal blood flow (and glomerular filtration) within 2 to 24 hours. As a result, the renin-angiotensin system is activated, leading to increased resistance in

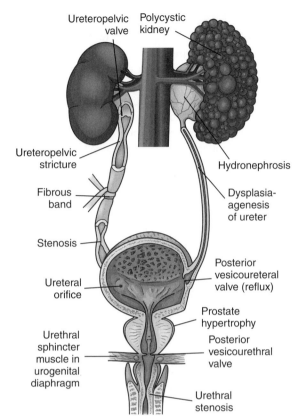

Fig. 7-1 Obstruction of the upper and lower urinary tract. (From McCance K, Huethner S: Pathophysiology: The Biologic Basics for Disease in Adults and Children, 5th edition. St Louis: Mosby, 2006.)

arteriolar pressure and a further decrease in glomerular filtration that may fall to as little as 20% of preobstruction levels. In addition, adverse changes in the renal interstitium occur. The interstitial response to obstruction is partially regulated by transforming growth factor beta (TGF-β), which controls the rate that the kidney manufactures new matrix and degrades older matrix.[8] Within approximately 7 days, the distal tubule begins to atrophy and dilate, followed by glomerular damage within 28 days.[7]

If the obstruction is not corrected, the kidney may be irreversibly damaged, even if the obstruction is subsequently corrected. The precise cause of irreversible renal failure is unknown, but impaired perfusion, cellular atrophy, and local inflammatory changes are hypothesized to gradually destroy nephrons and the supportive interstitium, which is ultimately replaced by a fibrous, thinned parenchyma supporting too few functioning nephrons necessary for the maintenance

of internal homeostasis. Even with complete obstruction of a kidney, some urine flows from the renal pelvis. Urine exits the completely obstructed kidney by several routes, including extravasation, pyelovenous backflow, or pyelolymphatic backflow.

If bilateral obstruction occurs and is subsequently alleviated, reversed, or bypassed by means of a stent catheter or nephrostomy tube, the patient may experience a transient period of brisk diuresis.[7] Although postoperative diuresis is usually mild and self-limiting, it is occasionally severe, leading to life-threatening fluid loss with postural hypotension and fluid and electrolyte imbalances unless fluid losses are replaced parenterally. Hypertension may occur during acute obstruction, owing to fluid and sodium retention and activation of the renin-angiotensin system. The nature of the relationship (if any) between acute or chronic obstruction and long-term hypertension is not clear.

When obstruction impairs renal function, the urinary system responds in several ways. If a single kidney is obstructed, the unaffected (contralateral) kidney undergoes a process called compensatory renal hypertrophy. This process is characterized by hypertrophy and hyperplasia that are most pronounced early in life and gradually diminish as the individual ages. The glomeruli increase in size but not in number; the precise mechanisms that regulate this response are not entirely understood. It may be attributable to stretch-induced cell death[7] and intracellular mechanisms.[9] Compensatory hypertrophy may be reversed if the obstruction is alleviated and the affected kidney regains normal function.

CAUSES OF OBSTRUCTION

Multiple taxonomies have been proposed for classifying the etiologies of obstruction based on the underlying cause, location, pathophysiology, or source of obstruction (extrinsic versus intrinsic). This chapter will review major causes of obstruction listed in Table 7-1. Clinical manifestations, assessment, and management of specific obstructive lesions are arranged based on the level of obstruction, beginning with the upper urinary tract and progressing to the lower. In addition, the reader is referred to Chapters 6, 8, 12, 13, 14, 15, and 16 for discussions of obstruction associated with congenital anomalies, urologic tumors, voiding dysfunction, vesicoureteral reflux, and urinary retention.

TABLE 7-1 Causes of Obstruction in Adults[7,210,211]

LEVEL OF OBSTRUCTION	OBSTRUCTIVE LESION
Upper urinary tract: kidney and renal pelvis	Infundibular stenosis
	Parenchymal or peripelvic cysts
	Ureteropelvic junction (UPJ) obstruction
	Renal tumor
	Urinary calculi
	Trauma
Upper urinary tract: ureter	Ureteral stricture
	Ureteral valve
	Retrocaval ureter
	Prune-belly syndrome
	Ureterocele
	Pregnancy
	Urinoma
	Tumor (transitional cell carcinoma of ureteral lining or compression from extramural tumor)
	Infection (tuberculosis, schistosomiasis, endometriosis, abscess)
	Retroperitoneal fibrosis
	Pelvic lipomatosis
	Aortic aneurysm
	Radiation therapy
	Lymphocele
Lower urinary tract: bladder, urethral and pelvic floor support	Posterior urethral valves or polyps
	Phimosis
	Urethral stricture
	Tumor (carcinoma of bladder or penis)
	Prostatic enlargement (benign prostatic hyperplasia, prostatitis, prostate cancer)
	Neurogenic bladder dysfunction (vesicosphincter dyssynergia, low bladder wall compliance)

INFUNDIBULAR STENOSIS

Stenosis of one or more infundibula is a relatively rare condition that is either congenital[10] or acquired.[11] Congenital cases may be attributable to cystic dysplasia, possibly resulting from abnormal ureteral budding,[12,13] possibly representing an uncommon variant of renal cystic disease. Up to 37% of patients with congenital infundibular stenosis will ultimately develop renal insufficiency or end-stage renal disease, usually accompanied by widespread areas of dysplasia not localized to the stenotic infundibulum. This observation forms the basis of the hypothesis that congenital stenosis represents a rare form of renal cystic disease and not an isolated obstructive lesion. Among adults, infundibular stenosis may occur after open or endourologic procedures, such as percutaneous nephrolithotomy, urinary diversion, or pyelolithotomy. In 1 study of 223 patients, stenosis developed in 5 (2%), and 1 case was associated with severe obstruction and compromised renal function.[11] In addition, 40% of patients with infundibular stenosis had diabetes mellitus as compared with 16% of patients without narrowing, suggesting the possibility that diabetic microangiopathy may increase the risk for scarring and stenosis.

Among infants and children, infundibular stenosis is often detected as an incidental finding on an imaging study. Clinical manifestations of infundibular stenosis include flank pain or constitutional signs and symptoms of renal insufficiency. Because of the possibility of progressive renal disease, infants or children with congenital infundibular stenosis should be referred to a pediatric nephrologist for long-term follow-up of renal function.[10] Patients with acquired stenosis may be observed by annual ultrasonic imaging, urinalysis, and measurement of serum creatinine and electrolytes.[11] Patients with moderate stenosis and good renal function may be managed by endoscopic dilation or incision of the stenotic infundibulum, but those with impaired or progressive renal insufficiency may require open reconstruction or partial nephrectomy.

PARENCHYMAL OR PERIPELVIC CYSTS

Simple renal cysts are frequently detected when the urinary system is imaged, and it is estimated that they are present in approximately 20% of adults in the fourth decade of life and 33% of adults in the sixth decade of life.[14] The majority of cysts do not compromise urinary system function in any way, but a small proportion is associated with clinically relevant uropathology, including obstruction. Parenchymal or peripelvic renal cysts produce obstruction when they compress the pelvicalyceal system (Figure 7-2).

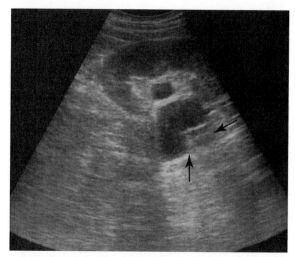

Fig. 7-2 Ultrasound of a peripelvic cyst *(arrows)* compressing the renal pelvis and resulting in hydronephrosis. (From O'Neill WC: Atlas of Renal Ultrasonography. Philadelphia: Saunders, 2001.)

Assessment

Although most cysts remain asymptomatic, others will produce clinically relevant signs and symptoms such as pain, hematuria, obstruction, recurring urinary tract infection, or (rarely) hypertension.[15,16] The location and size of the cyst and associated obstructive uropathy are usually diagnosed by abdominal computed tomography (CT) scan or ultrasonography. Although simple cysts are typically benign, malignancy is suspected particularly when the cyst is multilocular or lacks distinct borders. Urine cytology is obtained, and a retrograde pyelogram may be completed when a malignancy is suspected. In addition, fluid may be aspirated from a symptomatic cyst and cytologic analysis completed to detect malignant cells.

Nursing Management

Traditionally managed by surgical ablation, simple cysts may also be managed by a variety of techniques including unroofing during an open surgical procedure, insertion of a needle with percutaneous aspiration (with or without injection of a sclerosing agent), or laparoscopic resection.[15,17,18] The nursing management of patients with symptomatic parenchymal or peripelvic cysts includes preparation and education for surgery or percutaneous intervention and postprocedural care in the inpatient and outpatient settings.

The patient undergoing percutaneous drainage is counseled that the procedure is completed with the patient under local anesthesia. Using fluoroscopic guidance, an interventional radiologist will place an 18-gauge needle into the cyst to drain fluid that will be examined by a pathologist for malignant cells. Because fluid tends to reaccumulate in the cyst within 2 years, aspiration is often followed by injection of a sclerosing agent, such as ethanol, tetracycline, bismuth phosphate, autologous blood, or povidone-iodine (Betadine), to reduce this risk. Following the procedure, the patient is advised that he or she may experience mild to moderate discomfort at the site of the needle puncture but the discomfort is expected to resolve within several days. Flank pain or fever is not anticipated and should be reported promptly to the urologist or urologic nurse. Teaching about the possibility of cyst recurrence should be reinforced, emphasizing that even with the injection of a sclerosing agent the risk for fluid reaccumulating in the cyst within 40 months is approximately 50%[19] and that the risk for symptom recurrence (including pain) is about 25%.[18]

Laparoscopic resection of parenchymal or peripelvic cysts may be completed using an abdominal or transperitoneal approach.[16] Laparoscopic surgery may be undertaken when percutaneous procedures fail to achieve symptom relief or adequate reduction of the cyst in order to relieve obstruction or when the cyst is located in an area that cannot be safely aspirated using a percutaneous, fluoroscopic-guided approach. The patient is advised that brief hospitalization is necessary and that the procedure is expected to require three small incisions for laparoscopic ports. Patients with peripelvic cysts are counseled that hospitalization may be longer and that the risk for complications is higher when a peripelvic cyst requires treatment.[15] Patients are also counseled that approximately 50% will have a recurrence of the cyst within 40 months, although the risk for recurrence of symptoms is far less (refer to Chapter 11 for a detailed discussion of laparoscopic surgery in the adult). Open surgical resection also may be undertaken but is now less commonly performed because of the success achieved by less invasive methods.

Percutaneous drainage also may be used to relieve obstruction or other symptoms associated with polycystic or multicystic kidney disease, but overall management requires a coordinated effort of a urologist and nephrologist, and the course of the disease may lead to end-stage renal disease and transplantation. Refer to Chapter 11 for an in-depth discussion of the management of renal diseases.

URETEROPELVIC JUNCTION OBSTRUCTION

Whereas most cases of ureteropelvic junction (UPJ) obstruction in neonates result from an intrinsic or extrinsic congenital defect, UPJ obstruction in adults is typically associated with benign tumors such as fibroepithelial polyps, malignant ureteral tumors, stone disease, or inflammation and scarring from a urinary calculus or a urologic procedure.[17] This chapter provides a brief overview of the evaluation and management of UPJ obstruction in adults; refer to Chapter 12 for a detailed discussion of UPJ obstruction in infants and children.

Assessment

Unlike UPJ obstruction in infants, most adult cases are associated with flank pain that may occur after an episode of brisk fluid intake. Such an episode can result in a physiologic diuresis that overwhelms the urinary system's ability to adequately drain urine from the affected renal pelvis, leading to distention and colicky type pain. Alternatively, UPJ obstruction may present as a chronic or recurring flank pain. Urologic evaluation must address three goals: determine the cause and severity of the obstruction, assess the function of the affected and contralateral kidney, and identify the underlying cause of UPJ obstruction.[2] Several imaging studies may be employed to achieve these goals. As in the evaluation of neonates or children, a radionuclide scan is usually the principal imaging study used to assess the severity of UPJ obstruction and the function of the affected and contralateral kidneys. A diethylenetriamine pentaacetic acid (DTPA) or mertiatide (MAG3) scan, combined with administration of furosemide, allows the clinician to distinguish obstructive from nonobstructive hydronephrosis and to measure the differential function of the obstructed and contralateral kidneys. The Whitaker test allows direct measurement of pressures within the obstructed urinary tact but requires placement of a large-bore needle or nephrostomy tube in the kidney and does not evaluate renal function. Therefore it is limited to cases in which massive

dilation renders the results of a radionuclide study inconclusive when attempting to differentiate between obstructive and nonobstructive hydronephrosis. Spiral computed tomography may be obtained, particularly if a crossing vessel is suspected as a cause of UPJ obstruction.

Ultrasonography can be used to evaluate the severity of hydronephrosis associated with UPJ obstruction, but it cannot differentiate obstructive from nonobstructive dilation of the renal pelvis. An intravenous pyelogram (IVP) can be used to assess the severity of UPJ narrowing and the excretory function of the affected kidney. However, its ability to accurately differentiate obstructive from nonobstructive dilation is also limited, with reported sensitivity rates of 50% and a specificity rate of only 63%.[20] Voiding cystourethrography may be useful when UPJ obstruction is associated with higher-grade vesicoureteral reflux, and a retrograde pyelogram is completed in order to more accurately define the obstructive lesion itself, particularly if acute obstruction occurs in the presence of infection or compromised renal function.

Nursing Management

Urologic management of symptomatic UPJ obstruction typically focuses on surgical correction of the anatomic defect.[17] Pyeloplasty using an open surgical technique remains the gold standard that other procedures are measured against, but advances in laparoscopic and ureteroscopic techniques offer significant advantages when compared with open procedures, including avoidance of a surgical incision, reduced time spent in the hospital, and less postoperative pain.[17,21] Refer to Chapter 18 for a detailed discussion of open surgical endourologic techniques for managing UPJ obstruction.

RENAL TUMOR

Malignant tumors of the renal parenchyma (e.g., a renal cell carcinoma) or a cancer of the urothelium (e.g., a transitional cell carcinoma) may cause obstruction by compressing or directly growing into and blocking the lumen of the upper urinary tract or the ureterovesical junctions. Treatment is directed at the underlying tumor and may involve tumor resection or removal of the affected urinary organs. Refer to Chapter 8 for a detailed discussion of the evaluation and management of renal malignancies.

URINARY CALCULI

Urinary calculi (stones) are solid concretions that form in the urinary tract. Smaller calculi may form, pass through the tract, and be expelled during micturition, causing few or no symptoms, but larger stones become clinically relevant when they obstruct the urinary tract or harbor pathogens leading to persistent infection despite appropriate antimicrobial therapy.

Epidemiology

The prevalence of urinary stones varies significantly based on geography. For example, the overall prevalence of urinary calculi requiring hospitalization in the United States is 1.64 persons per 1000, but the rate for individual states varies from as high as 3 persons per 1000 in North Carolina to as few as 0.43 persons per 1000 in Missouri.[22] Similarly, the prevalence of urinary calculi among Canadians is comparatively lower than that of the United States at an estimated 0.5 per 1000 adults.[23] Although these estimates provide an indication of the frequency of stones causing severe obstruction and necessitating hospital-based care, they underestimate true prevalence. For example, a study of 798 adults living in Minnesota over a period of 25 years revealed that 51% were treated for urinary calculi on a strictly outpatient basis, a significant cohort not included in epidemiologic studies based on hospital admissions.[24]

Although supporting evidence is limited, existing research strongly indicates that the prevalence of urinary stones has increased over the past several decades in the United States[25] and in western Europe.[26-28] In the United States the prevalence has increased by approximately 37%.[25] This increase has been found to include men as well as women. Occurrences have risen in whites but not in African Americans. The reasons for this trend are not known, but increases in food portion sizes and total food intake; higher salt, protein, and calcium intake; and obesity itself have been hypothesized as possible contributing factors.[29,30]

Less is known about the incidence of urinary stones. The peak incidence has been reported as the second, third, and fourth decades of life,[31] although Johnson and colleagues[24] reported a peak incidence between ages 30 and 60 years. The annual incidence in this adult cohort living in Minnesota is 1.1 per 1000 for men and 0.36 per 1000 for women. Pearle and Lotan[31] estimate the likelihood of stone formation for a 70-year-old white male living in the United States as 1:8.

Multiple factors have been associated with the likelihood of developing a urinary stone (Table 7-2). The surprisingly wide variety of associated factors may reflect the multiple etiologies of stone formation as well as the variety of factors affecting the chemical composition of human urine.

Etiology and Pathophysiology

An understanding of the etiology and pathophysiology of urinary calculus formation requires a review of basic aspects of crystal formation and growth within a liquid medium. A urinary stone or calculus begins its existence when salt crystals (solutes) precipitate from a liquid medium (solvent). The chemical principles that govern this process can be illustrated by a simplistic experiment (Figure 7-3). In this experiment a liquid medium (pure or distilled water) is poured into a container and a salt (e.g., sodium chloride or table salt) is slowly added. At first, the salt dissolves into its constituent ions (a negatively charged chloride ion and a positively charged sodium ion) and the water remains undersaturated or capable of dissolving more salt. Eventually, however, the addition of more salt leads to a point where the solution becomes saturated. At this point, adding any more salt will lead to precipitation, defined as reformation of the salt into sodium chloride and the formation of visible salt crystals in the bottom of the beaker. The point at which salt precipitates is called the saturation point. However, by altering the physical or chemical properties of the solution in some way, such as by heating it, it is possible to create a solution that is *supersaturated*, or one that retains a higher concentration of solutes (ions capable of forming salts) than would be possible under normal conditions. As long as these conditions are maintained, the solution will remain supersaturated. If the properties of the supersaturated solution are changed, by allowing the solution to cool, precipitation of salt crystals will occur.

Applied to the clinical setting, the solvent in urine remains water as it was in the experiment described above, but the salts include a wide variety of positively and negatively charged ions capable of forming multiple salts that may, under the right conditions, precipitate and form crystals in the urine. Therefore, unlike the simplistic experiment

TABLE 7-2 Epidemiology of Urinary Calculus Formation: Associated and Risk Factors

FACTOR	INFLUENCE ON LIKELIHOOD OF URINARY CALCULUS FORMATION
Gender[30,31]	Men are more likely to form symptomatic stones than women: ratio of men/women approximately 3:1
Race[30,31,212]	Caucasians and Asians are at higher risk than African Americans and Native Americans; ratio of Caucasians/African Americans in the United States approximately 4:1
Genetics[69,213]	Approximately 25% of patients with urinary calculi have a family history of stone formation. First-degree relatives of persons with urinary calculi have a threefold risk compared with persons with a negative family history. As much as half of an individual's risk is estimated to arise from genetic factors and half from environmental factors. Approximately 2% of persons with urinary calculi have an underlying disorder with a clearly genetic etiology, such as cystinuria or xanthinuria.
Osteoporosis[214]	Osteoporosis is associated with an increased occurrence of urinary calculus formation, possibly owing to mutations in the *NPT2a* gene thought to be responsible for hypophosphatemia and hyperphosphaturia.
Climate[215,216]	The incidence of renal calculi tends to rise 1-2 mo following the maximum mean temperature of the year, typically in July, August, and September in North America.
Water[31]	Conflicting data exist that suggest that water supplies with higher mineral content may increase the risk for urinary calculi.
Occupation[217]	Persons with sedentary occupations may be at higher risk for urinary stones.
Stress[218]	The incidence of urinary calculus formation increased during and immediately following a distressing life event persisting for 1 wk or longer.
Inflammatory bowel disease[219,220]	Crohn disease and ulcerative colitis are associated with a high occurrence of urinary calculi, possibly because of higher excretion of urinary oxalate and lower citrate in the urine.
Diabetes mellitus[221,222]	Diabetes is associated with a higher risk for stone formation and recurrence than in a case control population; the precise mechanism for this increased risk is unknown, but one study has demonstrated that persons with insulin resistance tend to have low urinary ammonium and pH, resulting in a higher risk for uric acid stones.
Medullary sponge kidney[223]	A medullary sponge kidney is associated with a high risk for stone formation, usually calcium oxalate, but the nature of this relationship remains unclear.
Polycystic kidney disease[224]	Urinary calculi occur in approximately 20% of patients with polycystic kidney disease; uric acid stones are most common; urinary stasis and metabolic disorders including hypocitraturia and hyperuricosuria are hypothesized to cause the high risk for stone formation.
Urinary diversion[30]	Urinary diversion is indirectly associated with stone formation because of changes in gastrointestinal metabolism when bowel is isolated from the fecal stream and incorporated into the urinary tract and when a urinary diversion becomes colonized with urease-producing bacterial strains.
Cystic fibrosis[225]	Persons with cystic fibrosis have a higher prevalence of urinary stones than case control populations; the reasons for this association are unknown.

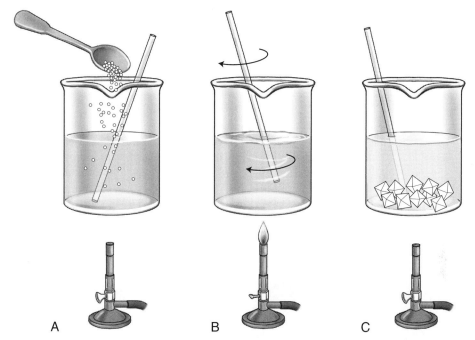

Fig. 7-3 A, Water in a beaker acts as a solvent. **B,** Addition of a salt leads to crystal formation, but altering the solution by heating allows the formation of a *supersaturated* solution, resulting in dissolution of crystals present when the solution is at room temperature. **C,** Altering the supersaturated solution (in this case by allowing to cool to room temperature) causes massive crystallization.

described above, it is not possible to define a saturation point of human urine or to predict precisely what conditions will lead to precipitation of a specific crystal or obstructing calculus. Multiple factors account for the complexity of supersaturation precipitation and crystal formation in the urine, including the influence of various ions within the urine, its temperature, its pH, and the existence of substances that inhibit or promote precipitation. Among these factors, only the temperature of human urine remains relatively constant.

In contrast to its temperature, the pH of the urine varies significantly, and this profoundly influences the likelihood that two salts commonly present in urine, uric acid and calcium phosphate, will precipitate.[30] Increasing the pH (raising its alkalinity) of urine that is supersaturated with calcium phosphate results in a rise in the concentration of hydroxyl ions (OH^-) and a reduction in hydrogen ion (H^+) activity. As a result, the concentration of phosphate ions (PO_4^-) increases and the likelihood of precipitation of calcium phosphate crystals from the urine is enhanced. In contrast, lowering the pH (raising its

acidity) to levels of 5.5 increases hydrogen ion activity and increases the likelihood that urate uric acid crystals will precipitate from the urine.

Similarly, the likelihood of crystal formation and growth is also affected by the presence of inhibiting or promoting substances in the urine (Table 7-3). These substances influence both the chemical properties of the urine itself and the response of the urinary epithelium to ions and salts within the urine.[31]

Crystal formation in supersaturated urine is only the first step toward the creation of an obstructing stone. In the laboratory setting, growth occurs by means of a process called crystallization (Figure 7-4). This process requires the urine to reach a point of supersaturation sufficient for the precipitation of crystals and to remain in this state until the crystals grow. Crystalline growth occurs at screw dislocations, imperfections that allow the crystal to bond with more salt molecules. The crystal grows by means of a process called lattice formation in which the crystal twists itself into a spiral shape whose center lies at the point of the original screw dislocation. Growth also occurs when crystals collide with one another in a

TABLE 7-3 Crystal Inhibitors and Promoters in the Urine[30,31]

SUBSTANCE	EFFECT OF PRECIPITATION AND CRYSTALLIZATION
Magnesium Nephrocalcin Pyrophosphate RNA fragments	Inhibit calcium phosphate precipitation
Citrate	Inhibits calcium phosphate precipitation; prevents epithelial damage associated with hyperoxaluria; exerts its maximum beneficial effects at a pH of 6.5
Uropontin	Protein that inhibits calcium oxalate monohydrate formation and crystallization, but it may promote crystal adherence to urinary epithelial cells under certain circumstances
Glycosaminoglycans (GAGs) Tamm-Horsfall glycoprotein	Potent inhibitors of calcium monohydrate crystal formation, they promote precipitation of other crystals but inhibit aggregation and growth of these crystals

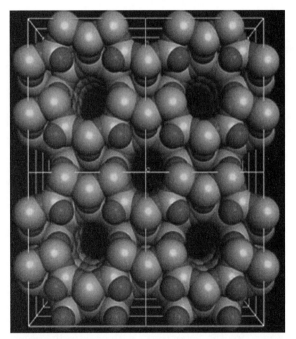

Fig. 7-4 Urinary stones grow by means of a process called crystallization, where ions form lattices or aggregations that grow in a somewhat predictable manner. (Image courtesy of Accelrys, www.accelrys.com.)

process called aggregation. Growth by way of lattice formation results in particularly dense calculi, whereas growth by way of aggregation leads to stones that are more easily disrupted by shock wave lithotripsy or other technologies.

Whereas stone formation through crystallization is somewhat predictable, calculus growth in human urine is more complex and less predictable than crystals created in an experiment because of the presence of proteinaceous material (matrix) and the complexity of ions in the ever-changing chemical solution produced by glomerular filtration. The role of matrix in urinary calculus formation has been the focus of a number of studies.[30,31] Matrix is a proteinaceous substance originating from organic materials in the urinary tract, such as cell membranes. It is not known whether matrix acts as the nidus of urinary stones or whether it allows additional growth in stones originally formed through crystallization. Regardless, it is known that crystals and epithelial cells in the urinary system interact and stimulate complex cytokine-mediated cellular responses and that stones containing substrate grow through a process called agglomeration, producing a complex concretion that may contain both mineralized crystals and proteinaceous components (Figure 7-5).

Crystal formation is hypothesized to occur initially at the papillary collecting ducts.[30] Fortunately, the vast majority of these crystals traverse the urinary tract without forming an obstructive stone. For example, only 5% to 10% of persons with excessive cystine molecules in the urine will experience symptomatic stones. Two hypotheses, free particle growth and fixed particle mechanism, attempt to explain the process of crystal retention and stone growth. The free particle growth hypothesis postulates that crystallization, aggregation, and/or agglomeration occur in the open lumen and that retention occurs only when a calculus grows rapidly enough to become entrapped in a collecting duct or similar structure

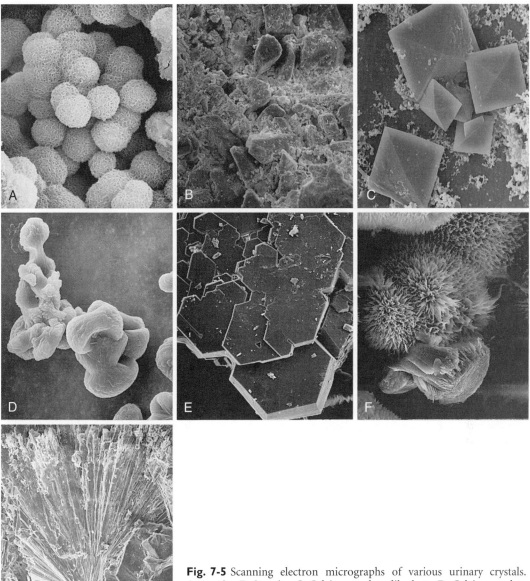

Fig. 7-5 Scanning electron micrographs of various urinary crystals. **A,** Apatite. **B,** Struvite. **C,** Calcium oxalate dihydrate. **D,** Calcium oxalate monohydreate. **E,** Cystine. **F,** Ammonium acid urate. **G,** Brushite. (From Wein AJ, Kavoussi LR, Novick AC, Partin AW, Peters CA: Campbell-Walsh Urology, 9th edition. Philadelphia Saunders, 2007.)

before traveling to the wider lumina of the mid and lower urinary tract. The fixed particle hypothesis asserts that while precipitation occurs in a lumen of the urinary tract, further growth occurs only when the crystal adheres to epithelium in the lining of the urinary system. The principal location of such adherence remains unknown, but possible sites include the loop of Henle, lymphatic vessels in the renal pelvis, and distal collecting ducts. Observations that hyperoxaluria promotes epithelial damage in the urinary tract provide some evidence for the existence of stone growth because of a fixed particle mechanism.[32,33]

Because of the complexity of the multiple solutes present in urine, the presence of matrix, and multiple substances known to inhibit or promote crystal growth, it is not possible to accurately predict the likelihood that a given urine or specific patient will form an obstructing stone within a given time frame. Nevertheless, research has led to increased understanding of how the human body metabolizes and excretes major ions within the urine, and various metabolic products are associated with a substantial risk of urinary calculus formation.

Calcium, Phosphate, and Magnesium. Approximately 85% of all urinary stones contain significant amounts of calcium, which is usually bound to phosphate or oxalate.[30,31] Persons living in North America typically eat a diet that is quite rich in calcium, often consuming as much as 600 to 1200 mg/day. The body retains 30% to 45% of this calcium to meet metabolic demands, but an additional 100 to 300 mg is secreted into the stool, yielding a net absorbed volume of 100 to 300 mg/day. Calcium is principally absorbed in the jejunum and proximal ileum, where pH levels are relatively low (below 6.0), but some calcium is absorbed throughout the entire length of the intestinal tract. The amount of calcium absorbed by way of the gut is primarily influenced by 1,25-dihydroxy–vitamin D_3. Parathyroid hormone (PTH) stimulates the conversion of vitamin D into this highly metabolically active form. Once formed, 1,25-dihydroxy–vitamin D_3 stimulates an enzyme (1α-hydroxylase) found in the renal tubules and macrophages to produce calcitriol. This substance promotes calcium absorption from the gut, reabsorption of calcium from bones (leading to their demineralization), and reabsorption within the kidney in exchange for phosphate, which is excreted into the urine. About 60% of phosphate is absorbed through the gut, and 65% is excreted by the kidney.

Magnesium is particularly important to calcium and phosphate metabolism. Magnesium is absorbed in the gut and principally excreted in the kidney, mainly within the loop of Henle. Magnesium influences calcium and phosphate concentrations in the urine by inhibiting PTH secretion.[30]

The most common disorder found in persons forming calcium phosphate or calcium oxalate stones is idiopathic hypercalciuria, which occurs in 30% to 60%. It is characterized by increased serum levels of calcium, leading to enhanced excretion into the urine.[30,31] As implied in the name, the precise cause of idiopathic hypercalciuria is not known, although a growing body of evidence supports a possible genetic etiology.[34,35] Several important

observations underpin this theory. Approximately half of patients with idiopathic hypercalciuria have a family history of urinary calculi. In addition, a number of genetic disorders have been identified leading to abnormal calcium metabolism by the bones, gut, or kidney. Nevertheless, no apparent genetic link has been identified that accounts for hypercalciuria, and additional research is needed to unlock the complex and as yet undefined inheritance patterns leading to this important risk factor for urinary stone disease.

Ongoing genetic research and current clinical management of idiopathic hypercalciuria are partially founded on pioneering work by Pak and associates,[36] who identified three primary sources of hypercalciuria in the human: absorptive, resorptive, and renal. *Absorptive hypercalciuria* is characterized by abnormally high absorption of calcium from the intestinal lumen. Several subtypes of absorptive hypercalciuria have been described that involve an intestinal defect leading to hyperabsorption or secondary excesses of absorption because of increased production of 1,25-dihydroxy–vitamin D_3. *Resorptive hypercalciuria* is caused by excessive production of PTH, resulting in bone demineralization and secondary hyperabsorption of calcium from the gut under the influence of high serum levels of PTH. *Renal hypercalciuria* occurs when the kidneys excrete abnormally high levels of calcium into the urine. PTH is elevated in patients who have renal hypercalciuria, but in this case the elevation is caused by the body's need to absorb additional calcium from the gut to compensate for abnormally high losses from the kidneys as they filter the blood to make urine. Additional factors that may produce hypercalcemia and secondary hypercalciuria are listed in Table 7-4.

Renal tubular acidosis (RTA) is an inherited disorder characterized by abnormal renal acidification leading to a hypokalemic, hyperchloremic metabolic acidosis. Specifically, the individual with RTA experiences excessive loss of potassium, calcium, and phosphorus with abnormally high retention of chloride, ultimately leading to a sustained metabolic acidosis and an increased risk for calcium phosphate urinary calculi. Two defects have been identified in persons with RTA. Type 2 RTA is characterized by a defect in reabsorption of the bicarbonate ion (HCO_3^-), which is essential for buffering the bloodstream. In contrast, persons with type 1 (classic) RTA retain the ability to

TABLE 7-4 Causes of Hypercalcemia-Induced Hypercalciuria[31]

CONDITION	LINK TO URINARY STONE RISK
Primary hyperparathyroidism	Abnormally high levels of parathyroid hormone lead to hypercalcemia and increased excretion of calcium in the urine.
Malignancy	Primary tumors of bony metastases may lead to hypercalcemia when they produce a bone-resorbing substance called PTH-related polypeptide.
Sarcoidosis	Sarcoid granulomas produce excessive 1,25-dihydroxy–vitamin D_3, leading to excessive intestinal absorption of calcium.
Cushing's disease	Excess glucocorticoids lead to excessive bone resorption, secondary hypercalcemia, and hypercalciuria.
Immobilization	Prolonged bed rest leads to increased bone turnover; when complicated by Paget's disease this can lead to hypercalcemia and hypercalciuria.
Thiazides	Use of thiazide diuretics can unmask primary hyperparathyroidism by increasing resorption of calcium from the proximal tubule.

PTH, Parathyroid hormone.

reabsorb filtered bicarbonate ion from the proximal tubule. Nevertheless, bicarbonate ions are lost because of a defect in the distal renal tubule that renders the person unable to excrete adequate hydrogen ions in the urine. Urinary calculi are seen in approximately 70% of patients with type 1 RTA. Excretion of high levels of calcium and phosphorus in the urine also leads to depletion from the bones, which has been linked to the slow growth patterns seen in children with type 1 RTA.

Oxalate. Oxalate is the ion created when oxalic acid loses two hydrogen ions when dissolved in a solution. Oxalic acid abounds in many plants, including rhubarb, spinach, black pepper, coffee, many nuts, most berries, and chocolate. The average Western diet contains approximately 100 to 150 mg/day, and some persons consume up to 900 mg/day.[30,37] Nevertheless, only 6% to 14% of this amount is absorbed from the gut. The vast majority is manufactured endogenously through oxidative metabolism of ascorbic acid. Several disorders are known to produce hyperoxaluria and increase the risk for calcium oxalate stone formation. Primary hyperoxaluria is a rare genetic disorder affecting glyoxylate metabolism. Type 1 primary hyperoxaluria is caused by a defect of peroxisomal alanine-glyoxylate aminotransferase enzyme production in the liver. Type 2 primary hyperoxaluria is caused by a deficiency of the glyoxylate reductase.

Enteric absorption may lead to hyperoxaluria in certain individuals. Multiple factors affect the amount of oxalate absorbed from dietary sources, including the amount of oxalic acid consumed in the diet, its structural form in specific food items, its digestibility, intestinal transit time, absorptive properties of the intestinal wall, and presence of oxalate-degrading microflora.[37] Oxalates that are consumed in the diet are released by the acid medium of the stomach.[30] The vast majority is bound to calcium and excreted in the stool as calcium oxalate. However, a number of gastrointestinal conditions may alter absorption, resulting in increased serum levels, increased excretion by the kidneys, and an elevated risk for crystallization and stone formation. They include inflammatory bowel disease, ileostomy, extensive surgical resection of the small bowel, and chronic pancreatitis. The presence of other foods in the diet also affects oxalate absorption from the gut. For example, fatty acids bind calcium and reduce its ability to bind oxalate. Ascorbate also may be converted into oxalate, and persons collecting a 24-hour urine specimen are advised to refrain from taking large quantities of vitamin C. Other factors associated with an increased risk of hyperoxaluria include dehydration and high protein intake.

Oxalobacter formigenes is a gram-negative obligate anaerobe responsible for degrading oxalates in many mammals, including humans. In humans it is mainly found in the colon and hypothesized to be the single most important bacterial strain required for the degradation of oxalates in the gut.[38] Nevertheless, a second bacterial species, *Providencia rettgeri,* has also been identified that demonstrates a potent ability to degrade oxalate in the gut.[39] Deficits in either of these bacterial species are thought to increase oxalate excretion by the kidney and the associated risk for calcium oxalate stone formation.

The presence of calcium oxalate monohydrate crystals in the urine is relevant to the risk for calcium stones and to the long-term health of the kidney. Calcium oxalate monohydrate crystals provoke the production of multiple inflammatory cytokines and prostaglandin E_2 that may contribute to fibrosis, nephron death, and compromised renal function.[40]

Cystine. Cystine is an amino acid used for protein synthesis, vitamin B_6 synthesis, wound healing, and the breakdown of mucous deposits. Cystinuria is an uncommon autosomal recessive genetic disorder affecting the metabolism of multiple amino acids including ornithine, lysine, and arginine.[41] Whereas normal individuals tend to excrete less than 30 mg of cystine per day, those with cystinuria excrete more than 400 mg, greatly increasing the risk for crystal formation and precipitation. Cystine is relatively insoluble in urine, particularly when the pH rises to 7.0 or higher. Because of its insolubility, more than half of patients with cystinuria will develop urinary calculi, and the risk for recurrence is approximately 60%. Cystinuria should be differentiated from cystinosis, an unrelated autosomal recessive inherited disorder characterized by intracellular accumulation of cystine crystals in the conjunctivae, bone marrow, lymph nodes, and internal organs.

Uric Acid. Uric acid is a product of purine metabolism (an essential element of nucleic acids).[30] Three factors determine the risk of uric acid crystal formation in the urine: acidic urine, low urine volume, and hyperuricosuria.[42] Approximately 10% of all stones are primarily made up of uric acid, and an additional 12% contain some portion of uric acid.[43] Most patients with uric acid stones have normal uric acid secretion but a low urinary pH with secondary crystal precipitation because of its relative insolubility when the pH of the urine is below 6.5 and especially when it is 5.4 or lower. Diarrhea can both reduce urine volume and lower its pH, although obesity and diabetes mellitus lead to a lower urinary pH without coexisting dehydration. Consumption of a diet rich in animal protein and low in carbohydrates, such as that advocated in the Atkins diet, lowers urinary pH and increases the risk for uric acid stones.

Multiple factors influence the risk of uric acid stone formation.[30] Approximately 25% of persons with primary gouty arthritis (i.e., joint inflammation, swelling and pain caused by formation of uric acids crystals in the synovial fluid) will experience uric acid stones. A minority of patients with uric acid stones have hypouricosuria caused by one of a number of rare genetic disorders, such as Lesch-Nyhan syndrome. These syndromes are caused by an X-linked chromosome defect that impairs or ablates the manufacture and actions of the enzyme hypoxanthine-guanine-phosphoribosyltransferase (HGPRT). However, many other patients repeatedly form uric acid stones without an identifiable underlying metabolic disorder other than acidic urine. Whether these stones are caused by a subclinical gouty diathesis or an as yet undefined genetic predisposition remains unclear.

Xanthine. Xanthine is a product of purine metabolism that ultimately yields uric acid under the influence of the enzyme xanthine oxidase.[30] Xanthine is even less soluble than uric acid in acidic urine, but its solubility rises sharply as the urinary pH rises. Genetic defects affecting the body's ability to manufacture the enzyme xanthine oxidase are associated with xanthuria and an increased risk of xanthine stones.

Crystallization and Urinary Tract Infection. Certain strains of bacteria have the ability to produce urease, an enzyme that catalyzes ammonia and carbon dioxide from urea. The result is a significant rise in urinary pH.[30,89] In the presence of alkaline urine, dissociation of phosphate occurs, resulting in formation of magnesium-phosphate-ammonium, commonly called struvite. Struvite stones account for 15% to 20% of urinary stones, and, unlike other calculi, they are more prevalent in women. Struvite stones may form a staghorn calculus that occupies a large portion of the pelvicalyceal system. Bacterial species associated with magnesium-phosphate-ammonium crystallization include almost all strains of *Proteus* and some strains of *Klebsiella, Staphylococcus,* and *Pseudomonas.* Of note, *Escherichia coli,* the most common cause of urinary tract infection in community-dwelling women, does not produce urease. Although infection-related stones tend to contain primarily struvite, multiple other elements are often present in these typically large calculi, including carbonate apatite, formed by the dissociation of carbonic acid, phosphate, and calcium ions in alkaline urine, and hydroxyapatite, formed when phosphate and calcium ions bind to two hydroxyl (OH^-) ions. Struvite stones are also likely to contain matrix, the proteinaceous substance discussed earlier.

Crystallization Caused by Pharmacologic Agents. The metabolic effects of certain drugs increase the risk for urinary calculus formation.[30] Fortunately, such stones are rare, collectively accounting for less than 1% of all urinary calculi.[31,44] Sulfonamides have long been known to carry the potential to precipitate in the urinary system, prompting advice to patients to take these drugs with a "full glass of water." Among adults, multiple cases of stones forming from the crystallization of sulfonamide medications or their metabolites have been reported in patients with human immunodeficiency virus (HIV) infection[45-47] or inflammatory bowel disease.[44] Sulfa-based stones have been reported in children and may lead to acute renal failure.[45] Acetazolamide, a carbonic anhydrase inhibitor used to treat glaucoma or certain types of seizures, produces changes in the urine similar to those seen in RTA, including urolithiasis.[46] Several cases of stones formed by triamterene and furosemide (both diuretics) or their metabolites also have been reported.[47,49] Indinavir is a protease inhibitor used to treat HIV infection. Indinavir crystals may precipitate in alkaline urine. The resulting stones are not visible on helical CT scan unless contrast is used.[50]

Crystallization Caused by Dietary and Health Supplements. High doses of ascorbic acid (more than 1 g/day) have been implicated as a possible risk factor for stone formation. Ascorbic acid indirectly influences the risk for calcium oxalate stones by increasing oxalate excretion into the urine.[51,52] In addition, case studies have found stones that form when certain individuals ingest significant dosages of dietary and health supplements, including calcium carbonate, magnesium oxide, and sodium citrate bicarbonate.[53] Regular laxative use has been associated with ammonium acid urate stone formation.

Assessment

The initial evaluation of a stone usually occurs when an obstructing stone causes renal colic, followed by referral to a urologist for definitive diagnosis and management. Renal colic is the pain produced by dilation of the urinary system and distention of

afferent nerves in the mucosa. The associated pain has a sudden onset, often awakening the person from sleep. It usually originates in the flank and extends laterally around the abdomen as the pain crescendos; it may be referred to the groin and scrotum in the male and labia or round ligament in the female depending on the level of obstruction. Renal colic is experienced as a cycle of recurring waves of pain that increase over a period of minutes, reach a peak, and subside slowly. The intensity of the pain varies, but it is often quite severe. Peritoneal signs, caused by acute abdominal infection, cause the patient to lie still in order to alleviate the pain caused by stretching or moving the peritoneum. In contrast, the patient with renal colic moves from marked restlessness to writhing from pain caused by unsuccessful attempts to relieve the discomfort by changing positions. Costovertebral angle tenderness is often present, but fever is absent unless the obstruction is complicated by urinary tract infection. Nausea and vomiting may be present, and bothersome lower urinary tract symptoms, including acute urgency or urge urinary incontinence, may be present if the stone is located in the lower ureter near the ureterovesical junction or in the bladder. The patient also may experience grossly visible hematuria. Refer to Chapter 3 for a detailed description of renal colic, its assessment, and its differential diagnosis.

Because patients with urinary calculi often present to an emergency department or urgent care facility with severe flank pain, the diagnostic approach varies depending on the age and gender of the patient, the character of the pain, the availability of a CT scanner, a prior history of urinary stones resulting in an ongoing relationship with a urologist, and the presence of associated factors, such as fever or peritoneal signs.[54] The initial evaluation routinely includes a history, physical examination, and urinalysis. An obstructing urinary calculus is strongly suspected when the history and physical examination are consistent with renal colic, peritoneal signs are absent, and the urinalysis reveals hematuria. Hematuria may be absent in as many as 10% to 15% of patients with obstructing urinary calculi, but this number drops to approximately 5% when dipstick analysis is combined with microscopy.[55] When a strong suspicion of an obstructing urinary calculus is present and complicating factors are absent, emergency department personnel may elect to manage the pain and nausea associated with renal colic without completing additional imaging studies and assist the patient in seeking prompt urologic care, typically within 24 hours. Additional diagnostic studies will be obtained in the urgent care setting when signs and symptoms are less convincing, complicating factors exist, or the patient's clinical scenario indicates a reasonable possibility of another condition, such as an ectopic pregnancy or ruptured abdominal aortic aneurysm.[54,56]

Urologic Evaluation. Urologic evaluation begins with assessment of existing stone burden and proceeds to the identification of physiologic or environmental factors contributing to the current calculus or increasing the risk for recurrence.[30] The clinical history begins with a determination of whether this is a first episode of renal colic or a recurrence. The patient's age at the onset of renal colic or a family history of urinary stone disease provides a clue to possible underlying metabolic abnormalities requiring additional evaluation. The person's geographic residence and occupation are queried, as are physical activities that may lead to prolonged dehydration, such as long-distance running or related activities. The patient is also asked about recent illnesses that may have led to periods of prolonged immobility with subsequent bone demineralization and hypercalciuria. A dietary history is obtained, focusing on intake of beverages or foods containing calcium oxalate or protein and the volume of fluid consumed on a daily basis. A review of systems is completed that concentrates on the urologic system and any known history of urinary tract infections. Particular attention is also paid to any previous history of urinary stone formation, the number of previous episodes, the results of any stone analysis, previous procedures to remove or crush obstructing stones, and the presence of known contributing conditions. Current medications are reviewed because of their association with certain atypical stones, as are vitamins and dietary supplements.

Physical Examination. The physical examination helps to characterize the nature and location of acute pain. The abdominal examination should reveal absence of peritoneal signs, although costovertebral angle tenderness may be present. Referred pain to the groin may mimic vulvitis or an acutely inflamed scrotum, but physical examination will reveal no signs of erythema or edema. The general examination may reveal underlying metabolic disorders.

Imaging Studies. Definitive diagnosis of a urinary calculus requires an imaging study. A plain abdominal film (kidney, ureter, and bladder [KUB]) followed by IVP is traditionally preferred for definitive diagnosis, but this approach has been largely replaced by an unenhanced helical CT scan.[30,31] The helical CT scan is preferred because it can be performed rapidly (less than 10 minutes), has a higher sensitivity than IVP (96% versus 87%), and has a comparable specificity (100% versus 96%) without the risk of hypersensitivity responses associated with intravenous injection of iodine-based contrast materials.[57] Identification of a stone on helical CT scan relies on visualization of a calcification within the course of the urinary tract as well as associated obstructive uropathy.[58] The calculus itself will appear as a brighter (lighter gray to white) structure visualized within the urinary tract (Figure 7-6). Stones that are formed by crystallization will appear brighter than those containing a higher portion of matrix, which appear darker because of soft attenuation when the proteinaceous materials are visualized. In addition to searching for a specific calcification, images will reveal signs of obstructive uropathy,

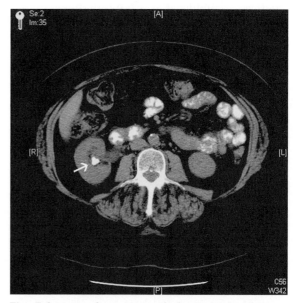

Fig. 7-6 Image of a urinary calculus (*arrow*). All stones (with the exception of some medication calculi) appear as dense, white objects within the urinary collecting system. (From Wein AJ, Kavoussi LR, Novick AC, Partin AW, Peters CA: Campbell-Walsh Urology, 9th edition. Philadelphia Saunders, 2007.)

including ureteral dilation, hydronephrosis, and asymmetric inflammation of the perinephric fat. Although helical CT will visualize approximately 98% of all urinary calculi, it is important to remember that even this study will not visualize indinavir stones in persons undergoing treatment for HIV infection. The search for a calculus on the helical CT scan concentrates on areas immediately proximal to a dilated ureter and known narrow areas within the course of the ureteral tract, including the UPJ, the point where the ureter crosses the iliac arteries, and the ureterovesical junction.

The plain abdominal film, or KUB, also may be used to visualize specific urinary calculi (Figure 7-7). For example, calculi that are composed of a radiopaque substance such as calcium phosphate or calcium oxalate stones are seen as white structures similar to bone. Struvite stones, because of their calcium content, and cystine calculi, because of their sulfur content, are also visible, but they will have a darker (grayer) appearance. Uric acid, indinavir, triamterene, or matrix stones are radiolucent and not visible on KUB films. Although the KUB provides an inexpensive method for visualizing stones, the lack of contrast highlighting the urinary tract, combined with overlying shadows from bone, bowel, and other abdominal organs, yields a low diagnostic rate of less than 40% when used as the sole imaging study, even in the hands of experienced clinicians.[59]

As noted earlier, the IVP was traditionally considered the gold standard for imaging urinary stones before the rise of the helical CT scan. Instead, its role has now evolved to use in selected patients in order to determine whether aggressive stone removal or ablation is indicated.[31]

Ultrasound may be used to identify urinary stones. They typically appear as bright (light gray or white) objects associated with long shadows caused by their significant density (Figure 7-8). When performed by a skilled technician, ultrasound can provide a reliable tool for diagnosis, but its sensitivity remains less than the helical CT at approximately 95%.[60] Nevertheless, it offers distinct advantages, including absence of radiation exposure and ready access in certain facilities, and it remains a viable option for imaging urinary stones in selected cases.

Retrograde pyelography is the visualization of one or both upper urinary tracts by means of retrograde

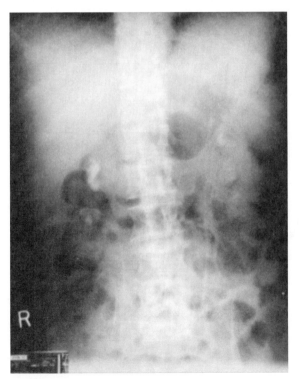

Fig. 7-7 Kidney, ureter, and bladder (KUB) film with large radiopaque calculi in the right kidney.

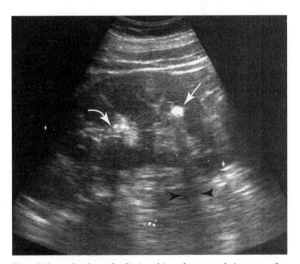

Fig. 7-8 Multiple calculi in this ultrasound image of a kidney (*white arrows*). The *left arrow* identifies multiple smaller stones in the upper pole of the kidney, while the *arrow to the right* indicates a single, larger calculus in the lower pole. The *small black arrowheads* at the bottom of the figure indicate the characteristic shadows produced by urinary calculi. (From O'Neill WC: Atlas of Renal Ultrasonography. Philadelphia: Saunders, 2001.)

injection of contrast material through a ureteral stent. It is occasionally used to detect radiolucent stones that are difficult to visualize using other imaging techniques. Magnetic resonance imaging (MRI) has not been widely used to diagnose urinary calculi because of poor visualization using traditional methods. However, a more recent technique that combines KUB with MRI demonstrated greater sensitivity than helical CT in visualizing certain aspects of obstructive uropathy but less sensitivity in direct visualization of the calculus itself. [61]

Urinalysis. Urinalysis detects the presence of blood, rules out complicating conditions such as infection, and identifies crystalluria. A dipstick analysis is obtained initially, followed by microscopy. Microscopy is essential to a complete urinalysis when evaluating for a urinary calculus, because it increases the likelihood of detecting hematuria, and it provides an opportunity to detect crystals in the urine that may provide clues to underlying metabolic disorders such as hypercalciuria, hyperoxaluria, hyperuricosuria, or cystinuria. Table 7-5 summarizes the appearance of common crystals using light microscopy.

Stone Analysis. Chemical analysis of stones forms the basis for subsequent medical therapy aimed at preventing recurrence. In order to obtain stone material, the patient is provided with a stone basket (straining device) and taught to urinate in the device, being careful to retain any stone material (including small particles resembling sand). Stone material is typically sent by registered courier to a certified laboratory for analysis.

Additional Evaluation. Based on the history, physical examination, urinalysis, and imaging studies, it is possible to classify patients as high or low risk for recurrence. Patients classified as low risk for stone recurrence typically undergo limited laboratory testing for associated metabolic disorders and are counseled about generalized measures to reduce the risk of recurrence. In contrast, those classified as high risk undergo a more extensive evaluation, sometimes referred to as an evaluation for metabolic stone disease or metabolic workup, and are placed on a preventive program based on the results of this evaluation. [30,31,56] A simplified evaluation typically includes a history; dietary history; stone analysis; SMA 20 testing for serum calcium, phosphorus, potassium, carbon dioxide, and uric acid; urinalysis; and urine culture when indicated. Elements of a detailed metabolic evaluation are outlined in Table 7-6.

Nursing Management

Acute management focuses on pain relief, alleviation of obstruction, and restoration of renal function in the affected kidney. Medical therapy focuses on prevention of recurrence by alleviating underlying metabolic disorders and long-term preservation of renal function. The urologic nurse is involved in both phases of management.

Urgent Interventions. Urgent and aggressive interventions are indicated for patients with infection of an obstructed urinary tract and those with impending renal deterioration. Infection of an obstructed urinary tract is likely to intensify renal colic, provoke fever, and greatly increase the risk of urosepsis. Because obstruction reduces effective renal blood flow and the glomerular filtration rate, administering an antibiotic alone will not eradicate infection. Instead, pharmacotherapy should be combined with immediate decompression of the affected kidney, typically by placement of a percutaneous nephrostomy tube or ureteral stent. Antimicrobial

TABLE 7-5 Appearance of Urinary Crystals Under the Microscope

CRYSTAL	SHAPE UNDER OPTICAL MICROSCOPE
Calcium oxalate monohydrate	Dumbbell or hourglass
Calcium oxalate dihydrate	Envelope or bipyramidal
Calcium phosphate-apatite	Amorphous
Calcium phosphate (brushite)	Needle shaped
Cystine	Hexagonal
Struvite (magnesium-ammonium-phosphate)	Coffin lid
Uric acid	Amorphous

From Menon M, Resnick MI: Urinary lithiasis, etiology diagnosis, and medical management. In Walsh PC, Retik AB, Vaughan DE, Wein AJ (eds): Campbell's Urology, 8th edition. Philadelphia: Saunders, 2002; p 3268.

therapy using broad-spectrum drugs capable of eradicating gram-negative and gram-positive pathogens is indicated until culture results are known. An oral fluoroquinolone, such as ciprofloxacin or levofloxacin, may be prescribed in selected cases or parenteral therapy initiated using a penicillamine (e.g., ampicillin or amoxicillin) and aminoglycoside (e.g., gentamicin or tobramycin) for patients with significant nausea and vomiting who are unable to tolerate oral medications. Close monitoring of the patient with an infection of an obstructed system is critical to preserve renal function and to ensure an adequate response to antimicrobial treatment. Failure of the fever to resolve within 1 to 3 days, increasing pain despite placement of a nephrostomy tube or ureteral stent, or significant hematuria should be promptly reported to a healthcare provider.

The intense pain associated with renal colic may be managed by opioid analgesics or nonsteroidal antiinflammatory drugs.[56] Table 7-7 lists analgesics commonly used for renal colic, dosages, and adverse side effects. Although opioid analgesics are traditionally used to manage renal colic, a systematic review comparing opioid analgesics with nonsteroidal antiinflammatory drugs (NSAIDs), such as ketorolac, found that many patients achieve adequate pain relief with fewer side effects when managed by NSAIDs.[62,63] Nevertheless, the intensity of the pain associated with renal colic often requires initial use of an opioid analgesic or a combination agent, such as acetaminophen plus codeine (Tylenol #3) or hydrocodone plus acetaminophen (Lortab), to provide adequate pain relief until obstruction is relieved and the pain subsides.

Desmopressin has been used alone and in combination with analgesic agents for the management of pain associated with renal colic. Lopes and colleagues[64] randomized 61 patients with acute renal colic to one of three treatments: the NSAID diclofenac (Voltaren), intranasal desmopressin (DDAVP), or combination therapy. Patients randomized to combination therapy (desmopressin plus diclofenac) had lower pain scores than those receiving desmopressin alone or diclofenac alone, and they had statistically significantly lower scores than those treated by desmopressin alone. An earlier study[65] found similar results when desmopressin was added to diclofenac therapy in 18 consecutive patients; but this study lacked a comparison group, thus severely limiting the ability to determine whether desmopressin truly increased the efficacy of NSAID therapy alone. Although these studies provide insufficient evidence

TABLE 7-6 Extensive Evaluation for Metabolic Disorders Contributing to Recurrent Urinary Stone Risk

DIAGNOSTIC TEST	PURPOSE
History	Family history of urinary stone disease, genetic or acquired diseases leading to underlying metabolic disorders, identification of modifiable factors influencing the risk of recurrence
Urinalysis	Evidence of underlying infection or bacteriuria
Fluid and dietary log	Low fluid intake leading to low urine volume; dietary intake for protein, calcium, sodium, oxalate, fiber, and phosphate; blood or urine tests may be repeated following dietary alterations
Bone density testing	Identification of resorptive hypercalciuria in patients with hypercalcemia or hypercalciuria
Urinalysis	Crystalluria, identification of the character of crystals, bacteriuria followed by culture when an infection-related stone (struvite) is suspected or confirmed
SMA 20	Measurement of serum calcium, alkaline phosphatase, phosphorus, potassium, bicarbonate, carbon dioxide, chloride, uric acid, and creatinine
24-hr urine test	Quantification of 24-hr urine volume, calcium, phosphorus, uric acid, oxalate, cystine, citrate, sodium, and magnesium
Fasting urine pH	Determination of effect of protein load on urinary pH
Automated stone risk analysis	Combination of data from multiple tests to provide a quantitative analysis of the risk for recurring urinary calculi

TABLE 7-7 Analgesics for the Management of Renal Colic

	DOSAGE	ADVERSE SIDE EFFECTS
Opioid Analgesics		
Meperidine (Demerol)	3 mg/kg IM every 3-4 hr	Nausea, vomiting, sedation, agitation, disorientation, constipation, flushing, dry mouth, urinary retention; respiratory and/or circulatory depression in rare cases
Morphine sulfate (MS)	0.05-0.2 mg/kg IM or IV every 4 hr	Similar to meperidine
Nonsteroidal Antiinflammatory Drugs		
Ketorolac	30-60 mg IV or IM every 4 hr	Dyspepsia, nausea, vomiting, abdominal pain, diarrhea, dizziness, anaphylactic reactions, acute renal failure, interstitial nephritis, gastrointestinal bleeding in rare cases
Diclofenac (Voltaren or Voltaren-XR)	50 mg PO two or three times daily, 100 mg daily (XR formulation)	Abdominal pain or cramps, constipation, diarrhea, headache, indigestion, nausea, anaphylactic reactions, acute renal failure, interstitial nephritis, gastrointestinal bleeding in rare cases
Combination Drugs		
Acetaminophen with codeine (Tylenol #3: containing 300 mg acetaminophen and 30 mg codeine)	One or two tablets PO every 4-6 hr	Sedation, drowsiness, dizziness, constipation, nausea, vomiting, respiratory depression, liver damage, hemolytic anemia in rare cases
Acetaminophen with hydrocodone (Lortab tablets containing 500 mg of acetaminophen plus 2.5, 5, 7.5, or 10 mg of hydrocodone)	One or two tablets PO every 4-6 hr	Sedation, dizziness, constipation, itching, mood changes, urinary retention

to recommend the addition of desmopressin to routine analgesia in the management of acute renal colic, they do provide a basis for considering therapy in selected patients who do not achieve adequate relief from analgesic agents alone and for further study of the role of desmopressin in this challenging clinical scenario.

Fluid intake must be managed judiciously. Increasing fluids augments urine volume, reduces supersaturation and the risk of additional crystallization, diminishes the likelihood of stone growth, and acutely raises intraluminal urinary tract pressure, promoting stone passage. However, it can also exacerbate the pain associated with acute renal colic,

especially in the presence of a very large or entrapped stone. Patients who are dehydrated or have low urine volume because of nausea and vomiting may require intravenous fluids, and all patients should be encouraged to consume adequate fluids to meet daily needs. However, advising patients to "force fluids" should be applied to patients with a reasonable chance of spontaneous passage rather than routinely dispensed as dogma. Refer to Clinical Highlights for Advanced and Expert Practice: Fluid Intake in the Management of Urinary Calculi for a more detailed discussion of this topic.[66-70]

Watchful Waiting. In the context of urinary stone management, watchful waiting (sometimes described

Clinical Highlights for Advanced and Expert Practice: Fluid Intake in the Management of Urinary Calculi[66-70]

Epidemiologic and chemical research clearly demonstrates that consumption of a low volume of fluids reduces urine volume; increases the osmolarity of multiple ions in the urine, including calcium, phosphate, oxalates, and uric acid; and enhances the risk for crystallization and stone growth. Because of this risk, clinicians commonly advise patients to increase fluid intake or "force fluids" in a variety of clinical scenarios. However, increasing fluid intake exerts a variety of effects on the urinary system, urine production, and its composition that may or may not assist the patient and clinician in what they wish to achieve. Therefore it is necessary to be judicious when advising patients to change patterns of fluid and to provide lucid and clear instruction that is based on clinical evidence or a research-based rationale. This clinical highlight provides recommendations for fluid intake in several common clinical scenarios that urologic nurses face when managing patients with urinary calculi. These recommendations apply to general scenarios; consultation with the urologist in individual cases is strongly recommended.

Acute Renal Colic

Acute renal colic occurs when a urinary stone blocks the urinary tract, resulting in distention of proximal urinary structures as the body attempts to remove the obstruction. Increasing fluid intake is frequently recommended in order to assist the body to "flush" the stone from the system. However, a systematic review by the Cochrane Renal Group found no evidence supporting or refuting the popular belief that increasing fluid intake promoted urinary stone passage. In addition, increasing fluid intake has been associated with exacerbation of the pain associated with renal colic, particularly when the stone is lodged within the urinary tract. Therefore all patients should be advised to consume adequate fluids to meet daily needs (½ oz per pound of body weight per day, or 2 to 2.5 L/day), and forcing fluids should be reserved for patients with a reasonable chance of passing stones spontaneously. Patients who are dehydrated because of nausea and vomiting may require intravenous hydration to reverse the deleterious effects on the urinary system and entire body.

Following Extracorporeal Shock Wave Lithotripsy or Percutaneous Nephrolithotomy

Increasing fluid intake is generally encouraged following extracorporeal shock wave lithotripsy (ESWL) or percutaneous nephrolithotomy to encourage the passage of stone fragments from the urinary tract. Consumption of approximately 3 L/day for the average adult may be recommended. Fluid intake may be particularly recommended when a ureteral stent is placed before the procedure, since this device is anticipated to ensure adequate drainage in the affected urinary tract and it may reduce some of the bothersome symptoms associated with a stent.

Preventing Recurrence

Consuming adequate fluids remains a mainstay in any treatment plan aimed at preventing urinary stone recurrence. Patients may be advised to consume adequate fluids to produce at least 2 L of urine per day, although some urologists recommend adequate intake to produce 3 L/day in selected cases. Fluids should be consumed throughout the day and particularly during the 1 to 2 hours following a protein-rich meal in order to reduce the effects of foods on urinary composition. Patients also may be encouraged to consume a glass of water when awakening at night. The influence of water "hardness" (mineral content) on stone risk remains unknown. Higher levels of calcium, magnesium, or bicarbonate in drinking water have been shown to influence urinary excretion of calcium, oxalate, and citrate (a stone inhibitor) in the urine. Nevertheless, epidemiologic studies have not revealed definitive evidence that consumption of hard water influences the overall risk for stone recurrence, regardless of underlying metabolic disorder or stone type. Therefore it is reasonable to counsel patients who voice concern about water hardness that filtration of drinking water or the purchase of bottled water provides an alternative to consuming more mineral-rich water, combined with counseling that there is insufficient evidence to determine whether these actions will have any significant effect on the risk of a recurring stone.

Consumption of water is strongly encouraged, but existing research does not support traditional recommendations that fluid intake should be restricted to water alone. Rather, several studies have demonstrated that consumption of a moderate volume of beer or wine (i.e., one bottle of beer or 8 oz of wine) exerts a protective effect, whereas consumption of high volumes of apple or grapefruit juice may increase the risk for stone formation. Cola consumption should be reduced or eliminated to less than 5 oz/day since it has been shown to increase both crystal formation and the rate of stone recurrence. In contrast, moderate consumption of coffee and tea was found to diminish stone formation when combined with an overall increase in fluid consumption.

as conservative management) is defined as symptomatic treatment of pain and nausea in anticipation of spontaneous passage of a urinary calculus. The likelihood that a stone will pass spontaneously is directly proportional to its size (small stones are more likely to pass than larger stones) and position within the ureter (stones in the lower ureter or at the ureterovesical junction are more likely to pass than those found in the proximal ureter or pelvicaliceal system). Specifically, the likelihood of spontaneously passing a stone that is 2 to 4 mm is 91% to 98% as compared with 48% for stones 7 to 9 mm and less than 25% for those greater than 9 mm.[71,72] Similarly, only 48% of stones located in the proximal ureter (irrespective of size) are likely to pass spontaneously, whereas 75% to 79% are likely to pass when located at the distal ureter or ureterovesical junction at the time of diagnosis.[72] Stone size and location also affect the mean time required for spontaneous passage. Calculi less than 4 mm spontaneously pass within a mean time of 8 to 12 days as compared with a mean passage time of 22 days for 4- to 6-mm stones. Stones that did not pass within 60 days are unlikely to pass spontaneously.

Because of the pain associated with renal colic, it is important to predict a patient's ability to spontaneously pass a specific stone with maximal accuracy. Fortunately, the ever-increasing sophistication of fast computers and advances in statistical techniques have enabled the development of an artificial neural network that has been designed to, among other things, predict the likelihood of spontaneous passage of a urinary calculus. Based on 17 input variables, Cummings and colleagues[73] reported on a neural network that achieved a 100% accuracy rate for predicting spontaneous stone passage.

Although stone passage is typically painful, watchful waiting offers several advantages for patients, including avoidance of invasive instrumentation, anesthesia, and the associated risk of adverse events. Nevertheless, these advantages must be carefully weighed against potential risks, including adverse effects of analgesics and loss of productivity owing to the pain associated with a ureteral calculus.[74] Regardless of its tolerability, aggressive interventions are indicated when urinary tract obstruction worsens; the stone fails to pass spontaneously after 60 days; the calculus produces significant pain, rendering watchful waiting intolerable; infection or significant hematuria occurs; and the calculus continues to grow despite appropriate medical management.

Patients managed by watchful waiting should be given a thorough explanation of the goals of this management strategy and indications that more aggressive treatment may be needed, such as the onset of significant hematuria, failure of passage after 1 to 2 months, or a sudden exacerbation of renal colic. Increasing fluid intake is generally encouraged since this will raise urine volume and pressures within the urinary tract. Although no evidence exists to determine the efficacy of this strategy, patients are generally encouraged to engage in light physical activity (move around) in an attempt to dislodge the stone and promote passage. α-Adrenergic blockers and calcium channel blockers have also been administered in an attempt to promote stone passage. Dellabella and colleagues[75] compared tamsulosin (Flomax), nifedipine (Procardia), and phloroglucinol (an herbal agent) in a group of 210 patients with distal ureteral stones 4 mm or greater in diameter. Patients managed with tamsulosin were more likely to spontaneously pass stones, and they passed stones quicker than did either of the other two groups. Yilmaz and colleagues[76] compared spontaneous passage rates using three α-adrenergic blockers (tamsulosin, doxazosin, and terazosin) in a randomized trial involving 114 patients with distal ureteral stones 4 mm or greater and found that all three groups were more likely to achieve spontaneous passage when compared with a control group. In addition, they did not find any differences in efficacy when comparing outcomes among the three groups. In a recent systematic review on the topic, there was supportive evidence in favor of either alpha blockers or calcium channel blockers in improved stone expulsion rates.[77]

Aggressive Interventions. Several techniques may be used to remove a stone or pulverize it into small particles, thus allowing spontaneous passage. The most commonly used techniques are extracorporeal lithotripsy, percutaneous lithotomy, and ureteroscopic manipulations.

Extracorporeal shock wave lithotripsy (ESWL) describes a number of electronic systems combining three essential components: a mechanism that generates and focuses a shock wave, a coupling medium, and an imaging system capable of localizing calculi.[30,78] Three generators are used to produce a shock wave capable of disrupting a calculus: electrohydraulic, piezoelectric, and electromagnetic.

The electrohydraulic generator uses a bath filled with degassed water as a coupling medium (Figure 7-9). A high-voltage spark plug is placed inside an ellipsoidal reflector that focuses the shock wave at the base of the water bath. A high-voltage spark plug causes very rapid evaporation of water, generating a shock wave as it expands surrounding fluids. The piezoelectric generator creates a shock wave by a sudden expansion of ceramic elements when excited by a high-frequency, high-voltage pulse. Although each individual element moves only slightly, excitation of thousands of elements creates a high-energy shock wave that is focused on a very specific point using a water-filled bag or small water basin as a coupling medium. The electromagnetic generator generates a shock wave when an electrical impulse moves a thin circular membrane housed in a cylindric shock tube. Acoustic lenses focus the shock wave, and a water-filled cushion and gel are used as coupling media.

Localization of the stone requires either fluoroscopy or ultrasonography; each modality offers specific advantages and disadvantages. Fluoroscopy generates images of radiopaque stones that are familiar to both urologists and radiologists, and the injection of contrast may be used to localize radiolucent stones. Disadvantages of fluoroscopy include the generation of ionizing radiation in order to generate image and the size and cost of the equipment. Ultrasonography avoids ionizing radiation and may be used to image radiolucent stones. However, this technique is more operator dependent than ultrasound, sometimes rendering the localization of small stones (less than 4 mm) difficult, and equipment is expensive.[30]

Regardless of their design, ESWL machines are designed to comminute (crush or pulverize) stones by four principal mechanisms.[78] Compression fracture occurs when shock waves travel through the stone, leading to a fracture of that aspect of the calculus that faces away from the incoming wave. Fragmentation (often referred to by endourologists as spallation) occurs when the shock wave reflects off imperfections in the stone, such as cavities or the border between crystalline and matrix materials, or the interface between the distal stone surface and urine. As a result, a negative wave is created that exerts a considerable tensile force against these impedance imperfections, resulting in stone disruption at multiple locations. Acoustic cavitation occurs when cavitation bubbles are formed by the shock waves that fragment the stone using the mechanisms described previously. Finally, dynamic fatigue may occur within the stone, particularly at the borders between crystalline growth and matrix, initially leading to microscopic cracks within the stone and ultimately to fragmentation.

As experience and expertise for ESWL have grown, the list of relative contraindications to treatment has narrowed significantly. They now include very large stones, significant dilation of the collecting system, untreated coagulopathy, urinary tract infection, calcified aortic aneurysm that is proximal to the stone, renal artery aneurysm, or pregnancy.

Although increasing experience with ESWL has limited the number of contraindications, a number of factors continue to influence its efficacy in certain clinical scenarios. For example, larger calculi require a comparatively high number of shocks to pulverize.

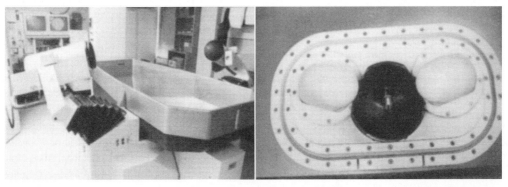

Fig. 7-9 Electrohydraulic extracorporeal shock wave lithotripsy (ESWL) system uses a high-voltage spark to create a shock wave and degassed water as a coupling medium. Stones are located using fluoroscopy.

In addition, they leave a comparatively large volume of fragments in the urinary tract, raising the risk of steinstrasse (obstructing column of stones) that may require ureteroscopic removal. The location of the calculus within the urinary tract influences the operator's ability to accurately localize and pulverize stones in a single session. Thus, whereas 85% to 92% of patients with urinary calculi will be rendered stone free by a single session of ESWL, only 75% to 80% of midureteral stones and less than 60% of stones located below the pelvic brim are eradicated by a single session of ESWL.[78] In addition, stones primarily consisting of oxalate monohydrate or cystine are "harder" and more difficult to comminute than "softer" stones primarily made up of calcium phosphate or calcium oxalate.

Preprocedural preparation includes anatomic and functional evaluation of the urinary system. Patients are advised that good-quality imaging studies are needed to determine the location of calculi and that functional studies (usually requiring injection of contrast or a radionuclide marker) are needed to define the function of the obstructed and contralateral renal units. Because many stones harbor bacteria that are released into a traumatized urinary tract during lithotripsy, a urine specimen is obtained and infection is eradicated *before* ESWL is completed. Stone analysis is completed before ESWL whenever possible, particularly when cystine or oxalate monohydrate calculi are suspected. Patients with struvite stones and those suspected of having calculi harboring bacteria are counseled that up to 2 weeks of suppressive antimicrobial therapy may be undertaken before ESWL to reduce the risk of serious infection when the stones are crushed by shock wave lithotripsy.[79]

Patients are advised that although ESWL is noninvasive, the procedure is associated with discomfort and pain control measures will be needed. Analgesia requirements are influenced by three technical factors: the size of the focal point, the area of shock wave entry, and the power (pressure) generated by the shock wave. These factors are largely determined by the type of lithotripter and the technology used to generate and focus a shock wave. Generally, the electrohydraulic generators use higher-energy shock waves with a limited focal point, resulting in the need for regional or general anesthesia. Although reducing the power of the shock waves delivered to the calculi may diminish the need for anesthesia, it

also lowers the likelihood of achieving stone-free status following a single treatment. Lithotripters using piezoelectric generators provide a larger skin entry zone and less powerful shock waves, eliminating the need for general or regional anesthesia to control pain in most cases. However, they are also associated with a higher re-treatment rate.[80] Lithotripters using electromagnetic generators have a smaller skin entry site, and power intensity lies between the electrohydraulic and piezoelectric generators in the pain associated with shock wave generation. As a result, patients may or may not require anesthesia when undergoing treatment. In addition to these considerations, the patient's medical and neurologic status and his or her ability to remain relatively still during the procedure as well as the desires and preferences of the patient, anesthesiologist, and urologist influence this important decision. Because of these and other considerations, a variety of approaches, including general or regional anesthesia, parenteral analgesics, and/or topical anesthetics, may be used to control pain during ESWL. The urologic nurse should consult with the urologist and lithotripsy staff to determine the type of analgesia or anesthesia in a specific case or facility. Prior knowledge about the type of anesthesia is important since this will profoundly affect preprocedural preparation.

Patients are also advised to consult the urologist about discontinuing or altering the dosage of prescriptive anticoagulant medications for a short period before surgery as directed. Patients are also counseled to discontinue over-the-counter drugs with anticoagulant actions, such as aspirin products, and dietary supplements, including high-dose vitamin E.

Because ESWL may affect cardiac firing and transmission[81] and the need for regional or general anesthesia in some cases, it is essential that the patient undergo a thorough integrated history and physical that includes a cardiovascular examination. Ganem and Carson[82] compared 933 patients undergoing fixed-rate ESWL and found that patients with a history of preexisting cardiac disease requiring medications were more likely to experience arrhythmias than those without a cardiac history. Shock waves are usually timed based on the electrocardiogram (ECG), avoiding the risk for arrhythmias. Nevertheless, clearance from a cardiologist is essential for the patient with a history of cardiovascular disease, and arrangements to temporarily turn off defibrillating pacemakers must be made before ESWL is undertaken.

Patients are counseled that a ureteral stent may be placed before the procedure. Placement is not routine and depends on multiple factors, including total stone burden, urinary system function, and physician preference. Refer to Clinical Highlights for Advanced and Expert Practice: Caring for Ureteral Stents for a more detailed description of the care of ureteral stents.[83-86] Patients may be further counseled that a parenteral fluid line may be placed and that the procedure is expected to last from 45 to 120 minutes.

Following ESWL, the patient is transferred to a postanesthesia recovery area for a brief period, usually no more than 1 to 3 hours. Patients managed by an electrohydraulic lithotripter, requiring partial submersion in water, are dried and damp bed clothing is changed.[87] The flank is assessed for ecchymosis, erythema, or petechiae, indicating soft tissue damage. Application of an ice pack to the flank may diminish edema and offer transient pain relief when theses signs occur.[88]

The urine is monitored for gross hematuria, a common sequela of ESWL. Patients are advised that grossly visible hematuria is anticipated during the first several voids following ESWL and should gradually clear within 1 to 5 days unless a ureteral stent is present. Bright red bleeding or passage of clots after this time is not anticipated and should prompt a call to the urologist or urologic nurse. Patients with a ureteral stent are advised that hematuria may persist until the stent is removed but that passage of bright red urine or blood clots is not expected.

Analgesic medications are usually required following ESWL, and patients should be advised that passage of stone fragments frequently causes pain. Patients are typically prescribed an analgesic and advised to avoid taking over-the-counter aspirin or NSAID medications that may exacerbate hematuria or bleeding within traumatized renal tissue.

Struvite and carbone apatite stones develop from a urease positive UTI[89]; to prevent or treat post UTI from stone fragmentation and release of organisms, an antimicrobial drug is usually prescribed post ESWL. The patient is advised to rest for the first 24 hours following ESWL, maintain good fluid intake, and restrict driving. Patients are taught to monitor for hematuria and infection, and they may be asked to strain the urine for stone fragments for chemical analysis.

Patients are counseled that complications of ESWL are uncommon but may be serious and require additional intervention. Renal trauma causes hematuria, interstitial edema and hemorrhage, renal tubular necrosis, damage to local nephrons, damage to renal vessels, or a generalized hematoma of the renal cortex and medulla.[90] The impairment to renal function is typically transient and directly related to the total number of shock waves delivered to the kidney. Pretreatment with aminophylline or nifedipine and allopurinol can block acute interstitial changes of the renal parenchyma.[91,92] Untreated hypertension and use of aspirin also enhance this risk. Long-term renal effects include permanent impairments in renal function, hypertension, and an increased rate of stone recurrence. Gastric or duodenal erosion or damage to the lungs or pancreas is a rare occurrence following ESWL.[93-95]

Percutaneous nephrolithotomy allows the urologist to gain access to the upper urinary tract by a percutaneous approach through the overlying flank.[96] Indications include the treatment of larger stones (more than 2 cm), struvite stones, lower pole stones, and stone management in selected persons with congenital renal defects, such as a horseshoe kidney. The patient is given appropriate anesthesia and placed in a prone position (Figure 7-10). Fluoroscopy is used to image the upper urinary tract and ensure safe access to the pelvicalyceal lumen. Once safe access is obtained, the nephrostomy tract is dilated and the stone is localized (Figure 7-11). Larger stones may be fragmented using intracorporeal electrohydraulic lithotripsy or a holmium laser; alternative techniques include ultrasonic or pneumatic lithotripters or pulse dye laser energy. Stone fragments may be removed under rigid or flexible nephroscopic visualization. Nevertheless, flexible nephroscopy is recommended to visualize the entire pelvicalyceal system so that all stone fragments are identified and removed. The collecting system is irrigated throughout the procedure with a physiologic solution to reduce the risk of dilutional hyponatremia. Following manipulations, a nephrostomy tube is placed in order to prevent excessive bleeding, to promote healing of the renal puncture site, to allow subsequent access to the kidney if needed, and to ensure adequate drainage of the kidney.

Clinical Highlights for Advanced and Expert Practice: Caring for Ureteral Stents[83-86,227]

A ureteral stent is a thin catheter or tube inserted into the ureter in order to ensure flow in an obstructed urinary tract. Stents come in a variety of diameters (4F to 10F), lengths (24 to 30 cm), and configurations; they are designed so that one or both ends have a J configuration, or they are coiled in a "pigtail" configuration. Ureteral stents are placed into the ureter using endoscopic guidance, usually with the patient under general or regional anesthesia, so that the proximal end opens in the renal pelvis and the distal end drains into the lower urinary tract. Ureteral stents are placed for a variety of indications, including ureteroscopy, surgical interventions involving extensive manipulation of the ureteropelvic junction or ureteral course, ensuring drainage across a ureteral stricture, and in the palliative care setting when a tumor leads to external compression of the ureter and subsequent obstruction. A stent may be placed in the patient with severe obstruction and renal colic caused by an obstructing stone or when pyelonephritis is present. It is frequently placed in the obstructed ureter immediately before extracorporeal shock wave lithotripsy (ESWL) to prevent obstruction and renal colic from stone fragments (steinstrasse). Placement of a stent has been shown to alleviate severe pain associated with renal colic and reduce rehospitalization rates and visits to the emergency department following ESWL (especially when stones larger than 2 cm are treated).

Although ureteral stents provide an effective means to drain an obstructed urinary tract, 20% to 70% of patients also experience distressing symptoms. A study of 135 patients with indwelling ureteral stents noted the following symptoms: voiding frequency (50%), urgency (55%), dysuria (40%), flank pain (32%), gross hematuria (2%), and fever (15%). Additional problems included impaired sleep (45%) and impaired libido (42% of men and 86% of women). Symptoms associated with ureteral stents are severe enough that approximately 70% of patients will require analgesia, 40% will restrict activities, and 50% will report an overall reduction in quality of life while the stent remains in place.

Management of bothersome symptoms associated with stents is individualized and influenced by the underlying reason for stent placement. Voiding frequency, urgency, and dysuria may be alleviated by increasing fluid intake while avoiding caffeinated beverages known to irritate the bladder. Antimuscarinic medications, such as oxybutynin (Ditropan), tolterodine (Detrol), solifenacin (VESIcare), darifenacin (Enablex), or trospium (Sanctura), may be prescribed to reduce urgency and voiding frequency. Alternatively, a prescriptive or over-the-counter urinary analgesic, such as phenazopyridine (Pyridium), or a combination agent containing a urinary analgesic and antispasmodic, such as Urised, may be prescribed when dysuria and lower urinary tract pain are particularly bothersome.

Patients are advised that hematuria is common when a ureteral stent is in place. They are further counseled that mild hematuria, resulting in lightly tinged urine, is anticipated. In contrast, passage of bright red urine or passage of clots is not expected and should be managed by promptly contacting a urologic care provider.

Flank pain is frequently associated with the presence of a ureteral stent, but its etiology may be multifactorial. For example, flank pain may indicate passage of ureteral fragments following ESWL or percutaneous lithotomy, or inflammation following surgical manipulation of the upper urinary tract or ureteroscopy. Analgesic medications are frequently required to manage pain observed in patients with indwelling ureteral stents. The type and potency of the analgesic rely on multiple factors, including the underlying condition and the severity of associated pain. Opioid analgesics are commonly required, particularly when a ureteral stent is placed during ESWL, and patients are advised to temporarily avoid nonsteroidal antiinflammatory drugs (NSAIDs) because of their anticoagulant side effects. Intravesical ketorolac has been found to reduce ureteral stent–related discomfort in one randomized study that compared its efficacy with oxybutynin or alkalinized lidocaine.

Pain associated with fever raises a strong suspicion of infection that requires treatment with an appropriate antibiotic. Similar to urethral catheters, long-term indwelling ureteral catheters may form a biofilm rendering them resistant to antimicrobial therapy and prone to recurring infection. The presence of a biofilm may lead to encrustation of the stent with calcium oxalate, rendering removal particularly difficult. Suppressive antibiotics may be used for short-term ureteral stents (2 weeks or less), but colonization with resistant bacterial strains occurs when long-term drainage is required.

Ureteral stent manufacturers are investigating changes in product design in an effort to reduce or prevent associated symptoms. Ongoing research is focusing on the material of construction, the application of various coatings, and changes in the stent's configuration.

Preoperative preparation focuses on obtaining imaging studies needed to carefully elucidate the anatomy of the affected urinary tract and to plan the optimal approach.[79,97] Intravenous urography, KUB, and a bladder scan are usually obtained. A CT scan is preferred when a renal anomaly is suspected. The CT scan also provides valuable anatomic information in morbidly obese patients, persons with orthopedic anomalies, and persons with a retrorenal colon. Any prescription or over-the-counter medicine, herbal supplement, or dietary supplement

with anticoagulant properties is discontinued 14 days before the procedure because of the risk of blood loss during the procedure (refer to Chapter 11). A urine culture is obtained, and bacteriuria is eradicated because of the potential risk of sepsis. Suppressive antibiotics are administered, particularly when a struvite stone is treated.

Donor or autologous blood should be available. Although significant bleeding during percutaneous lithotomy is uncommon (about 1%), it may occur quickly and requires rapid blood replacement after blood loss has been controlled.

Postoperative management focuses on urinary drainage, control of bleeding, and prevention of infection. Percutaneous drainage is almost always accomplished by a drainage tube. Common alternatives include a nephrostomy tube, self-retaining catheter, Foley catheter, Malecot tube, or circle nephrostomy tube. The catheter is connected to an appropriate drainage system, and the patient is taught to care for the catheter until it is removed, no sooner than 1 or 2 days following the procedure. The patient is also taught to monitor for signs and

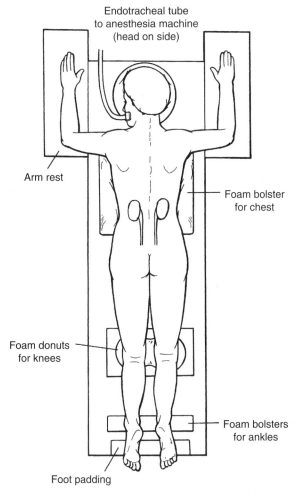

Fig. 7-10 The patient is placed in a prone position for percutaneous nephrolithotomy. Bolsters are placed on either side of the chest to ensure adequate respiration, and additional bolsters are placed under the head, knees, and feet to prevent pressure injury and promote ventilation and peripheral circulation. (From Walsh PC, Retik AB, Vaughan ED, Wein AJ (eds): Campbell-Walsh Urology, 8th edition. Philadelphia: Saunders, 2002.)

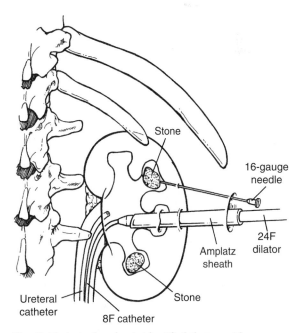

Fig. 7-11 A single calyx is identified that provides reasonable access to the calculi. A dilator and sheath are used to ensure percutaneous access to the affected kidney. (From Walsh PC, Retik AB, Vaughan ED, Wein AJ (eds): Campbell's Urology, 8th edition. Philadelphia: Saunders, 2002.)

symptoms of urinary tract infection, including fever and flank pain. Contrast is typically injected through the tube before its removal to ensure patency of the urinary tract, absence of extravasation, and absence of residual stone fragments.

Ureteroscopic manipulation of stones is used in selected cases, including removal of steinstrasse following ESWL, removal of selected stones lodged in the lower ureter, or manipulation of stones in the upper urinary tract.[98] Transurethral endoscopy is used to visualize the ureteral orifice, which is then dilated. Flexible or rigid endoscopes are used to visualize and manipulate stones. A large variety of instruments are now available to retrieve stones, including wire pronged graspers and stone baskets. Newer stone baskets have been designed that are able to disengage stones in a comparatively atraumatic fashion and to prevent retrograde stone migration. Working ports in the ureteroscope can be used to fragment stones using intracorporeal lithotripsy or laser energy. Ureteroscopy also may be used to pass a guidewire up the ureter in order to place a ureteral stent. Ureteral stents are commonly placed after ureteroscopic stone manipulation.

Preparation is similar to that described for percutaneous lithotomy, although imaging studies focus on endoscopic rather than percutaneous access. The patient is advised that intravenous sedation or light anesthesia will be necessary during the procedure. Postprocedural nursing management concerns are similar to those following any transurethral endoscopic procedure and include ensuring urinary drainage, ongoing monitoring of hematuria, prevention of infection, and pain management. Patients are counseled about other potential complications of ureteroscopic management, such as ureteral perforation or avulsion, strictures, or loss of a stone. Ureteral avulsion is a rare complication that occurs when the ureter becomes entrapped along with the stone during manipulation.[79] It is typically managed by open surgical repair of the ureter. Ureteral perforation occurs when ureteral integrity is compromised, often because of trauma incurred during electrohydraulic lithotripsy. It is managed by immediate discontinuation of the procedure, placement of a ureteral stent, and careful monitoring for 3 to 4 weeks until the ureter has a chance to heal. Ureteral perforation increases the risk for formation of a ureteral stricture; its management is discussed later in this chapter.

Open surgery was once standard aggressive treatment for obstructing urinary stones, but it is now used only in highly selected cases. Surgical approaches include nephrolithotomy (incision of the kidney with open surgical removal of a staghorn stone from the pelvicalyceal system), pyelolithotomy (open surgical removal of a stone from the renal pelvis), and ureterolithotomy (open surgical removal of a stone from the ureter) (Figure 7-12). Current indications are extremely large staghorn calculi (pyelolithotomy), salvage surgery for ureteral stones not adequately managed or amenable to less invasive techniques (ureterolithotomy), or because of

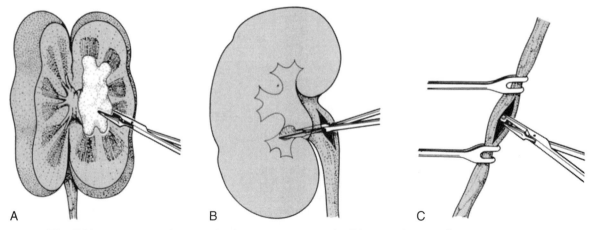

Fig. 7-12 Open surgery for removing large stones. **A,** Nephrolithotomy for a staghorn stone requires surgical incision of the parenchyma. **B,** Pyelolithotomy requires incision of the renal pelvis. **C,** Ureterolithotomy, with removal of a large stone from the ureter.

technical considerations, such as infundibular steno-sis or ureteropelvic obstruction, when an open pro-cedure allows the urologist to achieve multiple goals with a single procedure.

Preventing Recurrence. The overriding goal of nursing and medical management of stone disease is the prevention of recurrence. For the purposes of this discussion, prevention strategies include advice about fluid intake, meant for *all* patients at risk for recurring urolithiasis, and other methods based on specific underlying metabolic disorders.

Fluid intake. Increasing fluid intake reduces the osmolarity of all solutes in the urine, resulting in a diminished likelihood of crystal formation and growth. In a randomized clinical trial by Borghi and colleagues[99] increasing fluid intake alone reduced 5-year recurrence rates when compared with a con-trol group who were managed without formal fluid or dietary advice. Refer to Clinical Highlights for Advanced and Expert Practice: Fluid Intake in the Management of Urinary Calculi for a more detailed discussion of fluid intake for preventing urinary stone recurrence.

Idiopathic hypercalciuria. In addition to maintain-ing robust fluid intake, dietary modifications are typ-ically recommended for patients with idiopathic hypercalciuria and recurring calcium oxalate or cal-cium phosphate urinary stones. These interventions can be broadly summarized as favoring moderation in the intake of multiple foods or beverages known to influence calcium, phosphate, and oxalate excretion in urine. Dietary calcium is known to contribute to urine excretion by the kidneys. Nevertheless, it has been shown that consumption of a restrictive, low-calcium diet leads to resorption of calcium from bones, paradoxically raising calcium excretion in the kidney while demineralizing bones.[100] In addi-tion, epidemiologic data have shown that patients who form stones tended to ingest *less* calcium in their diet than did subjects who do not experience urinary stones.[101,102] Therefore individuals at risk for recurring stone formation should be advised to con-sume a well-balanced diet, including moderate con-sumption of foods rich in calcium, based on the daily recommended allowance of 1 g/day. Further, patients should be counseled to avoid consuming excessive amounts of calcium through either dietary sources or consumption of calcium-based antacids or dietary supplements, such as Tums.

The consumption of dietary sodium (table salt) is associated with an increase in both sodium and cal-cium excretion in the urine. Therefore patients with idiopathic hypercalciuria should be advised to mod-erate sodium in the diet to no more than the recom-mended daily allowance of 2.4 g/day (about 1 teaspoon). Patients are also advised that protein intake should be moderated, particularly among those pursuing an Atkins diet that advocates high protein intake and sharply reduced carbohydrate consumption. Consumption of a meal high in pro-tein is a concern for patients with idiopathic hyper-calciuria because it creates an "acid wash" in the urine characterized by a drop in urinary pH and sub-sequent increase in calcium excretion.

Oxalate intake also should be moderated, because individuals who form calcium oxalate stones have been shown to have as much as three times the normal load of oxalate excretion when compared with patients who remain stone free.[30] Diets that severely restrict oxalates are available, but most patients find them unpalatable, rendering long-term adherence difficult. Instead, persons at risk for recur-ring calcium oxalate or oxalate monohydrate stones may be counseled that foods rich in oxalic acid, which has no established recommended daily allow-ance, should be consumed in moderation. Table 7-8 lists dietary sources of oxalic acid.

In addition to diet, a number of medications may be administered to reduce the risk of calculus recurrence among patients with idiopathic hypercalciuria. Routine administration of thiazide diuretics, such as hydrochlorothiazide (HCTZ) or trichlormethiazide, has been found to reduce the risk of stone recur-rence.[103,104] HCTZ is administered as a 50-mg tablet twice daily, and trichlormethiazide is given as a 2-mg tablet twice daily. The pharmacologic mechanism altering stone risk is not known. These medications are hypothesized to promote calcium reabsorption in the proximal renal tubule. Thiazides have been hypothesized to affect oxalate excretion, but a recent study found no measurable effect on 24-hour urinaly-sis in 537 patients with a history of idiopathic recurring calcium stones.[105] Common side effects associated with thiazide diuretics include fatigue, muscle cramp-ing, hypokalemia or hypomagnesemia, diminished libido, or erectile dysfunction. A thiazide diuretic may be combined with potassium citrate, resulting in further reductions in calcium excretion in the urine,

TABLE 7-8 Dietary Sources of Oxalates[226]

Fruits	Blackberries
	Blueberries
	Raspberries
	Strawberries
	Currants
	Kiwi
	Grapes
	Figs
	Tangerines
	Plums
Vegetables	Spinach*
	Collard greens
	Okra
	Parsley
	Leeks
	Celery
	Green beans
	Rutabagas
	Summer squash
Nuts	Almonds
	Cashews
	Peanuts
Grains	Wheat germ
	Wheat bran
Legumes	Soy beans
	Tofu
Other sources	Cocoa
	Chocolate
	Black tea

*Spinach is a particularly rich source of oxalate, containing 750 mg/100 g serving.

while reducing the risk of hypokalemia and avoiding hypochloremic metabolic acidosis.[103] Patients are further counseled that a high sodium intake will nullify the therapeutic effect of thiazides. Regular use of a thiazide diuretic, combined with moderate dietary sodium intake, can reduce the risk of urolithiasis by approximately 90%.[104] Nevertheless, long-term follow-up is necessary because some patients will experience a recurrence of hypercalciuria within 30 to 120 months despite documented reductions in urine calcium levels with initial treatment.[106]

Orthophosphate, administered as 1.5 to 2 g daily, is frequently used to treat recurring calcium oxalate or calcium phosphate stones in patients who are normocalciuric.[30] It diminishes calcium excretion in the urine and free calcium ionic activity by altering urinary pH, reducing urinary phosphate levels and citrate levels, and by inhibiting the synthesis of 1, 25-dihydroxy–vitamin D. Orthophosphates reduce the risk of calcium phosphate but not calcium oxalate stones. In addition to preventing stone recurrence, previously formed small calculi within the urinary tract may dissolve or reduce in size during the first 3 to 6 months after therapy is begun. The most common adverse side effect associated with orthophosphate administration is diarrhea; its use is contraindicated in cases of renal insufficiency.

Cellulose phosphate is used to reduce stone recurrence in patients with absorptive hypercalciuria.[30] Whereas orthophosphate influences urinary excretion, cellulose phosphate binds calcium in the intestinal lumen and renders it unavailable. It is used exclusively in persons with absorptive hypercalciuria; it may paradoxically increase calcium crystal formation in those patients with resorptive or renal hypercalciuria. The typical dose is 5 g two or three times daily. It has also been advocated for the treatment of infantile hypercalcemia and nephrocalcinosis.[107] Because cellulose phosphate also binds magnesium, it is necessary to combine its administration with magnesium gluconate (1 to 1.5 g/day).

Potassium citrate reduces the risk of stone formation in patients with idiopathic hypercalciuria by increasing urinary pH and urinary citrate excretion. Citrate inhibits calcium oxalate crystallization and the concentration of ionic calcium in the urine. Whereas potassium citrate reduces the risk of stone formation, sodium citrate does not.[108] Magnesium has also been advocated for the prevention of stone recurrence because of several potential benefits, such as inhibition of calcium crystallization and absorption of dietary oxalate from the bowel. Early trials reported reductions in stone recurrence among patients using magnesium oxide or hydroxide, but no difference was found when a more carefully controlled randomized double-blind clinical trial was completed.[109] In contrast, a clinical trial that combined magnesium with potassium citrate demonstrated a reduction in stone recurrence and a reduction in the frequency of gastrointestinal upset seen when potassium citrate was administered alone.[110] A study in 25 normal men by Kato and colleagues[111] found that potassium citrate when combined with magnesium inhibited magnesium oxalate crystallization better than either agent when given alone.

Pentosan polysulfate has been advocated for the prevention of stone recurrence in patients with idiopathic hypercalciuria, but it has not enjoyed widespread use in the clinical setting.[30] Pentosan inhibits calcium oxalate crystallization, and it may promote repair of injured urothelium, thus inhibiting adhesion of crystals to epithelial defects in the urinary tract.[112] As of 2008, the randomized clinical trials needed to provide definitive answers to its potential role have not been completed or reported in the literature. However, an open label trial involving 121 subjects found that 48% remained stone free while on treatment, and urinary calculi produced while patients were taking the drug tended to be smaller and were more likely to pass spontaneously.[113]

Hyperoxaluria. Considerable research has focused on the management of hypercalciuria, but comparatively little has focused on oxaluria. Ingestion of large quantities of ascorbic acid (vitamin C) has been shown to increase oxalate excretion and stone formation, but significant increases occur only with consumption of very high doses of ascorbic acid (more than 2 grams a day.[114] In contrast, no research exists that has shown an increased risk for idiopathic hypercalciuria when adults consume the recommended daily allowance of vitamin C, whether it is obtained from foods or a multivitamin.

Moderation of dietary ingestion of oxalate including colas, combined with robust fluid intake, is advised for patients with idiopathic hypercalciuria. Bacteria in the gut have been shown to bind with oxalic acid, reducing both absorption from dietary sources and excretion of oxalates in the urine. One study found that administration of a highly concentrated preparation of freeze-dried lactic acid bacteria, containing *Lactobacillus acidophilus*, *L. plantarum*, *L. brevis*, *Streptococcus thermophilus*, and *Bifidobacterium infantis*, over a 4-week period significantly reduced oxaluria.[115] However, it is not yet known whether this strategy will significantly reduce the risk of recurring calcium oxalate or oxalate monohydrate stones.

As noted previously, primary hyperoxaluria is a genetic disorder characterized by overproduction and accumulation of oxalate in the body. Stone risk in patients with type 1 or type 2 primary hyperoxaluria is typically managed by administration of vitamin B$_6$ (given as 50 mg four times daily), calcium oxalate crystallization inhibitor, and ongoing fluid

management.[116] Although children with primary hyperoxaluria are at high risk for stone formation, it is important to remember that the condition is also associated with a very high risk of end-stage renal disease as well as deleterious effects on the bones, joints, retinas, cardiovascular system, and peripheral nerves. Therefore aggressive early treatment and ongoing follow-up by a multidisciplinary healthcare team including urology, nephrology, and pediatrics are essential.

Hyperuricosuria. In contrast to the medical management of most other stone types, conservative management of uric acid stones is used to both reduce the risk for recurrence and dissolve existing stones.[117] Treatment focuses on three immediate goals: increasing urine volume, alkalinizing the urine, and reducing the production of uric acid in the urine by administration of allopurinol (Zyloprim). Fluid intake should be boosted sufficiently to ensure a daily urine output of 1.5 to 3 L. Urinary alkalinization may be managed by administration of sodium bicarbonate, 650-mg tablets, or 1 to 2 teaspoons of baking soda taken two or three times daily. Patients are taught to measure the pH of their urine using litmus paper and to titrate bicarbonate so that their urine pH is approximately 6.0 to 6.5. Patients are further advised to avoid attempting to raise the pH much higher, since this may cause precipitation of calcium phosphate, preventing stone dissolution. Although clearly effective, alkalinization combined with robust fluid consumption increases sodium and water retention and therefore may not be tolerable to patients with congestive heart failure, cirrhosis of the liver, or poorly controlled hypertension. Acetazolamide (Diamox) has been used as an alternative, but it increases the risk for calcium phosphate crystallization. Therefore many clinicians prefer to alkalinize the urine with potassium citrate (given as 30 to 60 mEq/day), which avoids sodium and water retention while raising urinary pH to approximately 6.2.

Allopurinol is a xanthine oxidase inhibitor that is administered in a daily dose of 300 mg. It reduces urinary excretion of uric acid. When allopurinol is administered in combination with robust fluid intake and urinary alkalinization, pure uric acid stones can be dissolved, usually within 12 weeks.[117] In addition to teaching the dosage and scheduling of allopurinol, patients are taught to monitor for adverse side effects, including a skin rash, nausea and vomiting, and precipitation of an episode of gouty arthritis pain. Counseling should emphasize discontinuing allopurinol if a rash occurs and promptly contacting the urologist or urologic nurse since this may indicate a hypersensitivity response.

Xanthinuria. Xanthine stones rarely occur as an adverse side effect of allopurinol therapy, justifying immediate discontinuation of the drug. Others experience xanthinuria because of an inherited deficiency of xanthine oxidase. These individuals are managed by maintaining high fluid intake and urine output while restricting consumption of foods known to be rich in adenine, such as lentils.[30]

Cystinuria. Prevention of cystinuric stones focuses on four strategies: increasing urine volume, urine alkalinization, moderating dietary intake of methionine, and pharmacotherapy to convert cystine to its more soluble form, cysteine.[41] High urine volumes are generally recommended, varying from 3 to 5 L in adults and 3 L in children.[31,41] Patients should be counseled to maintain high water intake in particular and to drink both while awake and when arising at night to void. Water may be supplemented with beverages likely to alkalinize the water, such as mineral water, citrus juices, and herbal teas. Alkalinization is usually achieved by administration of potassium citrate, but the goal of treatment is a pH of 7.5. Consumption of orange juice is encouraged because it contains additional potassium citrate. As when managing patients at risk for uric acid stones, overzealous alkalinization is avoided because of the risk of provoking calcium phosphate crystallization.

Dietary modification concentrates on moderating intake of methionine.[41] Dietary sources of methionine include protein-laden foods, such as meat, fish, eggs, and soy. Unfortunately, the resulting diet is restrictive and unpalatable, reducing long-term compliance. In addition, strict protein restriction is contraindicated in growing children and adolescents. Therefore a diet that moderates the intake of methionine combined with high urine volume and alkalinization may be more realistic than a strict dietary regimen.

Chelating drugs are administered when nonpharmacologic agents fail to control stone recurrences.[41] Options include D-penicillamine (DP) and α-mercaptopropionylglycine (Thiola). Both agents cleave the disulfide bond of cystine into cysteine, a compound that is 50 times more soluble in urine. Thiola may have fewer side effects than DP, but even it is associated with significant adverse side effects, such as rash, arthralgias, thrombocytopenia, proteinuria, and nephritic syndrome. The usual dosage is 1.193 g/day. Captopril (Capoten) is a first-generation angiotensin-converting enzyme inhibitor. It converts cystine to captopril-cysteine, which is 200 times more soluble than cystine in urine. Its clinical efficacy is not yet established, and adherence to therapy is sometimes limited by the occurrence of orthostatic hypotension when given to normotensive individuals.

Struvite stones. Because struvite stones are associated with urea-splitting pathogens, medical therapy focuses on eradicating bacteria from the urinary system.[30] A urine culture is obtained, and an appropriate antibiotic is begun at least 48 hours before aggressive treatment. If a staghorn struvite stone is removed surgically, the renal pelvis is irrigated with hemiacidrin in an attempt to dissolve any residual particles. Following stone removal, antimicrobial therapy is continued for at least 2 months and sometimes considerably longer. Ammonium chloride (1.5 to 3 g/day) may be administered to acidify the urine and promote dissolution of stone fragments of small stones. Aceto-hydroxamic acid (Lithostat) is a urease inhibitor that reduces the risk of recurrent struvite stone formation. Up to 1.5 g/day is given in three or four divided doses. Patients taking Lithostat are taught to take the medication on an empty stomach and to self-monitor for side effects. Adverse side effects affect up to half of all patients taking the drug, and they include nausea and loss of appetite, headache, trembling or weakness, and deep vein thrombosis.

TRAUMA

Trauma to the urinary system or adjacent organs and iatrogenic injury during surgery may result in obstruction of the upper or lower urinary tract. Treatment focuses on correction of the underlying injury and often involves surgical reconstruction. Refer to Chapter 10 for a more detailed discussion of genitourinary trauma.

URETERAL STRICTURE

Ureteral strictures, defined as a narrowing in the course of the ureter, are usually the result of iatrogenic trauma associated with open or endoscopic urologic procedures, pelvic or gynecologic procedures, or laparoscopic surgery (Figure 7-13).[118] Other etiologies include the passage of stones, radiation therapy, periureteral fibrosis caused by abdominal aortic aneurysm or endometriosis, parasitic infection (i.e., tuberculosis or schistosomiasis), trauma, and congenital anomaly (rare).[17,119] Little is known about the epidemiology of ureteral stricture; the prevalence may be rising slightly because of the increase in endoscopic manipulation of the upper urinary tracts. Ureteral strictures occur in approximately 1% of diagnostic ureteroscopic procedures,[120] between 3% and 11% of interventional endoscopic procedures involving the ureters,[121,122] 4% of supravesical urinary diversions,[123] and 4% of renal transplantations.[124] Although rare in patients who spontaneously pass urinary stones or those undergoing ESWL, they occur in as many as 24% of patients with impacted ureteral stones that fail to pass within 60 days.[125]

A majority of ureteral strictures are discovered incidentally on imaging studies. Flank pain is the most common clinical manifestation associated with a ureteral stricture.[126] The pain resembles renal colic, but it is intermittent rather than ongoing and usually less intense than the pain associated with a calculus. Flank pain may be exacerbated by diuresis following consumption of a large volume of fluids, use of a diuretic medication, or suppression of vasopressin (antidiuretic hormone). Diagnosis is based on identification of a persistently narrowed area in the ureter during intravenous or retrograde pyelography, combined with evidence of obstructive uropathy. In addition to identifying the stricture, the

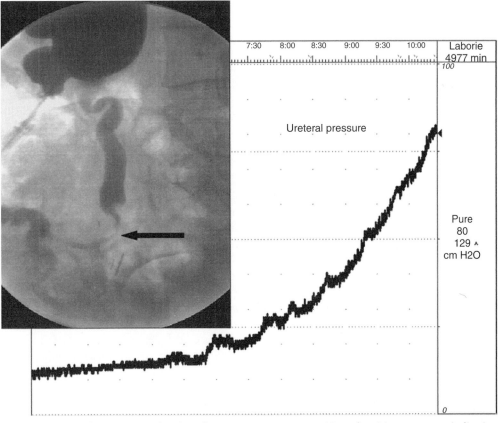

Fig. 7-13 Ureteral stricture at the site of a ureteroureterostomy. Note the rising pressures indicating severe obstruction on Whitaker testing. (From Gupta M, Ost MC, Shah JB, McDougall EM, Smith AD. Percutaneous management of the upper urinary tract. In: Wein AJ, Kavoussi LR, Novick AC, Partin AW, Peters CA (eds): Campbell-Walsh Urology. 9th edition. Philadelphia: Saunders, 2007; p. 1536.)

diagnostic evaluation is used to exclude the possibility of a malignant tumor. During antegrade studies such as the intravenous pyelogram, it is important to differentiate the stenotic area of a stricture from functional narrowing of the ureter caused by peristalsis. In contrast to ureters obstructed by urinary calculi, the MRI accurately identified ureteral obstruction caused by stricture or tumor in 83% of a group of 65 patients, whereas the non–contrast-enhanced helical CT scan identified the level of obstruction in only 28%.[127] Occasionally, a radionuclide scan or Whitaker test may be performed to identify the magnitude of obstruction associated with a ureteral stricture.

Because the stricture is an anatomic lesion, endoscopic or open surgical dilation or repair is required. Catheter or balloon dilation followed by insertion of a ureteral stent is often favored as an initial approach.[17,118] A retrograde pyelogram is performed, and a guidewire is passed in a retrograde fashion (from lower to upper urinary tract) into the pelvicalyceal system. An open-end catheter is advanced along the wire and ultimately replaced with a high-pressure balloon that is 4 cm long and 4 to 6 mm in diameter when inflated. Radiopaque markers are used to position the balloon within the stricture that is progressively dilated. A stent is left in the ureter for 2 to 4 weeks to promote healing and prevent stricture recurrence. Although a ureteral stent is an effective means for preventing obstruction, its presence is associated with adverse side effects including hematuria and bothersome lower urinary tract symptoms, such as urgency, voiding frequency, and urge urinary incontinence. Alternatively, an antegrade approach may be used in selected cases when the preferred retrograde approach is not technically feasible. In this case, percutaneous nephrostomy must be established to ensure adequate drainage of the affected upper urinary tract. Although this approach is minimally invasive when compared with open surgical repair, success rates vary from 50% to 85%.[17]

Other endoscopic approaches include endoureterotomy by means of a ureteroscopic or antegrade approach and cautery wire balloon incision. These approaches evolved from endoscopic balloon dilation and share multiple features. Ureteroscopic endoureterotomy begins with a retrograde pyelogram, followed by advancement of a guidewire through the stricture and into the affected pelvicalyceal system. However, the ureter is incised rather than merely dilated using a cold knife, cutting electrode, or holmium laser passed through a working port of the ureteroscope. Occasionally, a cautery wire balloon incision routinely used for endopyelotomy is adapted to incision of a ureteral stricture. Following incision, the largest ureteral stent that can be easily passed through the ureteral lumen is left in place in order to minimize the risk for recurrence. Alternative approaches include an antegrade or combined retrograde/antegrade approach. Indications for these approaches are technical, based on the location of the stricture, its proximity to great vessels, and its length.

Open surgical repair includes ureteroureterostomy, transureteroureterostomy, or intubated ureterostomy. Ureteroureterostomy is completed by resecting the ureteral stricture and forming a primary anastomosis of the two ends of the same (ipsilateral) ureter. In contrast, the transureteroureterostomy requires resection of the stricture and anastomosis of the affected ureter into the contralateral (unobstructed) ureter. If the ureteral stricture affects the distal 3 to 4 cm of the ureter (closest to the bladder wall), the stricture is resected and the remaining ureter is reimplanted into the bladder wall, usually by means of a Boari flap (a tubularized structure created from bladder tissue). Alternatives to these procedures include ileal ureteral substitution, where the proximal ureter is replaced with a segment of ileum isolated from the fecal stream, or a Davis intubated ureterotomy that relies on reepithelialization or variations on this procedure using a buccal mucosal graft or tissue from the renal pelvis.

Nursing management initially focuses on providing emotional support during diagnostic evaluation and subsequent treatment and management of flank pain when present. Many ureteral strictures are asymptomatic and diagnosed incidentally, but their presence may coexist with a metastatic tumor, such as cervical cancer, or a primary tumor of the ureteral epithelium. Other ureteral strictures are associated with flank pain. The pain tends to be mild to moderate in intensity and intermittent in nature. Imaging studies may reveal ureterohydronephrosis, but they may provide equivocal results when attempting to localize the stricture, leading to uncertainty and frustration for both patient and clinician. In these cases, patients may be encouraged to maintain a pain diary to help characterize and localize the pain and elucidate exacerbating and alleviating factors. Patients are further advised that functional tests, including a radionuclide scan or Whitaker test, are sometimes needed to localize the obstruction, determine its severity, and evaluate whether intervention is likely to resolve flank pain. Occasionally, a ureteral stricture is associated with acute obstruction with persistent and more severe flank pain. Acute obstruction may indicate the presence of an underlying malignant tumor or undetected calculus. When acute obstruction occurs, an NSAID, opioid analgesics, or combination agent may be required to manage pain. A percutaneous nephrostomy tube will be placed when the obstruction is compromising renal function or it is complicated by infection.

The preprocedural and postprocedural care for patients undergoing ureteral stricture repair varies according to the approach and type of procedure. Patients undergoing ureteroscopic repairs are advised that a transurethral approach will be used to gain access to the urinary system, followed by ureteral dilation, ureteroscopy, and dilation or incision of the stricture. A ureteral stent is almost always left in place, and patients are taught about commonly associated symptoms and their management. Emphasis is placed on self-monitoring for signs or symptoms of recurring obstruction, infection, or excessive hematuria. Those undergoing endoscopic manipulation using an antegrade approach or combination antegrade-retrograde approach are advised of the need for establishing access to the pelvicalyceal system and the possibility that a nephrostomy tube will be inserted. Patients undergoing open surgical repair are counseled about the need for general anesthesia, brief hospitalization, and placement of a ureteral stent following surgery. Patients who have a section of ileum incorporated into the ureter are advised about the need for bowel preparation before surgery and a nasogastric tube following the procedure.

URINOMA

A urinoma is an encapsulated mass of urine extravasated from the urinary tract.[128] Urinomas typically arise following renal injury secondary to blunt or penetrating abdominal trauma, although they are sometimes associated with ureteral injury. Urinomas have also been associated with endoscopic, laparoscopic, or open surgical manipulation. As fluid collects, the perirenal fat is replaced by inflammatory tissues within 2 to 5 days, and the urine is encapsulated within a fibrous sac within 3 to 6 weeks. Clinical manifestations include progressive abdominal pain and distention, fever, vomiting, and elevated white blood cell counts. Initial diagnosis is based on an imaging study such as a CT scan or intravenous pyelogram, but definitive diagnosis relies on aspiration of fluid and confirmation that it is urine. Obstruction arises because of local inflammation or compression of the adjacent ureter. Urinomas are treated by percutaneous drainage under ultrasonic or CT guidance and placement of a ureteral stent when indicated.

TUMORS

Urologic tumors may produce obstruction as they grow and fill the lumen of a ureter or by encroaching on the ureterovesical junction. Abdominopelvic tumors arising from adjacent organs such as the bowel or reproductive system also may produce obstruction when they grow large enough to compress the ureter or bladder outlet. Treatment is aimed at eradicating or debulking the underlying malignancy, although a ureteral stent may be placed in the palliative care setting to relieve ureteral colic.

INFECTIONS

Bacterial infections rarely cause urinary tract obstruction, but two pathogens (*Mycobacterium tuberculosis* and *Schistosoma haematobium*) invade the walls of the urinary tract, leading to fibrosis, low compliance, and obstruction. *S. haematobium* is a parasite that dwells in the rivers and lakes of Africa and the Middle East. The adult worm enters the body through the urethra and lays eggs in the urinary bladder, ureters, and kidneys. This process leads to inflammation and fibrosis of the walls of the urinary tract, resulting in low compliance, obstruction, and obstructive uropathy.[129] *M. tuberculosis* is a rod-shaped bacterium with a particularly thick cell wall. Infection of the urinary tract leads to lymphocytic infiltration, macrophages, and granuloma formation. The resulting inflammation and fibrosis frequently lead to ureteral scarring, stenosis of the ureterovesical junction, low bladder wall compliance, and/or urethral strictures. Both schistosomiasis and urinary system tuberculosis produce hematuria. Ultrasonography may be obtained to evaluate the character and severity of obstructive uropathy. Treatment initially focuses on eradication of the underlying infection, but surgical reconstruction including urinary diversion or creation of a neobladder may be necessary when extensive fibrosis occurs.

RETROPERITONEAL FIBROSIS

Retroperitoneal fibrosis is characterized by fibrosis of the retroperitoneum around the aorta and below the level of the renal arteries.[130] Its cause is unknown; but it has been compared with other fibrotic conditions, such as sclerosing cholangitis, mediastinal fibrosis, and large bowel strictures. Possible etiologic factors include an autoimmune process or an idiosyncratic response to specific drugs, such as methysergide, hydralazine, β-adrenergic blockers, or ergot alkaloids. Symptoms occur when fibrosis leads to ureteral obstruction and include abdominal or flank pain and fever. Ureteral obstruction is typically treated by surgical ureterolysis. Care is taken to ensure that a tissue specimen is obtained to rule out malignancy, which occurs in approximately 8% of all cases of retroperitoneal fibrosis. Although surgery has proved effective for relieving obstruction, progression of fibrosis resulting in obstruction of the affected or contralateral ureter may occur. In addition, large blood vessels coursing through the retroperitoneum or the duodenum may be affected. Long-term corticosteroid administration (up to 2 years) may be undertaken to prevent disease progression and recurring obstruction, but the benefits of ongoing corticosteroid treatment must be carefully weighed against potential adverse side effects including leukocytopenia with increased risk for infection, hyperglycemia with increased risk for steroid-induced diabetes mellitus, thinning of the bones, and relapse of fibrosis when steroid therapy is discontinued.

PELVIC LIPOMATOSIS

Deposition of mature, encapsulated fat in the retroperitoneal space is called pelvic lipomatosis.[4] Its etiology is unknown; it may be associated with obesity, but the response to weight loss or gain is variable. It has also been linked to Dercum's disease (characterized by painful subcutaneous fat deposits), cystitis glandularis, and chronic venous obstruction. It normally occurs in young adults, ages 25 to 55 years, with predominance in African American men. Men are at greater risk than women, but children are occasionally affected. Clinical manifestations include a nonlocalized pelvic discomfort, hematuria, suprapubic mass, hypertension, and lower urinary tract symptoms associated with cystitis glandularis, such as frequent urination and nocturia. Imaging studies will reveal a pear-shaped bladder whose base is elevated (Figure 7-14). The upper urinary tracts are normal in some cases, whereas others will have significant ureterohydronephrosis. Diagnosis requires abdominopelvic CT scan or an MRI. Weight loss may be recommended, but patients should be counseled that results will vary. Excessive pelvic fat may be removed surgically, but complications including excessive blood loss because of large veins in the fat and bowel or urinary tract injury because of obliteration of normal tissue planes may occur. Ureteral stents may be placed to relieve upper urinary tract obstruction, and ureteral reimplantation is indicated in certain cases.

AORTIC ANEURYSM

An aortic aneurysm is abnormal dilation of the aortic wall. Its estimated annual incidence is 6 cases per 100,000 people, and it typically affects patients in the sixth or seventh decades of life. A majority of thoracic aneurysms are associated with atherosclerosis, but some are associated with inflammatory disorders or an autoimmune process.[131] Inflammatory aortic aneurysms are often associated with ureteral obstruction that was managed by insertion of a ureteral stent preoperatively. Ureterolysis may be completed when the aneurysm is repaired, but the patient should be counseled that this procedure is technically demanding and sometimes associated with complications including renal failure.[132]

RADIATION THERAPY

Various forms of radiation therapy may lead to urinary tract obstruction. The location and character of obstruction are influenced by the total dose, mode of delivery, and associated malignancy. For example, brachytherapy of the prostate leads to acute congestion and bladder outlet obstruction that slowly subsides over a period of 12 months. Alternatively, external beam radiation therapy delivered to the pelvis may result in lower compliance and obstruction of the bladder or ureter. Treatment varies based on the location and character of the

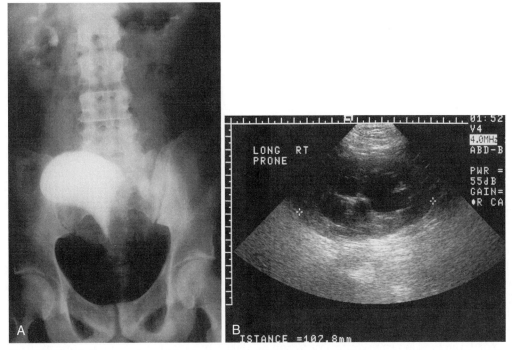

Fig. 7-14 Pelvic lipomatosis resulting in elevation of bladder base and obstruction of the urinary tract. **A,** The hydronephrosis on the intravenous pyelogram. **B,** The renal ultrasound. (From Walsh PC, Retik AB, Vaughan ED, Wein AJ (eds): Campbell's Urology, 8th edition. Philadelphia: Saunders, 2002.)

radiotherapy and the severity of the associated obstruction. The reader is referred to Chapter 8 for a detailed discussion of adverse side effects associated with radiation therapy for urologic malignancies.

LYMPHOCELE

A lymphocele is a cystic mass that is caused by damage to the lymphatic system. It occurs in approximately 5% to 6%[133] of renal transplantations and 3% to 4%[134] of patients undergoing radical prostatectomy. Lymphoceles occasionally result in upper urinary tract obstruction with hydronephrosis, a nontender mass of the lower abdomen, swelling of the scrotum, or ipsilateral edema of the leg.[133] Although rare, lymphocele may also cause bladder outlet obstruction.[135] Initial diagnosis is based on an imaging study, such as a CT scan, but definitive diagnosis requires aspiration of fluid from the mass and confirmation that it is lymph. Treatment options include percutaneous aspiration, usually accompanied by injection of a sclerosing agent such as povidone-iodine, tetracycline, fibrin glue, or bleomycin.[133] Combination therapy is often preferred because it reduces the risk of recurrence, but sclerosing therapy is associated with uncommon but significant complications, including acute renal failure. Surgical management requires wide drainage of fluid into the abdominal cavity, usually accomplished by a laparoscopic approach.

URETHRAL VALVES AND POLYPS

Urethral valves are thin membranes of tissue that occlude the urethral lumen and obstruct urinary outflow in male infants.[136] They are comparatively uncommon, occurring in between 1 in 8000 and 1 in 25,000 live births. Urethral polyps are even rarer. They occur most commonly in boys, but six cases have been reported in girls.[137] Because the obstructive lesion is located in the urethra, the resulting obstruction affects the entire urinary system. The obstructive uropathy seen with these lesions is often quite severe, especially when the valve or polyp occurs in the posterior urethra. Renal dysplasia or hypoplasia may occur, and the deleterious effects on the developing lower urinary tract may lead to lifelong voiding dysfunction. Refer to Chapter 12 for a detailed discussion of urethral valves and polyps.

PHIMOSIS

Phimosis is an abnormal stenosis of the penile foreskin that prevents it from being retracted to uncover the glans penis. The phimotic foreskin is characterized by indurated white plaques or scar tissue at the preputial orifice. Phimosis is associated with lichen sclerosus, forcible premature retraction, or repeated infections resulting in scarring of the foreskin. In severe cases, phimosus may produce obstruction of the distal urethra. Treatment options include partial or complete circumcision or treatment with topical steroids.[138]

URETHRAL STRICTURE

Strictly defined, the term *urethral stricture* usually refers to a narrowing of the anterior urethral lumen caused by scarring.[139] However, it also may be used to refer to congenital narrowing of the urethra or an iatrogenic process affecting the posterior urethra. Regardless of its cause or location, urethral strictures become clinically relevant when they cause sufficient narrowing of the urethral lumen to create obstruction.

Any process that injures the urethral epithelium so severely that the resulting inflammation and tissue repair result in scarring is capable of producing a stricture. Anterior urethral strictures are characterized by fibrous (scar) tissue that encroaches on the lumen and may extend throughout the underlying urethral wall. Kochakarn and coworkers[140] reviewed more than 300 cases of anterior urethral strictures treated over a period of 29 years and attributed 73% to trauma (including urethral instrumentation) and 16% to infection. Refer to Chapter 10 for a detailed discussion of urethral strictures caused by genitourinary trauma. Infections associated with an increased risk of stricture formation include gonococcal and nongonococcal urethritis[139] as well as lichen sclerosus.[141]

Posterior anastomotic strictures are also characterized by scar formation, but they arise from an obliterative process as a result of trauma or urethral surgery.[139] The most common surgical intervention associated with posterior urethral strictures is radical prostatectomy. Hu and associates[142] reviewed records of 12,079 American men who underwent radical prostatectomy over a 7-year period and found that 28% to 33% had urethral strictures that were severe enough to require treatment. The vast majority of these occurred at the site of the anastomosis following removal of the malignant prostate.

In contrast to these, congenital strictures contain a significant amount of smooth muscle and are thought to be caused by abnormal canalization of the urethra during embryogenesis.[143] The incidence is unknown, but reports in the literature are limited to single case studies or relatively small case series. For example, Nonomura and colleagues[144] identified only 74 boys with congenital strictures affecting the anterior urethra (sometimes referred to as Cobb's collar) over a period of 11 years.

Clinical manifestations of anterior or posterior urethral strictures include lower urinary tract symptoms associated with obstruction such as spraying, split stream, reduction in the force of the stream, and feelings of incomplete bladder emptying. Some patients will present with a bacterial prostatitis or epididymitis caused by the turbulence created by the narrowed urethral lumen.[139] Alternatively, a stricture is discovered in some patients who present with acute urinary retention when a urethral catheter cannot be passed beyond the level of the stricture. Signs and symptoms of upper urinary tract distress are rare. Lower urinary tract symptoms are also common with congenital urethral strictures, but the specific manifestations differ.[144] They include overactive bladder symptoms and nocturnal enuresis. Febrile urinary tract infections are common, and upper urinary tract distress (vesicoureteral reflux) may be found in more than half.

Diagnosis is based on localization of the stricture, identification of contributing factors, and evaluation of associated obstructive uropathy.[139] A retrograde urethrogram (RUG) provides a minimally invasive method for visualizing the urethra and stricture. The patient is placed in a supine position and the pelvis rotated slightly to create an oblique view. A catheter-tipped syringe or specially designed adapter is attached to the urethral meatus. The penis is extended to maximize visualization of the urethral course, and contrast is injected into the urethra in a retrograde fashion (Figure 7-15). Alternatives to the RUG include ultrasonography of the urethra, which is particularly useful for anterior urethral strictures, or urethroscopy.

Immediate treatment (i.e., urethral dilation using a urethral sound or filiforms and followers) is initiated after the location and basic characteristics of the stricture are evaluated. Most cases ultimately require surgical reconstruction. Multiple techniques have been developed; refer to Chapter 11 for a

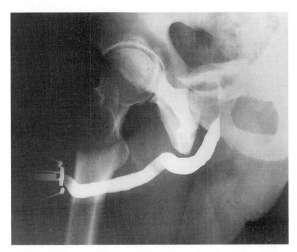

Fig. 7-15 Retrograde urethrogram in a male patient. Note that the patient has been moved to an oblique position and the penis extended to optimally visualize the entire urethral course. (From Walsh PC, Retik AB, Vaughan ED, Wein AJ (eds): Campbell-Walsh Urology, 8th edition. Philadelphia: Saunders, 2002.)

detailed discussion of the surgical and nursing management of urethral strictures.

BENIGN PROSTATIC HYPERPLASIA

Benign prostatic hyperplasia (BPH) is characterized by a nonmalignant enlargement of the prostate gland associated with aging. Technically, the term *BPH* refers to microscopic changes in the prostatic tissue, but it rises to clinical relevance when these microscopic changes lead to macroscopic changes in the organ that produce bothersome lower urinary tract symptoms or significant obstructive uropathy. Microscopically, BPH is characterized by proliferation (hyperplasia) of the stromal and epithelial cells within the periurethral zone of the prostate gland. Over time, microscopic changes lead to glandular enlargement and obstruction of the bladder outlet, along with the bothersome lower urinary symptoms associated with BPH. Clinicians tend to assume that the number and severity of lower urinary tract symptoms caused by BPH are directly related to the severity of the underlying obstruction. However, urodynamic studies have demonstrated that these phenomena are only weakly correlated,[145-147] and the natural epidemiology and natural history of BPH remain topics of continuing research. Historically, lower urinary tract symptoms seen in men with BPH were conceptualized as evidence of "prostatism"

(a term used to describe urinary symptoms associated with BPH as well as the underlying histologic changes). However, the 4th International Consultation on BPH recommends that clinicians and researchers use a more global term, namely, lower urinary tract symptoms (Table 7-9), because they are associated with multiple disorders affecting both women and men.[148,149]

Epidemiology

The incidence of BPH is approximately 15 per 1000 man-years, and it increases with age from 3 cases per 1000 in men younger than 49 years of age to 38 cases per 1000 man-years in men aged 75 years or older. Indeed, as many as 50% of men aged 60 years and 80% of 80-year-olds[150] will experience bothersome lower urinary tract symptoms associated with BPH. As the proportion of men living 70 years or more grows, the prevalence of BPH will continue to grow. The clinical relevance of BPH is principally associated with the negative impact associated lower urinary tract symptoms exert on health and health-related quality of life.[151]

Few modifiable risk factors for BPH have been identified. One study of Asian men noted that alcohol and smoking appeared to reduce BPH risk,[152] but other studies have found an *increased* risk. For example, a survey of African American men found an increased risk of lower urinary tract symptoms and BPH among men who were currently smoking; those who reported significant alcohol consumption; and those with a history of hypertension, heart disease, or diabetes mellitus.[153] Similarly, a survey of Finnish men found that smokers had a higher prevalence of lower urinary tract symptoms than those who did not.[154] Smoking is a sympathetic nervous system stimulant and may theoretically increase smooth muscle tone at the bladder neck and sphincter.[155] Men with fecal incontinence, neurologic disease, constipation, or arthritis are also more likely to experience moderate to severe lower urinary tract symptoms, but these conditions may affect the neurologic modulation of the detrusor muscle directly rather than influencing prostatic enlargement per se.[156]

Race influences BPH risk; African Americans tend to experience symptoms earlier than whites, while Japanese and Asian men tend to present somewhat later.[152] Numerous additional factors affect risk, presumably because of their influence on prostatic conversion of testosterone to dihydrotestosterone, or the

TABLE 7-9 Lower Urinary Tract Symptoms as Defined by the International Continence Society[149]

	DESCRIPTION
Storage Symptoms	
Increased daytime frequency	Complaint of voiding too frequently while awake
Nocturia	Arising from sleep because of the need to urinate
Urgency	The complaint of a sudden and compelling desire to urinate that is difficult to defer
Urinary incontinence	The complaint of any involuntary leakage of urine
Voiding Symptoms	
Slow stream	Patient's perception of reduced urine flow when compared with previous performance or when compared with others
Splitting or spraying of stream	Urine stream that is expressed in two identifiable streams (splitting) or multiple streams (spraying)
Intermittent stream	Urinary stream stops and starts on one or more occasions during micturition
Hesitancy	Difficulty initiating micturition that results in delay between readiness to urinate and onset of stream
Straining	Perception that abdominal straining is required to initiate, maintain, or enhance the force of the urinary stream
Terminal dribble	Prolonged end to micturition, when the stream has slowed to a trickle or dribble
Postvoid Symptoms	
Feelings of incomplete emptying	Perception of incomplete bladder evacuation despite micturition
Postvoid dribble	Involuntary urine loss immediately after urination, often occurring when male patients begin to move away from the toilet or when a woman arises from the toilet

production of growth factors and stromal-epithelial signaling.[157] The typical symptoms of decreased stream, hesitancy, intermittency, nocturia, terminal dribbling, frequency, and urgency are caused by gradually increasing prostate size. Approximately two thirds to three fourths of patients with clinical signs of BPH are found to have obstructed voiding,[158] but whether these symptoms will progress to complete urinary retention is unclear.[159] The primary risk factors for acute urinary retention in men with BPH include increasing symptom severity, perceptions of incomplete bladder emptying despite micturition, frequent urge to void (2 hours or less), and a weak urinary stream.[160] Objective measures of BPH associated with an increased risk of acute urinary retention are greater prostate volume and uroflowmetry parameters (maximum and average flow rates). In rare cases, BPH is associated with few or no bothersome lower urinary tract symptoms and is discovered only when a serious urologic complication, such as renal insufficiency, occurs. Nevertheless, the vast majority of men seek help because of the presence of bothersome lower urinary tract symptoms, leading BPH to be classified as a "quality of life disorder." As a result most cases are guided by the patient's perceptions of symptom severity and how symptoms impact his life rather than the size of the prostate or severity of the underlying obstruction.

Pathophysiology

The processes that regulate prostatic hyperplasia in the aging man have not yet been well defined. It has long been known that prostatic hyperplasia is testosterone dependent and that the process does not occur among men who were castrated as children.[161] Nevertheless, BPH is most prevalent in aging men who are also known to have a steady decline in bioavailable testosterone. Further research into this apparent paradox revealed that prostatic hyperplasia is primarily influenced by dihydrotestosterone, an androgenic hormone manufactured in the prostate under the influence of the 5α-reductase enzyme. Dihydrotestosterone is a powerful stimulator of cellular reproduction in the prostatic stroma, but its actions alone do not account for age-related BPH. Additional processes known to influence prostatic growth include nonandrogenic growth factors, stromal-epithelial cell interactions, and endogenous estrogens.[161] Cellular growth factors affect both new cell production and programmed cellular death (apoptosis). They are believed to function synergistically with androgens to stimulate stromal cell hyperplasia. The growth factors most relevant to BPH are EGF (epidermal growth factor), TGF-β (transforming growth factor-beta), KGF (keratinocyte growth factor), and bFGF (basic fibroblast growth factor). A synergistic effect involving androgens and growth factors helps to explain stromal cell hyperplasia in the presence of reduced androgen levels; however, it does not explain epithelial cell hyperplasia, since these cells are unresponsive to androgens.

The mitotic response of epithelial cells seen in BPH is believed to be mediated by stromal-epithelial cell interactions. Although epithelial cells are unresponsive to androgenic stimulation, they are very responsive to growth factors produced by the stromal cells, and these growth factors are produced in greater quantities when the stromal cells are stimulated by androgens. Thus androgenic stimulation is thought to indirectly affect epithelial hyperplasia. Finally, the testes may produce a nonandrogenic substance that acts to sensitize the prostatic tissues to the effects of androgens. The role of endogenous estrogens in BPH remains unknown; they are thought to play an as yet undefined supportive or synergistic role that may promote (rather than inhibit) prostatic growth.[161]

Although our understanding of the pathophysiologic processes that produce the lower urinary tract symptoms associated with BPH remains incomplete, it is known that bladder outlet obstruction is the central feature.[158,162,163] Obstruction arises from both static and dynamic components. Nevertheless, the lower urinary tract symptoms associated with BPH are also influenced by multiple other factors, including detrusor overactivity, sensory urgency, and detrusor contractility.

Obstruction: Static Component. Static factors in the hyperplastic prostate contribute to obstruction when they compress the urethral lumen. For example, the nonelastic prostatic capsule restricts the direction in which an enlarging prostate can spread, ultimately leading to increasing compression of the urethral lumen.[146] Therefore men with a total prostatic volume more than 30 g are three times more likely to experience acute urinary retention than men

whose prostatic volume remains below 30 g.[163] Growth of the median lobe is particularly important to obstruction because it can directly encroach on the urethral lumen, even in the absence of a significant increase in prostatic volume. In an attempt to quantify this discrepancy, some clinicians use the results of prostatic ultrasound to calculate the equation (transition zone volume divided by total prostate volume) because it has been shown to be more predictive of acute urinary retention risk than estimates of total prostatic volume alone.[164] Administration of 5α-reductase inhibitors may alleviate lower urinary tract symptoms associated with BPH and lowers the risk of acute urinary retention by reducing transition zone volume and overall prostate volume,[164,165] although the effect on nocturia is less pronounced.

Dynamic Component. Dynamic factors also contribute to bladder outlet obstruction.[162,163] In addition to increasing prostatic size, hyperplasia also raises sympathetic tone.[145,162,163] Stimulation of the sympathetic nerves excites α-adrenergic receptors located in the bladder neck and proximal urethra, resulting in increased urethral resistance. BPH also leads to smooth muscle hypertrophy (thus the use of the term benign prostatic hypertrophy), but its significance in promoting bladder outlet obstruction remains unclear.[163] Medications that enhance α-adrenergic tone, such as over-the-counter decongestants, increase sympathetic tone in the proximal urethra and the concomitant risk for urinary retention, whereas α-adrenergic blocking agents reduce sympathetic tone and ameliorate obstruction and associated lower urinary retention.[165]

Phases of Prostatic Obstruction. Tanagho[166] details two phases of obstruction in men with BPH. A *compensatory phase* is characterized by an increase in the contraction force of the detrusor muscle. Initially, the man may perceive a diminished force in the urinary stream, often accompanied by increased daytime voiding frequency, nocturia, and urgency. However, these symptoms may diminish or disappear as the detrusor muscle compensates for the increased urethral resistance by a more powerful contraction. In as many as 83% of men with BPH, their lower urinary tract symptoms are stable for 10 years or longer.[167] Urodynamic testing during this phase of BPH reveals elevated voiding pressures accompanied by a diminished maximum and average flow rate, with a low residual volume (Figure 7-16).

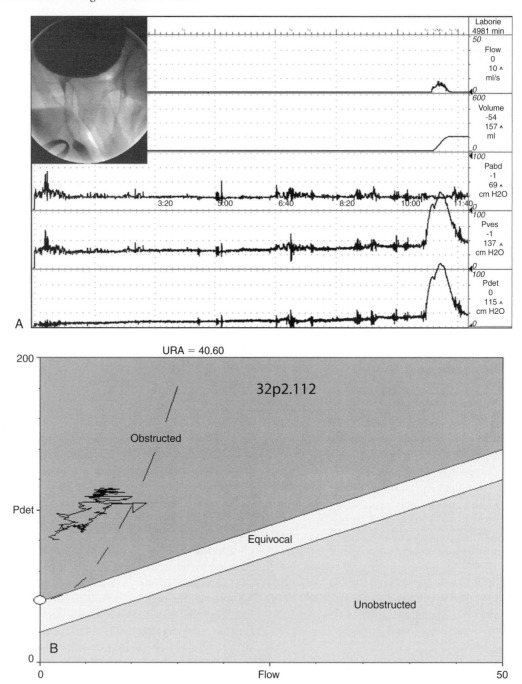

Fig. 7-16 A, Urodynamic evaluation of a 67-year-old male with benign prostatic hyperplasia (BPH) in the compensatory phase. **B,** The prolonged flow pattern and high-pressure detrusor contraction indicate obstruction, and this impression is quantitatively expressed on the ICS nomogram. Despite the obstruction, the postvoid residual volume is 10 ml, indicating compensation for obstruction by way of a stronger detrusor contraction.

The second stage of BPH is characterized by decompensation of the detrusor muscle and rising residual volumes.[166] Histologic analysis of the *decompensatory phase* reveals deposition of collagen in the smooth muscle of the bladder wall and a swollen submucosa infiltrated with plasma cells, lymphocytes, and polymorphonuclear cells. Cellules, or small pockets, are formed when the mucosa is pushed between superficial muscle bundles, and visible diverticula are formed when these cellules push their way through the entire musculature of the bladder. Diverticula may not empty effectively; instead they may act as a reservoir for debris, bacteria, or calculi. Visible trabeculation of the bladder wall is caused by collagen deposition in the detrusor muscle; severe trabeculation is associated with detrusor overactivity and lowered bladder wall compliance.[168,169] Trigonal hypertrophy contributes to ureteric obstruction and upper urinary tract obstruction by distorting the ureteral orifices. Urodynamic testing during the decompensatory phase reveals lowered bladder wall compliance, diminishing detrusor contraction strength, and elevated postvoid urinary residual volumes (Figure 7-17). If the obstruction is not relieved, upper urinary tract function is compromised and urinary residual volumes may reach 1000 ml or higher. Progression to this latter stage of BPH sometimes occurs when men fail to experience or perceive the significance of lower urinary tract symptoms associated with the earlier compensatory phase. This condition, often called silent prostatism, is mercifully rare.[170]

Benign Prostatic Hyperplasia and Overactive Bladder. Research in both human and animal models demonstrates that BPH, urgency, and detrusor overactivity are closely linked. Laboratory experiments in animal models show that both acute and progressive chronic obstruction cause increased voiding frequency and detrusor hyperactivity. Research in human subjects also reveals a close link between detrusor overactivity and symptoms of the overactive bladder in men with BPH.[171,172] Although the precise mechanisms that link these conditions are not entirely clear, this growing body of evidence suggests that bladder outlet obstruction acts as a cause of BPH and that chronic obstruction alters the neurologic mechanisms that moderate lower urinary tract function, ultimately leading to irreversible changes that may account for the persistent overactive bladder

dysfunction seen in some men even after bladder outlet obstruction has been alleviated.

Assessment

BPH usually presents in one of two scenarios. By far the most common scenario is a complaint of bothersome lower urinary tract symptoms, usually including reduced stream, terminal dribble, hesitancy, and intermittency of stream, which are reported by 80% or more of men with BPH.[173] Between 70% and 80% will report nocturia and daytime voiding frequency, and about half will report urgency or urge urinary incontinence. The International Prostate Symptom Score (AUA-7 instrument) is a well-accepted and widely used instrument that provides a rapid and valuable assessment of pertinent lower urinary tract symptoms commonly associated with BPH (Figure 7-18).[174,175] Although it is tempting to associate these lower urinary tract symptoms with BPH, it is essential to remember that they are not specific to prostatic enlargement. Instead, they may be caused by a variety of conditions, including bladder or prostate cancer; neurologic disorders such as stroke, Parkinson's disease, or dementia; metabolic disorders, such as diabetes mellitus; or a urethral stricture. Therefore a more detailed history and physical examination must be performed to determine the likely cause (or causes) of lower urinary tract symptoms. The routine evaluation includes a complete medical history that emphasizes a comprehensive review of systems. This review particularly focuses on the urologic, neurologic, gastrointestinal, and male reproductive systems. In addition to these systems, the patient is queried about sleep apnea or chronic obstructive pulmonary diseases that may be associated with polyuric nocturia and detrusor overactivity and about cardiovascular diseases that may increase nocturnal urine production, such as congestive heart failure or hypertension.

A sexual symptom inventory also may be obtained, such as the International Index of Erectile Function (IIEF) of Sexual Health Inventory for Men (SHIM). A study of more than 12,600 men revealed that erectile dysfunction (ED) and BPH are strongly correlated, suggesting that shared etiologic factors may predispose men to both conditions.[176] The nature of this relationship remains unclear, but five primary shared factors have been implicated: alterations in the nitric oxide and nitric oxide synthase

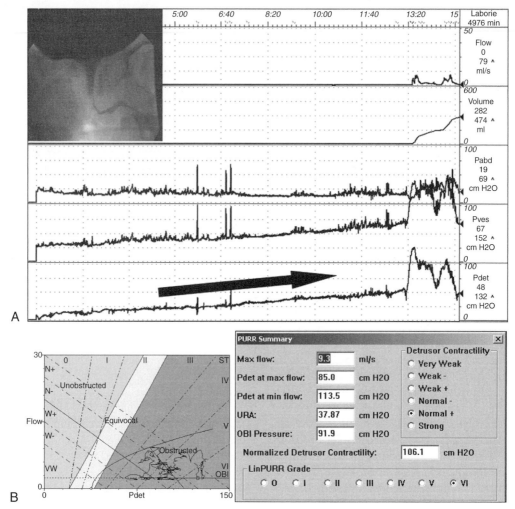

Fig. 7-17 Urodynamic evaluation of a 72-year-old male with benign prostatic hyperplasia (BPH) who has progressed to the decompensatory phase and presents for evaluation and management following an episode of acute urinary retention. **A,** Bladder wall compliance is now compromised due to thickening of the bladder wall *(arrow)*. Detrusor contraction strength is now compromised, and his residual volume has risen to 490 ml. **B,** Note the compromised detrusor contraction strength combined with bladder outlet obstruction quantified by the Schafer linear passive urethral resistance *(linPURR)* nomogram.

levels in the prostate and cavernosal bodies of the penis, increased autonomic tone within the lower urinary tract, prostate growth and cavernosal bodies, increased Rho-kinase activation and endothelin activity, and/or compromised blood flow to the prostate and penile bodies.[177,178]

Less common scenarios include acute urinary retention, urinary tract infection, or hematuria. Each of these scenarios is characterized by a relatively sudden onset of symptoms that typically prompts men to seek urgent care. Men who have passed into the decompensatory stage of BPH may experience acute urinary retention in response to a change in medications, following surgery, or for no apparent reason. Refer to Chapter 6 for a detailed discussion of the evaluation and management of acute urinary retention.

A final scenario can be described as constitutional signs and symptoms associated with renal insufficiency.

International Prostate Symptoms Score						
	Not at all	Less than 1 time in 5	Less than half the time	About half the time	More than half the time	Almost always
Scale	0	1	2	3	4	5
Over the past month, how often have you had a sensation of not emptying your bladder completely after you finished urinating?						
Over the past month, how often have you had to urinate again less than two hours after you finished urinating?						
Over the past month, how often have you found you stopped and started several times when you urinated?						
Over the past month, how often have you found it difficult to postpone urination?						
Over the past month, how often have you had a weak urinary stream?						
Over the past month, how often have you had to push or strain to begin urination?						
Over the past month, how many times did you most typically get up to urinate from the time you went to bed at night until the time you got up the next morning?	NONE	1 time	2 times	3 times	4 times	5 times or more

SCORE:_____ out of 35*

0-8 indicates mild LUTS

8-19 indicates moderate LUTS

19-35 indicates severe LUTS

Fig. 7-18 International Prostate Symptom Score (sometimes referred to as the AUA-7). *LUTS,* Lower urinary tract symptoms.

This condition, historically called *silent prostatism,* occurs when men do not perceive as bothersome, or fail to report or respond to, changes in lower urinary tract function as BPH progresses.[179] The incidence of renal insufficiency in men presenting with silent prostatism is unknown, but approximately 13.6% of men presenting to the urologist for evaluation of BPH will have evidence of renal insufficiency characterized by a serum creatinine of 2 to 3 mg/dl or greater.[180] Risk factors for renal insufficiency are not known, but post-void residual urine volumes above 300 ml, low bladder wall compliance, and detrusor overactivity have been implicated, as have recurring episodes of acute urinary retention, urinary tract infection, and secondary hypertension. Patients often experience significant improvement in renal function following prostatectomy, but the percentage who ultimately progress to end-stage renal disease is not known.

All men presenting with lower urinary tract symptoms should have a digital rectal examination and focused neurologic examination assessing the S2 to S4 dermatomes, presence of stool (and consistency) in rectum, and anal sphincter tone. In addition, the advanced practice nurse should assess the patient's mental status, ambulatory ability, and, if the patient is frail, living arrangements and support system. Support systems are particularly important for the older patient with slight cognitive impairment who may be prescribed medications for voiding symptoms or undergo a transurethral resection of the prostate (TURP) or minimally invasive prostatectomy.

Routine laboratory studies include a urinalysis to exclude urinary tract infection or hematuria. The presence of hematuria may indicate a malignant process, but it also may indicate bleeding from the enlarging prostate. A urine cytology is typically obtained to rule out bladder cancer, especially in men with predominantly irritative lower urinary tract symptoms.[159] Prostate-related, nonmalignant hematuria is prevalent among men with BPH, but a retrospective review of 3000 men undergoing TURP revealed that 12% underwent the procedure primarily to control recurring hematuria.[181] Because of the small but substantial risk of progressive renal insufficiency associated with BPH, a serum creatinine should be measured and more detailed evaluation of renal function completed when indicated.

Prostate-specific antigen (PSA) is not recommended as a routine test for all men with lower urinary tract symptoms, but it should be completed in certain men. Specifically, men with a life expectancy more than 10 years and those whose management will be altered by results of a PSA should be evaluated.[182] In addition, several trials have shown that PSA is a proxy for prostate volume and can be useful in predicting symptom progression and the response to therapies (5α-reductase inhibitors).[183] Men with lower urinary tract symptoms with a PSA above 1.5 ng/ml are more likely to have a prostate volume of at least 30 ml and are at higher risk of progressing to obstruction than men whose PSA is less than 1.5 ng/ml.[184] Thus men whose PSA is raised and who are symptomatic should have therapy directed to reducing prostate volume with 5α-reductase inhibitors (possibly in combination with α-blockers). On the other hand, men whose PSA is less than 1.5 ng/ml are much less likely to progress to obstructive symptoms and can be treated symptomatically as indicated with α-blockers.[184]

The optimal role of urodynamic testing in BPH remains somewhat controversial. Uroflowmetry testing is a noninvasive measure that characterizes the extent to which urinary flow has been compromised, but it fails to differentiate poor detrusor contraction strength from bladder outlet obstruction. Filling cystometry combined with a voiding pressure flow study will identify detrusor overactivity and bladder wall compliance. The voiding pressure flow study will characterize detrusor contraction strength and the magnitude of obstruction.[185,186] Routine urodynamics may be performed prior to an invasive procedure such as TURP or as a diagnostic evaluation when complicating factors such as neurologic disease or diabetes mellitus exist. Depending on patient age, medical history, and family history, PSA may be done to rule out prostate cancer.

Imaging studies of the upper urinary tracts or cystourethroscopy are not routinely indicated for the evaluation of BPH. Transurethral ultrasound of the prostate is sometimes recommended when prostate size is important in determining treatment.

Treatment

The introduction of pharmacologic agents and minimally invasive prostate procedures has significantly changed treatment options for BPH. Men can now be offered a comparatively wide range of treatment options, depending on symptom severity and complicating conditions, such as renal insufficiency or significant hematuria. These treatments include the following: watchful waiting, pharmacotherapy, prostate tissue ablation by means of a minimally invasive procedure, transurethral resection of the prostate, and open prostatectomy. Since most cases of BPH are associated with lower urinary tract symptoms in the absence of serious urologic complications, treatment choices are usually based on how bothersome symptoms and their impact on quality of life are perceived to be rather than on considerations of existing or likely complications. Based on a longitudinal study of men in the midwestern United States, treatment preferences during the late twentieth century include a diminished popularity of watchful waiting and surgery, while the number of men seeking pharmacotherapy has increased.[187]

Watchful Waiting. Patients who are relatively asymptomatic may be managed with a strategy called watchful waiting. It is characterized by avoidance of invasive interventions such as pharmacotherapy or surgery. Instead, the patient is taught to self-monitor himself for progression of symptoms and to watch for possible complications.

Initial instruction focuses on the location and functions of the prostate gland and its relationship to the bladder and urethra. The patient is reassured of the nonmalignant nature of BPH and its relationship to normal aging. Nevertheless, the patient is also counseled about potential sequelae associated with BPH, such as bothersome lower urinary tract symptoms, and possible complications, such as acute urinary retention, urinary tract infection, and hematuria. Education about lower urinary symptoms includes advice about the relationship between BPH and overactive bladder and behavioral strategies to minimize urgency or urge urinary incontinence, such as fluid and dietary alterations, scheduled toileting or bladder training, or urge suppression techniques. Men are also taught techniques to prevent or manage acute urinary retention by avoiding over-the-counter medications with α-adrenergic or antimuscarinic effects, by avoiding intake of large volumes of fluid over a brief period, and by warming up when attempting to urinate following prolonged exposure to a cold climate. Depending on the results of an initial evaluation, the patient is reevaluated every 1 to 2 years.

Pharmacotherapy. Two principal classes of drugs may be used to treat BPH: 5α-reductase inhibitors and α-adrenergic blockers. Two 5α-reductase inhibitors are currently available in North America: finasteride (Proscar) and dutasteride (Avodart). A larger number of α-adrenergic drugs are available, but four agents (i.e., doxazosin [Cardura], terazosin [Hytrin], tamsulosin [Flomax], and alfuzosin [Uroxatral]) are most commonly prescribed. Refer to Clinical Highlights for Advanced and Expert Practice: Pharmacotherapy for Benign Prostatic Hyperplasia for a detailed description of their use.[188-197]

Because of the close relationship between BPH and overactive bladder syndrome, a growing number of clinicians and researchers are beginning to explore whether combination therapy may be beneficial for men with BPH and urgency or urge incontinence.[198] Several studies have found that combining an antimuscarinic and α-adrenergic blocking agent provides greater symptom relief than use of an α-adrenergic blocking drug alone.[199-201] A persistent concern is whether the addition of an antimuscarinic medication will increase urinary residual volumes or possibly provoke an episode of acute urinary retention. No episodes of acute urinary retention occurred during three randomized clinical trials,[199-201] and a fourth study that evaluated urodynamic responses (including postvoid residual volumes) of men with detrusor overactivity and prostatic obstruction did not find a significant rise in residual volumes following administration of an antimuscarinic agent.[202]

Phytotherapy. The use of herbal remedies continues to rise among patients, and one agent, saw palmetto, is widely used for the management of BPH. Saw palmetto *(Serenoa repens)* is an extract of the American dwarf palm that has been found to inhibit 5α-reductase isoenzymes, lower dihydrotestosterone levels, interfere with prolactin receptor signal transduction, and increase apoptosis of prostatic tissues.[203] Multiple studies have shown that saw palmetto reduces lower urinary tract symptoms associated with BPH; it slightly improves urinary flow rates in some studies although no differences were found in others.[203,204] It has not been shown to influence PSA readings, and it does not significantly alter prostate volumes when compared with a placebo in clinical trials. The usual dosage is 160 to 320 mg daily. Adverse effects include mild gastrointestinal distress, rhinitis, headache, and a mild anticoagulant effect.

The nursing management of patients taking herbal preparations such as saw palmetto differs from that associated with a prescription or over-the-counter medication because of significant differences in the evidence base required to market the agent, the quality controls applied to its manufacture, and the variability in recommended dosages and dosages consumed by patients. Counseling begins with a factual and unbiased description of differences between herbal preparations and medications regulated by a governmental agency. Patients are further advised that the quality of herbal preparations varies and that concentrations of saw palmetto contained in these preparations also vary. Nevertheless, men taking saw palmetto can also be advised that existing evidence supports efficacy and demonstrates that adverse side effects tend to be mild and occur no more frequently than those reported by patients taking a placebo. It is particularly important to advise any patient using an herbal preparation that these substances do interact with prescription medications and to inform all healthcare providers that they are taking *Serenoa repens*. Possible drug interactions associated with saw palmetto include increased antiandrogenic effect if combined with a 5α-reductase inhibitor; enhanced anticoagulant effect if taken

Clinical Highlights for Advanced and Expert Practice: Pharmacotherapy for Benign Prostatic Hyperplasia

Pharmacotherapy for benign prostatic hyperplasia (BPH) provides relief from bothersome lower urinary tract symptoms, and it reduces the risk of certain complications, such as acute urinary retention. Two classes of drugs may be used to manage BPH symptoms, 5α-reductase inhibitors and α-adrenergic blocking drugs. Although each class has been shown to be effective when given individually, a large randomized clinical trial has shown that combination therapy is more effective than monotherapy.[188]

5α-Reductase Inhibitors

Two 5α-reductase inhibitors have been approved for use in the United States and Canada, finasteride and dutasteride. They work by blocking the production of dihydrotestosterone in the prostate. As a result, they block progression of hyperplasia, reduce the risk for acute urinary retention, reduce the need for surgical resection or ablation of prostatic tissue, and prevent or alleviate BPH-related hematuria.[189] They also affect prostate-specific antigen (PSA) levels and may adversely influence prostate cancer detection rates.[192] Because their primary action is blockade of glandular growth, they are most effective when given to men with larger prostatic volumes. A growing number of studies provide evidence that 5α-reductase inhibitors may reduce the risk for prostate cancer.[190,191] A large, multinational trial (REDUCE) is underway to provide more definitive answers to this question.[193]

Agent: Dutasteride (Avodart, Duagen)
Action: Inhibits both type 1 and type 2 isoenzymes of 5α-reductase, reducing prostatic concentrations of dihydrotestosterone (DHT) by 85% to 90% following 1 month of therapy
Dosage and administration: 0.5 mg daily
Nursing management: Patients are counseled that clinically relevant symptom relief usually occurs within 3 months of administration. Serum concentrations of the drug may be elevated when taken with ciprofloxacin, but no dose adjustment has been deemed necessary. No adverse interactions have been detected when the drug is taken with tamsulosin or terazosin. Patients should be counseled that common adverse reactions include erectile dysfunction, diminished libido, gynecomastia, and ejaculatory dysfunction. Nausea and itching have also been reported. Patients and partners are further advised that the drug should not be handled by women who are pregnant or may become pregnant because of the risk to a developing male fetus.

Agent: Finasteride (Proscar)
Action: Inhibits type 2 isoenzyme of 5α-reductase, reducing serum dihydrotestosterone concentrations by 70%
Dosage and administration: 5 mg daily
Nursing management: Patients are counseled that clinically relevant symptom relief usually occurs within 3 months of initiating therapy. No adverse drug-drug interactions have been reported. Patients should be counseled that common adverse side effects include erectile dysfunction, diminished libido, diminished ejaculatory volume, ejaculatory dysfunction, and breast enlargement or tenderness. Rashes have been reported in men taking the drug. Patients and partners are further advised that the drug should not be handled by women who are pregnant or may become pregnant because of the risk to a developing male fetus.

α-Adrenergic Blockers

Although a number of α-adrenergic antagonists are available in North America, four drugs (alfuzosin, doxazosin, tamsulosin, and terazosin) are commonly used for the management of BPH.[194] These drugs act by blocking α₁-adrenoreceptors in the proximal urethra and prostate. Their pharmacologic actions are not entirely understood, but clinically relevant outcomes are thought to include (1) reduction of urethral resistance, (2) alleviation of urinary urgency, and (3) promotion of apoptosis (programmed cellular death) in the prostate.[195-197] Two of these drugs, terazosin and doxazosin, are also used in the management of hypertension.

Agent: Terazosin (Hytrin)
Action: Selective α₁-adrenergic blocker
Dosage and administration: Begin with 1 mg, and gradually titrate to 5 or 10 mg daily

Clinical Highlights for Advanced and Expert Practice: Pharmacotherapy for Benign Prostatic Hyperplasia—cont'd

* *

Nursing management: Patients are instructed that adherence to the dosing and administration regimen is essential to avoid adverse side effects, particularly postural hypotension. The drug is initially given as 1 mg at bedtime in order to reduce the likelihood of first-dose postural hypotension or syncope. The dosage is gradually titrated by the patient's physician or nurse practitioner to 5 to 10 mg based on magnitude of symptom relief versus occurrence of adverse side effects. The risk for postural hypotension is exacerbated if the patient misses one or more doses, and repeated titration may be necessary if two or more doses are missed. The most common side effect is postural hypotension, which occurs in approximately 28% of cases. Patients are counseled to take the medication at night, to sit on the side of the bed before rising in the morning, and to exercise the legs for several moments if dizziness is encountered on arising. Patients are counseled that other potential adverse side effects include headache, asthenia (generalized weakness), and nasal congestion. Men with coexisting erectile dysfunction are advised to speak with their physician or nurse practitioner before taking a phosphodiesterase type 5 inhibitor, such as vardenafil, because of a risk of decreased blood pressure.

Agent: Doxazosin (Cardura)
Action: Selective α_1-adrenergic blocker
Dosage and administration: Begin with 1 mg, and gradually titrate to 4 or 8 mg daily
Nursing management: Patients are instructed that adherence to the dosing and administration regimen is essential to avoid adverse side effects, particularly postural hypotension. The drug is initially given as 1 mg at bedtime in order to reduce the likelihood of first-dose postural hypotension or syncope, and the dosage is gradually titrated by the patient's physician or nurse practitioner to 4 to 8 mg based on magnitude of symptom relief versus occurrence of adverse side effects. The risk for postural hypotension is exacerbated if the patient misses one or more doses, and repeated titration may be necessary if two or more doses are missed. The most common side effect is postural hypotension, which occurs in approximately 19% of cases. Patients are counseled to take the medication at night, to sit on the side of the bed before rising in the morning, and to exercise the legs for several moments if dizziness is encountered on arising. Patients are counseled that other potential adverse side effects include headache and drowsiness. Men with coexisting erectile dysfunction are advised to speak with their physician or nurse practitioner before taking a phosphodiesterase type 5 inhibitor, such as tadalafil, because of a risk of decreased blood pressure.

Agent: Alfuzosin (Uroxatral)
Action: Uroselective α_{1A}-adrenergic blocker
Dosage and administration: 10 mg daily
Nursing management: Patients are instructed to take their medication immediately following the same meal daily. Titration is not necessary, but patients should be counseled that dizziness remains the most common side effect, followed by headache. Patients are advised that the drug is metabolized in the liver and to seek advice from their physician or nurse practitioner before taking antihypertensives. Men with coexisting erectile dysfunction are advised to speak with their physician or nurse practitioner before taking a phosphodiesterase type 5 inhibitor, such as sildenafil, because of a risk of decreased blood pressure.

Agent: Tamsulosin (Flomax)
Action: Uroselective α_{1A}-adrenergic blocker
Dosage and administration: 0.4 to 0.8 mg daily
Nursing management: Patients are instructed to take their medication about 30 minutes following the same meal daily. Titration is not necessary, but patients should be counseled that dizziness remains a common side effect. Patients are counseled to seek advice from a physician or nurse practitioner before taking with an antihypertensive drug. Men with coexisting erectile dysfunction are advised to speak with their physician or nurse practitioner before taking a phosphodiesterase type 5 inhibitor, such as sildenafil, because of a risk of decreased blood pressure. The most common adverse side effect reported by patients taking tamsulosin is headache. Other side effects include asthenia, back pain, nasal congestion or rhinitis, and abnormal ejaculation.

with warfarin, ibuprofen, or naproxen; and nausea and vomiting if taken with metronidazole or disulfiram (Antabuse).

Surgery. Before the age of effective medications for BPH, surgery was the only effective treatment option. Historically, open prostatectomy was replaced by TURP. More recently, the predominance of TURP has been challenged by a growing variety of minimally invasive procedures designed to reduce bladder outlet obstruction while reducing the morbidity associated with TURP. A variety of open, transurethral, and minimally invasive procedures have been developed for the management of BPH (Table 7-10).[205,206] Despite an ever-increasing proliferation of such procedures, TURP remains the gold standard against which all other procedures are compared. Refer to Chapter 11 for a detailed discussion of the nursing management of the patient undergoing open prostatectomy, TURP, and some of the more commonly performed minimally invasive procedures.

Indications for surgery for BPH include significant complications such as acute urinary retention, uncontrolled bleeding, or renal insufficiency. In addition, prostatic resection may be undertaken as a voluntary procedure in order to relieve bothersome lower urinary tract symptoms or reduce the risk of urologic complications. Although open prostatectomy, TURP, or the minimally invasive procedures will relieve obstruction, careful evaluation is indicated to determine the likely outcome of prostatic tissue resection. Specifically, prostatic resection has been found to provide no benefit to patients experiencing bothersome lower urinary tract symptoms but no bladder outlet obstruction.[207] In addition, it may exacerbate urge incontinence with detrusor overactivity by reducing urethral resistance, and it is unlikely to benefit patients whose retention is caused primarily by poor detrusor contraction strength.[186] Risk factors for poor voiding function after TURP or similar procedures include age greater than 80 years, urinary retention of more than 1500 ml, diminished awareness of bladder filling or the need to urinate, and poor detrusor contraction strength (maximum detrusor pressure below 28 cm H_2O during micturition).[208] A urodynamic evaluation including a voiding-pressure-flow study is essential to differentiate between outlet obstruction and impaired contractility.[186,209]

TABLE 7-10 Alternative Procedures for Prostate Tissue Removal[23,37-39,61,101,112,113,150,151,165]

PROCEDURE	DESCRIPTION	ADVANTAGES	DISADVANTAGES	POSTPROCEDURAL CARE*
Transurethral vaportrode	Resection of prostatic tissue under direct, endoscopic visualization. Tissue is removed using a "roller ball" or "roller bar" and electrocautery energy.	Superior visualization of prostate Less risk of bleeding Possibly less risk of transurethral resection (TUR) syndrome Procedure may be performed as outpatient Prostate tissue available for pathologic analysis to determine presence of prostate cancer Additional equipment costs are relatively low	None yet identified	Indwelling catheter for 24 h; patient may experience some hematuria for several days; passage of scabs with transient hematuria in 7–10 days

TABLE 7-10 Alternative Procedures for Prostate Tissue Removal[23,37-39,61,101,112,113,150,151,165]—cont'd

PROCEDURE	DESCRIPTION	ADVANTAGES	DISADVANTAGES	POSTPROCEDURAL CARE*
Transurethral incision of the prostate (TUIP)	Incision of the prostatic capsule under direct endoscopic visualization. A small cutting loop and electrocautery energy are used to incise the prostatic capsule.	Local anesthesia may be used to reduce risk of spinal or general anesthesia Reduced hospital stay (1–2 days shorter when compared with TURP) Less risk of bleeding, retrograde ejaculation, bladder neck contracture Lower risk of TUR syndrome Additional equipment relatively inexpensive	Limited to smaller glands Marked enlargement of median lobe comprises relative contraindication Risk of incontinence, erectile dysfunction similar to TURP Prostate tissue not available for pathologic analysis	Brief hospital stay may be necessary; indwelling catheter for 24 h; three-way irrigation not typically required, but catheter is placed under gentle traction
Laser prostatectomy (transurethral incision of the prostate, visual laser ablation of the prostate [VLAP])	Ablation of prostate tissue using laser energy (Nd:YAG). The visualization technique varies; VLAP is generally preferred because of the ability to visualize the prostate using direct endoscopy.	Hospitalization not required Low risk of bleeding Less risk of retrograde ejaculation Reduced mortality rate	Prolonged period of tissue slough (7 days; may persist up to 30 days) Postoperative discomfort and irritation occur with prolonged edema Long-term efficacy as compared with TURP has not been established Prostate tissue not available for pathologic analysis Additional equipment costs are significant	Indwelling (suprapubic or urethral) catheter for at least 7 days; postprocedure discomfort may occur during period of edema and tissue slough
Intraurethral stent insertion	A medical-grade steel is placed in the prostatic urethra to widen the prostatic urethra and mechanically alleviate obstruction.	Less risk of bleeding No risk of TUR syndrome Procedure is reversible (limited window of opportunity)	Does not correct bladder neck obstruction Occasionally causes discomfort requiring removal Urethral tissue may fail to reepithelialize around stent, necessitating removal	Performed as outpatient; suprapubic catheter up to 30 days after insertion; initial irritative voiding symptoms may require antispasmodic therapy
Interstitial laser therapy	Ablation of prostate tissue using a transurethral,	Similar to laser prostatectomy	Degree of postprocedure	Indwelling catheter, otherwise unknown

Continued

TABLE 7-10 Alternative Procedures for Prostate Tissue Removal[23,37-39,61,101,112,113,150,151,165]—cont'd

PROCEDURE	DESCRIPTION	ADVANTAGES	DISADVANTAGES	POSTPROCEDURAL CARE*
	transrectal, or transperineal approach. Prostatic size and location are determined using ultrasonic techniques. Laser energy is used to ablate prostate tissue without disrupting integrity of rectal or urethral wall.	Preservation of urothelium may reduce postprocedure discomfort, irritative voiding symptoms	discomfort has not been determined Tissue not available for pathologic analysis	
Transurethral ultrasonic aspiration	Destruction of prostate tissue, using ultrasonic energy (0–700–micron vibration) at an excursion rate of 39 kHz; maximum power 100 W. Prostatic size and location are determined using ultrasound imaging.	Lower risk for significant bleeding Incontinence rate may be reduced Impotence risk is comparable to TURP	Procedure will not correct significant bladder neck hypertrophy obstruction	Indwelling catheter for 18–24 h; in-hospital stay 2–3 days
Transurethral needle ablation of the prostate (TUNA)	Ablation of prostatic tissue under indirect endoscopic visualization (the surgeon will see the prostatic urethra, but does not see the needles penetrate the prostatic capsule). Low-level radiofrequency energy is used to heat the prostate, causing tissue destruction.	Lower risk of significant blood loss Lower risk of postprocedure irritative voiding symptoms Lower risk of impotence Lower risk of retrograde ejaculation	Tissue not available for tissue analysis Prolonged time for symptom improvement (> 1 month) Transient urinary retention, approximately 3 days (range 1–21 days) Urethral stricture may occur	Hematuria and dysuria persist for 2–3 days; indwelling catheter may be left in place for 7–10 days
High-intensity focused ultrasound (HIFU)	Coagulative destruction of prostate tissue using high-intensity, focused ultrasonic energy. The ultrasonic energy is delivered via a transrectal route, and the prostate is	Less risk of bleeding Low postoperative discomfort No risk of TUR syndrome	Transient retention lasting 6 days (range 1–42 days) Hematospermia, mild hematuria Urinary tract infection Moderate symptom improvement only	PSA values are transiently elevated (12–24 h); suprapubic catheter for 6–7 days; symptom improvement generally requires 6 months

TABLE 7-10 Alternative Procedures for Prostate Tissue Removal[23,37-39,61,101,112,113,150,151,165]**—cont'd**

PROCEDURE	DESCRIPTION	ADVANTAGES	DISADVANTAGES	POSTPROCEDURAL CARE*
	localized using ultrasonic imaging techniques.			
Transurethral microwave thermotherapy (TUMT)	Microwave (radiating heat energy) is used to destroy prostate tissue while conductive cooling is used to prevent urethral injury. The microwave energy is delivered via a 20F balloon type of catheter, and a temperature probe is then placed to measure anterior rectal wall temperature.	Performed as an outpatient Less risk of significant bleeding No risk of TUR syndrome Low risk of retrograde ejaculation	Multiple treatments may be required Rectal wall injury may occur Long-term efficacy (> 12 months postprocedure) has not been established Effect of therapy on the bladder neck is not known	PSA values are transiently elevated following procedure (up to 3 months); transient urinary retention occurs, and suprapubic catheter drainage is required
Cryotherapy	Prostate tissue is destroyed by rapid freezing. A cryotherapy probe is inserted into the prostate, and the adjacent tissue is rapidly cooled to −180° to −190° C.	Less risk of bleeding Reduced risk of TUR syndrome	Risk of impotence and incontinence may be significant when compared with TURP Urethrorectal, urethrocutaneous fistulae may occur Tissue not available for pathologic analysis	Indwelling catheter for several weeks; sloughing of tissue will occur during this period; primarily used for prostate cancer

*Refined nursing care plans may not be available, primarily because of a lack of clinical experience with these techniques.

SUMMARY

Obstructive uropathies are among the most common disorders encountered in urologic practice. Successful management of the patient with an obstructive uropathy is based on identification of the cause of the obstruction, its severity and impact on renal function, and its association with bothersome symptoms.

REFERENCES

1. Freeman IM: Physics Made Simple. New York: Doubleday, 1990.
2. Wolf JS Jr, Siegel CL, Brink JA, Clayman RV: Imaging for ureteropelvic junction obstruction in adults. Journal of Endourology, 1996; 10(2):93-104.
3. Whitaker RH: The Whitaker test. Urologic Clinics of North America, 1979; 6:529-39.
4. Pais VM, Strandhoy JW, Assimos DG: Pathophysiology of urinary tract obstruction. In Wein AJ, Kavoussi LR, Novick AC, Partin AW, Peters CA (eds): Campbell-Walsh Urology, 9th edition. Philadelphia: Saunders, 2007; pp 1195-1226.
5. Wein AJ: Pathophysiology and classification of voiding dysfunction. In Wein AJ, Kavoussi LR, Novick AC, Partin AW, Peters CA (eds): Campbell-Walsh Urology, 9th edition. Philadelphia: Saunders, 2007; pp 1973-85.
6. George NRJ: Interactive obstructive uropathy: observations and conclusions from studies on humans. In Mundy AR, Fitzpatrick JM, Neal DE, George NJR (eds): The Scientific Basis of Urology. UK: Isis Medical, 1999; pp 124-41.
7. Gillenwater JY: Hydronephrosis. In Gillenwater JY, Grayhack JT, Howards SS, Mitchell ME (eds): Adult and Pediatric Urology, 4th edition. Philadelphia: Lippincott, Williams & Wilkins, 2002; pp 879-905.

8. Roth KS, Koo HP, Spotswood S, Chan J: Obstructive uropathy: an important cause of renal failure in children. Clinical Pediatrics, 2002; 41(5):309-14.

9. Nguyen HT, Hsieh MH, Gaborro A, Tinloy B, Phillips C, Adam RM: JNK/SAPK and p38 SAPK-2 mediate mechanical stretch-induced apoptosis via caspase-3 and -9 in NRK-52E renal epithelial cells. Nephron. Experimental Nephrology, 2006; 102(2):e49-e61.

10. Nurzia MJ, Constantinescu AR, Barone JG: Childhood infundibular stenosis. Urology, 2002; 60(2):344xi-xiii.

11. Parsons JK, Jarrett TW, Lancini V, Kavoussi LR: Infundibular stenosis after percutaneous nephrolithotomy. Journal of Urology, 2002; 167:35-8.

12. Kelalis PP, Malek RS: Infundibular stenosis. Journal of Urology, 1981; 125:568-71.

13. Husmann DA, Kramer SA, Malek RS, Allen TD: Infundibulopelvic stenosis: a long-term followup. Journal of Urology, 1994; 152(3):837-40.

14. Laucks SP, McLachlan MSF: Aging and simple renal cysts of the kidney. British Journal of Radiology, 1981; 54:12-4.

15. Roberts WW, Bluebond-Langner R, Boyle KE, Jarrett TW, Kavoussi LR: Laparoscopic ablation of symptomatic parenchymal and peripelvic renal cysts. Urology, 2001; 58(2):165-9.

16. Wilson PD, Goilav B: Cystic disease of the kidney. I Annual Review of Pathology, 2007; 2:341-68.

17. Hsu THS, Streem SB, Nakada SY: Management of upper urinary tract obstruction. In Wein AJ, Kavoussi LR, Novick AC, Partin AW, Peters CA, editors: Campbell-Walsh Urology, 9th edition. Philadelphia: Saunders, 2007; pp 1227-73.

18. Paananen I, Hellstrom P, Leinonen S, Merikanto J, Perala J, Paivansalo M, Lukkarinen O: Treatment of renal cysts with single-session percutaneous drainage and ethanol sclerotherapy: long-term outcome. Urology, 2001; 57(1):30-3.

19. Plas EG, Hubner WA: Percutaneous resection of renal cysts: a long-term followup. Journal of Urology, 1993; 149(4):703-5.

20. Whitfield HN, Britton KE, Hendry WF, Wickham JEA: Furosemide intravenous pyelography in the diagnosis of pelviureteric junction obstruction. British Journal of Urology, 1979; 51:445-8.

21. Munver R, Sosa RE, del Pizzo JJ: Laparoscopic pyeloplasty: history, evolution, and future. Journal of Endourology, 2004; 18(8):748-55.

22. Sierakowski R, Finlayson B, Landes R: Stone incidence as related to water hardness in different geographical regions of the United States. Urological Research, 1979; 7(3):157-60.

23. Statistics by Country for Urinary Stones. Retrieved Jan 15, 2008 from http://www.wrongdiagnosis.com/u/urinary_stones/stats-country.htm.

24. Johnson CM, Wilson DM, O'Fallon WM, Malek RS, Kurland LT: Renal stone epidemiology: a 25-year study in Rochester, Minnesota. Kidney International, 1979; 16(5):624-31.

25. Curhan GC: Epidemiology of stone disease. Urologic Clinics of North America, 2007; 34(3):287-93.

26. Hesse A, Brandle E, Wilbert D, Kohrmann KU, Alken P: Study on the prevalence and incidence of urolithiasis in Germany comparing the years 1979 vs. 2000. European Urology, 2003; 44(6):709-13.

27. Trinchieri A, Coppi F, Montanari E, Del Nero A, Zanetti G, Pisani E: Increase in the prevalence of symptomatic upper urinary tract stones during the last ten years. European Urology, 2000; 37(1):23-5.

28. Amato M, Lusini ML, Nelli F: Epidemiology of nephrolithiasis today. Urologia Internationalis, 2004; 72(suppl):1-5.

29. Goldfarb DS: Increasing prevalence of kidney stones in the United States (editorial). Kidney International, 2003; 63:1951-2.

30. Seiner R: Impact of dietary habits on stone incidence. Urological Research 2006; 34(2):131-3.

31. Pearle MS, Lotan Y: Urinary lithiasis, etiology, epidemiology, and pathogenesis. In Wein AJ, Kavoussi LR, Novick AC, Partin AW, Peters CA (eds): Campbell's Urology, 9th edition. Philadelphia: Saunders, 2007; pp 1363-92.

32. Khan SR, Hackett RL: Hyperoxaluria, enzymuria and nephrolithiasis. Contributions to Nephrology, 1993; 101:190-3.

33. Byer K, Khan SR: Citrate provides protection against oxalate and calcium oxalate crystal induced oxidative damage to renal epithelium. Journal of Urology, 2005; 173(2):640-6.

34. Gambaro G, Vezzoli G, Casari G, Rampoldi L, D'Angelo A, Borghi L: Genetics of hypercalciuria and calcium nephrolithiasis: from the rare monogenic to the common polygenic forms. American Journal of Kidney Diseases, 2004; 44(6):963-86.

35. Moe OW, Bonny O: Genetic hypercalciuria. Journal of the American Society of Nephrology, 2005; 16(3):729-45.

36. Pak CY, Oata M, Lawrence EC, Snyder W: The hypercalciurias. Causes, parathyroid functions, and diagnostic criteria. Journal of Clinical Investigation, 1974; 54(2):387-400.

37. Holmes RP, Assimos DG: The impact of dietary oxalate on kidney stone formation. Urologic Research, 2004; 32:311-6.

38. Stewart CS, Duncan SH, Cave DR: Oxalobacter formigenes and its role in oxidative metabolism in the human gut. FEMS Microbiology Letters, 2004; 230:1-7.

39. Hokama S, Toma C, Iwanaga M, Morozumi M, Sugaya K, Ogawa Y: Oxalate-degrading Providencia rettgeri isolated from human stools. International Journal of Urology, 2005; 12(6):533-8.

40. Khan SR: Crystal induced inflammation of the kidneys: results from human studies, animal models, and tissue-culture studies. Clinical and Experimental Nephrology, 2004; 8:75-88.

41. Knoll T, Zollner A, Wendt-Nordahl G, Michel MS, Alken P: Cystinuria in childhood and adolescence: recommendations for diagnosis, treatment, and follow-up. Pediatric Nephrology, 2005; 20(1):19-24.

42. Maalouf NM, Cameron MA, Moe OW, Sakhaee K: Novel insights into the pathogenesis of uric acid nephrolithiasis. Current Opinion in Nephrology and Hypertension, 2004; 13(2):181-9.

43. Miller NL, Evan AP, Lingeman JE: Pathogenesis of renal calculi. Urologic Clinics of North America, 2007; 34(3):295-313.

44. Russinko PJ, Agarwal S, Choi MJ, Kelty PJ: Obstructive nephropathy secondary to sulfasalazine calculi. Urology, 2003; 62(4):748.

45. Colebunders R, Depraetere K, De Droogh E, Kamper A, Corthout B, Bottiau E: Obstructive nephropathy due to sulfa crystals in two HIV seropositive patients treated with sulfadiazine. Organe de la Societe Royale de Belge de Radiologie, 1999; 82(4):153-4.

46. Diaz F, Collazos J, Mayo J, Martinez E: Sulfadiazine-induced multiple urolithiasis and acute renal failure in a patients with AIDS and Toxoplasmosis encephalitis. Annals of Pharmacotherapy, 1996; 30(1):41-2.

47. Alpert SA, Noe HN: Furosemide nephrolithiasis causing ureteral obstruction and urinoma in a preterm neonate. Urology, 2004; 64(3):589.

48. Catalano-Pons C, Bargy S, Schlecht D, Tabone MD, Deschenes G, Bensman A, Ulinski T: Sulfadiazine-induced nephrolithiasis in children. Pediatric Nephrology, 2004; 19(8):928-31.

49. Parikh JR, Nolan RL: Acetazolamide-induced nephrocalcinosis. Abdominal Imaging, 1994; 19(5):466-7.

50. Kalaitzis C, Dimitriadis G, Tsatidis T, Kuntz R, Touloupidis S, Kelidis G: Treatment of indinavir sulfate induced urolithiasis in HIV-positive patients. International Urology and Nephrology, 2002; 34(1):13-5.

51. Baxmann AC, De OG, Mendonca C, Heilberg IP: Effect of vitamin C supplements on urinary oxalate and pH in calcium stone-forming patients. Kidney International, 2003; 63(3):1066-71.

52. Traxer O, Huet B, Poindexter J, Pak CY, Pearle MS: Effect of ascorbic acid consumption on urinary stone risk factors. Journal of Urology, 2003; 170(2, p. 1):397-401.

53. Allie S, Rodgers A: Effects of calcium carbonate, magnesium oxide and sodium citrate bicarbonate health supplements on the urinary risk factors for kidney stone formation. Clinical Chemistry and Laboratory Medicine, 2003; 41(1):39-45.

54. Brown J: Diagnostic and treatment patterns for renal colic in US emergency departments. International Urology & Nephrology, 2006; 38(1):87-92.

55. Press SM, Smith AD: Incidence of negative hematuria in patients with acute urinary lithiasis presenting to the emergency room with flank pain. Urology, 1995; 45:753-7.

56. Teichman JM: Clinical practice: acute renal colic from ureteral calculus. New England Journal of Medicine, 2004; 350(7):684-93.

57. Miller OF, Rineer SK, Reichard SR, Buckley RG, Donovan MS, Graham IR, Goff WB, Kane CJ: Prospective comparison of unenhanced spiral computed tomography and intravenous urogram in the evaluation of acute flank pain. Urology, 1998; 52(6):982-7.

58. Rucker CM, Menias CO, Bhalla S: Mimics of renal colic: alternative diagnoses at unenhanced helical CT. RadioGraphics, 2004; 24(supp 1):S11-S33.

59. Ramakumar S, Patterson DE, LeRoy AJ, Bender CE, Erickson SB, Wilson DM, Segura JW: Prediction of stone composition from plain radiographs: a prospective study. Journal of Endourology, 1999; 13(6):397-401.

60. Haddad MC, Sharif HS, Abomelha MS, Riley PJ, Sammak BM, Shahed MS: Management of renal colic: redefining the role of the urogram. Radiology, 1992; 184(1):35-6.

61. Regan F, Kuszyk B, Bohlman ME, Jackman S: Acute ureteric calculus obstruction: unenhanced spiral CT versus HASTE MR urography and abdominal radiograph. British Journal of Radiology, 2005; 78(930):506-11.

62. Holdgate A, Pollock T: Systematic review of the relative efficacy of non-steroidal anti-inflammatory drugs and opioids in the treatment of acute renal colic. British Medical Journal, 2004; 328(7453):1401.

63. Holdgate A, Pollock T: Nonsteroidal anti-inflammatory drugs (NSAIDs) versus opioids for acute renal colic. Cochrane Database of Systematic Reviews, 2007; 4.

64. Lopes T, Dias JS, Marcelino J, Varela J, Ribeiro S, Dias J: An assessment of the clinical efficacy of intranasal desmopressin spray in the treatment of renal colic. BJU International, 2001; 87(4):322-5.

65. el-Sherif AE, Salem M, Yahia H, al-Sharkawy WA, al-Sayrafi M: Treatment of renal colic by desmopressin intranasal spray and diclofenac sodium. Journal of Urology, 1995; 153(5):1395-8.

66. Heilberg IP: Update on dietary recommendations and medical treatment of renal stone disease. Nephrology Dialysis and Transplantation, 2000; 15:117-23.

67. Rodgers A: Effect of cola consumption on urinary biochemical and physicochemical risk factors associated with calcium oxalate urolithiasis. Urological Research, 1999; 27(1):77-81.

68. Siener R, Hesse A: Fluid intake and epidemiology of urolithiasis. European Journal of Clinical Nutrition, 2003; 57(supp 2):S47-S51.

69. Curhan GC, Willett WC, Speizer FE, Stampfer MJ: Beverage use and risk for kidney stones in women. Annals of Internal Medicine, 1998; 128(7):534-40.

70. Worster A, Richards C: Fluids and diuretics for acute ureteric colic. Cochrane Renal Group Cochrane Database of Systematic Reviews; 4 Retrieved Jan 2008, last substantive update May 2005, from http://gateway.ut.ovid.com/gw1/ovidweb.cgi

71. Segura JW, Preminger GM, Assimos DG, Dretler SP, Khan RI, Lingeman JE, Macalusco JN: Ureteral stones clinical guidelines panel: panel summary report on the management of ureteral calculi. Jouranl of Urology, 1997; 158(5):1915-21.

72. Coll DM, Varaneli JM, Smith RC: Relationship of spontaneous passage of ureteral calculi to stone size and location revealed by unenhanced helical CT. American Journal of Roentgenology, 2002; 178:101-3.

73. Cummings JM, Boullier JA, Izenberg SD, Kitchens DM, Kothandapani RV: Prediction of spontaneous ureteral calculus passage by an artificial neural network. Journal of Urology, 2000; 164(2):326-8.

74. Anagnostou T, Tolley D: Management of ureteric stones. European Urology, 2004; 45(6):714-21.

75. Dellabella M, Milanese G, Muzzonigro G: Randomized trial of the efficacy of tamsulosin, nifedipine and phloroglucinol in medical expulsive therapy for distal ureteral calculi. Journal of Urology, 2005; 174(1):167-72.

76. Yilmaz E, Batislam E, Basar MM, Tuglu D, Ferhat M, Basar H: The comparison and efficacy of 3 different alpha1-adrenergic blockers for distal ureteral stones. Journal of Urology, 2005; 173(6):2010-2.

77. Singh A, Alter HJ, Littlepage A: A systematic review of medical therapy to facilitate passage of ureteral calculi. Annals of Emergency Medicine, 2007; 50(5):552-63.

78. Kim HH, Lee JH, Park MS, Lee SE, Kim SW: In situ extracorporeal shockwave lithotripsy for ureteral calculi: investigation of factors influencing stone fragmentation and appropriate number of sessions for changing treatment modality. Journal of Endourology, 1996; 10(6):501-5.

79. Lingeman JE, Matlaga BR, Evan AP: Surgical management of upper urinary tract calculi. In Wein AJ, Kavoussi LR, Novick AC, Partin AW, Peters CA (eds): Campbell-Walsh Urology, 9th edition. Philadelphia: Saunders, 2007; pp 1431-1507.

80. Preminger GR: Sonographic piezoelectric lithotripsy: more bang for your buck. Journal of Endourology, 1989; 3:321.

81. Zanetti G, Ostini F, Montanari E, Russo R, Elena A, Trinchieri A, Pisani E: Cardiac dysrhythmias induced by extracorporeal shock wave lithotripsy. Journal of Endourology, 1999; 13(6):409-12.

82. Ganem JP, Carson CC: Cardiac arrhythmias with external fixed-rate generators in shock wave lithotripsy with the Medstone lithotripter. Urology, 1998; 51(4):548-52.

83. Leibovici D, Cooper A, Lindner A, Ostrowsky R, Kleinmann J, Velikanov S, Cipele H, Goren E, Siegel YI: Ureteral stents: morbidity and impact on quality of life. Israel Medical Association Journal, 2005; 7(8):491-4.

84. Rana AM, Sabooh A: Management strategies and results for severely encrusted retained ureteral stents. Journal of Endourology, 2007; 21(6):628-32.

85. Beiko DT, Watterson JD, Knudsen BE, Nott L, Pautler SE, Brock GB, Razvi H, Denstedt JD: Double-blind randomized controlled trial assessing the safety and efficacy of intravesical agents for ureteral stent symptoms after extracorporeal shockwave lithotripsy. Journal of Endourology, 2004; 18(8):723-30.

86. El-Nahas AR, El-Assmy AM, Shoma AM, Eraky I, El-Kenawy MR, El-Kappany HA: Self-retaining ureteral stents: Analysis of factors responsible for patients' discomfort. Journal of Endourology, 2006; 20(1):33-7.

87. DeLeskey KL, Massi-Ventura G: Management of the extracorporeal shock wave lithotripsy patient. Journal of PeriAnesthesia Nursing, 2000; 15(2):94-101.

88. Lafrades AR, Madrid S: Ice pack therapy after extracorporeal shock wave lithotripsy. Urologic Nursing, 1996; 16(3):103-4.

89. Bichler KH, Eipper E, Naber K, Braun V, Zimmermann R, Lahme S: Urinary infection stones. International Journal of Antimicrobial Agents, 2002; 19(6):488-98.

90. Labanaris AP, Kuhn R, Schott GE, Zugor V: Perirenal hematomas induced by Extracorporeal Shock Wave Lithotripsy (ESWL). Therapeutic management. TheScientificWorldJournal, 2007; 7:1563-6.

91. Chan AJ, Prasad PV, Priatna A, Mostafavai MR, Sunduram C, Saltzman B: Protective effect of aminophylline on renal perfusion changes induced by high-energy shockwaves identified by Gd-DTPA-enhanced first-pass perfusion MRI. Journal of Endourology, 2000; 14(2):117-21.

92. Li B, Zhou W, Li P: Protective effects of nifedipine and allopurinol on high energy shock wave induced acute changes of renal function. Journal of Urology, 1995; 153(3, pt 1):596-8.

93. Vimalraj V, Surendran R, Sekar KS, Rajendran N: Massive hemoptysis in a patient with chronic pancreatitis. Journal of Thoracic and Cardiovascular Surgery, 2005; 130(3):910-1.

94. Maker V, Layke J: Gastrointestinal injury secondary to extracorporeal shock wave lithotripsy: a review of the literature since its inception. Journal of the American College of Surgeons, 2004; 198(1):128-35.

95. Tiede JM, Lumpkin EN, Wass CT, Long TR: Hemoptysis following extracorporeal shock wave lithotripsy: a case of lithotripsy-induced pulmonary contusion in a pediatric patient. Journal of Clinical Anesthesia, 2003; 15(7):530-3.

96. Skolarikos A, Alivizatos G, de la Rosette JJ: Percutaneous nephrolithotomy and its legacy. European Urology, 2005; 47(1):22-8.

97. Wong MY: An update on percutaneous nephrolithotomy in the management of urinary calculi. Current Opinion in Urology, 2001; 11(4):367-72.

98. Bagley DH, Kuo RL, Zeltser IS: An update on ureteroscopic instrumentation for the treatment of urolithiasis. Current Opinion in Urology, 2004; 14:99-106.

99. Borghi L, Meschi T, Amato F, Briganti A, Novarini A, Giannini A: Urinary volume, water and recurrences in idiopathic calcium nephrolithiasis: a 5-year randomized prospective study. Journal of Urology, 1996; 155(3):839-43.

100. Tugcu V, Ozbek E, Aras B, Ozbay B, Islim F, Tasci AI: Bone mineral density measurement in patients with recurrent normocalciuric calcium stone disease. Urologic Research, 2007; 35(1):29-34.

101. Sowers MR, Jannausch M, Wood C, Pope SK, Lachance LL, Peterson B: Prevalence of renal stones in a population-based study with dietary calcium, oxalate, and medication exposures. American Journal of Epidemiology, 1998; 147(10):914-20.

102. Leonetti F, Dussol B, Berthezene P, Thirion X, Berland Y: Dietary and urinary risk factors for stones in idiopathic calcium stone formers compared with healthy subjects. Nephrology Dialysis Transplantation, 1998; 13(3):617-22.

103. Odvina CV, Preminger GM, Lindberg JS, Moe OW, Pak CY: Long-term combined treatment with thiazide and potassium citrate in nephrolithiasis does not lead to hypokalemia or hypochloremic metabolic alkalosis. Kidney International, 2003; 63(1):240-7.

104. Yendt ER, Cohanim M: Absorptive hyperoxaluria: a new clinical entity—successful treatment with hydrochlorothiazide. Clinical and Investigative Medicine—Medecine Clinique et Experimentale, 1986; 9(1):44-50.

105. Parks JH, Coe FL: Thiazide does not affect urine oxalate excretion. Journal of Urology, 2003; 170(2, pt 1):393-6.

106. Preminger GM, Pak CY: Eventual attenuation of hypocalciuric response to hydrochlorothiazide in absorptive hypercalciuria. Journal of Urology, 1987; 137(6):1104-9.

107. Mizusawa Y, Burke JR: Prednisolone and cellulose phosphate treatment in idiopathic infantile hypercalcaemia with nephrocalcinosis. Journal of Pediatrics and Child Health, 1996; 32(4):350-2.

108. Park GD, Spector R: Hypocitraturic calcium-oxalate nephrolithiasis. Annals of Internal Medicine, 1986; 104(5):723-4.

109. Massey L: Magnesium therapy for nephrolithiasis. Magnesium Research, 2005; 18(2):123-6.

110. Ettinger B, Pak CY, Citron JT, Thomas C, Adams-Huet B, Vangessel A: Potassium-magnesium citrate is an effective prophylaxis against recurrent calcium oxalate nephrolithiasis. Journal of Urology, 1997; 158(6):2069-73.

111. Kato Y, Yamaguchi S, Yachiku S, Nakazono S, Hori J, Wada N, Hou K: Changes in urinary parameters after oral administration of potassium-sodium citrate and magnesium oxide to prevent urolithiasis. Urology, 2004; 63(1):7-12.

112. Jones M, Monga M: Is there a role for pentosan polysulfate in the prevention of calcium oxalate stones? Journal of Endourology, 2003; 17(10):855-8.

113. Fellstrom B, Backman U, Danielson B, Wikstrom B: Treatment of renal calcium stone disease with the synthetic glycosaminoglycan pentosan polysulfate. World Journal of Urology, 1994; 12(1):52-4.

114. Massey LK, Liebman M, Knysat-Gales SA: Ascorbate increases human oxaluria and kidney stone risk. Journal of Nutrition, 2005; 135(7):1673-7.

115. Campieri C, Campieri M, Bertuzzi V, Swennen E, Matteuzzi D, Stefoni S, Pirovano F, Centi C, Ulisse S, Famularo G, De Simone C: Reduction of oxaluria after an oral course of lactic acid bacteria at high concentration. Kidney International, 2001; 60(3):1097-1105.

116. Cochat P, Basmaison O: Current approaches to the management of primary hyperoxaluria. Archives Diseases in Childhood, 2000; 82:470-3.

117. Shekarriz B, Stoller ML: Uric acid nephrolithiasis: current concepts and controversies. Journal of Urology, 2002; 168(4, pt 1):1307-14.

118. Goldfischer ER, Gerber GS: Endoscopic management of ureteral strictures. Journal of Urology, 1997; 157(3):770-5.

119. Hwang AH, McAleer IM, Shapiro E, Miller OF, Krous HF, Kaplan GW: Congenital mid ureteral strictures. Journal of Urology, 2005; 174(5):1999-2002.

120. Harmon WJ, Sershon PD, Blute ML, Patterson DE, Segura JW: Ureteroscopy: current practice and long-term complications. Journal of Urology, 1997; 157(1):28-32.

121. Geavlete P, Georgescu D, Nita G, Mirciulexcu V, Cauni V: Complications of 2735 retrograde semirigid ureteroscopy procedures: A single-center experience. Journal of Endourology, 2006; 20(3):179-85.

122. Tal R, Sivan B, Kedar D, Baniel J: Management of benign ureteral strictures following radical cystectomy and urinary diversion for bladder cancer. Journal of Urology, 2007; 178(2):538-42.

123. Regan JB, Barrett DM: Stented versus nonstented ureteroileal anastomoses: is there a difference with regard to leak and stricture? Journal of Urology, 1985; 134(6):1101-3.

124. Sellers MT, Velidedeoglu E, Bloom RD, Grossman RA, Markmann JW, Naji A, Frank AM, Kass AB, Nathan HM, Hasz RD, Abrams JD, Markmann JF: Expanded-criteria donor kidneys: a single-center clinical and short-term financial analysis—cause for concern in retransplantation. Transplantation, 2004; 78(11):1670-5.

125. Roberts WW, Cadeddu JA, Micali S, Kavoussi LR, Moore RG: Ureteral stricture formation after removal of impacted calculi. Journal of Urology, 1998; 159(3):723-6.

126. Karod JW, Danella J, Mowad JJ: Routine radiologic surveillance for obstruction is not required in asymptomatic patients after ureteroscopy. Journal of Endourology, 1999; 13(6):433-6.

127. Shokeir AA, El-Diasty T, Eassa W, Mosbah A, El-Ghar MA, Mansour O, Dawaba M, El-Kappany H: Diagnosis of ureteral obstruction in patients with compromised renal function: the role of noninvasive imaging modalities. Journal of Urology, 2004; 171(6, pt 1):2303-6.

128. Gupta M, Ost MC, Shah JB, McDougall EM, Smith AD: Percutaneous management of the upper urinary tract. In Wein AJ, Kavoussi LR, Novick AC, Partin AW, Peters CA (eds): Campbell-Walsh Urology, 9th edition. Philadelphia: Saunders, 2007; pp 1526-34.

129. Jyding Vennervald B, Kahama AI, Reimert CM: Assessment of morbidity in *Schistosoma haematobium* infection: current methods and future tools. Acta Tropica, 2000; 77(1):81-9.

130. Kardar AH, Kattan S, Lindstedt E, Hanash K: Steroid therapy for idiopathic retroperitoneal fibrosis: dose and duration. Journal of Urology, 2002; 168(2):550-5.

131. Klein DG: Thoracic aortic aneurysms. Journal of Cardiovascular Nursing, 2005; 20(4):245-50.

132. Lacquet JP, Lacroix H, Nevelsteen A, Suy R: Inflammatory abdominal aortic aneurysms: a retrospective study of 110 cases. Acta Chirurgica Belgica, 1997; 97(6):286-92.

133. Bailey SH, Mone MC, Holman JM, Nelson EW: Laparoscopic treatment of postrenal transplant lymphoceles. Surgical Endoscopy, 2003; 17:1896-9.

134. Pepper RJ, Pati J, Kaisary AV: The incidence and treatment of lymphoceles after radical retropubic prostatectomy. BJU International, 2005; 95(6):772-5.

135. Katz R, Landau EH, Pikarsky AJ, Eid A: Bladder outlet obstruction by a lymphocele following kidney transplantation. Urologia Internationalis, 1997; 59(3):186-7.

136. Close CE: The valve bladder. In Gillenwater JY, Grayhack JT, Howards SS, Mitchell ME: Adult and Pediatric Urology, 4th edition. Philadelphia: Lippincott Williams & Wilkins, 2002; pp 2311-8.

137. Ben-Meir D, Yin M, Chow CW, Hutson JM: Urethral polyps in prepubertal girls. Journal of Urology, 2005; 174(4, p. 1):1443-4.

138. Berdeu D, Sauze L, Ha-Vinh P, Blum-Boisgard C: Cost-effectiveness analysis of treatments for phimosis: a comparison of surgical and medicinal approaches and their economic effect. BJU International, 2001; 87(3):239-44.

139. Jordan GH, Schlossberg SM: Surgery of the penis and urethra. In Wein AJ, Kavoussi LR, Novick AC, Partin AW, Peters CA (eds). Campbell-Walsh Urology, 9th edition. Philadelphia: Saunders, 2007; pp 1023-97.

140. Kochakarn W, Muangman V, Viseshsindh V, Ratana-Olarn K, Gojaseni P: Stricture of the male urethra: 29 years experience of 323 cases. Journal of the Medical Association of Thailand, 2001; 84(1):6-11.

141. Barbagli G, Palminteri E, Balo S, Vallasciani S, Mearini E, Constantini E, Mearini L, Zucchi A, Vivacqua C, Porena M: Lichen sclerosus of the male genitalia and urethral stricture diseases. Urologia Internationalis, 2004; 73(1):1-5.

142. Hu JC, Gold KF, Pashos CL, Mehta SS, Litwin MS: Temporal trends in radical prostatectomy complications from 1991 to 1998. Journal of Urology, 2003; 169(4):1443-8.

143. Andrich DE, Mundy AR: Urethral strictures and their surgical treatment. BJU International, 2000; 86(5):571-80.

144. Nonomura K, Kanno T, Kakizaki H, Koyama T, Yamashita T, Koyanagi T: Impact of congenital narrowing of the bulbar urethra (Cobb's collar) and its transurethral incision in children. European Urology, 1999; 36(2):144-9.

145. Dobosy JR, Roberts JL, Fu VX, Jarrard DF: The expanding role of epigenetics in the development, diagnosis and treatment of prostate cancer and benign prostatic hyperplasia. Journal of Urology, 2007; 177(3):822-31.

146. Jacobsen SJ, Girman CJ, Lieber MM: Natural history of benign prostatic hyperplasia. Urology, 1998; 58(6 Supp 1):5-16.

147. Madersbacher S, Marszalek M, Lackner J, Berger P, Schatzi G: The long term outcome of medical therapy for BPH. European Urology, 2007; 51(6):1522-33.

148. Denis L, McConnell O, Yoshida S, et al. Recommendations of the International Scientific Committee. In Denis L, Griffiths K, Khoury S et al (eds): 4th International Consultation on Benign Prostatic Hyperplasia (BPH). Plymbridge, UK: Health Publication Ltd, 1998; pp 669-84.

149. Abrams P, Cardozo L, Fall M, Griffiths D, Rosier P, Ulmsten U, van Kerrebroeck P, Victor A, Wein A: The standardization of terminology of lower urinary tract function: report from the Standardization Sub-committee of the International Continence Society. American Journal of Obstetrics and Gynecology, 2002; 187(1):116-26.

150. Verhamme KM, Dieleman JP, Bleumink GS, van der Lei J, Sturkenboom MC, Artibani W, Begaud B, Berges R, Borkowski A, Chappel CR, Costello A, Dobronski P, Farmer RD, Jimenez Cruz F, Jonas U, MacRae K, Pientka L, Rutten FF, van Schayck CP, Speakman MJ, Sturkenboom MC, Tiellac P, Tubaro A, Vallencien G, Vela Navarrete R, Triumph Pan European Expert Panel: Incidence and prevalence of lower urinary tract symptoms suggestive of benign prostatic hyperplasia in primary care—the Triumph project. European Urology, 2002; 42:323.

151. Koskimaki J, Hakama M, Huhtala H, Tammela TL: Is reduced quality of life in men with lower urinary tract symptoms due to concomitant diseases? European Urology, 2001; 40:661.

152. Kang D, Andriole GL, Van De Vooren RC, Crawford D, Chia D, Urban DA, Reding D, Huang WY, Hayes RB: Risk behaviors and benign prostatic hyperplasia. BJU International, 2004; 93:1241.

153. Joseph MA, Harlow SD, Wei JT, Sarma AV, Dunn RL, Taylor JM, James SA, Cooney KA, Doerr KM, Montie JE, Schottenfeld D: Risk factors for lower urinary tract symptoms in a population-based sample of African-American men. American Journal of Epidemiology, 2003; May 157(10):906-14.

154. Koskimaki J, Hakama M, Huhtala H, Tammela TL: Association of smoking with lower urinary tract symptoms. Journal of Urology, 1998; 159:1580.

155. Haass M, Kubler W: Nicotine and sympathetic neurotransmission. Cardiovascular Drugs and Therapy, 1997; 10:657.

156. Koskimaki J, Hakama M, Huhtala H, Tammela TL: Association of non-urological diseases with lower urinary tract symptoms. Scandinavian Journal of Urology and Nephrology, 2001; 35:377.

157. Foley CL, Bott SR, Shergill IS, Kirby RS: An update on the use of 5-alpha reductase inhibitors. Drugs of Today, 2004; 40:213.

158. Blaivas JG: Obstructive uropathy in the male. Urologic Clinics of North America, 1996; 23:373.

159. AUA Practice Guidelines Committee: AUA guideline on management of benign prostatic hyperplasia. Journal of Urology, 2003; 170:530.

160. Meigs JB, Barry MJ, Giovannucci E, Rimm EB, Stampfer MJ, Kawachi I: Incidence rates and risk factors for acute urinary retention: the health professionals followup study. Journal of Urology, 1999; 162:376.

161. Djavan B, Remzi M, Erne B, Marberger M: The pathophysiology of benign prostatic hyperplasia. Drugs of Today, 2002; 38(1):867-76.

162. Bosch J, Kranse R, Van Mastrigt R, Schroder FH: Reasons for the weak correlation between prostate volume and urethral resistance parameters in patients with prostatism. Journal of Urology, 1995; 153:689.

163. Girman CJ: Natural history and epidemiology of benign prostatic hyperplasia: Relationship among urologic measures. Urology, 1998; 51:8.

164. Sandhu JS, Te AE: The role of 5-alpha-reductase inhibition as monotherapy in view of the MTOPS data. Current Urology Reports, 2004; 5(4):274-9.

165. Johnson TM 2nd, Burrows PK, Kusek JW, Nyberg LM, Tenover JL, Lepor H, Roehrborn CG: Medical Therapy of Prostatic Symptoms Research Group: The effect of doxazosin, finasteride and combination therpy on nocturia in men with benign prostatic hyperplasia. Journal of Urology, 2007; 178(5):245-50.

166. Tanagho EA: Urinary obstruction and stasis. In Tanagho EA, McAninch JW (eds): Smith's General Urology, 16th edition. New York: Lange Medical Books/McGraw-Hill, 2004; pp 175-87.

167. Thomas AW, Cannon A, Bartlett E, Ellis-Jones J, Abrams P: The natural history of lower urinary tract dysfunction in men: minimum 10-year urodynamic follow-up of untreated bladder outlet obstruction. BJU International, 2005; 96(9):1301-6.

168. Levin RM, Monson FC, Haugaard N, Buttyan R, Hudson A, Roelofs M, Sartore S, Wein AJ: Genetic and cellular characteristics of bladder outlet obstruction. Urologic Clinics of North America, 1995; 22:263.

169. Gosling JA, Gilpin SA, Dixon JS, Gilpin CJ: Decrease in the autonomic innervation of human detrusor muscle in outflow obstruction. Journal of Urology, 1986; 136:501.

170. Roehrborn CG, McConnell JD: Benign prostatic hyperplasia: etiology, pathophysiology, epidemiology, and natural history. In Wein AJ, Kavoussi LR, Novick AC, Partin AW, Peters CA (eds): Campbell-Walsh Urology, 9th edition. Philadelphia: Saunders, 2007; pp 2727-65.

171. Chai TC, Gray M, Steers WD: The incidence of a positive ice water test on bladder outlet obstructed patients: evidence for altered innervation. Journal of Urology, 1998; 160:34-8.

172. Hirayama A, Fujimoto K, Matsumoto Y, Hirao Y: Nocturia in men with lower urinary tract symptoms is associated with both nocturnal polyuria and detrusor overactivity with positive response to ice water test. Urology, 2005; 65(6):1064-9.

173. Peters TJ, Donovan JL, Kay HE, Abrams P, de la Rosette JJ, Porru D, Thuroff JW: The International Continence Society "Benign Prostatic Hyperplasia" Study: the bothersomeness of urinary symptoms. Journal of Urology, 1997; 157(3):885-9.

174. Barry MJ, Fowler FJ Jr, O'Leary MP, Bruskewitz RC, Holtgrewe HL, Mebust WK, Cockett AT: The American Urological Association symptom index for benign prostatic hyperplasia. Journal of Urology, 1992; 148:1549.

175. Gray M: Psychometric analysis of the international prostate symptom score. Urologic Nursing, 1998; 18:175-83.

176. Barqawi A, O'Donnell C, Kumar R, Koul H, Crawford ED: Correlation between LUTS (AUA-SS) and erectile dysfunction (SHIM) in an age-matched racially diverse male population: data from the Prostate Cancer Awareness Week (PCAW). International Journal of Impotence Research, 2005; 17(4):370-4.

177. Berger AP, Deibl M, Leonhartsberger N, Bektic J, Horninger W, Fritsche G, Steiner H, Pelzer AE, Bartsch G, Frauscher F: Vascular

damage as a risk factor for benign prostatic hyperplasia and erectile dysfunction. BJU International, 2005; 96(7):1073-8.

178. McVary KT: Erectile dysfunction and lower urinary tract symptoms secondary to BPH. European Urology, 2005; 47(6):838-45.

179. Finestone AJ, Rosenthal RS: Silent prostatism. Geriatrics, 1971; 26(5):89-92.

180. Rule AD, Lieber MM, Jacobsen SJ: Is benign prostatic hyperplasia a risk factor for chronic renal failure? Journal of Urology, 2005; 173(3):691-6.

181. Kashif KM, Foley SJ, Basketter V, Holmes SA: Hematuria associated with BPH—natural history and a new treatment option. Prostate Cancer Prostatic Disease, 1998; 1:154-6.

182. Kirby R, Lepor H: Evaluation and nonsurgical management of benign prostatic hyperplasia. In Wein AJ, Kavoussi LR, Novick AC, Partin AW, Peters CA (eds): Campbell-Walsh Urology, 9th edition. Philadelphia: Saunders, 2007; pp 2766-2802.

183. Roehrborn CG, Boyle P, Bergner D, Gray T, Gittelman M, Shown T, Melman A, Bracken RB, deVere White R, Taylor A, Wang D, Waldstreicher J: Serum prostate-specific antigen and prostate volume predict long-term changes in symptoms and flow rate: results of a four-year, randomized trial comparing finasteride versus placebo. PLESS Study Group. Urology, 1999; 54(4):662-9.

184. Bartsch G, Fitzpatrick JM, Schalken JA, Isaacs J, Nordling J, Roehrborn CG: Consensus statement: the role of prostate-specific antigen in managing the patient with benign prostatic hyperplasia. BJU International, 2004; 93:27.

185. Comiter CV, Sullivan MP, Schacterle RS, Cohen LH, Valla SV: Urodynamic risk factors for renal dysfunction in men with obstructive and nonobstructive voiding dysfunction. Journal of Urology, 1997; 158:181.

186. Javle P, Jenkins SA, West C, Parsons KF: Quantification of voiding dysfunction in patients awaiting transurethral prostatectomy. Journal of Urology, 1996; 156:1014.

187. Sarma AV, Jacobson DJ, McGree ME, Roberts RO, Lieber MM, Jacobsen SJ: A population based study of incidence and treatment of benign prostatic hyperplasia among residents of Olmsted County, Minnesota: 1987 to 1997. Journal of Urology, 2005; 173(6):2048-53.

188. Kaplan SA, McConnell JD, Roehrborn CG, Meehan AG, Lee MW, Noble WR, Kusek JW, Nyberg LM Jr: Medical Therapy of Prostatic Symptoms (MTOPS) Research Group: Combination therapy with doxazosin and finasteride for benign prostatic hyperplasia in patients with lower urinary tract symptoms and a baseline total prostate volume of 25 ml or greater. Journal of Urology, 2006; 175(1):217-21.

189. Foley CL, Kirby RS: 5 alpha-reductase inhibitors: what's new? Current Opinion in Urology, 2003; 13(1):31-7.

190. Brawley OW, Barnes S, Parnes H: The future of prostate cancer prevention. Annals of the New York Academy of Sciences, 2001; 952:145-52.

191. Reid P, Kantoff P, Oh W: Antiandrogens in prostate cancer. Investigational New Drugs, 1999; 17(3):271-84.

192. Andriole GL, Roehrborn C, Schulman C, Slawin KM, Somerville M, Rittmaster RS: Effect of dutasteride on the detection of prostate cancer in men with benign prostatic hyperplasia. Urology, 2004; 64(3):537-43.

193. Schulman C: Use of 5-alpha-reductase inhibitors in the prevention of prostate cancer. Annales d Urologie, 2004; 38(Suppl 2) pp S35-S42.

194. Schwinn DA, Price DT, Narayan P: Alpha1-adrenoceptor subtype selectivity and lower urinary tract symptoms. Mayo Clinic Proceedings, 2004; 79(11):1423-34.

195. Kyprianou N: Doxazosin and terazosin suppress prostate growth by inducing apoptosis: clinical significance. Journal of Urology, 2003; 169(4):1520-5.

196. Ruggieri MR Sr, Braverman AS, Pontari MA: Combined use of alpha-adrenergic and muscarinic antagonists for the treatment of voiding dysfunction. Journal of Urology, 2005; 174(5):1743-8.

197. Kortmann BB, Floratos DL, Kiemeney LA, Wijkstra H, de la Rosette JJ: Urodynamic effects of alpha-adrenoceptor blockers: a review of clinical trials. Urology, 2003; 62(1):1-9.

198. Reynard JM: Does anticholinergic medication have a role for men with lower urinary tract symptoms/benign prostatic hyperplasia either alone or in combination with other agents?. Current Opinion in Urology, 2004; 14:3.

199. Athanasopoulos A, Gyftopoulos K, Giannitsas K, Fisfis J, Perimenis P, Barbalias G: Combination treatment with an alpha-blocker plus an anticholinergic for bladder outlet obstruction: a prospective, randomized, controlled study. Journal of Urology, 2003; 169(6):2253-6.

200. Lee KS, Choo MS, Kim DY, Kim JC, Kim HJ, Min KS, Lee JB, Jeong HJ, Lee T, Park WH: Combination treatment with papaverine hydrochloride plus doxazosin controlled release gastrointestinal therapeutic system formulation for overactive bladder and coexisting benign prostatic obstruction: a prospective, randomized, controlled multicenter study. Journal of Urology, 2005; 174(4, pt 1):1334-8.

201. Lee JY, Kim HW, Lee SJ, Koh JS, Suh HJ, Chancellor MB: Comparison of doxazosin with or without tolterodine in men with symptomatic bladder outlet obstruction and an overactive bladder. BJU International, 2004; 94(6):817-20.

202. Abrams P, Kaplan S, De Koning Gans HJ, Millard R: Safety and tolerability of tolterodine for the treatment of overactive bladder in men with bladder outlet obstruction. Journal of Urology, 2006; 175(3, pt 1):999-1004.

203. De Smet PA: Herbal remedies. New England Journal of Medicine, 2002; 347(25):2046-55.

204. Gordon AE, Shaughnessy AF: Saw palmetto for prostate disorders. American Family Physician, 2003; 67(6):1281-3.

205. de la Rosette JJ, Froeling FM, Debruyne FM: Clinical results with microwave thermotherapy of benign prostatic hyperplasia. European Urology, 1993; 23(supp 1):68-71.

206. de la Rosette JJ, de Wildt MJ, Alivizatos G, Froeling FM, Debruyne FM: Transurethral microwave thermotherapy (TUMT) in benign prostatic hyperplasia: placebo versus TUMT. Urology, 1994; 44(1):58-63.

207. Nitti VW, Adler H, Combs AJ: The role of urodynamics in the evaluation of voiding dysfunction in men after cerebrovascular accident. Journal of Urology, 1996; 155:263.

208. Djavan B, Madersbacher S, Klingler C, Marberger M: Urodynamic assessment of patients with acute urinary retention: is treatment failure after prostatectomy predictable? Journal of Urology, 1997; 158:1829.

209. Comiter CV, Sullivan MP, Schacterle RS, Yalla SV: Prediction of prostatic obstruction with a combination of isometric detrusor contraction pressure and maximum urinary flow rate. Urology, 1996; 48:723.

210. Joseph DV: Vesicoureteral reflux. In Gearhart JP (ed): Pediatric Urology. Totowa, NJ: Humana Press, 2003; pp 51-82.

211. Koff SA, Mutabagani KH: Anomalies of the kidney. In Gillenwater JY, Grayhack JT, Howards SS, Mitchell ME (eds): Adult and Pediatric Urology, 4th edition, vol 3. Philadelphia: Lippincott Williams & Wilkins, 2002; pp 2129-54.

212. Sarmina I, Spirnak JP, Resnick MI: Urinary lithiasis in the black population: an epidemiological study and review of the literature. Journal of Urology, 1987; 138(1):14-7.

213. Griffin DG: A review of the heritability of idiopathic nephrolithiasis. Journal of Clinical Pathology, 2004; 57(8):793-6.

214. Prie D, Huart V, Bakouh N, Planelles G, Dellis O, Gerard B, Hulin P, Benque-Blanchet F, Silve C, Grandchamp B, Friedlander G: Nephrolithiasis and osteoporosis associated with hypophosphatemia caused by mutations in the type 2a sodium-phosphate cotransporter. New England Journal of Medicine, 2002; 343(7):983-91.

215. Prince CL, Scardino PL, Wolan CT: The effect of temperature, humidity and dehydration on the formation of renal calculi. Journal of Urology, 1956; 75(2):209-15.

216. Prince CL, Scardino PL: A statistical analysis of ureteral calculi. Journal of Urology, 1960; 83:561-5.

217. Sutor DJ, Wooley SE: Composition of urinary calculi by X-ray diffraction. Collected data from various localities. XV-XVII. Royal Navy; Bristol, England; and Dundee, Scotland. British Journal of Urology, 1974; 46(2):229-32.

218. Najem GR, Seebode JJ, Samady AJ, Feuerman M, Friedman L: Stressful life events and risk of symptomatic kidney stones. International Journal of Epidemiology, 1997; 26(5):1017-23.

219. Buno Soto A, Torres Jimenez R, Olveira A, Fernandez-Blanco Herraiz I, Montero Garcia A, Mateos Anton F: Lithogenic risk factors for renal stones in patients with Crohn's disease. Archivos Espanoles de Urologia, 2001; 54(3):282-92.

220. Trinchieri A, Lizzano R, Castelnuovo C, Zanetti G, Pisani E: Urinary patterns of patient with renal stones associated with inflammatory bowel disease. Archivio Italiano di Urologic, Andrologia, 2002; 74(2):61-4.

221. Meydan N, Barcuta S, Caliskan S, Camasari T: Urinary stones in diabetes mellitus. Scandinavian Journal of Urology and Nephrology, 2003; 37(1):64-70.

222. Abate N, Chandalia M, Cabo-Chan AV Jr, Moe OW, Sakhaee K: The metabolic syndrome and uric acid nephrolithiasis: novel features of renal manifestation of insulin resistance. Kidney International, 2004; 65(2):386-92.

223. Yagisawa T, Kobayashi C, Hayashi T, Yoshida A, Toma H: Contributory metabolic factors in the development of nephrolithiasis in patients with medullary sponge kidney. American Journal of Kidney Diseases, 2001; 37(6):1140-3.

224. Torres VE, Wilson DM, Hattery RR, Segura JW: Renal stone disease in autosomal dominant polycystic kidney disease. American Journal of Kidney Diseases, 1993; 22(4):513-9.

225. Gibney EM, Goldfarb DS: The association of nephrolithiasis with cystic fibrosis. American Journal of Kidney Disease, 2003; 41(10):1-11.

Urologic oncology includes tumors affecting the urinary or male reproductive systems. Urinary system tumors affect the kidneys, ureters, bladder, and urethra; and male reproductive system tumors involve the prostate, testes, and penis. Although the general principles of urologic oncology presented here apply to any tumor of the genitourinary tract, this chapter is limited to detailed reviews of renal, bladder, prostate, testicular, and penile cancer.

RENAL TUMORS

Renal tumors arise as primary or metastatic malignancies; the most common is the adenocarcinoma (renal cell carcinoma, or hypernephroma) (Figure 8-1). Primary renal tumors are relatively rare, accounting for only 6% of all cancer cases in adults. Approximately 38,890 new cases of renal cancer are reported annually in the United States and 12,840 deaths from this disease.[1] It most commonly affects persons in the sixth and seventh decades of life, and men are at greater risk than women (men/women 2:1). Age-specific incidence demonstrates a small, temporary peak in early childhood because of Wilms tumor; occurrence rates then decline and remain low until they again rise during the fourth decade of life to reach their peak during the sixth and seventh decades. The racial/ethnic patterns for ages 55 to 69 years and 70 years and over are similar to those for all ages combined.

Although epidemiologic reports generally combine cancers affecting the renal parenchyma with tumors of the pelvicalyceal system, it is important to remember that these tumors are histologically and clinically distinct. About one in five kidney cancers occurs in the renal pelvis.[2] Internationally, the highest incidence rates occur in the United States, Canada, Northern Europe, Australia, and New Zealand. These rates are eight times higher than those reported in developing countries such as Thailand, China, and the Philippines. Differences may reflect environmental exposures specific to more industrialized countries,

or they may echo the impact of modern imaging techniques, such as magnetic resonance imaging (MRI), computed tomography (CT), and ultrasonography, not as readily available in developing countries.[3]

Etiology and Risk Factors

Although the etiology of renal cell carcinoma is unknown, a number of environmental and genetic factors have been identified. Cigarette smoking consistently emerges as a risk factor for renal cell carcinoma.[3-5] Whereas the precise relationship between cigarette smoking and the onset of kidney cancers is not understood, it is known that cigarette and cigar smoking are associated with statistically significant risks of developing renal cell carcinoma that is not associated with the use of pipes or smokeless tobacco. It has also been observed that smoking cessation for a period of 10 years or more reduces the risk of renal cell carcinoma by 30% and the risk of renal pelvis cancers by approximately 50%.[4,5]

Analgesic use and hypertension are also associated with an increased risk of renal cell carcinoma.[3,6,7] It is not known whether the relationship between renal cell carcinoma and hypertension arises from the disorder itself or from medications used to treat hypertension, such as the diuretics.[8] Obesity is associated with an increased risk for renal cancer[7]; this risk occurs irrespective of fat distribution patterns in women, although it appears to be greater among men with lower hip circumference (usually associated with greater abdominal girth).[9] Alcohol consumption increases the risk of renal cell carcinoma, but this effect is greater among women as compared with men for unclear reasons.[10]

Occupational exposures linked to kidney cancer risk include chlorinated solvents and asbestos. A study of Canadian workers revealed an association between exposure to benzene, benzidine, creosote, asphalt, herbicides, mustard gas, pesticides, and vinyl chloride and kidney cancer.[11] Of note, these exposures carried a higher risk for men compared with women.

Genetic factors may play a role in the etiology of renal cell carcinoma.[3] The defect is most likely located on chromosomes 3, 7, or 17.[12] Although it remains unclear what proportion of the sporadic occurrences of renal cell carcinoma is attributable to genetic factors, clear cell renal cell carcinoma has long been linked to hereditary disorders such as von Hippel–Lindau disease, which carries a lifetime risk for renal cell carcinoma of 23% to 45%.[13]

Pathophysiology

The pathophysiologic significance of a renal cell carcinoma arises from its propensity for local invasion and metastasis to distant sites. Renal cell carcinoma is such an aggressive neoplasm that many patients have distant metastasis, and even with aggressive treatment, significant morbidity and death occur.[6,14] The tumor originates from the proximal renal tubular epithelial cells, and it grows from the inner aspect (cortex) of the kidney toward the periphery, producing the characteristic bulging mass noted on imaging studies. Tumor growth also distorts normal pelvicalyceal architecture, resulting in calyceal splaying noted on intravenous pyelography. Tumors often contain cystic structures, areas of necrosis, and fat, and they may obstruct one or more calices. Renal cell carcinomas tend to invade adjacent structures including the renal vein and the inferior vena cava (15%). Thrombi created by these invasive extensions may reach the right atrium.

Tumors also may invade the perirenal fat before disrupting the renal capsule, increasing the risk of metastasis to adjacent organs.

In addition to its propensity for local invasion, a renal cell carcinoma is likely to spread by metastasis.[6] The lungs and bones are the most common sites, but other sites are the paraaortic and other regional lymph nodes, adrenal gland, brain, and other adjacent organs, including the liver, pancreas, and colon. Metastatic spread occurs by hematogenous and lymphatogenous routes.

Clinical Manifestations

Early-stage renal cancer is usually asymptomatic and discovered incidentally. As a result, many patients present with advanced-stage disease. The classic triad of hematuria (intermittent or gross), flank pain, and palpable mass is associated with advanced disease. In addition, patients may experience anemia and fatigue. Because the renal tumor excretes parathyroid hormone and erythropoietin, hypercalcemia and erythropoiesis may be present.[15] Box 8-1 summarizes paraneoplastic syndromes frequently associated with advanced renal carcinoma.

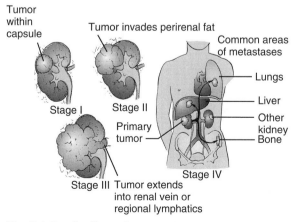

Fig. 8-1 Renal cell carcinoma. (Black J, Hank J: Medical-Surgical Nursing-Clinical Management for Positive Outcomes, 8th edition. Philadelphia-Saunders, 2009.)

BOX 8-1 Paraneoplastic Syndromes Associated with Renal Carcinomas[15]

Syndromes
Hypercalcemia
Nonmetastatic hepatopathy
Hypertension
Erythrocytosis
Pyrexia
Galactorrhea
Gynecomastia
Serum glucose abnormalities

Serologic Factors and Other Syndromes
Prostaglandins
Alkaline phosphatase
Neuromyopathy
Amyloidosis
Coagulation factors
Iron metabolism
γ-Enolase
α-Fetoprotein
Vasculitis
Fibroblast growth factor

Diagnosis and Staging

The diagnosis of renal cell carcinoma is often made on incidental findings, such as an ultrasound, abdominal CT, or MRI. Advanced-stage disease is typically symptom driven, although it also may be diagnosed as the result of an episode of gross hematuria in the absence of other bothersome signs or symptoms.[6] The diagnostic evaluation should determine the stage of the tumor (Table 8-1) and the presence of paraneoplastic syndromes. Common diagnostic tests obtained during the evaluation of a renal mass are outlined in Table 8-2.

Medical Management of Renal Carcinoma

Traditionally, radical nephrectomy provided the only hope for a long-term cure for early-stage renal cell carcinomas. Fortunately, since advances in imaging techniques have led to increasing diagnosis of early-stage tumors, the number of patients who can be managed by partial (i.e., nephron-sparing) surgery has grown.[6] In contrast, advanced-stage renal cell carcinoma remains difficult to treat, and the prognosis for patients with one or more distant metastases, in particular, remains poor.

Treatment

Because of the highly aggressive nature of renal cell carcinomas associated with symptoms, the concept of watchful waiting has not been a realistic option. However, with advances in imaging studies, the question of watchful waiting has become a reality. In the twenty-first century, watchful waiting may be considered in patients who have a very small (less than 3 cm), solitary T1 tumor. This tumor should be well marginated, solid, and homogenous and found in a patient who is aging or is considered a poor surgical risk.[16-18] Since the majority of these lesions ultimately grow to a point that metastasis is likely, this strategy is *not* a viable option for the young, otherwise healthy patient with a small, early-stage renal cell carcinoma.[6,17]

Clearly, the majority of patients diagnosed with lower-stage tumors will require surgical resection. Traditionally, all renal cell carcinomas were treated with radical nephrectomy, but less invasive procedures, referred to as nephron-sparing techniques, have gained popularity in the last decade.[19] Nephron-sparing techniques include open partial nephrectomy, laparoscopic partial nephrectomy, robot-assisted partial nephrectomy, and cryosurgery.[6,20,21] Indications for these procedures include patients with a solitary kidney or bilateral tumors and those with a unilateral tumor but a contralateral kidney damaged by renal artery stenosis, severe hydronephrosis, or parenchymal scarring. A nephron-sparing procedure also may be considered

TABLE 8-1 Robson and TNM Staging Systems for Renal Cell Carcinoma[6,124]

STAGE CLASSIFICATION	TNM CLASSIFICATION (AJCC)	N	M
Stage I: confined to renal capsule	T1a: tumor ≤ 4 cm, confined within renal capsule without distortion of pelvicalyceal system	N0	M0
	T1b: tumor > 4 cm < 7 cm, confined within renal capsule but distorts the pelvicalyceal system		
Stage II: extends into perirenal fat and/or ipsilateral adrenal; contained by Gerota's fascia	T2: tumor > 7 cm, extends into the perirenal fat and ipsilateral adrenal gland; not beyond Gerota's fascia	N0	M0
Stage IIIA: renal vein or vena caval involvement	T3: tumor extends into major veins or invades adrenal or perinephric tissues but not beyond Gerota's fascia	N0	M0
	T3a: perinephric or adrenal extension		
	T3b: spread to renal vein or vena cava below diaphragm		
	T3c: involves renal vein and inferior vena cava above the diaphragm		
Stage IIIB: lymphatic involvement	T4: tumor invades beyond Gerota's fascia	N1-4	M0
Stage IIIC: vein and node involvement			
Stage IVA: contiguous organ involvement	T1-T4	N0-4	M0
Stage IVB: metastasis to lungs, bones	T4	N0-4	M1

AJCC, American Joint Cancer Committee; *TNM,* tumor-nodes-metastasis.

in patients with a systemic disease such as diabetes mellitus or long-term hypertension associated with nephrosclerosis likely to have compromised function of both kidneys. More recently, these techniques have been applied to low-stage (T1) tumors and a normal contralateral kidney. Arguments against this include the possibility that early-stage renal cell carcinoma is a multifocal tumor leading to incomplete tumor eradication. Arguments for it include the relatively low risk of multifocal disease (5%) when an isolated T1 tumor is resected, and at least one study has reported equivocal 10-year disease-free survival rates (73% versus 74%) with a lower risk for renal insufficiency in those managed by nephron-sparing techniques (11% versus 22%).[22]

Although the indications for nephron-sparing surgeries are increasing, radical nephrectomy remains the principal surgical approach when managing a patient with renal cell carcinoma.[6] The kidney, its surrounding fascia (including Gerota's fascia), ipsilateral adrenal gland, and proximal half of the ureter are removed. Some clinicians advocate regional lymphadenectomy, but others argue that removal of the hilar nodes is sufficient. Potential advantages of a regional lymphadenectomy include more accurate tumor staging, but the value of this information has been questioned given the lack of effective treatment options based on identification of a precise stage. As discussed above, radical nephrectomy remains a primary treatment option for early-stage, localized renal cell carcinoma. In more advanced disease, tumor resection also may require resection of a tumor that has extended into the renal vein, inferior vena cava, liver, bowel, or other adjacent structures. In some cases the entire tumor cannot be removed, and the tumor is debulked rather than resected.

Effective treatment options for metastatic renal cell carcinoma remain elusive. Metastatic renal cell carcinomas are almost always nonresponsive to hormonal therapy and resistant to chemotherapy, possibly because of the tumor's ability to overexpress a multidrug resistance gene. Therefore they are managed with cytokine-based treatments, usually interferon-α or interleukin-2 administered alone or in combination. Unfortunately, a meta-analysis derived from 42 randomized clinical trials involving 4216 patients found a 10% partial response rate and a 3% total response that persisted for at least 24 months following therapy.[23]

TABLE 8-2 Diagnostic Evaluation of Renal Cell Carcinoma

TEST	FINDINGS
Complete blood count	Anemia related to blood loss or erythrocytosis related to excessive secretion of erythropoietin
Sedimentation rate	Elevated in many cases (limited assistance in differential diagnosis)
Serum electrolytes	Hypercalcemia caused by bone metastasis or paraneoplastic syndrome
Urinalysis	Gross or microscopic hematuria
Urine cytologic studies	Nonspecific findings (rarely helpful for diagnosis of renal cell carcinoma)
Intravenous pyelogram/urogram (IVP/IVU)	Distortion of the internal renal architecture with splaying of the calices; tumor may have calcified elements; obstructive uropathy may be present; IVP not sensitive or specific enough for small to medium tumors
Renal arteriography	Neovascularity of tumor and tumor invasion into renal vein or inferior vena cava; done only if renal-sparing surgery is anticipated
Renal ultrasound (especially for patients with contrast allergy)	Accurate differentiation between cystic and solid masses; needle aspiration of cyst may be done under ultrasound guidance and fluid sent for cytology
Chest x-ray	To rule out pulmonary involvement
Computed tomography (CT)	Differentiates normal renal parenchyma from tumor or fluid-filled cyst or stone; also useful for detecting regional lymph node involvement, invasion of the inferior vena cava, and larger distant metastases; used to stage primary tumor
Magnetic resonance imaging (MRI)	Advantages over CT include being able to move in multiple planes; more accurate than CT in determining the presence and level of tumor invasion into renal vein or inferior vena cava

Cytokine-based therapies are associated with significant adverse side effects, particularly in patients with higher-stage disease. Radiation and chemotherapy regimens have also been tried, but renal cell carcinoma has proven comparatively resistant to both of these modalities, even when multiple agents or combination regimens are employed.[6,14] Because metastatic tumors are capable of significant angiogenesis, treatment may include antiangiogenic drugs. Several agents have been tested in clinical trials or used in the clinical setting, including bevacizumab (Avastin), thalidomide, AE-941 (Neovastat), and SU11248.

Researchers are attempting to locate new targets for therapy. Possible targets include the Raf kinase pathway, which has been linked to uncontrolled cellular growth and production of cancer cells, and the mTOR pathway, which is associated with malignant cell proliferation and angioneogenesis. Alternative investigational therapeutic strategies include injection of monoclonal antibodies against G250/CA IX or tumor necrosis factor alpha (TNF-α), vaccinations designed to prevent the negative actions of dendritic cells within the tumor, and allogenic stem cell transplantation.

Nursing Management

The surgical technique; the presence, location, and size of the surgical incision; and the presence of local invasion determine the nursing management of the patient undergoing surgical resection of a renal cell carcinoma. A detailed discussion of the nursing care of the patient undergoing radical nephrectomy or a laparoscopic, nerve-sparing surgery is provided in Chapter 11.

Because of the poor prognosis associated with advanced-stage renal cell carcinoma, urologic nurses must be cognizant of the anxiety and fear that patients and their families may experience when a diagnosis of renal cell cancer is made. Assessing the patient's understanding of the disease and treatment is necessary before comprehensive care can be initiated. Patients who have had a nephrectomy will need assurance that they can function normally with one kidney. Normal postoperative recovery instructions will be given, such as eating well, drinking adequate fluids (30 ml/kg), walking, and avoidance of heavy lifting until at least 4 weeks after surgery. Follow-up will include routine monitoring of blood pressure. Patients are advised that uncontrolled pain,

changes in respiratory status, fever, wound drainage, decreased urine output, fluid retention, and hypertension should be reported immediately to their physician.[24]

Patient education will include instruction about the need for ongoing monitoring for tumor recurrence. Patients managed by watchful waiting are monitored with a chest x-ray, complete blood count (CBC), and physical examination every 6 months for 2 years and then annually. Abdominal CT scans are recommended annually for 2 years and then every 2 years.

BLADDER CANCER

Bladder cancer is the fourth most commonly diagnosed cancer in men and the ninth most common in women.[25] It is the second most commonly diagnosed urologic malignancy, but its incidence is significantly less than prostate cancer (61,240 versus 234,460 cases in 2006).[1,25] Bladder cancer receives far less public notice than prostate or breast cancer, and this trend is reflected in lower research funding. Nevertheless, urologic nurses maintain a keen interest in the prevention, diagnosis, and management of bladder cancer because of its proclivity for local invasion and metastasis, leading to subsequent morbidity and mortality unless successfully treated at an early stage.

Epidemiology

Approximately 69,000 U.S. citizens will be diagnosed with bladder cancer in 2008.[1] The ratio of men to women is approximately 3:1, and whites are more likely to experience bladder cancer than are African Americans or Latinos. Although the overall risk rises with aging,[26] young adults appear to have higher rates of disease progression, possibly indicating that tumors in these persons are more aggressive than bladder malignancies diagnosed in older adults.[27]

Bladder cancers tend to be aggressive, and it is rare to find an undetected malignancy on autopsy.[26] Approximately 13,600 Americans died of bladder cancer in 2006,[1] and multiple studies have shown that the anticipated prognosis for persons with advanced-stage, metastatic tumors is less than 1 year.[28] Whereas white males have the highest overall incidence of bladder cancer, genetic and epidemiologic evidence suggests that African Americans tend to experience more aggressive tumors, resulting in lower

5-year survival rates.[25,26] In addition, both white and African American males have a higher 5-year survival rates than do white or African American females. Epidemiologic studies of Hispanic Americans demonstrate incidence rates similar to those of African Americans, but their 5-year survival rates are higher than those of both African Americans and whites. Fortunately, mortality rates have declined in recent years, but this reduction is limited to men; women continue to have relatively low 5-year survival rates for unknown reasons.

Risk Factors

Cigarette smoking is the most important risk factor for bladder cancer because it increases the risk of developing a tumor twofold to fourfold, is associated with approximately one third of all cases of bladder malignancies, and is a modifiable behavior. The risk is related to both the number of cigarettes smoked per day and the duration of smoking.[25,26] It is diminished when the person stops smoking, but a period of 20 years must pass before the bladder cancer risk falls to that of nonsmokers. Some evidence suggests that cigarette smoking may be a more potent risk in women compared with men, but pooled data from 8316 persons in 14 case control studies demonstrated no clear difference in risk based on gender.[29] Pipe or cigar smoking is associated with a minimal increase in bladder cancer risk. The carcinogen most responsible for this risk is not known; 4-aminobiphenyl is undergoing intense scrutiny because it has been identified in cigarette smoke as well as multiple industrial chemicals associated with bladder cancer.[29,30]

Occupational factors also influence bladder cancer risk.[26,31] Arylamine compounds, used in synthetic dyes, are associated with an increased risk of bladder cancer. Other potential risk factors include biphenyls, naphthylamine, chlorinated hydrocarbons, coal soot, and aldehydes used in mining and the manufacture of rubber and textile products as well as aluminums, paints, and solvents and diesel engines. Prolonged exposure (30 to 50 years) is needed to significantly alter risk, but these factors are estimated to contribute to as many as 20% of bladder cancer cases in the United States.

Consumption of coffee and tea was implicated as a risk factor for bladder cancer in one study,[32] but this statistical relationship disappears when the confounding factor, smoking, is factored into the findings.[33] Self-medication with high doses of phenacetin, which has a similar structure to amine dyes, over a period of at least 5 years, may increase the risk of bladder cancer. However, use of phenacetin has been largely replaced by nonsteroidal antiinflammatory drugs (NSAIDs), which may *reduce* the risk of bladder cancer.[25,26] Consumption of large quantities of artificial sweeteners in animal models has been linked to an increased risk of bladder cancer,[34] but case control epidemiologic studies have failed to demonstrate a clinically relevant risk in humans.[32]

Chronic inflammation associated with long-term indwelling catheterization or schistosomiasis is associated with an increased risk of bladder cancer, but 80% of these tumors are squamous cell carcinomas as compared with the more common transitional cell carcinomas seen in noncatheterized patients.[26] Additional risk factors include cyclophosphamide chemotherapy, pelvic irradiation, and blackfoot disease (a disorder affecting the cardiovascular system and increasing the risk of multiple malignancies that is endemic to southern Taiwan). Renal transplant recipients are at increased risk for bladder cancer, possibly because of the chronic immunosuppression necessary to maintain the transplanted organ.

In 1999 Michaud and coworkers[35] examined the relationship between fluid intake and bladder cancer risk in 47,909 men over a period of 10 years. They found that a higher fluid intake reduced risk in men, possibly by diluting potentially carcinogenic urinary metabolites. Although limited to male participants, this study is particularly interesting to urologic nurses. It provides further evidence to support adequate fluid intake as an important component of bladder health in order to alleviate bothersome lower urinary tract symptoms without increasing the frequency of urinary incontinence (UI) episodes, reduce urinary tract infection (UTI) and constipation risk, and reduce the risk of bladder cancer without adverse side effects. Intake of dietary folate (water-soluble vitamin B), found in many fruits and vegetables, was reported to reduce bladder cancer risk in a relatively small case control study of 451 subjects, but additional research is needed before these results can be confirmed.[36]

Although familial clusters of bladder cancer have been reported,[37] a preponderance of the available evidence fails to implicate a strong genetic component in most bladder cancers.[25,26] In addition to specific substances known to affect cancer risk, regional variations in the incidence have been observed in the United States.[38] This risk is higher in the northeastern United States as compared with the West, and it persists even when known risk factors, such as smoking, or constructional factors, such as race or gender, are controlled.

Etiology and Pathophysiology

The cause of bladder cancer remains unknown.[25,26] Malignant degeneration in the bladder is postulated to arise from a complex (and poorly understood) interaction between host responses to carcinogenic agents, tumor suppression genes, or (in some cases) overexpression of genes that code for growth factors and receptors within the bladder wall. More than one cellular type may undergo neoplastic degeneration in the human bladder. Approximately 90% of all bladder cancers are transitional cell carcinomas, arising from the epithelium of the urothelium and forming a multilayered tumor with characteristic papillary folds. These tumors may coexist with the inflamed, flattened tumors of carcinoma in situ. The second most common form of bladder cancer is the squamous cell carcinoma.[26] Squamous cell tumors account for approximately 3% of all tumors in the United States, as compared with 30% of bladder cancer cases in Africa where schistosomiasis is endemic.[39] Rare types of bladder cancer include adenocarcinomas, which are typically associated with bladder exstrophy or cystitis glandularis.

Stage and Grade. Traditionally, bladder cancer was staged according to the Jewett-Strong-Marshall system, which contained five stages varying from stage 0 (benign papillomas or noninvasive carcinoma in situ) to stage D tumors (highly invasive tumors with metastases)[40] (Figure 8-2). Now the tumor-nodes-metastasis (TNM) grading system is preferred, and all subsequent discussion will use this taxonomy when referring to bladder cancer stage (Table 8-3).

Pathologic grading of bladder cancer continues to evolve. A consensus conference of bladder cancer experts convened by the World Health Organization has recommended several changes in bladder cancer grading that are slowly permeating practice in the early twenty-first century.[41] The conference recommends changing the term *transitional cell cancer of the bladder* to *urothelial cancer*, but this

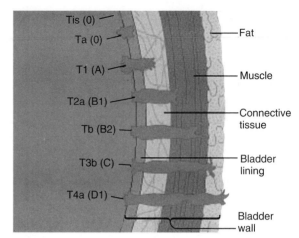

Fig. 8-2 Tumor-nodes-metastasis (TNM) staging system for bladder cancer.

latter term has not yet gained widespread use in the clinical setting or published literature. In contrast to traditional grading and staging systems that relied on depth of tumor invasion to determine progression risk, the conference now recommends classifying these tumors as high grade versus low grade and staging them as noninvasive versus invasive based on grade. Low-grade tumors with orderly cellular arrangements and minimal atypia should now be labeled papillary urothelial neoplasm of low malignant potential (PUNLMP). These tumors, previously labeled as low-grade transitional cell carcinoma, are now recognized as having such a small risk for local invasion or metastasis that they have been redefined as benign. Nevertheless, pathologists and clinicians are advised that recurrent lesions carry approximately a 3% risk of recurring as a high-grade urothelial cancer so that some follow-up is warranted. Similarly, low-grade papillary tumors (TNM stage Ta, grade 1) or tumors with a low pathologic grade should be labeled papillary cancer low grade. They carry a 5% to 10% risk of progression and warrant closer follow-up.

In contrast, papillary cancers with high grade (TNM stage Ta, grade 3) carry a high risk of progression (15% to 40%), and they warrant more aggressive treatment and very close follow-up. Carcinoma in situ (CIS) is classified as high grade, and it carries a 50% or higher risk of progression, indicating the need for aggressive treatment and very close follow-up, even though it presents as a flat malignancy

TABLE 8-3 Staging Systems for Bladder Cancer[25,40]

JEWETT-STRONG-MARSHALL	TNM (PREFERRED)	5-YEAR SURVIVAL
Stage 0: benign papilloma or carcinoma in situ	Ta: benign papilloma Tis: carcinoma in situ	90%
Stage A: tumor invades submucosa but not lamina propria	T1N0M0: N0 indicates absence of metastasis to lymph nodes, and M0 indicates no metastases to adjacent or distant organs	75%
Stage B1: tumor penetrates lamina propria and superficial detrusor muscle	T2N0M0: tumor invades only the inner half of the detrusor muscle	60%
Stage B2: tumor penetrates lamina propria and invades deep into detrusor muscle	T3aN0M0: tumor penetrates into outer half of detrusor muscle	40%
Stage C: tumor invades into fat surrounding bladder (perivesical fat)	T3bN0M0: tumor invades perivesical fat, invasion may be microscopic or form perivesical mass	30%
Stage D1: tumor penetrates bladder wall and invades adjacent organs (urethra, rectum, pelvic bones) or adjacent (pelvic) lymph nodes	T4a: tumor penetrates bladder wall and invades prostate, uterus, or vagina	5%
Stage D2: invasive tumor associated with metastases to distant organs	T4b: tumor penetrates bladder wall and invades pelvic or abdominal wall N1-3: lymph node metastases ranging from spread to single regional node to multiple nodes with enlargement > 5 cm M1: metastasis to organ outside urinary bladder	

TNM, Tumor-nodes-metastasis.

confined to the urothelium. High-grade T1 tumors (grade 3) also carry a high risk of progression (30% to 50%) despite their shallow depth, and they are also managed as a urothelial malignancy with high risk for progression, as are higher-stage tumors that have invaded the muscularis of the bladder wall.

Assessment

A discussion of bladder cancer assessment includes issues related to screening, early detection, and diagnosis and clinical staging procedures. The ongoing assessment that occurs as the patient undergoes treatment for bladder cancer will be discussed later in the chapter.

Clinical Manifestations

Painless hematuria is considered characteristic for bladder cancer. Approximately 85% will experience grossly visible hematuria, and nearly all will have microscopic hematuria.[25,26] It is usually intermittent in nature, and patients should be counseled that cessation of a spontaneous episode of hematuria does not imply resolution of the underlying disorder. In addition, the presence of one or more urine specimens free from blood in a patient with a history of gross, painless hematuria is not sufficient to exclude the possibility of a malignancy of the bladder (or upper urinary tracts). Nevertheless, whereas nearly all patients with bladder cancer experience hematuria, only about 20% of patients with gross hematuria will be diagnosed with bladder cancer. Therefore, although bladder cancer remains a possibility in any patient who presents with gross or microscopic hematuria, the index of suspicion is heavily influenced by the presence or absence of coexisting risk factors. Epidemiologic research demonstrates that relevant risk factors include males over 50 years of age, as well as women or men with a history of smoking, occupational or environmental exposure to carcinogens associated with bladder cancer, or specific risk factors such as pelvic radiotherapy or cyclophosphamide chemotherapy.

Although the hematuria associated with bladder cancer is characteristically painless, it is associated with bothersome (irritative) lower urinary tract symptoms including daytime voiding frequency, urgency, nocturia, and/or urge UI. These symptoms occur in papillary tumors, but they are particularly severe in patients with carcinoma in situ. Other clinical manifestations include flank pain indicating ureteral obstruction, swelling of the lower extremities, or unintentional weight loss. These manifestations are mercifully uncommon and usually indicate extensive local invasion or advanced-stage disease with metastasis.

Screening

Several arguments support the need to screen at-risk patients for bladder cancer. They include the following facts: cells and other debris from malignant tumors are shed into the urine and provide a noninvasive medium for screening, nearly all cases of metastatic bladder cancer begin with a localized tumor, localized disease is associated with a much higher survival rate compared with metastatic disease, and women tend to be diagnosed later than men and at higher stages of the disease and thus have an even greater potential to benefit from early detection than do men. Nevertheless, screening is only useful if it results in decreased mortality and morbidity when compared with those seen in a nonscreened population and when safe and accurate screening techniques are available.

Unfortunately, no widely accepted, accurate screening test is available to screen high-risk populations for bladder cancer.[26,42] Testing for hematuria using urinalysis, although cost-effective and free from adverse effects, is unreliable because of the intermittent nature of bleeding associated with bladder tumors and the myriad of other factors known to produce microscopic hematuria. Urine cytology relies on the histologic analysis of cells shed in the voided urine. Although it is reasonably specific (associated with few false positives), cytology has a low sensitivity (higher proportion of false negatives) and must be combined with cystoscopic examination before potentially lethal bladder malignancies can be diagnosed. Numerous attempts have been made to overcome these shortcomings, including the BTA (bladder tumor antigen) test, NMP22 (nuclear matrix protein) test, and TRAP (telomeric repeat amplification protocol) assay, but none has demonstrated adequate sensitivity or specificity to gain widespread use for screening for invasive bladder cancers in asymptomatic adults.[43-46] However, until one of these techniques demonstrates adequate sensitivity and specificity to replace traditional methods, bladder cancer screening continues to rely on urinalysis to detect hematuria, followed by urine cytology.[47]

Diagnosis

Definitive diagnosis of bladder cancer relies on cystoscopy and biopsy. Cytology is typically obtained from a voided specimen, although a bladder washing may be obtained in special circumstances.[25,26,47] A first morning specimen is avoided because of the risk of cellular degeneration when urine has remained in the bladder for a prolonged period of time during sleep. Cytology is deferred in the patient with a UTI, indwelling catheter, or recent urethral instrumentation and is avoided in patients undergoing intravesical chemotherapy or radiotherapy. Because of the risk of cellular degradation confounding pathologic analysis, the handling of cytology specimens is a particularly important consideration for the urologic nurse. Ideally a fresh specimen is collected in a plastic, lidded container and transported to the laboratory for prompt analysis. Refrigeration is necessary when transporting of the specimen is required, and the pathologist should be notified if a cytomegalovirus infection is present. Urine cytology is most likely to yield positive results when the patient has a higher-grade tumor, but its sensitivity is limited when detecting low-grade malignancies.

A bimanual examination and detailed cystoscopic examination are performed when the urine cytology is positive or when a bladder cancer is strongly suspected based on results of an imaging study or screening cytology.[25,26] The patient is placed in a lithotomy position while under anesthesia, and the clinician palpates the suprapubic area for evidence of a bladder mass. When a mass is present, its size and whether it is adhering to any pelvic structures are assessed. If a bladder tumor is palpable and transurethral resection is undertaken, the bimanual examination is repeated to determine whether a mass persists (indicating possible extravesical invasion). The cystoscopic examination is meticulous and focuses on identifying the number and character of visible tumors and their influence on urinary system function. The bladder mucosa is also inspected for areas of edema or irregularity. Retrograde pyelography (see Chapter 4) may be performed if an imaging study has not been completed to exclude the possibility of tumors affecting the upper urinary tract. Once inspection is complete, tissue is obtained for pathologic analysis by biopsy or during transurethral resection of bladder tumors. Biopsy specimens of any inflamed or irregular areas are also obtained since these are suspicious for carcinoma in situ. In addition to specimens from these areas, the urologist will obtain specimens from each of four routine sites: lateral to each ureteral orifice, the bladder dome, and the trigone. Biopsies of the prostatic urethra and stroma are done in men because as many as 30% with carcinoma in situ will have involvement of one or both of these areas.

Transurethral resection of superficial bladder tumors is completed at the time of cystoscopy, but resection of large or deeply invasive tumors is avoided when radical cystectomy is contemplated. Tumors may be resected, fulgurated, or ablated using a laser when adequate tissue specimens have been obtained for pathologic analysis. Resection or ablation continues until all visible tumors or suspicious areas have been treated. Treatment is typically followed by intravesical chemotherapy or immunotherapy in order to reduce the risk of tumor recurrence, which is approximately 50% when cystoscopy alone is used to treat superficial disease. The urologic nurse uses extraordinary care when retrieving, preserving, and labeling these specimens, since they are critical for accurate diagnosis and subsequent treatment.

Following transurethral resection of bladder tumors, the nurse instructs both the patient and family or partner about potential complications of the procedure. Bleeding is controlled during the procedure using cauterization or laser ablation, but occasionally bleeding worsens after the bladder is emptied at the end of the procedure when the indwelling catheter is left in place. Prolonged bleeding usually leads to clot formation and catheter blockage that must be promptly relieved in order to prevent excessive blood loss and/or bladder rupture. Rarely, the bladder is ruptured during the resection procedure; small ruptures will heal spontaneously with catheter drainage alone, but larger wounds may require surgical repair and prolonged drainage. Reflux or obstruction of a ureteral orifice may occur. Reflux typically resolves spontaneously, but obstruction may require placement of a ureteral stent until edema at the orifice subsides.

The patient's urine is monitored for patency and for signs of excessive bleeding. The patient and care providers are advised that pink-tinged urine is expected, but bright red urine or the passage of larger clots should be promptly reported to the physician. Blockage of the catheter with clots leads to urinary retention, suprapubic pain, and bladder spasms. It requires irrigation of the bladder and catheter under the supervision of a physician. Suprapubic discomfort is expected after tumor resection, but increasing flank pain indicates ureteral obstruction demanding prompt intervention.

Additional tests may be obtained when a patient is undergoing evaluation for bladder cancer. They include intravenous urography to identify upper urinary tract tumors, to assess excretory renal function, and to characterize obstructive uropathy. Abdominal CT or other studies also may be obtained if advanced disease is suspected to identify the location and extent of metastatic tumors.

Treatment

For purposes of treatment, bladder cancer can be divided into lower-stage (superficial) tumors and higher-stage (invasive) malignancies. Superficial disease is typically managed by resection and intravesical chemotherapy, but invasive tumors require more aggressive treatment, often including radical cystectomy.

Treatment of Superficial Tumors. For the patient with superficial (low-stage) bladder cancer, treatment begins at the time of initial diagnosis when visible tumors are resected, fulgurated, or ablated using a laser. This procedure is followed by regular cystoscopic surveillance and intravesical chemotherapy. Cystoscopy is completed every 3 months for the first 2 years after initial treatment. If there is no recurrence, surveillance is reduced to every 6 months for 1 year and annually thereafter. Both the urologist and urologic nurse should emphasize the importance of adherence to surveillance, since recurrence occurs 5 years or later in 20% of patients treated for superficial disease, including many who will have invasive disease at the time of recurrence. Imaging studies also may be undertaken on an annual basis, depending on physician judgment and the grade of the initial tumors.

Intravesical chemotherapy. Intravesical therapy is primarily used to prevent recurrence of superficial disease or progression to a more invasive tumor. In selected cases it is used to treat residual, nonresected bladder cancer or to prevent perioperative tumor implantation. Instillations may be repeated over a period of months to years. Intravesical therapy is often given by the urologic nurse, and knowledge of the administration, actions, and potential side effects of chemotherapy agents is essential to protect both the patient and the nurse. Refer to Clinical Highlights for Expert and Advanced Practice: Intravesical Chemotherapy for Superficial Bladder Cancer for a detailed discussion of intravesical therapy for superficial bladder cancer.

Intravesical immunotherapy. Intravesical chemotherapy with bacille Calmette-Guérin (BCG) has emerged as the gold standard against which all other treatment (e.g., thiotepa) is measured.[48-50] BCG is a live but attenuated tuberculosis vaccine that provokes an immunologic response when instilled into the urinary bladder. Its mechanism of action remains unclear, but it is postulated to activate macrophages, T- and B-lymphocytes, and cytokine production, ultimately resulting in enhanced natural killer cell activity. The optimal dosage remains unclear; it typically varies from 40 to 150 mg, representing an effective dose of 3 $\times$ 10^8 colony-forming units (CFUs) up to 1 $\times$ 10^9 depending on the underlying strain. It is administered weekly over a period of 4 to 6 weeks, and maintenance treatments may be given every 3 months. Special care is used when BCG is constituted to protect both the patient and nurse, and a number of manufacturers of BCG strains have developed special systems to enable rapid and safe reconstitution for administration. The patient is taught to refrain from fluid intake for 4 hours before instillation and to urinate immediately before treatment to minimize dilution with urine. In addition, the urologic nurse avoids using excessive lubricant on the catheter since it can interfere with BCG delivery and efficacy. Following instillation, the patient is asked to retain the solution for 2 hours and urinate in a sitting position to avoid unintentional splashing of solution. The patient is then advised to wash his or her hands and pour 2 cups of household bleach into the toilet and let the solution stand for 2 hours to eradicate any residual mycobacteria. The process is repeated for each micturition occurring during the first 6 hours after treatment. The patient is also advised to cleanse the perineum and genitalia after instillation.

Although BCG remains the most effective of the intravesical agents for the treatment of superficial bladder cancer and carcinoma in situ in particular, it can produce significant toxicity, and careful monitoring of all patients is mandatory. Contraindications to BCG therapy include significant immunosuppression, including human immunodeficiency virus (HIV), transplant patients, or persons undergoing treatment for leukemia or Hodgkin disease. Additional contraindications include pregnant women and patients with active tuberculosis (TB). In addition, UTI should be eradicated before therapy is started to both reduce the risk of systemic infection and maximize the efficacy of the mycobacterium itself.

The most common side effects are bothersome lower urinary symptoms, including daytime voiding frequency, urgency, and dysuria. These can occur in more than 90% of cases[26] and usually peak after the third treatment and do not respond particularly well to antimuscarinic therapy. Urinary analgesics may be prescribed in selected cases, and all patients are taught to consume adequate fluids following treatment and avoid bladder irritants, such as caffeine. Gross hematuria occurs in up to 34% of cases and is usually transient.[51] The patient is advised to inform the urologist if hematuria persists for more than 2 to 3 weeks since this may indicate tumor recurrence.

Common systemic side effects include low-grade fever, joint pain, cough, and malaise. The urologic nurse should advise the patient that these flulike symptoms typically appear after the third instillation and persist for approximately 48 hours. The patient may be advised to take acetaminophen or ibuprofen for mild systemic symptoms. Nevertheless, accidental absorption of BCG occurs in approximately 3% of patients, leading to more significant toxicity.[50] This condition, sometimes called BCG-osis, causes high and persistent fever (101°F [38.3°C] or greater), chills, joint pain, and malaise and may progress to a fatal sepsis unless promptly treated. Because of similarity of symptoms, BCG-osis must be differentiated from UTI related to catheterization. A urine culture is obtained, but empiric antibiotic therapy and triple antitubercular pharmacotherapy (isoniazid, rifampin, and ethambutol) are also begun. Preventive measures include deferral of therapy if urethral bleeding occurs before instillation and avoidance of instillation under any pressure greater than gravity.

Clinical Highlights for Expert and Advanced Practice: Intravesical Chemotherapy for Superficial Bladder Cancer[49,50,125-127]

. . . .

Agent: Triethylenethiophosphoramide (Thiotepa)

Action: Alkylating agent that binds with DNA in cancerous cells and inhibits protein synthesis

Dosage and administration: 30 to 60 mg in a concentration of 1 mg/ml mixed with sterile water or normal saline; weekly doses typically given over a period of 4 to 8 weeks, followed by monthly instillations for up to 1 year

Nursing management: The patient is advised to postpone urination for a period of 1 to 2 hours to allow sufficient time for the drug to interact with tumor cells in the bladder. Because the thiotepa molecule is relatively small, systemic absorption is significant and the risk of myelosuppression is relatively high, with leukopenia occurring in about 10% and thrombocytopenia in 9%. Therefore a complete blood count is obtained before treatment, and alterations in therapy are discussed with the physician if clinically relevant myelosuppression occurs. Myelosuppression may be managed by deferring treatment, altering dosage or frequency of therapy, or switching to another agent. Other systemic effects may include nausea, vomiting, or diarrhea. Bothersome lower urinary tract symptoms, which occur in approximately 25% of patients, rarely respond to antimuscarinic therapy. Instead, the patient is advised to maintain adequate intake of water and to urinate regularly and is reassured that irritative lower urinary tract symptoms are transient. When symptoms are very bothersome, the urologic nurse may discuss dosage reduction or consider switching to another agent. As with all intravesical therapy requiring catheterization, there is a low risk of urinary tract infection, and urinalysis or urine cultures should be completed when an infection is suspected.

Agent: Mitomycin C

Action: Alkylating agent that binds to DNA, inhibits its synthesis, and breaks existing bands, leading to death of rapidly proliferating tumor cells

Dosage and administration: 20 to 60 mg administered as 0.5 to 2 mg/ml of sterile water; given weekly over a course of 6 to 8 weeks, and maintenance doses may be given monthly or every 3 months for up to 1 year following initial treatment

Nursing management: Patients are advised to retain the drug for 1 to 2 hours following instillation. Mitomycin C can cause tissue necrosis, and the patient and nurse must avoid contact with the drug during preparation and administration. Strategies to ensure avoidance of contact include use of gloves when preparing the solution, careful draping of the patient with waterproof materials, tightly pinching the catheter to avoid dribbling the solution on the perineum when removing the catheter, and use of a moisture barrier at the urethral meatus if indicated. A number of strategies have been proposed to enhance drug efficacy; implementation of these strategies is completed in close consultation with the physician. Some have advocated acidification of the urine or instillation of mitomycin in a mildly acidic solution to enhance drug efficacy. Patients may be advised to refrain from consuming fluids for 4 to 6 hours before therapy or to take desmopressin before therapy in order to minimize dilution of mitomycin by means of natriuresis. Although acidification has been shown to enhance absorption in a laboratory setting and fasting or desmopressin to increase the concentration of mitomycin in the bladder, neither result has been linked to clinical effectiveness. Patients are warned of potential side effects, including drug-induced cystitis causing bothersome lower urinary tract symptoms. Symptoms occur in approximately 75% of patients, but fewer than 25% require treatment deferral. Bacterial cystitis may occur requiring antibiotic treatment, and hematuria occurs in approximately 5%. Refer to thiotepa for a description of irritative lower urinary tract symptoms. Allergic reactions occur in fewer than 5% of patients. Patients are advised that mitomycin C may cause a rash, redness, desquamation, or swelling affecting the palms and perineum. The incidence of these reactions is not known; reported occurrences vary from 4% to 12%. Patients are advised to immediately wash their hands and perineum when urinating intravesical chemotherapy solutions and to report rashes or dermatologic reactions before subsequent treatments. Dermatologic symptoms vary from mild to severe, necessitating treatment deferral in as many as one third of patients who experience cutaneous reactions.

Agent: Doxorubicin (Adriamycin) and Epirubicin

Action: Both are anthracyclines that bind with DNA, inhibiting its replication and protein synthesis; epirubicin is a derivative of doxorubicin with a reportedly improved side effect profile

Dosage and administration: Doxorubicin administered in doses of 30 to 100 mg in a concentration of 0.5 to 2 mg/ml mixed with sterile saline; it is instilled every 1 to 3 weeks over a period of 6 to 12 weeks; epirubicin given as 50 to 80 mg in a concentration of 1 to 1.6 mg/ml every 1 to 2 weeks for a period of 8 weeks

Continued

Clinical Highlights for Expert and Advanced Practice: Intravesical Chemotherapy for Superficial Bladder Cancer[49,50,125-127]—cont'd
. . . .

Nursing management: There is a risk of necrosis similar to that associated with mitomycin so care is taken to avoid contact with the skin of the patient or nurse. Both molecules are relatively large so the risk of myelosuppression is low (less than 1%). Nevertheless, the patient is advised that mild and transient systemic reactions may occur that include vomiting, diarrhea, and fever. Allergic reactions occur in less than 1% of cases. Bothersome lower urinary tract symptoms occur in about 20% and are similar to those seen with other chemotherapeutic agents. As with all intravesical therapies, the typically low-grade fever experienced as a drug side effect must be differentiated from a high-grade fever; dysuria occurring 12 to 24 hours after treatment indicates a strong suspicion of urinary tract infection.

Agent: Ethoglucid (Epodyl)
Action: Podophyllin derivative with mechanisms of action similar to the alkylating agents
Dosage and administration: 1 g ethoglucid diluted with 100 ml of sterile water and instilled intravesically; instillations completed weekly over a period of 4 to 12 weeks, and maintenance therapy may be continued up to 1 year
Nursing management: The patient is advised to retain the solution for 1 hour. Because the molecule is relatively large, the risk of systemic toxicity is relatively low. Only a single case of clinically relevant myelosuppression has been reported in the literature, but bothersome lower urinary tract symptoms occur in 3% to 56%. Management of these symptoms includes variability in the frequency of instillations as well as fluid and dietary measures discussed previously.

Although intravesical instillation of BCG does not cause systemic absorption, mycobacteria persist in the bladder wall.[52] This persistence probably accounts for the prolonged efficacy of BCG, but it also may lead to delayed complications, including granulomatous hepatitis, osteomyelitis, arthritis, or endophthalmitis in rare cases.[53-55]

Patients who do not respond to intravesical monotherapy may be managed by dual-agent therapy, often combining BCG with a chemotherapy agent such as epirubicin, or they may be managed by combination immunotherapy combining BCG and interferon alfa-2b (Intron A). Alternatively, radical cystectomy is considered, or radiation therapy may be completed when surgery is not feasible.

Treatment of Invasive Tumors. Radical cystectomy with pelvic lymph node dissection remains the principal treatment option for locally invasive bladder cancers.[26,50] When radical cystectomy is completed in patients with negative nodal involvement the 5- and 10-year recurrence rates are 8% and 14%, respectively, but they are 32% and 34% even when nodal metastases are present. For a detailed discussion of the nursing management of radical cystectomy, refer to Chapter 11. Alternatives to radical cystectomy are aggressive transurethral resection of tumors with intravesical and/or systemic chemotherapy, partial cystectomy, and radiation therapy. Although these treatment options may seem attractive to patients who are frightened by the prospect of bladder removal and urinary diversion, it must be remembered that they are only appropriate for highly selected patients and do not provide outcomes comparable to radical cystectomy.

Neoadjuvant Chemotherapy. Although radical cystectomy provides excellent local control for invasive bladder tumors, approximately 25% of patients will have evidence of nodal metastasis.[49,56] It remains controversial whether neoadjuvant chemotherapy may provide better long-term disease-free survival as compared with surgery alone.[57-59] Traditionally the M-VAC (methotrexate, vinblastine, Adriamycin [doxorubicin], and cisplatin) regimen was preferred, but its utility has since been abandoned because of associated toxicity. Alternatively, a dual- or triple-agent regimen, such as MCV (methotrexate, cisplatin, and vincristine), or regimens employing newer agents such as gemcitabine, carboplatin, paclitaxel, or ifosfamide have been evaluated and are associated with fewer adverse side effects, although no regimen has emerged that is clearly superior to M-VAC.[60]

The nursing management of patients undergoing neoadjuvant chemotherapy for bladder cancer begins with a careful explanation of the goals for therapy and common side effects. These effects may be severe (particularly if the M-VAC regimen is used) and usually include leukopenia, increased susceptibility to infection, nausea, vomiting, and fatigue. Patients are advised to minimize exposure to infections by avoiding crowds and prolonged contact with adults or children with a febrile or communicable illness, such as an upper respiratory infection or the flu. Because of the risk for gastrointestinal bleeding, the patient is also advised to promptly report black, tarry stools and to avoid aspirin or aspirin-containing products while undergoing treatments. The patient's nutritional intake is monitored and assisted to obtain up to six small meals daily, consisting of primarily bland foods palatable to that person. The urologic nurse typically administers chemotherapy in the evening to minimize the negative impact of nausea and vomiting. In addition, the patient is informed of the potential for hair loss and counseled about the potential for regrowth once therapy is completed.

Metastatic Bladder Cancer

Whereas surgery is the mainstay for muscle-invasive, localized bladder cancer, systemic chemotherapy is first-line therapy for metastatic tumors. Cisplatin-based regimens, usually M-VAC or MCV, have been the most commonly used, but they are associated with significant adverse side effects, including myelosuppression, nephrotoxicity, and severe nausea and vomiting.[61] In order to reduce toxicities, carboplatin-based regimens (carboplatin/gemcitabine/paclitaxel or carboplatin/gemcitabine) are being tested in clinical trials, and biologic agents such as trastuzumab (directed against *HER2/neu*) and gefitinib are in earlier stages of investigation. The nursing management of patients undergoing systemic chemotherapy is similar to that described for neoadjuvant treatments. However, while newer agents and novel regimens offer hope, it should be remembered that the 5-year survival rate for patients with metastatic bladder cancer remains low at approximately 5%.[56] Therefore nursing management of these patients incorporates fostering communication among the patient, significant others, and physician based on the realization that goals of management may shift from curative to palliative when aggressive treatments prove ineffective, particularly when they are associated with significant toxicity.

PROSTATE CANCER

Epidemiology

In 2008, more than 200,000 men in the United States will be diagnosed with prostate cancer (Figure 8-3).[1]

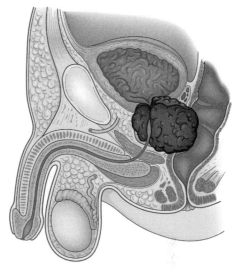

Fig. 8-3 Carcinoma of the prostate.

It has risen to the most commonly diagnosed malignancy in men and is a leading cause of cancer deaths in American males, accounting for an estimated 28,660 deaths in 2008.

Risk Factors

Multiple factors have been associated with prostate cancer risk.[62] Modifiable factors include dietary intake, although genetic predisposition, age, race, and ethnicity also influence overall risk and the likelihood that a malignancy is biologically aggressive (Table 8-4).

Prevention

Counseling men about prevention is an ideal role for the urologic nurse. Primary prevention focuses on reducing modifiable risk factors associated with prostate cancer while promoting protective factors. This includes identifying dietary and lifestyle factors.[63] Specifically, men may be counseled to reduce dietary intake of animal fats and cholesterol-rich foods. In contrast, they should be encouraged to increase intake of lycopenes, phytoestrogen, and catechin.[64] Foods rich in lycopenes include cooked and fresh tomatoes, apricots, grapefruits, and olive oil. Catechin is found in green tea, and foods rich in phytoestrogen include fishes rich in omega-3 fatty acids, leafy green vegetables, soy beans, and extra virgin olive oil. Exercising three times weekly can improve lipid and cholesterol profiles, and men who are not in a stable, monogamous relationship may be counseled about safer sex practices since sexually transmitted

TABLE 8-4 Risk Factors for Prostate Cancer[62]

Age	Under age 40 yr, risk 1:10,000
	Over age 60 yr, risk 1:7
Race/ethnicity	Highest in African American men; lowest in Asian men living in Asia
Family history	Doubled risk with one first-degree relative and quadrupled risk if two or more first-degree relatives
Hormones	Testosterone; early-onset male pattern baldness (associated with high levels of testosterone)
	Insulin-like growth factor I (possible link)
Diet	High fat, low fiber
Vasectomy	Implicated in one study; subsequent studies refute its role as risk factor

diseases also raise the risk for prostate cancer. Although the evidence base supporting the magnitude of effect associated with some protective factors is sparse, adaptation of these dietary and lifestyle recommendations is not associated with harmful side effects and they are generally thought to benefit overall health.

Ongoing research is examining the effect of selenium and vitamin E on prostate cancer prevention.[65] This multisite study began enrolling subjects in July 2001, and more than 32,000 men living in the United States and Canada are expected to participate. The results of this well-designed study are expected to lead to significant insights into our understanding of prostate cancer prevention strategies.

A growing body of research has examined whether long-term administration of a 5α-inhibitor will reduce prostate cancer risk.[66-69] Although Thompson's group[66] reported a 25% risk reduction after 7 years of administration of finasteride, they also noted that men taking the drug who did develop prostate cancer tended to experience higher-grade tumors and metastases more often than those in the control group. Other researchers[70] have concluded that long-term administration of a 5α-reductase inhibitor should not be advocated. Their arguments are primarily based on population-based analysis of risk versus benefit, long-term survival modeling, and cost. Based on research to date, it is not possible to counsel patients whether routine long-term administration of 5α-reductase inhibitors provides a significant reduction in prostate cancer risk.[71]

Etiology and Pathophysiology

The cause of prostate cancer is unknown.[72] It is unique from other urologic cancers, such as bladder or renal, because it occurs in two forms. A clinically latent or slow-growing form affects about 30% of men over 50 years of age and 60% to 70% of men over 80 years of age. The clinically aggressive form or evident form of prostate cancer is characterized by the potential for local invasion and metastases seen with other solid tumors.

About 9% of prostate cancers are inherited.[73] Genetic studies of men with hereditary prostate cancer have identified mutations on the long arm of chromosome 1 (1q24-25) as the probable location for this greatly increased susceptibility for prostatic malignancies.[72] Genetic factors affecting chromosome 8p may affect sporadic prostate cancers, but this observation must be considered in the context of the strong evidence that prostate cancer is significantly influenced by environmental factors, including diet. Since prostate cancer occurs in latent (slow-growing) and evident (aggressive) forms, considerable research has focused on factors leading to tumor growth and metastasis. Genetic alterations in chromosome 8q 10Q are often found in advanced-stage, aggressive tumors. These alterations may inhibit the effect of a suppressor gene (*PTEN/MNAC* or *MYC*) found on these chromosomes. Alteration in the expression of suppressor gene *p27*, located on chromosome 12, has also been associated with aggressive tumor behaviors. Additional factors undergoing intensive scrutiny for their potential roles in prostate cancer progression include the X chromosome, androgen-dependent factors regulating apoptosis (programmed cellular death) in the prostate, and vascular endothelial growth factor, thought to be involved in regulation of critical blood supply to the growing tumor.

Although the remaining 91% of prostate cancers are sporadic, genetic factors also play a role in these men. Several studies associate the elevated prostate cancer prevalence and death rates among African

TABLE 8-5 TNM Staging System for Prostate Cancer

Primary Tumor	
Tx	Primary tumor not assessed
T0	No evidence of primary tumor
T1	Not palpable or evident by imaging study alone
T1a	Incidental finding during TURP, malignant cells detected in < 5% of resected tissue
T1b	Incidental finding during TURP, malignant cells detected in > 5% of resected tissue
T1c	Nonpalpable tumor associated with elevated PSA; diagnosis based on results of needle biopsy
T2	Tumor confined within prostate
T2a	One lobe of prostate involved
T2b	Both lobes of prostate involved
T3	Tumor extends beyond prostatic capsule and into the seminal vesicles
T4	Tumor fixed or invades adjacent structures other than seminal vesicles, such as the bladder neck, external urethral sphincter, rectum, pelvic floor muscles, or pelvic wall
Regional Lymph Nodes	
Nx	Regional lymph nodes cannot be assessed
N0	No regional lymph nodes involved
N1	Metastasis to one or more regional lymph nodes
Distant Metastases	
M0	Presence of distant metastases cannot be assessed
Mx	No evidence of distant metastases
M1	Distant metastases involving nonregional lymph nodes (M1a), bones (M1b), or distant organs (M1c)

PSA, Prostate-specific antigen; *TNM*, tumor-nodes-metastasis; *TURP*, transurethral resection of the prostate.

American men with genetic factors,[74,75] and some data exist that the age of onset of prostatic cancer may be influenced by defects in two or three genetic loci yet to be identified.[76]

Staging and Grading. As with all cancers, pathologic staging and grading are clinically relevant because these factors determine the biologic aggressiveness of a particular tumor, the extent of local invasion or distant metastases, and treatment options.

Pathologic grade predicts the biologic aggressiveness of a tumor. For prostate cancer the Gleason system is used most commonly because of its high correlation with the pathologic extent of the disease.[73,77] Gleason grade X indicates a tumor that cannot yet be graded. Low Gleason grades (i.e., 1 to 4) indicate well-differentiated tumors with little potential for metastases (20%); moderately differentiated tumors (i.e., Gleason grades 5 to 7) have a higher risk for metastases (40%). In contrast, tumors with marked anaplasia (i.e., poor cellular differentiation, Gleason grades 8 to 10) carry a high risk for metastases of approximately 75%. A Gleason score is determined by adding the most common tumor

grade in a single specimen to the second most common grade contained in that specimen.

As with other urologic cancers, the TNM staging system is recommended; Table 8-5 summarizes the TNM staging system as applied to prostate cancers. From a clinical perspective, prostate cancer stage can be roughly divided into localized tumors that are contained within the prostatic capsule and advanced-stage tumors that have invaded adjacent structures or progressed to nodal or solid organ metastasis.

Clinical Manifestations

Localized prostate cancer is rarely associated with symptoms. It may be detected by digital rectal examination (DRE) but most frequently by measurement of the prostate-specific antigen (PSA) blood test. Occasionally, a localized tumor may produce bothersome lower urinary tract symptoms, such as an increase in episodes of nocturia, daytime voiding frequency, or a diminished force of the urinary stream. Advanced-stage prostate cancer is more likely to produce bothersome lower urinary tract symptoms and is often associated with bone pain affecting the pelvis or lower back, spontaneous (pathologic) fracture, or constitutional symptoms such as fatigue, nausea, vomiting, and weight loss.

Early Detection of Prostate Cancer

Although the American Cancer Society (ACS) and American Urological Association recommend routine prostate cancer screening, evidence to support the practice is limited.[78] An effective strategy program should not only detect disease, but also substantially reduce the mortality rate from that disease. Long-term data are not yet available on the mortality rate since the adoption of PSA and DRE screening. In the meantime, men over 50 years or men in high-risk groups at age 40 years may be advised to follow a healthy lifestyle and have annual prostate assessment.

The annual checkup always includes a DRE and usually a serum PSA. An abnormal DRE has a positive predictive value of 72% for the diagnosis of prostate cancer, but a negative DRE results in a positive predictive value of only 37%.[79] As a result, prostate cancer is suspected when the DRE reveals one or more discrete nodules, asymmetry between the size of the palpable lobes, induration, or a stony gland that is fixed to the rectal wall. Nevertheless, the absence of an abnormal finding does not necessarily exclude the presence of prostate cancer, especially when the serum PSA is elevated.

The serum PSA is influenced by age and prostate size (Table 8-6). Serum PSA levels typically vary from 2.05 to 2.66 ng/ml in adult men.[80] However, as the prostate grows because of benign prostatic hyperplasia (BPH), it may rise to a range of 2.56 to 3.9 ng/ml. A serum PSA level that is above 10 ng/ml indicates a high level of suspicion for prostate cancer unless there is evidence of acute prostatic inflammation. Values between 4 and 10 ng/ml indicate a moderate risk of prostate cancer, and three advanced techniques of PSA analysis are used to more accurately identify prostate cancer in these cases.[81] The percent of free PSA measures the percentage of free PSA versus the proportion bound to two proteins: α_1-antichymotrypsin and α_2-macroglobulin. The PSA velocity uses repeated measurements to determine patterns over time; a rapid rise increases the risk for prostate cancer whereas a more gradual rise is more likely to indicate benign hyperplasia. The PSA density is calculated by dividing the PSA value by the prostatic volume, obtained during transrectal ultrasound (TRUS) with biopsy.

Diagnosis

Although an elevated serum PSA or abnormal DRE creates suspicion of prostate cancer, definitive diagnosis relies on TRUS-guided biopsy. TRUS requires inserting a probe into the rectum in order to image the prostate gland. Tissue samples are obtained by a specialized biopsy needle delivery system incorporated into the TRUS equipment. Preparation for TRUS and needle biopsy includes careful explanation of the procedure to the patient, including the necessity of introduction of a transrectal probe. The probe and biopsy will produce mild to moderate discomfort and pressure in the rectal area that is relieved as soon as the probe is removed at the completion of imaging and biopsy. The patient is warned that obtaining a biopsy specimen produces a sudden noise (sometimes perceived as a bang or pop) as the specimen is obtained. All anticoagulant medications, including prescribed agents such as warfarin, over-the-counter drugs such as aspirin, or dietary supplements such as vitamin E taken in doses of 400 to 800 units should be discontinued 7 days before and 1 day following TRUS with biopsy. Bowel cleansing using an enema or stimulant is recommended in selected patients, and antimicrobial therapy with a fluoroquinolone is typically administered on the day of and for several days following the procedure, depending on physician judgment. Rare complications are septicemia or rectal bleeding. After the biopsy, patients should be advised to contact their urologist if they see fresh blood in their stool, have a raised temperature, or experience feelings of malaise.

TABLE 8-6 PSA Levels*

PSA	SUSPICION
<4 ng/ml	Normal (low suspicion)
4-10 ng/ml	Moderate suspicion
>10 ng/ml	High level of suspicion

PSA, Prostate-specific antigen.
*Consult facility laboratory for normal finding.
False-positive results: ejaculation 24-48 hr before test, prostatitis; recent catheterization; cystoscopy; or prostate biopsy.

Additional Evaluation

If the patient is asymptomatic with a life expectancy of less than 10 years, further staging workup may not be indicated. In contrast, patients who have a life expectancy of 10 years or longer and those who are symptomatic routinely undergo additional evaluation including a CBC, serum creatinine, and possibly alkaline phosphatase.[82,83] Bone scan is recommended for men who have a stage T1 to T4 tumor and who have a PSA less than 10 ng/ml or a Gleason score less than or equal to 8. Those with bulky tumors should undergo CT or MRI of the abdomen and pelvis to evaluate the extent of local tumor invasion or pelvic lymph node or abdominal metastases. Fine-needle aspiration is occasionally performed on suspicious-appearing lymph nodes.

Treatment

The optimal treatment plan for each man affected by prostate cancer is based on multiple considerations, including the tumor stage and grade, the patient's chronologic and physiologic age, and the preferences of the man and his partner, spouse, or family. For the purposes of this discussion, treatment options will be divided into two clinical categories: localized and advanced-stage tumors.

Localized Prostate Cancer. Treatment options for localized prostate cancer are watchful waiting, cryotherapy, radical prostatectomy, external beam radiotherapy, and interstitial radiotherapy (brachytherapy). Watchful waiting, also referred to as active surveillance, is based on growing recognition that latent (slow-growing) tumors may not require treatment, especially if a patient's life expectancy is less than 10 years.[84,85] Ongoing observation includes a DRE and serum PSA every 6 to 12 months and careful monitoring for the onset of bothersome lower urinary tract symptoms, acute urinary retention, or systemic signs or symptoms indicating potential metastases. Lower urinary tract symptoms may be monitored by regular administration of the International Prostate Symptom Score (IPSS); clinically relevant systemic signs and symptoms include unintended weight loss, hematuria, bone pain, or pathologic fracture.

Cryotherapy destroys prostate cancer cells through exposure to freezing temperatures that ultimately disrupt the cell membrane.[86] Although cryotherapy avoids the need for an incision, it is associated with a significant risk of urinary incontinence and erectile dysfunction (ED) and is not a widely used option for the management of localized prostate cancer.

Radical retropubic or perineal prostatectomy involves removal of the prostate, seminal vesicles, and adjacent tissues including overlying fat and pelvic sidewall and is described in detail in Chapter 11. Nerve-sparing radical retropubic prostatectomy reduces the risk of postoperative ED and may diminish the risk of postprostatectomy urinary incontinence. Contraindications to the nerve-sparing procedure include locally invasive disease (stage T3c tumors), palpable disease at the apex of the prostate, a Gleason score above 5, a serum PSA above 20 ng/ml, and pre-existing ED.[87] Long-term complications associated with radical prostatectomy are urinary incontinence and ED.

Prostate cancer may be treated by external beam radiation therapy (EBRT). The total dose delivered to the pelvic region is about 70 gray (Gy), administered over a period of 6 weeks.[88] Before starting EBRT, the patient will have the relevant structures marked by the radiation oncologist using indelible ink, typically in the shape of a box or rectangle so that the beam can be delivered exactly to the same location at each treatment. Alternatively, three-dimensional CT imaging with computer reconstruction (conformal radiation therapy) may be administered because it limits exposure of the pelvic organs[89] and allows higher overall doses of radiation. Conformal proton beam radiotherapy employs a technique similar to that of traditional conformal therapy, but it uses charged protons that are capable of traveling through superficial tissues, delivering only a relatively small dose of radiation at the termination of the particle's path. When combined with three-dimensional imaging, it is possible to treat the patient in a manner that the main energy delivered by the charged protons is delivered to the prostate while avoiding adjacent structures including the bladder and rectum.[90] Table 8-7 reviews potential complications associated with radiation therapy for prostate cancer and their management.

Radioactive seeds of palladium-103 and iodine-125 may be placed directly into the prostate gland under ultrasonic or CT guidance (Figure 8-4). These seeds emit relatively low levels of highly localized radiation energy intended to destroy malignant cells while producing no or minimal damage to adjacent tissues.

TABLE 8-7 Managing Complications Associated with External Beam Radiation Therapy for Prostate Cancer

COMPLICATION	NURSING MANAGEMENT
Acute Radiation Cystitis *Definition*: inflammation of bladder wall and urothelial lining *Symptoms*: daytime voiding frequency, urgency, suprapubic or lower back pain with bladder filling, dysuria, feelings of incomplete bladder emptying, hematuria	Reassure the patient that symptoms typically subside within 4-6 wk after treatment is completed. Advise the patient to consume an adequate volume of water on a daily basis while avoiding potential bladder irritants, such as caffeine. An antimuscarinic agent or urinary analgesic may be administered to reduce pain. Teach the patient to routinely monitor the urine for hematuria and to contact a healthcare provider if gross hematuria occurs, particularly when associated with passage of blood clots or inability to urinate. Hyperbaric oxygen therapy treatments may be administered for severe, persistent symptoms.
Proctitis *Definition*: inflammation of rectal mucosa *Symptoms*: frequent defecation, rectal urgency, cramping and passage of mucus or blood with stools	Encourage the patient to regularly defecate and avoid bowel irritants including caffeine and fatty or highly spiced foods. An antimuscarinic medication may be prescribed to relieve excessive rectal urgency and cramping. Teach the patient to routinely monitor stools for excessive bleeding or passage of clots. Counsel the patient to avoid rectal biopsy because of risk of bleeding or fistula formation. Advise the patient to consult a gastroenterologist if proctitis symptoms persist for more than 4-6 wk following treatment or if excessive rectal bleeding occurs.
Perineal Skin Irritation	Wash perineal skin with mild cleanser and lukewarm water (ensuring radiation markings are not removed during active therapy). Dust small amounts of talcum-based powder or cornstarch over affected area; wear loose-fitting, cotton clothing.
Fatigue, Loss of Appetite	Counsel the patient to eat six small meals daily, consuming foods high in protein and carbohydrates; avoid spicy, fatty foods; and take a daily multivitamin.

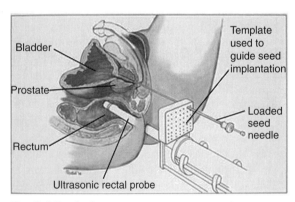

Fig. 8-4 Brachytherapy. (From Lewis SM, Heitkemper MM, Heitkemper M, Dirkson S: Medical-Surgical Nursing, 6th edition. St Louis: Mosby, 2004; p 1447.)

Preparation for brachytherapy begins with an imaging study to map the anatomy of the prostate, typically using TRUS. Bowel cleansing is not usually required for the preprocedural marking but will be necessary when the seeds are implanted. Preparation usually includes an oral bowel stimulant such as magnesium citrate, consumption of a clear liquid diet the day before the procedure, and a cleansing enema the morning of the procedure. A 7- to 10-day course of antibiotic prophylaxis with a fluoroquinolone is generally recommended.

Urinary retention may occur after brachytherapy. The catheter is removed within hours of the procedure, but an indwelling catheter may remain in place for up to 1 to 2 weeks until prostate congestion subsides in selected patients. Prostate congestion will also produce a change in lower urinary tract symptoms, typically including increases in voiding frequency, urgency, and difficulty initiating a urinary stream. Rectal bleeding is rare following prostatic brachytherapy, but patients should be advised to monitor their stool for passage of large volumes of bright red blood. Acute radiation proctitis may occur, and its management is outlined in Table 8-7. Because seeds are implanted during brachytherapy, patients and families are counseled about radiation safety. Men undergoing brachytherapy are taught that their semen will have a brownish discoloration that will persist for several months following seed implantation. Intercourse with the goal of bearing children is contraindicated unless cleared by the urologist or radiation oncologist, and patients should refrain from having children (or adults) sit in the lap for about 2 months following treatment.

Psychosocial implications. The urologic nursing care of men and their families with localized prostate cancer begins immediately following diagnosis. The diagnosis of cancer strikes fear and dread in most people, and typical emotions are anxiety in both the patient and his partner. The level of anxiety impedes the ability to retain information about treatment options or prognosis, and several supportive clinic visits or telephone calls may be required. Factual verbal, written, and video information should be provided to the patient along with credible website addresses so that the patient and partner can make an informed, considered decision before pursuing a given treatment option. Counseling by the urology nurse includes the importance of routine monitoring and symptoms of disease progression. In consultation with the urologist or medical oncologist, patients may wish to try alternative therapies such as dietary supplements.[91,92] Although unproven, these strategies may provide an important psychologic benefit and the nurse must balance objective information with ongoing support as the patient seeks to survive and thrive despite a diagnosis of prostate cancer.

Advanced-Stage Prostate Cancer. Management of advanced prostate cancers is either aggressive or palliative. Aggressive treatments are designed to eradicate cancer cells, prevent local invasion, and alleviate or prevent metastasis.[93,94] Palliative care is designed to alleviate pain or other bothersome symptoms associated with advanced-stage prostate cancer while assisting the patient and family to prepare for end of life rather than attempting to create a cure.

Aggressive treatment. Hormone deprivation is first-line treatment for advanced-stage prostate tumors.[62] Androgen (testosterone) deprivation destroys or arrests the growth of androgen-dependent and androgen-sensitive cells, but it has no effect on androgen-independent cells. As a result, a hormone-resistant tumor may emerge after initial treatment with androgen deprivation, often within 2 years of hormone therapy.[93,94] Androgen deprivation can be

achieved by a number of techniques. Orchiectomy removes the main site of testosterone production. Although the procedure is clearly effective, it carries a profoundly negative psychologic impact for most men. Alternatively, drugs can be administered to create a chemical castration without the need for a surgical orchiectomy (Table 8-8).

Side effects associated with androgen deprivation therapies may be significant. Adverse effects include loss of libido, nausea, vomiting, fatigue, mood changes, hot flushes, diarrhea, or gynecomastia. A hormone flare occurs with initial treatment that persists for 2 to 3 weeks. It may increase bone pain or provoke urinary retention if prostate cancer is widespread, but these initial symptoms tend to subside after 3 to 4 weeks and do not recur. Men with advanced local invasion or extensive bony metastases may require a steroidal antiandrogenic blocking agent to prevent complications of the initial androgenic flare. Reduced libido is an expected side effect of androgen deprivation therapy, and ED is very common.

Hot flushes occur in up to 68% of men managed by androgen deprivation therapy.[95] They are characterized by a sudden sensation of heat affecting the upper body and face, often associated with redness of the skin and sweating. Vitamin E (800 units/day) or soy powder (taken as 60 mg daily) provides relief in some men. The urologist or nurse practitioner may prescribe megestrol acetate (Megace), which reduces hot flushes by as much as 50%. Alternative drugs include venlafaxine (Effexor) or clonidine (Catapres), although these agents have not proved particularly effective in controlled studies.

Other adverse effects associated with hormone deprivation therapy include fatigue, mood swings, gynecomastia, and osteoporosis. Men with gynecomastia may be advised to wear loose shirts and avoid pressure against the breasts, particularly that associated with wearing overalls or suspenders. Tamoxifen or a short course of radiation therapy to the breasts is recommended when conservative measures do not provide adequate relief from breast tenderness. The risk of osteoporosis can be alleviated by regular exercise and daily calcium and vitamin D supplementation. Alendronate (Fosamax) combined with high-dose vitamin D (2000 units/day) is administered when osteoporosis is more advanced.

Estrogenic agents, including diethylstilbestrol, high-dose megestrol acetate, chlorotrianisene (TACE), or estramustine phosphate (EMP), are given in selected cases. These drugs suppress luteinizing hormone (LH) secretion from the pituitary, block androgen receptor activity, and inhibit androgen synthesis in the testes. However, estrogenic drugs are associated with significant adverse effects, including cardiovascular events and gynecomastia. PC-SPES is an herbal compound with eight principal ingredients: chrysanthemum, isatis, licorice, *Ganoderma lucidum, Panax pseudoginseng, Rabdosia rubescens*, saw palmetto, and skullcap.[96] It has estrogenic compounds distinct from

diethylstilbestrol (DES), estrone, and estradiol and may benefit some patients with advanced-stage tumors.[97]

Chemotherapy is given to highly selected men with advanced-stage hormone-independent prostate cancer.[98] Chemotherapy regimens vary; two- to three-drug protocols using estramustine with vinblastine, paclitaxel, docetaxel, etoposide, or vinorelbine have shown limited efficacy. Alternatively an anthracycline antibiotic such as doxorubicin may be combined with 5-fluorouracil and/or mitomycin C, or

TABLE 8-8 Androgen Deprivation Therapy for Advanced-Stage Prostate Cancer[62]

DRUG	PHARMACOLOGIC ACTION	NURSING CONSIDERATIONS
LH-RH Agonists Leuprolide (Lupron) Goserelin (Zoladex) Extended-release leuprolide implant (Viadur)	Act at hypothalamus to produce initial surge and then rapid decline in LH, FSH, and testosterone Implanted device uses osmotic releasing system to deliver low dose of leuprolide; actions similar to depot LHRH antagonist	Leuprolide is given as a deep intramuscular injection every 1-4 mo. Goserelin is administered as a subcutaneous injection every 1-3 mo. The Viadur implant is implanted in the upper arm every 12 mo. Adherence to therapy is critical to maintaining androgen levels at low (castrate) levels.
Nonsteroidal Antiandrogens Flutamide (Eulexin) Bicalutamide (Casodex) Nilutamide (Nilandron)	Block androgen receptors in the cancer cells to prevent testosterone and dihydrotestosterone from stimulating further tumor growth	Antiandrogenic drugs are administered orally once daily to three times daily. Monotherapy with these agents may avoid some of the long-term adverse events associated with LHRH agonists, but the long-term efficacy of this approach is not yet established.
Estrogens DES Conjugated estrogens (Premarin or ethinyl estradiol) Estrogens contained in PC-SPES (herbal agents with multiple active ingredients including estrogenic substances)	Precise mechanisms of actions in men with hormone-resistant prostate cancer remain unclear, known to directly kill certain cancer cells and to lower serum FSH, LH, and testosterone	These agents are administered orally, usually once daily. Serious side effects may occur with administration of estrogenic hormones.
Steroids Prednisone	Suppresses corticotropin-releasing hormone and ACTH, resulting in suppression of androgen production by adrenals	Prednisone is administered orally; dosages must be carefully titrated, and adverse effects may occur if therapy is abruptly discontinued.

ACTH, Adrenocorticotropic hormone; *DES,* diethylstilbestrol; *FSH,* follicle-stimulating hormone; *LH,* luteinizing hormone; *LH-RH,* luteinizing hormone–releasing hormone.

cyclophosphamide may be given with oral etoposide. The patient undergoing chemotherapy is at risk for bone marrow suppression, nausea, vomiting, hair loss, unintended weight loss, and complications associated with nutritional deficits.

Palliative care. When curative treatments are no longer effective, the goal of medical and nursing management switches from aggressive treatment to palliative care. At this point, the goals of care switch from tumor control to alleviation of pain, bothersome lower urinary tract symptoms, and systemic sequelae of the disease.[93,99]

Moderate to severe pain often occurs in late-stage prostate cancer, partly because of metastases to the bones and cytokines or prostaglandin release as the tumor grows and metastasizes.[100] Opioid analgesics, nonsteroidal antiinflammatory antidepressants, and anticonvulsants, such as gabapentin, are effective. Severe pain may be managed by steroids or opioid analgesics delivered by a continuous/on-demand intrathecal infusion system. EBRT or wide-field treatments relieve pain in up to 80% of patients, and as many as 30% may be rendered pain free at the termination of treatment. Strontium-89 chloride (Metastron) is a radioactive isotope that is preferentially absorbed by areas of bone with high mineral metabolism caused by the growth and spread of metastatic prostate cancer. It is subsequently washed out of healthy bone but retained in metastatic deposits for a prolonged period of time.

Palliative nursing also involves issues related to death and dying. It is important that the urologic nurse provide opportunities for the patient, his partner, and family members to speak about feelings of death and dying in a caring and supportive environment. The nurse also may be asked to assist with advanced directives, disposition of the patient's wishes following death, or arrangements for care during the terminal stages of prostate cancer. Providing opportunities to discuss these topics allows the patient and family time to make difficult and anxiety-provoking decisions. This is vital before events transpire in which decisions must be made on the family's best guess concerning the desires of the patient.

TESTICULAR TUMORS

Epidemiology

The incidence of testicular cancer is highest at three points in a man's life: during infancy, between ages 15 and 35 years, and late adulthood (age 60 years and older).[101,102] By far the highest risk period is in early adulthood, making testicular cancer the most common solid tumor of American men ages 20 to 34 years and second most common in ages 35 to 40 years. Approximately 8250 cases of testicular cancer were diagnosed in the United States in 2006.[1] The incidence is higher in white American males compared with African Americans.[101] Testicular cancer is highly curable if diagnosed at an early stage (Figure 8-5).

Classification

Between 90% and 95% of all primary testicular cancers arise from the germ cells (those directly responsible for spermatogenesis).[102] Their incidence has doubled in the past 40 years, and they continue to increase at a rate of 3% to 6%, presumably because of environmental factors.[103] Germ cell tumors are broadly classified into two subgroups: seminomas and nonseminomas. About 50% of testicular malignancies are pure seminomas and typically detected at a fairly early stage of development. They respond well to treatment when diagnosed early. Nonseminomas tend to be more aggressive tumors compared with seminomas; the remaining 5% of testicular cancers are nongerminal neoplasms from Leydig cells, Sertoli cells, or gonadoblastoma (Box 8-2).

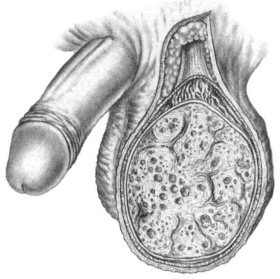

Fig. 8-5 Testicular cancer.

Etiology

The etiology of testicular cancer is unknown, but two risk factors have been repeatedly identified: atrophic or cryptorchid testes. Since cryptorchidism is slightly more common on the right, it has been posed as an explanation for the higher incidence of cancer involving the right testicle. The risk of developing testicular cancer is very high for boys with at least one intraabdominal testis (1:20) and slightly less elevated for boys with an inguinal testis (1:80).[104] Other factors sometimes associated with testicular cancer, including scrotal trauma and infection-induced atrophy (e.g., mumps orchitis), have not been directly linked with testicular cancer. Racial differences in testicular cancer risk have been noted. For example, the incidence of testicular cancer in African Americans is about 33% less than that seen in white, but nearly tenfold higher than in blacks living in Africa. Israeli Jews have an eightfold increase over non-Jewish Israelis. In Hawaii, Chinese, white, or native men are 10 times more likely to develop testicular cancer than Filipino or Japanese men.[102]

Little is known about the role that genetic factors play in the development of testicular cancer, although familial cases have been documented.[105] Specifically, 1% to 3% of patients with a germ cell tumor will have a first-degree relative with testicular cancer, and monozygotic twins have a higher risk than do dizygotic twins.[103] In addition, various syndromes associated with abnormal testicular embryogenesis and cryptorchidism are associated with an increased risk for testicular tumors, such as Down syndrome.

BOX 8-2 Types of Testicular Tumors[102]

Germ Cell Tumors (95%)
Seminomatous Tumors (40%)
Classic
Anaplastic
Spermatocytic (5%)

Nonseminomatous Germ Cell Tumors (NSGCTs)
Embryonal cell (60%)
Yolk sac
Teratocarcinoma
Teratoma
Choriocarcinoma

Non–Germ Cell Tumors (4% to 5%)
Leydig cell
Sertoli cell

Testicular Self-Examination

A testicular self-examination is an effective tool to ensure that testicular cancer can be diagnosed at an early stage.[106] A man should perform testicular self-examination once each month, following a warm bath or shower because the scrotum is soft and the testicles hang down and away from the body (Figure 8-6). While standing, each testicle should be rolled between the thumbs and fingers of both hands. A normal testicle should feel smooth and be egg shaped and about 1 to 1.5 inches long. One testicle may feel larger than the other, which is completely normal. It is important that the epididymis is also examined; it should feel rope-like, soft, and tender. Any abnormal findings, such as a lump or hard area in the testicle, or a scrotum that is swollen on one side, should be reported immediately to a clinician.

Clinical Manifestations

Several symptoms are associated with testicular cancer. The most common is a painless lump about the size of a pea found on the front or the side of the testicle. Additional symptoms include enlargement, change in consistency, and a sudden accumulation of blood or fluid in the scrotum. An individual with testicular cancer may present with a dull ache in the groin or perhaps swelling and tenderness in other parts of the body, such as the breast or neck.[15]

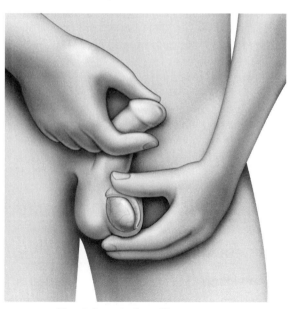

Fig. 8-6 Testicular self-examination.

Diagnosis

Not all testicular masses are cancerous, and the possibility of spermatic cord torsion, epididymitis, orchitis, hydrocele, hernia, hematoma, or spermatocele must be considered when evaluating a testicular mass. However, until proven otherwise, a firm, solid mass in the testicle is considered highly suspicious for a malignancy. In addition to a careful scrotal examination, ultrasonography provides a rapid and reliable method to exclude these causes of a testicular mass or enlargement. When a malignancy is detected, an abdominal CT scan is obtained to identify retroperitoneal lymph node involvement, and a chest x-ray is obtained to rule out involvement of the lung or mediastinal structures.

Two tumor markers are important to the evaluation of a testicular cancer: serum α-fetoprotein and human chorionic gonadotropin. They are most useful when evaluating patients with seminomas. In contrast, only 50% to 70% of patients with nonseminomatous tumors will have elevations of these markers.

Staging

Tumor staging is based on the results of multiple tests and orchiectomy (with or without retroperitoneal lymph node dissection). Table 8-9 outlines the TNM staging system for testicular tumors.

Treatment

Treatment is based on the tumor stage and type. Multimodal treatment, combining surgical resection, irradiation, and chemotherapy, is typically indicated.

Before aggressive treatment, men diagnosed with testicular cancer are provided counseling about parenthood, fertility, and erectile function and an opportunity to bank sperm. However, whereas spermatogenesis is greatly reduced or absent immediately following treatment, it improves with time and the potential for conception and pregnancy remains a strong possibility within 2 to 3 years following treatment for testicular cancer.[107] Sexual dysfunction, including absent or decreased ejaculate volume, loss of libido, decreased arousal, erectile dysfunction, or decreased orgasmic intensity, affects 25% of men treated for testicular cancer.[108] The risk for sexual dysfunction is greatest when a retroperitoneal lymph node dissection (RPLND) is performed. Fortunately, advances in RPLND techniques preserve the sympathetic nerve fibers on the contralateral side with respect to the tumor, allowing greater preservation of ejaculatory function and fertility potential. For example, one review of patients undergoing a nerve-sparing RPLND technique found that antegrade ejaculation was preserved in 89% and more than 50% had fathered children over a 5-year period.[109]

TABLE 8-9 TNM Staging System for Testicular Carcinoma[102]

T: Primary Tumor	
Tx	Cannot be assessed
T0	No evidence of primary tumor
Tis	Intratubular cancer (CIS)
T1	Limited to testis without vascular invasion
T2	Invades beyond tunica albuginea or into epididymis, or limited to testis with vascular invasion
T3	Invades spermatic cord
T4	Invades scrotum
N: Regional Lymph Nodes	
Nx	Cannot be assessed
N0	No regional lymph node metastasis
N1	Metastasis in a single lymph node ≤ 2 cm
N2	Metastasis in a single lymph note > 2 cm and < 5 cm or multiple nodes none > 5 cm
N3	Metastasis in lymph nodes > 5 cm
M: Distant Metastasis	
Mx	Cannot be assessed
M0	No distant metastasis
M1	Distant metastasis present

TNM2, Tumor-nodes-metastasis.

Orchiectomy and Lymph Node Dissection. Radical orchiectomy of the affected testis is first-line treatment for all stages of seminoma (Figure 8-7). Postoperatively, most patients will have a Penrose drain in a stab wound beside the inguinal incision and will require moderate pain control because of the extent of dissection. Early mobilization of the patient is strongly recommended. As with all surgeries in the inguinal area, patients are at risk for urinary retention; fluid intake and voiding should be monitored during the first 24 hours. Bilateral orchiectomy is performed if both testes are affected. A prosthetic implant may be placed at the time of surgery.

Patients with nonseminomatous germ cell testicular tumors also undergo orchiectomy and, depending on the stage, RPLND. Because the lymph nodes are the first site of metastasis an RPLND may be curative for some men. The RPLND is done through a transabdominal approach and takes approximately 2 to 3 hours; a nasogastric tube is inserted, and an indwelling catheter is inserted to ensure urinary drainage.

Radiation Therapy. Following orchiectomy, patients undergo radiation therapy, which comprises 25 Gy delivered to paraaortic nodes, over a period of 6 weeks. For patients with advanced-stage tumors, wider field radiotherapy involving the retroperitoneal lymph nodes is completed (Figure 8-8). However, irradiation of the kidney is avoided because of its sensitivity to radiation.

Side effects associated with radiation therapy include diarrhea, fatigue, nausea, fertility issues, myelosuppression, gastric ulcers, and radiation cystitis. A low-residue diet and antidiarrheal medications typically control diarrhea, but the patient is advised to consult the radiation oncologist if diarrhea persists or excessive rectal bleeding occurs. Nausea and vomiting are also common; an antiemetic may be given approximately 1 hour before radiotherapy to prevent subsequent vomiting. Some patients experience

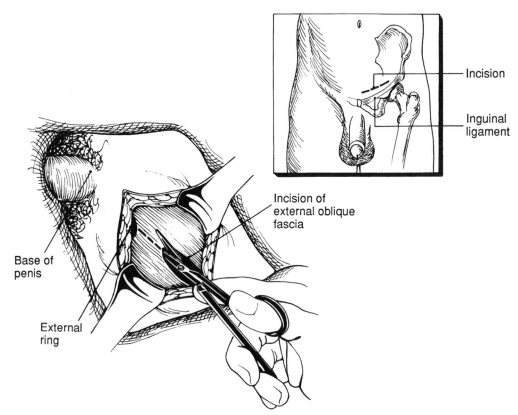

Fig. 8-7 Approach for radical inguinal orchiectomy, showing division of the external oblique fascia down to the external inquinal ring. (From Walsh P, Retik AB, Vaughan ED, Wein AJ (eds): Campbell-Walsh Urology, 8th edition. Philadelphia: Saunders, 2002.)

dyspepsia that may be relieved by the use of antacids and consumption of small, low-fat meals. Myelosuppression occurs when the paraaortic and pelvic lymph nodes are irradiated. Blood counts are usually monitored weekly, and neutropenic patients are advised to avoid medications that may mask a fever and rapidly seek medical assistance if they develop a fever, bruising, or bleeding. Fatigue is particularly common in patients with myelosuppression, and counseling about activity regulation, interspersed with appropriate rest periods, is particularly helpful for the young adult previously accustomed to few if any restrictions in physical activity.[110]

Chemotherapy. Carboplatin may be used as a single agent to treat lower-stage seminomas.[102,111] In contrast, cisplatin-based chemotherapy regimens, such as the three-agent regimen of bleomycin, etoposide, and cisplatin, provide a 70% to 80% cure rate in men with metastatic germ cell tumors.[112] The latter regimen is also used for men with nonseminomatous tumors; alternative regimens have been advocated that incorporate multiple agents such as vinblastine, actinomycin D, and cyclophosphamide. Refer to the treatment of advanced bladder cancer for a detailed review of the nursing management of patients undergoing multiple-agent chemotherapy.

Psychosocial Considerations

In addition to counseling the patient and his family on the side effects of radiation and chemotherapy, the nurse will need to be sensitive to the psychologic issues associated with the diagnosis of testicular cancer. Sexual function and perception of self may be affected by the orchiectomy.[110] As many as 30% of previously sexually active men report long-term sexual problems after orchiectomy.[113] Once concerns of survival are addressed, issues of fertility and sexual function become integral to comprehensive patient care both preoperatively and in the follow-up months after initial treatment. Technologic advances in reproductive medicine are important but should not take the place of assisting the patient and his partner in openly discussing their concerns.

PENILE CANCER

Penile cancer is rare in North America and Europe but far more common in certain areas of Africa, South America, and Asia.[114] This discussion is limited to premalignant (possessing a high likelihood of evolving into a neoplasm) or malignant lesions most commonly encountered by urologic nurses in North America or Europe (Figure 8-9).

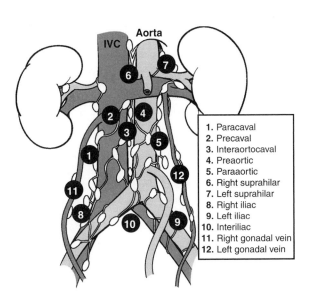

1. Paracaval
2. Precaval
3. Interaortocaval
4. Preaortic
5. Paraaortic
6. Right suprahilar
7. Left suprahilar
8. Right iliac
9. Left iliac
10. Interiliac
11. Right gonadal vein
12. Left gonadal vein

Fig. 8-8 Anatomic regions of the retroperitoneum. (From Walsh P, Retik AB, Vaughan ED, Wein AJ (eds): Campbell-Walsh Urology, 8th edition. Philadelphia: Saunders, 2002.)

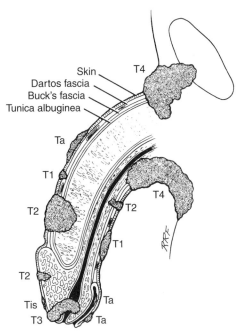

Fig. 8-9 Penile cancer. (From Walsh P, Retik AB, Vaughan ED, Wein AJ (eds): Campbell-Walsh Urology, 8th edition. Philadelphia: Saunders, 2002.)

Premalignant Lesions. Approximately 42% of men diagnosed with squamous cell penile cancer have a history of a premalignant lesion.[115] Although the likelihood that premalignant lesions will progress to malignant tumors is unknown, their detection justifies patient education concerning possible progression and consultation with a urologist or dermatologist concerning the need to resect the lesion. Table 8-10 describes common premalignant penile lesions.

Penile Malignancies. Squamous cell carcinoma is the most common malignant tumor affecting men in North America and Europe.[114] Slightly more than 1500 men in the United States were diagnosed with penile cancer in 2006.[1] It accounts for less than 1% of malignancies in men in North America and is decreasing in the United States, as compared with 10% in Asia and Africa.[114] In addition to the premalignant lesions described above, risk factors for penile cancer include phimosis, penile injury, genital warts, inflammation or chronic itching of the penile skin, and tobacco use (both smoked and smokeless forms increase the risk).[116,117] Circumcision reduces the risk of invasive squamous cell carcinoma, but it exerts a less protective effect on penile squamous cell carcinoma in situ.[118] Nevertheless, based on the lifetime risk of invasive

penile cancer, routine neonatal circumcision is not advocated as a preventive measure against penile cancer.[119] It is also important to note that adult circumcision does not provide the protection associated with neonatal circumcision. Modifiable risk factors of particular interest to the urologic nurse include meticulous and ongoing perineal hygiene to prevent phimosis, refraining from cigarette smoking, and safer sex practices in order to avoid human papillomavirus (HPV) infection, genital warts, syphilis, or other sexually transmitted disease associated with ulcerative lesions of the penis.[114,120]

Because of the acquired immunodeficiency syndrome (AIDS) epidemic, Kaposi's sarcoma is an increasingly common form of penile cancer. Verrucous carcinoma of the penis (sometimes referred to as a Buschke-Löwenstein tumor or giant condyloma acuminatum) is similar to benign condyloma acuminatum except that it invades and destroys adjacent structures by compression. Lymph node metastasis is rare and probably represents expression of an invasive squamous cell carcinoma.

Etiology and Pathophysiology

The cause of squamous cell carcinoma remains unknown. However, although the majority of cases

TABLE 8-10 Premalignant Lesions of the Penis

LESION	ETIOLOGY AND DESCRIPTION	TREATMENT
Cutaneous horn	Hyperkeratotic protuberance forms over an existing lesion (wart, abrasion, nevus, malignant tumor)	Resection and pathologic analysis of lesion and biopsy from base to exclude underlying cancer
Keratotic balanitis	Hyperkeratotic growth on the glans penis, may represent verrucous carcinoma	Excision, laser ablation, or cryotherapy; close follow-up and pathologic analysis critical
Balanitis xerotica obliterans	Whitish patch on prepuce or glans penis that may extend into meatus and fossa navicularis; may cause local pain, pruritus, or urethral obstruction	Topical steroid creams, injectable steroids, or resection (particularly if associated with obstruction); follow-up and biopsy may be necessary
Leukoplakia	Single or multiple whitish plaques of urethral meatus may lead to squamous cell carcinoma or verrucous carcinoma	Resection with close follow-up and repeated biopsies when indicated
Condyloma acuminatum	Papillary lesions that may involve the meatus or urethra; they are caused by HPV and are communicable; some varieties associated with squamous cell carcinoma of penis and cervical cancer	Topical podophyllin or trichloroacetic acid, laser ablation; urethral lesions may be treated with 5-fluorouracil

HPV, Human papillomavirus.

occur in elderly men, it is postulated that exposure to etiologic agents probably occurs during infancy, childhood, or early adulthood. Two primary forms of penile cancer are described: carcinoma in situ and invasive carcinoma. Carcinoma in situ is also called erythroplasia of Queyrat; it presents as a red, circumscribed lesion of the glans penis or prepuce of the uncircumcised male. In some cases the lesion will ulcerate, causing discharge and pain. Invasive squamous cell carcinoma begins with a small macular or papillary lesion that involves the glans penis. However, unlike in situ tumors, invasive tumors invade the shaft and corpora, ultimately causing autoaugmentation of the penis unless early diagnosis and treatment occur.

Stage. No universal staging or grading system exists for squamous cell carcinoma.[114] For the purposes of this chapter, the American Joint Cancer Committee system, which combines historical classifications of penile tumors with the TNM system advocated for other genitourinary system tumors, is used (Table 8-11). When evaluating tumor stage in men with penile carcinoma, the urologic nurse should pay special attention to the presence of metastasis to the lymph nodes, since this is the most important prognostic factor in squamous cell penile cancer.

Clinical Manifestations

The principal clinical manifestation of penile cancer is a visible skin lesion.[114] These lesions vary from minimal induration to a warty growth or apparent papillary tumor. Ulceration is common, especially for invasive carcinomas, and it may vary from shallow erosion to a full-thickness ulcer with rolled borders. Approximately half are found on the glans penis, 10% on the glans and prepuce, and fewer than 2% on the penile shaft. Associated symptoms include pain (usually mild) or itching, often occurring with ulceration and exudate. Constitutional symptoms, such as unintentional weight loss, fatigue, or malaise, indicate advanced disease or chronic suppuration. Because of the location of the lesion and its association with guilt, fear, or embarrassment, men often delay seeking help.

Diagnosis

Physical examination focuses on careful inspection of the lesion, the glans penis, foreskin, urethral meatus, and fossa navicularis. The inguinal lymph nodes are palpated for enlargement and mobility. Biopsy of the lesion is obtained for definitive diagnosis, staging, and tumor grade. Imaging studies are obtained in selected cases; a contrast-enhanced MRI or ultrasound may be used to identify corporal invasion, particularly if a partial penectomy is under consideration. Palpation of lymph nodes is generally preferred to lymphangiography or pelvic CT scan.

Treatment

Small (2 cm or less) superficial penile cancers may be managed by surgical excision, provided a 2-cm circumferential margin can be achieved to prevent local recurrence.[121] However, partial or total penectomy is often preferred for invasive carcinomas because it provides better local control than does laser ablation, radiotherapy, or chemotherapy.[114,122] The reported recurrence rate for local disease following penectomy varies from 0% to 7%.[117] Nevertheless, penectomy is associated with a risk of adverse sexual and psychologic outcomes, and the magnitude of these effects is much greater for complete as compared with partial penectomy. In addition, the urologist must address the need for regional lymphadenectomy. Lymphadenectomy comprises the single most important prognostic factor relevant to long-term survival, and it is curative in some cases. The postoperative morbidity associated with bilateral lymph node dissection, in particular, may include lymphedema adversely affecting both legs and leading to chronic

---

TABLE 8-11 American Joint Cancer Committee Staging of Penile Cancer

Primary Tumor	
Tis	Carcinoma in situ
Ta	Noninvasive verrucous carcinoma
T1	Tumor invades subepithelial connective tissue
T2	Tumor invades corpus spongiosum
T3	Tumor invades urethra or prostate
T4	Tumor invades adjacent structures
Nodes	
N1	Unilateral lymph node involved but it remains movable
N2	Bilateral nodes remain movable
N3	Lymph nodes are involved and fixed
Metastases	
M1	Evidence of distant metastases

swelling, discomfort, and impaired mobility. Because of these considerations, a modified lymph node dissection or fine-needle biopsies may be undertaken before traditional inguinal or ilioinguinal lymphadenectomy is completed.

EBRT is useful in highly selected patients, but the risk of complications such as urethral fistula, stricture, or penile necrosis is significant. Alternatively, interstitial radiation therapy (brachytherapy) has been used in patients with superficial lesions.[123] Although initial results are promising, close follow-up is essential because of the risk for local recurrence (up to 64% at 5 years). Radiotherapy also may be applied to the inguinal area in an attempt to reduce metastatic disease. Nevertheless, it is also limited to a highly selected group of men who are not candidates for lymphadenectomy. Chemotherapy is also limited to selected men who cannot undergo surgical resection. Although as many as 60% experience partial responses, they are short lived, and chemotherapy should be combined with radiotherapy.[114]

In addition to caring for the patient undergoing surgery, radiotherapy, or chemotherapy, urologic nursing management focuses on enabling the man to express grief and receive support when coping with the adverse psychologic effects of penile cancer. These effects are most severe for the man with suppurative lesions of the penis leading to autoamputation or total penectomy. Psychosocial support includes the man and his partner whenever possible, and assessment extends well beyond the initial postoperative period when a focus on cancer eradication may overshadow the long-term adverse effects of partial or total penile amputation. In addition to these considerations, the urologic nurse should educate the patient undergoing lymphadenectomy about the risk for lymphedema. Early referral to a wound, ostomy, and continence (WOC) nurse or physical therapist with expertise in compression and lymphedema management is indicated *before* significant swelling of the lower extremities occurs.

SUMMARY

The urologic nurse plays a critical role in both localized and advanced-stage disease as well as in the early detection and management of prostate cancer. In localized disease, the primary focus of nursing management is early detection and management of the disease with the goal of cure. In advanced-stage tumors, the

urology nurse participates in therapies designed to cure or to arrest the disease. Even in tumors that have proved refractory to hormonal suppression and resistant to alternative treatments, the urologic nurse functions in a central role, providing palliative care designed to maximize comfort, relieve constitutional symptoms, and allow anticipatory grieving.

REFERENCES

1. American Cancer Society (ACS): Cancer Facts & Figures 2008. Retrieved May 15, 2008, from the American Cancer Society website: http://www.cancer.org/docroot/STT/STT_O.asp.
2. Pisani P, Parkin DM, Bray F, Ferlay J: Estimates of the worldwide mortality from 25 cancers in 1990. International Journal of Cancer, 1999; 83:18-29.
3. Godley P, Kim SW: Renal cell carcinoma. Current Opinion in Oncology, 2002; 14(3):280-5.
4. Miller BA, Kolonel LN, Bernstein L, Young JL Jr, Swanson GM, West D, Key CR, Liff JM, Glover CS, Alexander GA, et al (eds): Racial/Ethnic Patterns of Cancer in the United States 1988-1992, National Cancer Institute; 2007. NIH Pub. No. 96-4104. Bethesda, Md.
5. Nelson EC, Evans CP, Lara PN Jr: Renal cell carcinoma: Current status and emerging therapies. Cancer Treatment Reviews, 2007; 33(3):299-313.
6. Campbell SC, Novick AC, Bukowski RM: Renal tumors. In Wein AJ, Kavoussi LR, Novick AC, Partin AW, Peters CA (eds): Campbell-Walsh Urology, 9th edition. Philadelphia: Saunders, 2007; pp 1567-1637.
7. Chow WH, Gridley G, Fraumeni JF Jr, Jarvholm B: Obesity, hypertension, and the risk of kidney cancer in men. New England Journal of Medicine, 2000; 343(18):1305-11.
8. Rosenberg L, Stephenson WP, Rao RS, Palmer JR, Strom BL, Shapiro S: The diagnosis of renal cell cancer in relation to hypertension. Cancer Causes and Control, 1998; 9(6):611-4.
9. Pischon T, Lahmann PH, Boeing H, Tjonneland A, Halkjaer J, Overvad K, Klipstein-Grobusch K, Linseisen J, Becker N, Trichopoulou A, Benetou V, Trichopoulos D, Sieri S, Palli D, Tumino R, Vineis P, Panico S, Monninkhof E, Peeters PH, Bueno-de-Mesquita HB, Buchner FL, Ljungberg B, Hallmans G, Berglund G, Gonzalez CA, Dorronsoro M, Gurrea AB, Navarro C, Martinez C, Quiros JR, Roddam A, Allen N, Bingham S, Khaw KT, Kaaks R, Norat T, Slimani N, Riboli E: Body size and risk of renal cell carcinoma in the European Prospective Investigation into Cancer and Nutrition (EPIC). International Journal of Cancer, 2006; 118(3):728-38.
10. Parker AS, Cerhan JR, Lynch CF, Ershow AG, Cantor KP: Gender, alcohol consumption, and renal cell carcinoma. American Journal of Epidemiology, 2002; 155(5):455-62.
11. Hu J, Mao Y, White K: Renal cell carcinoma and occupational exposure to chemicals in Canada. Occupational Medicine (Oxford), 2002; 52(3):157-64.
12. Young AN, Dale J, Yin-Goen Q, Harris WB, Petros JA, Datta MW, Wang MD, Marshall FF, Amin MB: Current trends in molecular classification of adult renal tumors. Urology, 2006; 67(5):873-80.
13. Herring JC, Enquist EG, Chernoff A, Linehan WM, Choyke PL, Walther MM: Parenchymal sparing surgery in patients with hereditary renal cell carcinoma: 10-year experience. Journal of Urology, 2001; 165(3):777-81.
14. Atkins MB, Garnick MB: Renal neoplasia. In Brenner BM (ed): The Kidney, 6th edition. Philadelphia: Saunders, 2000; pp 1844-8.
15. Minai FN, Monem A: Paraneoplastic syndrome of renal cell carcinoma. Journal of the College of Physicians & Surgeons - Pakistan, 2006; 16(1):81-2.

16. Bosniak MA: The use of the Bosniak classification system for renal cysts and cystic tumors. Journal of Urology, 1997; 157(5):1852-3.
17. Bosniak MA, Birnbaum BA, Krinsky GA, Waisman J: Small renal parenchymal neoplasms: further observations on growth. Radiology, 1995; 197(3):589-97.
18. Bosniak MA: Observation of small incidentally detected renal masses. Seminars in Urologic Oncology, 1995; 13(4):267-72.
19. Tomita Y: Early renal cell cancer. International Journal of Clinical Oncology, 2006; 11(1):22-7.
20. Kaouk JH, Aron M, Rewcastle JC, Gill IS: Cryotherapy: clinical end points and their experimental foundations. Urology, 2006; 68(1, suppl):38-44.
21. Janetschek G: Laparoscopic partial nephrectomy: How far have we gone?. Current Opinion in Urology, 2007; 17(5):316-21.
22. Lau WK, Blute ML, Weaver AL, Torres VE, Zincke H: Matched comparison of radical nephrectomy vs nephron-sparing surgery in patients with unilateral renal cell carcinoma and a normal contra-lateral kidney. Mayo Clinic Proceedings, 2000; 75(12):1236-42.
23. Coppin C, Porzsolt F, Kumpf J, Coldman A, Wilt T: Immunotherapy for advanced renal cell cancer. Cochrane Prostatic Diseases and Urologic Cancers Group Cochrane Database of Systematic Reviews, 2003; 1.
24. Monaghan M: Renal cell cancer. In Miaskowski C, Buchsel P (eds): Oncology Nursing: Assessment and Clinical Care. St Louis: Mosby, 1999; pp 1089-105.
25. Skinner DG, Stein JP, Ross R, Nichols P, Bochner B, Raghavan D: Cancer of the bladder. In Gillenwater JY, Grayhack JT, Howards SS, Mitchell ME (eds): Adult and Pediatric Urology, 4th edition. Philadelphia: Lippincott Williams & Wilkins, 2002; pp 1297-362.
26. Flanigan RC: Urothelial tumors of the upper urinary tract. In Wein AJ, Kavoussi LR, Novick AC, Partin AW, Peters CA (eds). Campbell-Walsh Urology, 9th edition. Philadelphia: Saunders, 2007, pp 1638-85.
27. Yossepowitch O, Dalbagni G: Transitional cell carcinoma in young adults: presentation, natural history and outcome. Journal of Urology, 2002; 168:61-6.
28. Dreicer R: Locally advanced and metastatic bladder cancer. Current Treatment Options in Oncology, 2001; 2:431-6.
29. Puente D, Hartge P, Greiser E, Cantor KP, King WD, Gonzalez CA, Cordier S, Vineis P, Lynge E, Chang-Claude J, Porru S, Tzonou A, Jockel KH, Serra C, Hours M, Lynch CF, Ranft U, Wahrendorf J, Silverman D, Fernandez F, Boffetta P, Kogevinas M: A pooled analysis of bladder cancer case-control studies evaluating smoking in men and women. Cancer Causes and Control, 2006; 17(1):71-9.
30. Grimmer G, Dettbarn G, Seidel A, Jacob J: Detection of carcinogenic aromatic amines in the urine of non-smokers. Science of the Total Environment, 2000; 247:81-90.
31. Band PR, Le ND, MacArthur AC, Fang R, Gallagher RP: Identification of occupational cancer risks in British Columbia: a population-based case-control study of 1129 cases of bladder cancer. Journal of Occupational and Environmental Medicine, 2005; 47(8):854-8.
32. Morrison AS: Advances in the etiology of urothelial cancer. Urologic Clinics of North America, 1984; 11:557-66.
33. Cohen SM, Johansson HL: Epidemiology and etiology of bladder cancer. Urologic Clinics of North America, 1992; 19:421-8.
34. Sontag JM: Experimental identification of genitourinary carcinogens. Urologic Clinics of North America, 1980; 7:803-14.
35. Michaud DS, Spiegelman D, Clinton SK, Rimm EB, Gurhas GC, Willett WC, Giovannucci EL: Fluid intake and risk of bladder cancer in men. New England Journal of Medicine, 1999; 340:1390-97.
36. Schabath MB, Spitz MR, Lerner SP, Pillow PC, Hernandez LM, Delclos GL, Grossman HB, Wu X: Case-control analysis of dietary folate and risk of bladder cancer. Nutrition and Cancer, 2005; 53(2):144-51.
37. Kiemeney LA, Moret NC, Witjes JA, Schoenberg MP, Tulinius H: Familial transitional cell carcinoma among the population of Iceland. Journal of Urology, 1997; 157:1649-51.
38. Michaud DS, Clinton SK, Rimm EB, Willett WC, Giovannucci E: Risk of bladder cancer by geographic region in a US cohort of male health professionals. Epidemiology, 2001; 12:719-26.
39. el-Mawla NG, el-Bolkainy MN, Khaled HM: Bladder cancer in Africa: update. Seminars in Oncology, 2001; 28:174-8.
40. Syrigos KN, Skinner DG: Bladder Cancer: Biology, Diagnosis, and Management. New York: Oxford University Press, 1999.
41. Jones JS, Campbell SC: Non-muscle-invasive bladder cancer. In Wein AJ, Kavoussi LR, Novick AC, Partin AW, Peters CA (eds): Campbell-Walsh Urology, 9th edition. Philadelphia: Saunders, 2007; pp 2447-67.
42. Patton SE, Hall C, Ozen H: Bladder cancer. Current Opinion in Oncology, 2002; 14:265-72.
43. Gray M, Sims T: NMP-22 for bladder cancer screening and surveillance. Urologic Nursing, 2004; 24(3):171-9.
44. Sanchini MA, Gunelli R, Nanni O, Bravaccini S, Fabbri C, Sermasi A, Bercovich E, Ravaioli A, Amadori D, Calistri D: Relevance of urine telomerase in the diagnosis of bladder cancer. JAMA, 2005; 294(16):2052-6.
45. Davies B, Chen JJ, McMurry T, Landsittel D, Lewis N, Brenes G, Getzenberg RH: Efficacy of BTA stat, cytology, and survivin in bladder cancer surveillance over 5 years in patients with spinal cord injury. Urology, 2005; 66(4):908-11.
46. Smith SD, Wheeler MA, Plescia J, Colberg JW, Weiss RM, Altieri DC: Urine detection of survivin and diagnosis of bladder cancer. Journal of the American Medical Associations, 2001; 285:324-8.
47. Brown FM: Urine cytology. Is it still the gold standard for screening? Urologic Clinics of North America, 2000; 27:25-37.
48. Hall RR: Clinical Management of Bladder Cancer. London: Arnold, 1999.
49. Duque JLF, Loughlin KR: An overview of the treatment of superficial bladder cancer. Urologic Clinics of North America, 2000; 27:125-35.
50. O'Donnell MA: Advances in the management of superficial bladder cancer. Seminars in Oncology, 2007; 34(2):85-97.
51. Koya MP, Simon MA, Soloway MS: Complications of intravesical therapy for urothelial cancer of the bladder. Journal of Urology, 2006; 175(6):2004-10.
52. Durek C, Richter E, Basteck A, Rusch-Gerdes S, Gerdes J, Joacham D, Bohle A: The fate of bacillus Calmette-Guerin after intravesical instillation. Journal of Urology, 2001; 165:1765-8.
53. Aljada IS, Crane JK, Corriere N, Wagle DG, Amsterdam D: *Mycobacterium bovis* BCG causing vertebral osteomyelitis (Pott's disease) following intravesical BCG therapy. Journal of Clinical Microbiology, 1999; 37:2106-8.
54. Han DP, Simons KB, Tarkanian CN, Moretti ST: Endophthalmitis from *Mycobacterium bovis*-bacille Calmette-Guerin after intravesical bacille Calmette-Guerin injections for bladder carcinoma. American Journal of Ophthalmology, 1999; 128:648-50.
55. Rodevand E, Faxvaag A, Ostensen M, Brevik B: Arthritis after BCG treatment of bladder cancer: a rare complication. Tidsskrift for Den Norske Laegeforening, 1996; 116:3231-32.
56. Schoenberg M, Gonzalgo ML: Management of invasive and metastatic bladder cancer. In Wein AJ, Kavoussi LR, Novick AC, Partin AW, Peters CA (eds): Campbell-Walsh Urology, 9th edition. Philadelphia: Saunders, 2007; pp 2468-78.
57. Winquist E: Perioperative chemotherapy for localized bladder cancer. Canadian Journal of Urology, 2006; 13(suppl 1):77-80.
58. Garcia JA, Dreicer R: Adjuvant and neoadjuvant chemotherapy for bladder cancer: management and controversies. Nature Clinical Practice Urology, 2005; 2(1):32-7.
59. Advanced Bladder Cancer (ABC) Meta-analysis Collaboration: Adjuvant chemotherapy for invasive bladder cancer (indivicual patient data). Cochrane Database of Systematic Reviews, 2006; issue 4. Art. No.: CD006018. DOI: 10.1002/14621858.CD006018.
60. Akaza H: Advances in chemotherapy of invasive bladder cancer. Current Opinion in Urology, 2000; 10:453-7.
61. Chee KG, Cambio A, Lara PN Jr: Recent developments in advanced urothelial cancer. Current Opinion in Urology, 2005; 15(5):342-9.
62. Gray M: Prostate cancer primer. Urologic Nursing, 2002; 22:151-69.
63. Gray M, Sims T: Prostate cancer: an update for nurse practitioners. Prevention and management of localized disease. Nurse Practitioner, 2006; 31(9):14-29.

64. American Cancer Society (ACS): Cancer prevention and early detection worksheet for men. 2006. Retrieved Jan 15, 2008 from the American Cancer Society website: http://www.cancer.org/downloads/PED/Cancer%20Prevention%20and%20Early%20Detection%20Worksheet%20for%20Men.pdf.

65. Lippman SM, Goodman PJ, Klein EA, Parnes HL, Thompson IM, Kristal AR, Santella RM, Probstfield JL, Moinpour CM, Albanes D, Taylor PR, Minasian LM, Hoque A, Thomas SM, Crowley JJ, Gaziano JM, Stanford JL, Cook ED, Fleshner NE, Lieber MM, Walther PJ, Khuri FR, Karp DD, Schwartz GG, Ford LG, Coltman CA: Designing the Selenium and Vitamin E Cancer Prevention Trial (SELECT). Journal of the National Cancer Institute, 2005; 97(2):94-102.

66. Thompson IM, Klein EA, Lippman SM, Coltman CA, Djavan B: Prevention of prostate cancer with finasteride: US/European perspective. European Urology, 2003; 44(6):650-5.

67. Klein EA: Can prostate cancer be prevented? Nature Clinical Practice Urology, 2005; 2(1):24-31.

68. Unger JM, Thompson IM Jr, LeBlanc M, Crowley JJ, Goodman PJ, Ford LG, Coltman CA Jr: Estimated impact of the Prostate Cancer Prevention Trial on population mortality. Cancer, 2005; 103(7):1375-80.

69. Andriole G, Bostwick D, Brawley O, Gomella L, Marberger M, Tindall D: REDUCE Study Group: Chemoprevention of prostate cancer in men at high risk: rationale and design of the reduction by dutasteride of prostate cancer events (REDUCE) trial. Journal of Urology, 2004; 172:1314-7.

70. Zeliadt SB, Etzioni RD, Penson DF, Thompson IM, Ramsey SD: Lifetime implications and cost-effectiveness of using finasteride to prevent prostate cancer. American Journal of Medicine, 2005; 118(8):850-7.

71. Grover S, Lowensteyn I, Hajek D, Trachtenberg J, Coupal L, Marchand S: Do the benefits of finasteride outweigh the risks in the prostate cancer prevention trial? Journal of Urology, 2006; 175(3, pt 1):934-8.

72. Klein EA, Platz EA, Thompson IM: Epidemiology, etiology and prevention of prostate cancer. In Wein AJ, Kavoussi LR, Novick AC, Partin AW, Peters CA (eds): Campbell-Walsh Urology, 9th edition. Philadelphia: Saunders, 2007; pp 2854-73.

73. Carter HB, Allaf ME, Partin AW: Diagnosis and staging of prostate cancer. In Wein AJ, Kavoussi LR, Novick AC, Partin AW, Peters CA (eds): Campbell-Walsh Urology, 9th edition. Philadelphia: Saunders, 2007; pp 2912-31.

74. Chen L, Ambrosone CB, Lee J, Sellers TA, Pow-Sang J, Park JY: Association between polymorphisms in the DNA repair genes XRCC1 and APE1, and the risk of prostate cancer in white and black Americans. Journal of Urology, 2006; 175(1):108-12.

75. Hernandez J, Balic I, Johnson-Pais TL, Higgins BA, Torkko KC, Thompson IM, Leach RJ: Association between an estrogen receptor alpha gene polymorphism and the risk of prostate cancer in black men. Journal of Urology, 2006; 175(2):523-7.

76. Conlon EM, Goode EL, Gibbs M, Stanford JL, Badzioch M, Janer M, Kolb S, Hood L, Ostrander EA, Jarvik GP, Wijsman EM: Oligogenic segregation analysis of hereditary prostate cancer pedigrees: evidence for multiple loci affecting age at onset. International Journal of Cancer, 2003; 105(5):630-5.

77. Gleason DF: Classification of prostatic carcinoma. Cancer Chemotherapy Reports, 1966; 50:125-8.

78. Gwede CK, McDermott RJ: Prostate cancer screening decision making under controversy: implications for health promotion practice. Health Promotion Practice, 2006; 7(1):134-46.

79. Ng TK, Vasilareas D, Mitterdorfer AJ, Maher PO, Lalak A: Prostate cancer detection with digital rectal examination, prostate-specific antigen, transrectal ultrasonography and biopsy in clinical urological practice. BJU International, 2005; 95(4):545-8.

80. Punglia RS, D'Amico AV, Catalona WJ, Roehl KA, Kuntz KM: Impact of age, benign prostatic hyperplasia, and cancer on prostate-specific antigen level. Cancer, 2006; 106(7):1507-13.

81. Busby JE, Evans CP: Determining variables for repeat prostate biopsy. Prostate Cancer and Prostatic Diseases, 2004; 7(2):93-8.

82. National Comprehensive Cancer Network: NCCN practice guidelines in oncology. Prostate cancer 2007. Retrieved Jan 15, 2008 from http://www.nccn.org/professionals/physician_gls/PDF/prostate.pdf.

83. Algaba F, Trias I, Arce Y: Natural history of prostatic carcinoma: The pathologist's perspective. Recent Results in Cancer Research, 2007; 175:9-24.

84. Allaf ME, Carter HB: Update on watchful waiting for prostate cancer. Current Opinion in Urology, 2006; 14:171-5.

85. Klotz L: Active surveillance for prostate cancer: for whom? Journal of Clinical Oncology, 2005; 23(32):8165-9.

86. Lam JS, Pisters LL, Belldegrun AS: Cryotherapy for prostate cancer. In Wein AJ, Kavoussi LR, Novick AC, Partin AW, Peters CA (eds): Campbell-Walsh Urology, 9th edition. Philadelphia: Saunders, 2007; pp 3032-52.

87. Sokoloff MH, Brendler CB: Indications and contraindications for nerve-sparing radical prostatectomy. Urologic Clinics of North America, 2001; 28(3):535-44.

88. Fowler JF: Radiobiological principles of prostate cancer. In Greco C, Kelefsky MJ (eds): Radiotherapy of Prostate Cancer. Amsterdam: Harwood, 2000; pp 131-43.

89. Zelefsky MJ: Three-dimensional radiotherapy. In Greco C, Kelefsky MJ (eds): Radiotherapy of Prostate Cancer. Amsterdam: Harwood, 2000; pp 221-32.

90. Rossi CJ, Slater JD, Shipley WU: Conformal proton beam therapy of prostate cancer. In Greco C, Kelefsky MJ (eds): Radiotherapy of Prostate Cancer. Amsterdam: Harwood, 2000; pp 289-96.

91. Morton MS, Turkes A, Denis L, Griffiths K: Can dietary factors influence prostatic disease? BJU International, 1999; 84(5):549-54.

92. Allen NE, Sauvaget C, Roddam AW, Appleby P, Nagano J, Suzuki G, Key TJ, Koyama K: A prospective study of diet and prostate cancer in Japanese men. Cancer Causes & Control, 2004; 15(9):911-20.

93. Eisenberger MA, Carducci M: Treatment of hormone-refractory prostate cancer. In Wein AJ, Kavoussi LR, Novick AC, Partin AW, Peters CA (eds): Campbell-Walsh Urology, 9th edition. Philadelphia: Saunders, 2007; pp 3101-18.

94. Nelson JB: Hormone therapy for prostate cancer. In Wein AJ, Kavoussi LR, Novick AC, Partin AW, Peters CA (eds): Campbell-Walsh Urology. 9th edition. Philadelphia: Saunders, 2007; pp 3082-3100.

95. Baum NH, Torti DC: Managing hot flashes in men being treated for prostate cancer. Geriatrics, 2007; 62(11):18-21.

96. Hsieh T, Chen SS, Wang X, Wu JM: Regulation of androgen receptor (AR) and prostate specific antigen (PSA) expression in the androgen-responsive human prostate LNCaP cells by ethanolic extracts of the Chinese herbal preparation, PC-SPES. Biochemistry and Molecular Biology International, 1997; 42(3):535-44.

97. Small EJ, Frohlich MW, Bok R, Shinohara K, Grossfeld G, Rozenblat Z, Kelly WK, Corry M, Reese DM: Prospective trial of the herbal supplement PC-SPES in patients with progressive prostate cancer. Journal of Clinical Oncology, 2000; 18(21):3595-3603.

98. Smith DC: Chemotherapy for hormone refractory prostate cancer. Urologic Clinics of North America, 1999; 26(2):323-32.

99. Coyle N: Introduction to palliative nursing, In Ferrell BR, Coyle N (eds): Textbook of Palliative Nursing. 2nd edition. Oxford, England: Oxford University Press, 2006.

100. Esper P, Redman BG: Supportive care, pain management, and quality of life in advanced prostate cancer. Urologic Clinics of North America, 1999; 26(2):375-89.

101. Sonneveld DJ, Schaapveld M, Sleijfer DT, Meerman GJ, van der Graaf WT, Sijmons RH, Koops HS, Hoekstra HJ: Geographic clustering of testicular cancer incidence in the northern part of the Netherlands. British Journal of Cancer, 1999; 81:1262-7.

102. Ritchie JP, Steele GS: Neoplasms of the testis. In Wein AJ, Kavoussi LR, Novick AC, Partin AW, Peters CA (eds): Campbell-Walsh Urology, 9th edition. Philadelphia: Saunders, 2007; pp 893-935.

103. Horwich A, Shipley J, Huddart R: Testicular germ-cell cancer. Lancet, 2006; 367:754-65.

104. Stoller ML, Kane CJ, Meng MV: Urology. In McPhee SJ, Papadakis MA, Tierney LM: Current Medical Diagnosis and Treatment. New York: Lang Medical Books/McGraw-Hill, 2008. Retrieved Jan. 15, 2008 from http://www.accessmedicine.com/content.aspx?aID=11857.

105. Swerdlow AH, De Stavola BL, Swanwick MA, Maconochie NE: Risks of breast and testicular cancer in young adult twins in England and Wales: evidence on prenatal and genetic etiology. Lancet, 1997; 350:1723-8.

106. McCullagh J, Lewis G, Warlow C: Promoting awareness and practice of testicular self-examination. Nursing Standard, 2005; 19(51):41-9.

107. DeSantis M, Albrecht W, Holtl W, Pont J: Impact of cytotoxic treatment on long-term fertility in patients with germ-cell cancer. International Journal of Cancer, 1999; 83(6):864-5.

108. van Basten JP, Jonker-Pool G, van Driel MF, Sleijfer DT, Droste JH, van de Wiel HB, Schraffordt Koops H, Molenaar WM, Hoekstra HJ: Sexual functioning after multimodality treatment for disseminated nonseminomatous testicular germ cell tumor. Journal of Urology, 1997; 158:1411-6.

109. Jacobsen KD, Ous S, Waehre H, Trasti, Stenwig AE, Lien HH, Aass N, Fossa SD: Ejaculation in testicular cancer patients after post-chemotherapy retroperitoneal lymph node dissection. British Journal of Cancer, 1999; 80:249-55.

110. Poirier SM, Rawl SM: Testicular germ cell cancer. In Yarbro CH, Goodman M, Frogge MH, Growenwald SL (eds): Cancer Nursing: Principles and Practice, 6th edition. Boston: Jones and Bartlett, 2005; pp 1494-1510.

111. Shelley MD, Burgon K, Mason MD: Treatment of testicular germ-cell cancer: a Cochrane evidence-based systematic review. Cancer Treatment Reviews, 2002; 28(5):237-53.

112. Kollmannsberger C, Nichols C, Bokemeyer C: Recent advances in management of patients with platinum-refractory testicular germ cell tumors. Cancer, 2006; 106(6):1217-26.

113. Aass N, Grunfeld B, Kaalhus O, Fossa SD: Pre and post treatment sexual life in testicular cancer patients: a descriptive investigation. British Journal of Cancer, 1993; 67:1113-17.

114. Pettaway CA, Lynch DF, Davis JW: Tumors of the penis. In Wein AJ, Kavoussi LR, Novick AC, Partin AW, Peters CA (eds): Campbell-Walsh Urology, 9th edition. Philadelphia: Saunders, 2007; pp 2945-29[Chapter 31].

115. Bouchot O, Auvigne J, Peuvrel P, Glemain P, Buzelin JM: Management of regional lymph nodes in carcinoma of the penis. European Urology, 1989; 16:410-5.

116. Tseng HF, Morgenstern H, Mack T, Peters RK: Risk factors for penile cancer: results of a population-based, case-control study in Los Angeles County (United States). Cancer Causes and Control, 2001; 12:267-77.

117. Misra S, Chaturvedi A, Misra NC: Penile carcinoma: a challenge for the developing world. Lancet Oncology, 2004; 5(4):240-7.

118. Schoen EJ, Oehrli M, Colby C, Machin G: The highly protective effect of newborn circumcision against invasive penile cancer. Pediatrics, 2000; 105:627-8 (abstract).

119. Anonymous: Neonatal circumcision revisited. Fetus and Newborn Committee, Canadian Pediatric Society Canadian Medical Association Journal, 1996; 154:769-80.

120. Daling JR, Madeleine MM, Johnson LG, Schwartz SM, Shera KA, Wurscher MA, Carter JJ, Porter PL, Galloway DA, McDougall JK, Krieger JN: Penile cancer: importance of circumcision, human papillomavirus and smoking in in situ and invasive disease. International Journal of Cancer, 2005; 116(4):606-16.

121. Micali G, Nasca MR, Innocenzi D, Schwartz RA: Penile cancer. Journal of the American Academy of Dermatology, 2006; 54(3):369-91.

122. Mobilio G, Ficarra V: Genital treatment of penile carcinoma. Current Opinion in Urology, 2001; 11:299-304.

123. Crook JM, Jezioranski J, Grimard L, Esche B, Pond G: Penile brachytherapy: results for 49 patients. International Journal of Radiation Oncology, Biology, Physics, 2005; 62(2):460-7.

124. Gettman MT, Blute ML: Update on pathologic staging of renal cell carcinoma. Urology, 2001; 60:209-17.

125. Baselli EC, Greenberg RE: Intravesical therapy for superficial bladder cancer. Oncology (Huntington), 2000; 14(5):719-31, 734, 737.

126. Bohle A, Jocham D, Bock PR: Intravesical bacillus Calmette-Guerin versus mitomycin C for superficial bladder cancer: a formal meta-analysis of comparative studies on recurrence and toxicity. Journal of Urology, 2003; 169(1):90-5.

127. Masters JR: Re: methods to improve efficacy of intravesical mitomycin C: results of a randomized phase III trial. Journal of the National Cancer Institute, 2001; 93(20):1574-5.

Sexual and Reproductive Dysfunction

Male sexual dysfunction is a broad label applied to a wide variety of disorders affecting erectile or reproductive function. Although none of these disorders is associated with mortality, they exert a profound influence on the quality of life that negatively affects both the patient and his partner. This chapter will discuss disorders of sexual function that impair penile erection, ejaculation, and fertility.

ERECTILE FUNCTION DISORDERS

The most common disorders affecting erectile function are the inability to generate an erection adequate for sexual activity (erectile dysfunction [ED] or impotence), painful curvature of the penis (Peyronie's disease), and a prolonged painful erection (priapism).

ERECTILE DYSFUNCTION

ED is defined as the inability to achieve or sustain an erection adequate for sexual performance.[1-3] Mild ED is defined as the inability to achieve an erection adequate for sexual performance during approximately 20% of attempts, and severe ED is defined as a lack of success approaching 100%.[4] From a clinical perspective, ED is considered clinically relevant when it occurs during at least 50% of attempts at sexual activity or when it persists for more than 3 months.[1]

Epidemiology

Reports of the prevalence and incidence of ED vary widely, ranging from 10% to 69%, depending on the criteria used to identify ED and the characteristics of the population studied.[2] If the definition promulgated by the National Institutes of Health (NIH) Consensus panel is used,[3] it is estimated that by the year 2007, over 50 million American men between the ages of 40 and 70 years of age will have experienced at least occasional ED.[5] Global estimates of ED also vary widely, with a reported prevalence of 81% of Japanese[6] and 62% of Italian men[7] as compared with approximately 19% of German and Spanish men.[8]

Finally, the prevalence in the older person is even higher, and it tends to be underreported and undertreated.

Prevalence rates stratified by age group were examined in the Massachusetts Male Aging Study, completed in 1989.[9] It revealed a proportional increase in ED prevalence with rising age. Specifically, 39% of men experienced some degree of ED during the fourth decade of life, although 67% experienced at least occasional erectile problems during the seventh decade. When men with severe ED, defined as the total inability to achieve an adequate erection regardless of stimulus, were compared, the prevalence rose from 5% among men in their 40s to 15% of men affected in their 70s.

Pathophysiology

Traditionally, ED was characterized as psychogenic or organic. Psychogenic factors were hypothesized to account for nearly 90% of all cases of ED, although organic causes were thought to predominate in about 10%.[10] Advances in our understanding of erectile dysfunction now show that purely psychogenic factors account for only a small percentage of men with ED, although psychological distress is associated with almost all cases. Rather, it is now widely acknowledged that an erection is a neurovascular event and that ED occurs when one or more components of this complex cascade is impaired.[11] When erectile function is conceptualized as a neurovascular event, three principal impairments can be identified that lead to ED—failure to initiate an erection, failure to fill the corporal bodies with blood adequately, and failure to trap and store blood in the corporal bodies adequately during erection.[4]

Failure to initiate an erection occurs when there is a failure to stimulate or inhibit the peripheral nerves or central neuromodulatory centers needed. Contributing factors include neurologic disorders that interfere with afferent or efferent neurologic signals or psychological distress. Failure to fill the corporal bodies adequately usually occurs when endothelial function results in the inability to achieve an erection with the rigidity needed for sexual performance. Common contributing factors include diabetes mellitus, atherosclerosis, dyslipidemia, and heart disease. Failure to entrap and store blood in the corporal bodies leads to the inability to sustain an erection. Contributing factors include failure to achieve sufficient relaxation of smooth muscle within the corporal body because of psychological distress and fibrosis of the corporal bodies caused by trauma.

Effect of Aging. Although age does not cause ED, age-associated changes and a number of age-related diseases may cause erectile difficulties, such as age-related changes in the arterioles of the penis and cavernous bodies. These changes include an increase in α_1-adrenergic receptors, decrease in cholinergic receptors, and reduction in nitric oxide immunoreactive nerves. Collectively, these changes are postulated to diminish the frequency and rapidity of tumescence.[12,13] Age-related changes in endocrine function include diminished serum levels of total and bioavailable testosterone, a reduction in luteinizing hormone pulse frequency, and increased serum levels of estradiol and serum prolactin. Collectively, these tend to reduce libido—interest or desire to engage in sexual activity.[1] Thus, normal aging is associated with fewer nocturnal erections, prolongation of the period required to achieve sexual arousal, and an increased interval between successful erections. Nevertheless, it must be emphasized that *none* of these changes inevitably leads to ED and many older men enjoy successful erections and intercourse throughout their lifetimes.

Research into sexual dysfunction in older men has also shown an association between bothersome lower urinary tract symptoms (LUTS) and ED.[14] A multinational study of 12,815 men aged 50 to 80 years in North America and western Europe has revealed a strong association between LUTS and mild to severe ED. This relationship was positively correlated with age and severity of LUTS and was independent of common comorbidities, such as diabetes mellitus, hypertension, cardiac disease, and hypercholesterolemia. The precise mechanisms for this association remain unknown.

Cardiovascular System Disorders. Because erections are a neurovascular event, it follows that disorders of the cardiovascular system represent a major risk factor for ED.[5,15] ED occurs in approximately 75% of men with stable (treated) coronary heart disease, but most do not report the condition to their cardiologist or primary care physician. Other cardiovascular disorders specifically linked with ED include atherosclerosis, dyslipidemia, and coronary artery disease.

Hypertension and its treatment are also risk factors.[1] One study of 1412 men has revealed that duration of hypertension, age, and coexisting diabetes mellitus all influence the risk.[16] The relationship between ED and hypertension is not completely understood, but erectile function has been linked to arterial stenotic lesions and local vascular factors rather than to a rise in systemic blood pressure or the severity of this elevation. In addition, antihypertensive medications may produce reversible ED, particularly diuretics, beta blockers, and α-adrenergic blocking drugs. The use of two or more antihypertensive medications is associated with a greater risk in men than when a a single agent is used.

Cigarette Smoking. Although a cause and effect relationship has not been established, long-term cigarette smoking is strongly associated with ED.[17] Although the immediate effects of smoking a cigarette do not cause erectile failure, it is known to increase circulating norepinephrine levels. Long-term smoking adversely affects the endothelium of the penile vasculature and corporal bodies and clearly increases the risk of ED. These changes increase platelet and leukocyte adherence within the cavernosal bodies and lead to the release of inflammatory substances such as cytokines, thrombogens, chemotactics, and mitogens. Adherent platelets and leukocytes induce the endothelium to release the vasoconstrictors thromboxane A_2 and serotonin. Collectively, these processes compromise the function of nitric oxide, which is critical to the generation of a successful erection. Smoking further exacerbates ED risk by amplifying the deleterious effects of associated cardiovascular diseases.

Endocrine Disorders and Diabetes Mellitus. Diabetes mellitus is a particularly potent risk factor for ED, affecting 75% to 80% of men diagnosed with diabetes for 10 years or longer.[18,19] The pathogenesis of ED in men with diabetes mellitus is multifactorial and only partly understood. Both animal and human studies have demonstrated that nitric oxide synthase and nitric oxide levels are reduced in diabetes mellitus.

Specific aspects of diabetes associated with ED include autonomic and sensory polyneuropathies, vascular factors such as microangiopathies and veno-occlusive disease, and abnormal endothelial and platelet function. In addition, abnormal expression of a number of growth factors, including transforming growth factor-β (TGF-β), insulin-like growth factor, and vascular endothelial growth factor, have been associated with vasculopathies and retinopathy, and possibly with ED. Endocrine changes associated with diabetes mellitus may also exert an effect by adversely affecting serum testosterone levels and pituitary function, although the evidence for this association remains mixed.

A number of other endocrine disorders are associated with ED.[20] For example, reduction in circulating androgens reduces libido, the frequency of sexual fantasies, and the incidence of nocturnal and morning erections. Primary hypogonadism caused by Klinefelter's syndrome, prepubertal testicular trauma, orchitis, or orchiectomy leads to ED because of adverse effects on the development of the penis, prostate, and secondary male characteristics. Low androgen production also occurs in men with Cushing's syndrome, hyper- and hypothyroidism, hyperprolactinemia, and morbid obesity.

Hemachromatosis is an inherited disorder characterized by excessive absorption of iron from the gastrointestinal system.[21] Deposition of excess iron adversely affects pituitary function, causing suppression of follicle-stimulating hormone (FSH) and luteinizing hormone (LH) secretion, secondary hypogonadism, and ED. Symptoms occur during middle adulthood, and ED is likely to develop by the end of the fourth decade of life.

End-stage renal disease is frequently associated with ED.[22] The pathogenesis is probably endocrinologic; contributing factors include erythropoietin deficiency, hyperprolactinemia, diminished FSH and LH production, and anemia. Exogenous supplementation of erythropoietin frequently improves erectile function and libido by increasing testosterone, FSH, and LH levels and by correcting anemia.

Neurologic Disorders. Neurologic disorders produce ED when they adversely affect modulatory centers in the brain or spinal cord.[1] Spinal cord injury above S1 and S2 eliminates psychogenic erections, but tends to preserve reflexogenic erections. Sacral spine injuries tend to preserve psychogenic erections, but ablate reflexogenic erections. Nontraumatic disorders affecting the brain and spinal cord, such as multiple sclerosis, parkinsonism, Alzheimer's disease, and multisystem atrophy (Shy-Drager syndrome), are frequent causes of ED. For example, cerebrovascular accident (stroke) adversely influences a number of aspects of sexual function, including libido, frequency of intercourse, ejaculatory function, and erectile function, although the precise mechanisms that lead to ED remain unclear.[23]

Chronic Disease and Trauma. Chronic disease increases the risk of ED because of direct effects on erectile function or indirect sequelae, such as depression, fatigue, and functional limitations.[1] Prevalent examples include cancer,[24] chronic obstructive pulmonary disease,[25] advanced liver disease,[26] and AIDS.[27]

Pelvic or penile trauma may produce ED, probably because of local nerve damage or direct injury to the cavernosal tissue. Nerve entrapment may increase risk in long-distance cyclists,[28] and local denervation is postulated to produce the high prevalence of ED observed following pelvic fracture.[29] In addition, two penile disorders—Peyronie's disease and priapism—are associated with an increased risk of ED (see later).[30,31]

Drugs. Numerous drugs may cause reversible ED because of direct effects on the neurovascular events responsible for an erection or by reducing the desire for sexual activity (diminished libido).[32,33] Box 9-1 lists drug classes associated with ED. In addition to prescription or over-the-counter drugs, excessive intake of alcohol, as well as the misuse or abuse of illicit drugs such as opiates, marijuana, cocaine, or hallucinogens, can cause transient or ongoing loss of erectile function.

Surgery. Surgical procedures can result in central denervation, alteration of local blood flow, or changes in endocrine function. Major abdominopelvic surgery such as radical prostatectomy, radical cystectomy, anterior posterior resection, or other procedures requiring urinary or fecal diversion result in ED because of unavoidable local denervation.[34-36]

Genetic Factors. The role of genetic predisposition in ED remains unknown. However, a study of 890 pairs of male-male monozygotic and dizygotic twins has supported the hypothesis that a genetic predisposition exists for independent factors such as diabetes mellitus or hypertension.[37] Further research is needed to determine the extent to which genetic factors influence the risk of ED.

BOX 9-1 Commonly Used Medications for Erectile Dysfunction

α-Adrenergic Agonists
Ephedrine
Pseudoephedrine

Antianxiety Agents
Diazepam
Flurazepam

Antidepressants
Tricyclics
Selective serotonin reuptake inhibitors
Monoamine oxidase inhibitors

Antihypertensives
Nonselective Beta Blockers
Carvedilol
Bucindolol
Propranolol
Nadolol
Timolol

Selective Beta Blockers
Metoprolol
Atenolol
Esmolol
Bisoprolol

α-Adrenergic Blockers
Doxazosin
Terazosin

Calcium Channel Blockers
Amlodipine
Diltiazem
Nifedipine
Verapamil

Angiotensin-Converting Enzyme Inhibitors
Captopril
Enalapril

Cardiac Glycosides
Digoxin
Digitoxin

Diuretics
Thiazide Diuretics
Hydrochlorothiazide
Polythiazide

Potassium-sparing Diuretics
Amiloride
Spironolactone

Histamine-2 Antihistaminic Antacids
Cimetidine
Ranitidine

Nonsteroidal Anti-inflammatory Drugs
Indomethacin
Naproxen

Psychological Factors. Although essentially every case of ED produces secondary psychosocial distress in all men, psychological causes produce ED in some men.[38] Psychogenic ED is particularly common in younger men. Psychological factors frequently associated with ED in younger men include sexual abuse, paraphilia (atypical or unusual sexual fantasies), and gender identity problems. Among older men, death of a spouse, deterioration of a relationship or divorce, serious vocational problems, or a change in the partner's health status are common contributing factors.

Assessment

As therapeutic options for managing ED continue to expand, the setting for its evaluation and treatment has shifted from a urologic (specialty practice) environment to the primary care setting.[39] The urologic nurse, and the advanced practice nurse in particular, are likely to encounter men undergoing evaluation and management in both settings.

Initial Evaluation. Because of the embarrassment and negative psychosocial consequences associated with ED, active screening is critical to its initial evaluation.[40] Routine screening by primary care providers should be completed in men younger than 50 years with specific risk factors, including diabetes mellitus and cardiovascular disease, and in all men aged 50 years and older. A simple query such as, "Are you experiencing any problems with erections?" provides patients and their partners with permission to discuss this embarrassing and often hidden problem. Inclusion of the partner whenever feasible is important because the patient is likely to have discussed ED with the partner, and sexual partners often participate in the decision to seek health care.[41]

Key questions related to ED include the onset of the problem, its duration, and the most recent attempt at sexual activity.[39] These questions can provide valuable clues that allow initial differentiation between ED related to organic factors and ED primarily caused by psychological distress. A sudden onset of ED that is situational in nature and associated with rigid erections outside of sexual intercourse, in the context of an emotionally stressful event or circumstance, often indicates psychogenic ED. In contrast, a gradual onset of erectile difficulties, occurring with regularity despite varying circumstances and associated with poor erectile quality outside of attempts at intercourse, especially combined with medical risk factors, usually indicates a strong organic component.

The medical history includes prevalent risk factors, such as cardiovascular disorders, diabetes mellitus or related endocrine disorders, cigarette smoking, neurologic disease, and chronic illness such as cancer or chronic obstructive pulmonary disease. The clinician queries the patient about his surgical history, particularly focusing on major abdominopelvic surgery, neurosurgical procedures, and pelvic trauma.

The physical examination focuses on the male reproductive system, assessing normal and abnormal genital development. The perineal area is examined for hair distribution and the entire body for signs of secondary male characteristics. The penis is examined for size and evidence of chordee or Peyronie's disease, and the testes are evaluated for size and consistency. The breasts are examined for signs of gynecomastia and the male diabetic is assessed for evidence of peripheral or autonomic polyneuropathies. A neurologic examination is performed; this includes assessment of perineal and genital sensation, anal sphincter tone, and bulbocavernosus reflex. The blood pressure should be checked if a man presents to a physician or nurse practitioner with a specific complaint of ED who has not undergone routine physical assessment within the last 6 months or longer.

The use of laboratory tests in the evaluation of ED is strongly influenced by the patient's medical history, presence of known risk factors, and the results of a careful history and physical examination. For some patients, treatment may be initiated with limited testing, although men with no apparent risk factors or who have not sought regular health care may require more extensive evaluation prior to initiating treatment. Laboratory analysis is recommended to characterize or identify diabetes mellitus (fasting glucose or glycosylated hemoglobin level), hyperlipidemia (lipid profile), and hypothalamic-pituitary-gonadal function (free or bioavailable serum testosterone) unless these conditions have been recently evaluated. Optional testing recommendations include measurement of serum prolactin, LH, and thyroid-stimulating hormone levels. A complete blood count and urinalysis may prove useful screening for the man who has not had recent contact with any healthcare provider.[42]

Urologic Evaluation. In addition to these tests, evaluation of ED in a urologic clinic or office may include more complex or specialized testing and further exploration of symptoms of sexual dysfunction via a self-administered symptom score. Several instruments have been developed that possess reasonable reliability and validity, including the International Index of Erectile Function short form (IIEF-5) (Figure 9-1),[43] the Brief Male Sexual Function Inventory (Figure 9-2),[44] and the Erectile Dysfunction Intensity Scale[39,42] (Figure 9-3).

Urologic testing frequently includes intracavernous injection with alprostadil to determine the ability to generate an erection. Alprostadil is an analogue of prostaglandin E_1 (PGE_1), known to stimulate an erection when injected into the cavernosal body. Because testing is completed within a clinic setting, provision of maximal privacy and additional stimulation are strongly recommended to maximize the resulting erection.[45] Duplex ultrasonography or dynamic infusion cavernosometry and cavernosography may be obtained in selected cases when injection fails to produce an adequate erection (see Chapter 4). Dynamic infusion cavernosometry, cavernosography, radioisotopic penography, or arteriography is performed only in highly selected cases.

Complex testing for ED includes nocturnal penile tumescence testing. A RigiScan device is typically used because it allows evaluation of the number and duration of erections, as well as a measure of their rigidity. Neurologic testing may be used in highly selected cases, including biothesiometry, sacral evoked response testing, and bulbocavernosus reflex latency assessment.

International Index of Erectile Function (IIEF-5)

This questionnaire is designed to help you and your doctor determine if you may be experiencing ED. Knowing everything you can about ED means you're better prepared to make the most important step of all: getting treatment.

In answering the questions, the following definitions apply:
Sexual stimulation includes situations such as foreplay, erotic pictures, etc.
Sexual intercourse is defined as sexual penetration of your partner.

Over the past 6 months:

1. How do you rate your **confidence** that you could get and keep an erection?
   ☐ Very low
   ☐ Low
   ☐ Moderate
   ☐ High
   ☐ Very high

2. When you had erections with sexual stimulation, **how often** were your erections hard enough for penetration (entering your partner)?
   ☐ Almost never/never
   ☐ A few times (much less than half the time)
   ☐ Sometimes (about half the time)
   ☐ Most times (much more than half the time)
   ☐ Almost always/always

3. During sexual intercourse, **how often** were you able to maintain your erection after you had penetrated (entered) your partner?
   ☐ Almost never/never
   ☐ A few times (much less than half the time)
   ☐ Sometimes (about half the time)
   ☐ Most times (much more than half the time)
   ☐ Almost always/always

4. During sexual intercourse, **how difficult** was it to maintain your erection to completion of intercourse?
   ☐ Extremely difficult
   ☐ Very difficult
   ☐ Difficult
   ☐ Slightly difficult
   ☐ Not difficult

5. When you attempted sexual intercourse, **how often** was it satisfactory for you?
   ☐ Almost never/never
   ☐ A few times (much less than half the time)
   ☐ Sometimes (about half the time)
   ☐ Most times (much more than half the time)
   ☐ Almost always/always

Fig. 9-1 International Index of Erectile Function short form (IIEF-5) combines 4 items taken from the IIEF-15 (a longer form used primarily for research purposes) with a single item that queries the patient's satisfaction with intercourse. Scores of 5-7 indicate severe ED, scores of 8-11 indicate moderate ED, scores ranging from 12-16 indicate mild to moderate ED, and scores of 17-21 indicate very mild ED. Scores of 21 or higher indicate normal erectile function.[43]

Nursing Management

The management of ED changed forever during the last decade of the twentieth century when research revealed the role of nitric oxide and phosphodiesterases in erectile function, leading to the development of three oral agents used to manage ED.[46] However, it must be pointed out that the introduction of effective oral medications comprises only one component of a management plan necessary when men and their partners seek to overcome ED.

Brief Male Sexual Function Inventory

SEXUAL DRIVE

Let's define sexual drive as a feeling that may include wanting to have a sexual experience (masturbation or intercourse), thinking about having sex, or feeling frustrated due to lack of sex.

1. During the past 30 days, on how many days have you felt a sexual drive?

No days	A few days	Some days	Most days	Almost every day
0	1	2	3	4

2. During the past 30 days, how would you rate your level of sexual drive?

None	Low	Medium	Medium high	High
0	1	2	3	4

ERECTIONS

3. Over the past 30 days, how often have you had partial or full sexual erections when you were sexually stimulated in any way?

Not at all	A few times	Fairly often	Usually	Always
0	1	2	3	4

4. Over the past 30 days when you had erections, how often were they firm enough to have sexual intercourse?

0	1	2	3	4

5. How much difficulty did you have getting an erection during the past 30 days?

Did not get erections	A lot	Some	A little	No difficulty
0	1	2	3	4

EJACULATION

6. In the past 30 days, how much difficulty have you had ejaculating when you have been sexually stimulated?

No sexual stimulation	A lot	Some	A little	No difficulty
0	1	2	3	4

7. In the past 30 days, how much did you consider the amount of semen you ejaculated to be a problem for you?

Did not climax	Big problem	Medium problem	Small problem	No problem
0	1	2	3	4

PROBLEM ASSESSMENT

8. In the past 30 days, to what extent have you considered a lack of sex drive to be a problem?

Big problem	Medium problem	Small problem	Very small problem	No problem
0	1	2	3	4

9. In the past 30 days, to what extent have you considered your ability to get and keep erections to be a problem?

0	1	2	3	4

10. In the past 30 days, to what extent have you considered your ejaculation to be a problem?

0	1	2	3	4

OVERALL SATISFACTION

11. Overall, during the past 30 days, how satisfied have you been with your sex life?

Very dissatisfied	Mostly dissatisfied	Neutral or mixed	Mostly satisfied	Very satisfied
0	1	2	3	4

Fig. 9-2 The Brief Male Sexual Function Inventory comprises 11 items covering 5 domains: (1) erectile function, (2) ejaculation, (3) libido, (4) magnitude of bother associated with symptoms of erectile or ejaculatory symptoms, and (5) overall satisfaction with sexual function. Individual items are scored from 0-4. However, because the instrument queries multiple domains of sexual function, no meaningful summary score can be generated from this instrument.

Erectile Dysfunction Intensity Scale[39,42]

	Almost never or never	A few times (much less than half the time)	Sometimes (about half the time)	Most times (much more than half the time)	Almost always
How often were you able to get an erection during sexual activity?	1	2	3	4	5
When you had erections with sexual stimulation, how often were your erections hard enough for penetration (entering your partner)?	1	2	3	4	5
When you attempted intercourse, how often were you able to penetrate (enter) your partner?	1	2	3	4	5
During sexual intercourse, how often were you able to maintain your erection after you had penetrated (entered) your partner?	1	2	3	4	5
	Extremely difficult	Very difficult	Difficult	Slightly difficult	Not difficult
During sexual intercourse, how difficult was it to maintain your erection to completion of intercourse?	1	2	3	4	5

ED INTENSITY SCORE

Fig. 9-3 The Erectile Dysfunction Intensity Scale comprises five items that rate the ability to generate and maintain an erection adequate for vaginal penetration. A total score ranging from 5 to 10 indicates severe ED, scores ranging from 11 to 15 indicate moderate ED, and those between 16 to 20 indicate mild ED. Scores of 21 or more indicate normal erectile function.

Prevention. Little is known about primary prevention of ED, although studies of probable risk factors, such as smoking, alcohol consumption, obesity, and a sedentary lifestyle, have suggested several possible strategies. Data from the Massachusetts Male Aging Study have suggested that smoking cessation during middle adulthood, following a long history of smoking since late adolescence or early adulthood, may not reduce ED risk.[47] Similar results were observed in men who reduced alcohol intake after a long history of heavy consumption or those who reduced body weight after a long-term history of obesity. In contrast, initiating a program of regular exercise was found to reduce the risk of ED. Based on these relatively disappointing results, the researchers hypothesized that modification of these risk factors must occur earlier in life to reduce the risk of subsequent ED significantly.

Long-distance bicycling has also been associated with genital numbness, perineal compression, reduced penile blood flow, and reductions in local tissue oxygenation.[48] When four different seat designs were compared, it was found that absence of the anterior nose was most effective in reducing perineal compression

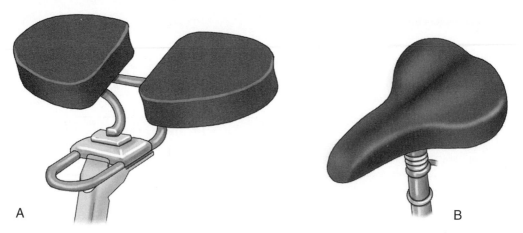

Fig. 9-4 An example of (**A**) a bicycle seat designed to reduce the risk of ED and (**B**) a traditional bicycle seat.

and declines in tissue oxygen pressure. Data from the Massachusetts Male Aging Study also found that prolonged bicycling (more than 3 hours/week) increased the risk of ED, although cycling for less than 3 hours/week was associated with a reduced incidence of ED.[49] These observations lend further support to arguments that cycling while in a seated position should be reduced to no more than 3 hours/week or the cyclist should equip the bicycle with a seat without an anterior nose, thus preventing direct compression of perineal and penile vessels (Figure 9-4).

Education and Counseling. For a small number of men, anxiety about ED occurs despite evidence of normal erectile function. Misconceptions may arise from cultural or personal perceptions about sexual function, such as false expectations that an erection is a merely mechanical event that a male should be able to generate, with little or no regard to psychosocial context. Others may define themselves as impotent if they do not engage in sexual activity on a regular basis, such as once a night or even more often. In these cases, counseling about normal male sexual function, and the highly variable frequency of sexual encounters, provides reassurance and avoids the risks associated with more aggressive treatments.

Men who experience ED may also suffer from significant psychological distress that causes or contributes to their dysfunction. Psychological counseling, ideally involving the man and his sexual partner, should be initiated first, because treatment may correct ED or alleviate psychological barriers that prevent an adequate response to other treatments.

Tailoring Medications. Because many drugs may influence erectile function, careful selection of medications may alleviate or relieve erectile failure. For example, nonselective beta blockers, statins, and[39] thiazide diuretics are associated with ED in men with cardiovascular disease and hypertension. In some cases, switching a patient to an alternative agent,[15] such as substituting an angiotensin-converting enzyme (ACE) inhibitor, may relieve ED in a man with hypertension. The urologic nurse can function effectively as a patient advocate through close consultation with the urologist and internist or primary care physicians when considering medication alterations for the management of ED.

Pelvic Floor Muscle Rehabilitation. Pelvic floor muscle rehabilitation has been shown to improve erectile function in many patients with ED and venous leakage.[50,51] Biofeedback techniques are used to teach the man to identify, isolate, contract, and relax the pelvic floor muscles. Muscle exercises may be completed daily or twice daily; many clinicians and researchers recommend completing exercises in different positions (e.g., supine, sitting, standing). Neuromuscular re-education (skill training) may include tightening the pelvic floor muscles rhythmically during sexual activity to maximize penile rigidity or forceful contraction of the pelvic muscles to delay premature ejaculation.[50] See Chapter 6 for a more detailed description of pelvic floor muscle rehabilitation.

Vacuum Erection Devices. Vacuum erection devices (VEDs) combine a cylinder to enhance

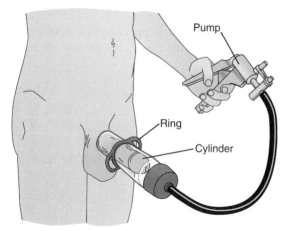

Fig. 9-5 A vacuum erection device combines a constrictive band and tube capable of creating negative pressure needed to promote blood flow. The constrictive device is placed at the base of the tube, which is placed over the penile shaft in an airtight fashion. Negative pressure is applied to the tube, promoting blood flow to the corpora cavernosa. When an erection is achieved, the constrictive bland is slipped off the base of the tube near the base of the penis, thus trapping blood within the cavernosal bodies. (From Lewis S, Heitkemper M, Dirksen S, et al: Medical Surgical Nursing, 7th edition. St. Louis: Mosby, 2008.)

penile blood flow mechanically and a flexible ring device placed at the penile base to trap blood in the penis and ensure an adequate erection (Figure 9-5). Long-term success relies on the patient's ability to become proficient with its use. VEDs appear to be preferred by persons with moderate ED, and they tend to use the device for prolonged periods.[52] As with many treatment options, the role of VEDs in ED management has evolved because of the introduction of oral agents. For example, in one study, a group of 52 men who had successfully managed ED by a VED agreed to switch to sildenafil therapy.[53] Although 67% preferred to continue oral therapy, 33% returned to the VED, primarily because they preferred to avoid the adverse side effects associated with oral agents.

Nursing management focuses on teaching the patient, and ideally the partner, to use the device, ensuring that the constriction ring is removed within about 30 minutes of application and monitoring for adverse events. Adverse effects associated with VED are uncommon and typically mild. The most common are duskiness, bruising, or ecchymosis of the penile skin. More severe complications are rare; these include single case reports of urethral bleeding, necrosis of the penile skin,

or inadvertent entrapment of a testis.[54,55] Ischemic complications are managed by teaching the patient to monitor the penis after application of the constriction ring and to ensure prompt removal after sexual activity. Entrapment of a testis is managed by promptly cutting the ring with a pair of scissors.

Hormonal Treatments. Hormonal supplementation is indicated only when an endocrine imbalance (e.g., deficit or hypersecretion of a hormone) is diagnosed.[56] Hypogonadism, characterized by loss of libido, depression, decreased lean body mass with increased visceral fat, changes in hair distribution, loss of skin turgor, and ED, is managed by testosterone replacement. Oral therapies are typically avoided because of the risk of long-term adverse effects. Instead, depot injections of testosterone may be given every 2 to 4 weeks. These preparations provide an initial surge of testosterone rising above physiologic needs, followed by a steady decline over a period of 2 to 3 weeks. Several transdermal formulations of testosterone are available, including several patches and a gel. One patch must be applied to the scrotum, but newer versions can be placed on the abdomen or hip. Because various factors may affect absorption, a serum testosterone level should be obtained 2 to 3 weeks after therapy is initiated and the dosage titrated accordingly. A transdermal testosterone gel is also available. It is applied daily and dries quickly, in less than 5 minutes. It may avoid some of the skin irritation associated with patch application but require rotations of application sites, as recommended for most transdermal patch delivery systems.

For the urologic nurse, patient teaching includes education about dosage and administration of specific testosterone preparations and about the recognition and management of potential adverse effects. Men are taught to rotate sites, inspect the underlying skin, and apply barrier creams to irritated skin as indicated; those using androgen gel are advised to wear an undershirt when likely to have close contact with a female partner. Men using parenteral testosterone supplementation are counseled about the varying serum levels associated with depot injections, including breast tenderness and gynecomastia. Men are also advised about the need for monitoring for vascular side effects with long-term therapy. Erythrocytosis is particularly common after 3 months or longer of treatment, and regular laboratory testing is indicated. Finally, men and their partners must be allowed to express any fears or concerns related to prostate cancer. Although existing prostate cancer is a strong contraindication to therapy, treatment has not been linked with the development of cancer in men with hypogonadism and a normal prostate.[57,58]

Oral Agents. As noted earlier, the development of the phosphodiesterase type 5 (PDE5) inhibitor reflects a significant advance in the treatment of ED, and this is the class of drugs most commonly used in North America.[39,59] Nevertheless, various other drugs have been prescribed for ED. This discussion will review a number of agents that may or may not posses a specific indication for the management of ED provided by the U.S. or Canadian Food and Drug Administration (FDA).

Yohimbine is an α_2-adrenergic agonist obtained from the bark of the *Corynanthe yohimbe* tree. It promotes erectile function by promoting adrenergic receptor activity and altering dopamine and serotonin activity in the central nervous system.[39] Clinical trials with yohimbine have shown modest efficacy when compared with a placebo in men with organic ED.[60] In contrast, yohimbine has shown greater efficacy when given to men with psychogenic ED (62% to 71%).[61,62] The urologic nurse can reassure men that side effects are typically mild, but may include headache, anxiety, and a slight increase in blood pressure.

Trazodone is a serotonin reuptake inhibitor typically prescribed as an antidepressant.[63] Because priapism is an occasional adverse event of trazodone, it has been tried as a treatment for ED. Unfortunately, there is little evidence supporting its efficacy in men with organic or psychogenic ED.[64]

As noted in the introduction of this chapter, the use of PDE5 inhibitors has revolutionized the management of ED. Three agents have been approved for the management of ED in the United States and Canada—sildenafil, vardenafil, and tadalafil. Refer to the box, Clinical Highlights for Advanced and Expert Practice: Phosphodiesterase Inhibitors in the Management of Erectile Dysfunction in Men, for a detailed discussion of PDE5 inhibitors for the management of ED.

Apomorphine is a dopaminergic agonist, with affinity for both D_1 and D_2 receptor subtypes. It acts on dopaminergic receptors in the paraventricular nucleus, an area known to modulate the sexual drive in animals. Like the phosphodiesterase inhibitors, clinical studies have shown that the drug enhances erectile function only when stimulation for sexual activity occurs. It has undergone clinical testing in the United States, the United Kingdom, and western Europe.[39]

Intraurethral Agents. Alprostadil may be administered by intraurethral insertion of a small pellet (Figure 9-6, *A*). The recommended dosage is 500 μg and the 1- × 3-mm pellet is administered into the distal urethra by a proprietary device. During clinical trials, 65% of subjects reported successful intercourse,[65] but the response rate observed with home use in a clinical setting is approximately 43%.[39] Nursing care of men treated with intraurethral alprostadil focuses on correct use of the insertion device and management of the most common adverse effect, urethral discomfort. The patient is advised to hold the penis in an upright position when inserting the pellet and to leave it in this position when the applicator is removed from the meatus. He is further taught to roll the penis firmly between his hands while maintaining the meatus in an upright position to ensure absorption and prevent inadvertent dislodgment. Discomfort associated with intraurethral injection may be perceived as a dull ache in the penis, scrotum, and lower extremities and is thought to arise from venous pooling. If burning occurs, urinating just prior to insertion of the urethral suppository and rubbing the penis for an additional 30 to 60 seconds may help. Hypotension or fainting occurs in 1% to 6% of cases and the patient is advised to administer the drug in a sitting position to prevent injury if these side effects occur.

Intracavernous Injections. Intracavernous injections have evolved from a first-line pharmacologic option to their current role as a second- or third-line treatment option, and their role in the urologic evaluation of ED.[39,66] Three principal agents are used in North America. Alprostadil is the only agent approved by the U.S. FDA for the management of ED. It is an analogue of prostaglandin E and stimulates an erection through interaction with cyclic adenosine monophosphate (cAMP), resulting in smooth muscle relaxation. Alprostadil is injected into a cavernosal body of the mid to distal penile shaft by the patient using a proprietary delivery system; this provokes an erection adequate for vaginal penetration in 70% to 80% of men.[39] Two additional agents, papaverine—a vasodilating agent that

Clinical Highlights for Advanced and Expert Practice: Phosphodiesterase Inhibitors in the Management of Erectile Dysfunction in Men

Introduction

Phosphodiesterases are a family of enzymes critical to a wide variety of human metabolic function. One member of this enzymatic family, phosphodiesterase type 5 (PDE5), breaks down an enzyme critical to erectile function, cyclic guanosine monophosphate (cGMP). PDE5 inhibitors inhibit the catabolism of cGMP in the sinusoids of the penile corpora cavernosa, thus potentiating the physiologic actions of nitric oxide, the primary neurotransmitter responsible for sinusoidal engorgement and tumescence.

Agent

Sildenafil (Viagra)

Action

Selectively inhibits phosphodiesterase typ. 5

Efficacy

56%-84% in a clinical trial of 4526 subjects receiving 25-100 mg[96]

Dosage and Administration

25-100 mg

Nursing Management

The initial dose is 25 to 50 mg; the total dosage may be titrated to 100 mg but no more than a single dose should be taken in a 24-hour period. Phosphodiesterase inhibitors are contraindicated in men taking nitrates, including any nitroglycerin, isosorbide, or amyl nitrate. Any exceptions to this contraindication are based on consultation with the patient, urologist, and cardiologist and should be accompanied by careful and thorough disclosures of accompanying risks for adverse effects related to very low blood pressure. An α_1-adrenergic blocker such as alfuzosin or tamsulosin may produce significant hypotension in some men and should not be taken within 4 hours of a single dose of sildenafil. The patient is also advised to discuss the use of prescriptive or over-the-counter drugs such as cimetidine, ketoconazole, mibefradil, rifampin, or itraconazole, which may produce adverse interactions if administered with sildenafil.

Sildenafil is typically administered 1 hour prior to anticipated sexual activity. Men are counseled to avoid a high-fat meal when taking sildenafil because it may slow absorption and the onset of its action. If a heavy meal is eaten, the patient is advised to take the medication 2 hours prior to sexual activity. Men are counseled that PDE5 inhibitors enhance erectile function, but they do not directly stimulate an erection. Therefore, stimulation within an appropriate psychosocial context for each man is necessary for the drug to be effective. Sildenafil should be taken no more than once daily and the patient should avoid strenuous physical activity for several hours following a dose, particularly if the activity occurs in a hot or humid climate. Men and their partners should be warned that sildenafil will not protect a female partner from impregnation or any partner from a sexually transmitted disease; therefore, birth control and safe sex methods must be used when engaging in sexual activity. All men should be warned of potential adverse effects, including headache; flushing of the face, neck, or upper chest; and visual effects such as a blue or green haze.

Agent

Vardenafil (Levitra)

Action

Selective inhibitor of PDE5

Dosage and Administration

5-20 mg

Efficacy

58%-62% satisfaction versus 23% (placebo) with 10 or 20 mg in a clinical trial of 805 subjects[97]

Continued

Clinical Highlights for Advanced and Expert Practice: Phosphodiesterase Inhibitors in the Management of Erectile Dysfunction in Men—cont'd

Nursing Management

The initial dose is usually 10 mg taken 25 to 60 minutes prior to sexual activity. Older patients and those with mild to moderate hepatic or renal function impairment should be given an initial dose of no more than 5 mg. No more than one dose should be taken within a 24-hour period. Similar to sildenafil, its use is contraindicated in patients receiving nitrates or nitric oxide donors, such as amyl nitrate. Any exceptions to this contraindication are based on consultation with the patient, urologist, and cardiologist and should be accompanied by careful and thorough disclosures of accompanying risks for adverse effects related to very low blood pressure. Concomitant use with an α_1-adrenergic blocker such as alfuzosin or tamsulosin may produce significant hypotension in some men and is contraindicated. Adverse effects include flushing, headache, nausea, dizziness, and rhinitis. The patient is also advised to discuss the use of prescriptive or over-the-counter drugs, including CYP3A4 inhibitors such as ritonavir or ketoconazole. Concomitant intake of grapefruit juice is also contraindicated because of the likelihood of increasing serum levels of vardenafil.

Agent
Tadalafil

Action
Selective inhibitor of PDE5 inhibitor

Dosage and Administration
5-20 mg

Efficacy
58% successful intercourse in a group of 4262 men receiving 20 mg on demand or three times weekly (some with diabetes)[98]

Nursing Management

Initial dosage is usually 10 mg given within 36 hours of anticipated sexual activity; no more than one dose of tadalafil should be taken within a 72-hour period. The half-life of tadalafil (17 hours) is significantly different than that of sildenafil or vardenafil, and men who have been managed by one or both of these agents should be carefully counseled about differences in dosage frequency and anticipated duration of effect. The initial dose is reduced to 5 mg in men with mild to moderate hepatic function impairment. No dose adjustment is required for men with mild renal function impairment, but those with moderate impairment should be started on a 5-mg dose. Administration of tadalafil is contraindicated for patients receiving nitrates or nitric oxide donors, such as amyl nitrate or butyl nitrate, which may cause a transient decrease in blood pressure. Therefore, patients taking these medications must do so only in close consultation with a urologist and cardiologist. In addition, treatment must be accompanied by careful and thorough disclosures of accompanying risks for adverse effects related to transient lowering of blood pressure. Concomitant use with an α_1-adrenergic blocker such as alfuzosin or tamsulosin also may produce significant hypotension in some men and is contraindicated. Adverse effects include flushing, headache, nausea, dizziness, and rhinitis. Similar to vardenafil, patients taking CYP3A4 inhibitors such as ritonavir or ketoconazole should take no more than 10 mg of tadalafil every 72 hours. Adverse effects include headache, dyspepsia, nasal congestion, and flushing. Unlike other drugs in this class, thoracolumbar back pain and myalgia affecting the lower extremities occur in 1% to 6% of patients. They are typically mild to moderate and occur within 12 to 24 hours of administration. If these adverse effects occur, the patient may be advised that they typically resolve within 48 hours. Subsequent clinical trials with tadalafil have revealed no associated neuromuscular inflammation or renal damage. These symptoms may be exacerbated when the patient lies down, and treatment with a nonsteroidal anti-inflammatory drug typically relieves back pain or general myalgia.

promotes erectile function through actions on cAMP and cyclic guanosine monophosphate (cGMP)—and phentolamine—an α-adrenergic agonist—also have been injected to stimulate erection. Mixtures of these agents, such as papaverine plus phentolamine or papaverine plus phentolamine plus alprostadil, have been used,[39,66,67] but have not undergone extensive clinical trials and represent off-label prescribing.

Nursing management of the man with ED undergoing injection therapy focuses on accurate preparation of

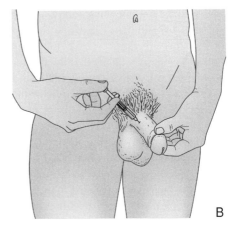

Pellet

A   B

Fig. 9-6 A, Intraurethral injection of alprostadil for ED. The penis is held upright and a small suppository or pellet is inserted into the urethra. Pressure must be applied to ensure adequate absorption of the drug. **B,** Intravenous injection of PGE1. (From Lewis S, Heitkemper M, Dirksen S, et al: Medical Surgical Nursing, 7th edition. St. Louis: Mosby, 2008.)

the 27- to 28-gauge syringe, filling the syringe with an accurate dose, injecting the drug into a cavernosal body while avoiding superficial veins or the urethra, and monitoring for adverse side effects (Figure 9-6, *B*).[68] After drawing the proper dosage of medication, the patient is advised to grasp the penis near its base and pull the skin taut. An injection site is chosen on the distal two thirds of the penile shaft and several centimeters proximal to the glans penis; rotation is recommended. Following injection, the patient is taught to apply pressure to the area. An erection will develop within several minutes of injection and should persist for 30 to 90 minutes.

Adverse effects associated with cavernosal injections include bleeding or pain at the injection site, flushing or dizziness, syncope, or prolonged and painful erection (priapism). Bleeding is managed by prolonged pressure against the injection site. This strategy also assists to manage pain, which typically subsides within 5 to 7 minutes of injection. Dizziness or facial flushing sometimes may progress to syncope. Therefore, the man is advised to lie down for about 10 minutes and alert his partner about the side effect. The management of priapism is discussed later in this chapter.

Surgery. Surgery is considered only after conservative or pharmacologic methods have been fully explored. With improved nonsurgical alternatives, the number of penile prostheses has declined, from approximately 29,000 in 1991 to 12,000 in 2000.[69,70] A number of prostheses are available that are

generally divided into two broad categories, malleable and inflatable.[71] Malleable prostheses, sometimes called semirigid devices, retain rigidity, but newer designs allow the patient to conceal the device under clothing more easily (Figure 9-7, *A*). Paired rods are constructed of silicone rubber or contain an intertwined metallic core or polytetrafluoroethylene rings connected via a spring-loaded cable and implanted into the corpora cavernosa.

Inflatable prostheses incorporate hydraulics into a two- or three-piece prosthesis that more closely mimics the erect and flaccid state than a malleable device. Two-piece systems are composed of self-contained paired cylinders that are implanted into the cavernosal bodies. The three-piece system also incorporates a scrotal pump and reservoir that is placed suprapubically (Figure 9-7, *B*).

Vascular procedures can also be classified according to two major categories—penile revascularization and repair of veno-occlusive disease.[71] Vascular surgery is highly individualized depending on the needs of the patient, and the indications for these procedures are limited. Relative contraindications to vascular surgery include diabetes mellitus, cigarette smoking, neurologic disease, and arterial disease. Younger patients with a history of trauma causing ED are often considered the best candidates for vascular surgery.

Nursing management of the patient undergoing implantation of a penile prosthesis begins with preoperative counseling, ideally involving both partners.[72]

The patient and partner are shown a model of the prosthesis and instructed about its use. They are further advised that the erection created following implantation of a prosthesis will be slightly shorter than erections obtained prior to the onset of ED and that the glans penis will not be as firm because of the limited cylinder length that can be safely implanted. In addition, they are warned that implantation will impair responsiveness to pharmacologic agents. There is also a rare possibility that it may need to be removed because of infection or mechanical problems. Following surgery, the patient is counseled that an indwelling catheter is typically left in place for the first postoperative day, depending on the type of implant and surgeon's preference. The patient is counseled to avoid any shaving of the groin area for 2 weeks before surgery and he may be asked to cleanse the groin with an antimicrobial soap such as chlorhexidine (Hibiclens) on the morning of surgery.

Infection is the principal complication associated with implantation of a penile prosthesis. Patients with diabetes mellitus or spinal cord injury are at greatest risk. Infection must be avoided because of the risk for colonization of the device and formation of a biofilm (see Chapter 5). Clinical symptoms associated with infection include fever, penile pain, and erythema or induration over the prosthesis, with subsequent erosion

through the skin. The incidence of prosthetic infection is about 1% to 9%,[71] and gram-positive pathogens are the most common organisms responsible. Symptomatic infection may be treated by explantation of the device, aggressive antibiotic treatment, and reimplantation at a future date. This approach is effective, but scarring of the corporal bodies may occur, and the patient may lose an additional 1 to 1.5 inches of effective erectile length.[73] Clinically apparent infection not associated with erosion through the skin may be managed by removal, irrigation of local tissues with an antiseptic solution, and immediate reimplantation of a new device. Chronic pain associated with a prosthesis may indicate subclinical colonization and may be managed with systemic antibiotics. Clearly, prevention is the best strategy and the patient is taught to monitor the penis and groin regularly for signs and symptoms of infection and to advise his physician, surgeon, or dentist of the presence of the implant prior to any invasive procedure so that suppressive antibiotics may be given.

Following implantation, pain may be managed by opioid analgesics, local application of an ice bag, and scrotal elevation using a supportive bridge. Prophylactic antimicrobial medications should be take for approximately 1 week as prescribed, and the patient is warned to avoid sexual activity for 6 to 8 weeks following surgery. Premature use of the

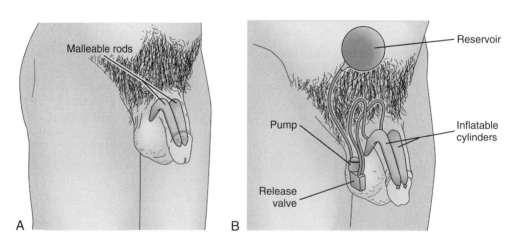

Fig. 9-7 A, Malleable penile prostheses use an intertwined metallic core or polytetrafluorethylene rings connected via a spring loaded cable to achieve sufficient rigidity for vaginal penetration and allow the patient to hide the device underneath clothing when not engaged in sexual activity. **B,** A three-piece inflatable penile prothesis more closely mimics the erect and flaccid states. To create an erection, the pump is squeezed several times, baffling fluid from the resevoir to the inflatable cylinders. Activation of the release valve moves fluid back into the resevoir, restoring a flaccid state. (From Lewis S, Heitkemper M, Dirksen S, et al: Medical Surgical Nursing, 7th edition. St. Louis: Mosby, 2008.)

device may interfere with proper healing and lead to infection or mechanical problems. The patient should also avoid lifting an object weighing more than 5 pounds for several weeks to prevent excessive tension against suture lines. The man and his partner also may be advised that the typical life span for a prosthesis, when subjected to regular use, is about 10 years.

Nursing management of patients undergoing vascular surgery for ED also begins with careful preoperative discussion concerning the goals of the procedure and realistic expectations for immediate and long-term outcomes. This counseling includes disclosure of two potentially adverse effects, hypesthesia and penile shortening caused by scar formation. The patient is advised to anticipate penile swelling that persists for 2 to 3 weeks following surgery.

PEYRONIE'S DISEASE

Peyronie's disease occurs when a penile plaque (induration) causes curvature and/or pain of sufficient magnitude to impair erectile function and sexual performance (Figure 9-8, A, B).[30,74] Little is known about its epidemiology; it typically occurs during the fifth decade of life and is estimated to affect less than 0.5% of men in North America. This estimate includes only men with sufficiently severe function to prompt them to seek help; autopsy studies have revealed an incidence as high as 22%.

The cause of Peyronie's disease is not well understood; blunt trauma is thought to lead to bleeding within the layers of the tunica albuginea. Plaque formation occurs when fibrin is trapped in inflammatory cells, leading to overexpression of specific cytokines and growth factors such as TGF-β and inhibition of metalloproteinases. Potential risk factors include Paget's disease, Dupuytren's contracture, and autoimmune disease.[75]

Assessment

During the early stages of plaque formation, a palpable nodule or plaque can be palpated and the patient will report pain associated with erection. This plaque will harden over time, with penile curvature and ED.[74] Palpation of the penile shaft usually reveals a hardened nodule or induration on the dorsal surface of the flaccid penis, although lateral and ventral plaques sometimes occur. Penile pain usually reaches a crescendo during erection or sexual activity in the earlier stages of plaque formation; this will gradually subside over the next 6 months. The diagnosis is based primarily on physical findings, although an ultrasound or color duplex ultrasonography following intracavernous injection may be performed to delineate vascular flow within the penis.

Nursing Management

Reassurance may be sufficient for certain men with a mild curvature that does not compromise erectile function. Men with more severe plaques and ED or chronic pain with erection are initially managed by

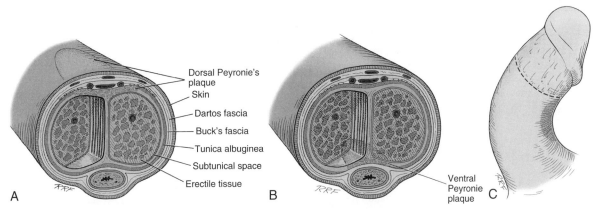

Fig. 9-8 Peyronie's disease plaque formation can form (**A**) dorsally or (**B**) ventrally. **C,** An erection demonstrates the dorsal curvature of the penis caused by the inelastic scar tissue in a dorsal plaque of Peyronie's disease. The incision to be made in the scar of the previous circumcision has been marked. (From Wein AJ, Kavoussi LR, Novick AC, Partin AW, Peters CA (eds): Campbell-Walsh Urology, 9th edition. Philadelphia: -Saunders, 2007.)

Labels in figure:
Dorsal Peyronie's plaque
Skin
Dartos fascia
Buck's fascia
Tunica albuginea
Subtunical space
Erectile tissue
Ventral Peyronie plaque

pharmacologic agents taken orally or injected directly into the penile lesion, such as potassium aminobenzoate, tamoxifen, acetyl-L-carnitine, colchicine, and vitamin E.[74,76] Table 9-1 summarizes the oral agents used to treat Peyronie's disease.

A number of pharmacologic agents have been injected directly into Peyronie's plaques, including steroids, calcium channel blockers, purified clostridial collagenase, orgotein (a metalloproteinase),[74] and interferon alfa-2.[77] Among these, the calcium channel blocker verapamil is most commonly used but the optimal dosage, technique for administration, and role of combination agents designed to reduce pain caused by its administration are not yet known. For example, electromotive administration of the calcium channel blocker verapamil, 5 mg, combined with 8 mg of dexamethasone, was found to be superior to the electromotive dispensation of 5 mg of verapamil combined with 2% lidocaine.[78]

Extracorporeal shock wave therapy has been used in an attempt to disrupt Peyronie's plaques.[79] Treatment appears to relieve the pain associated with the disease, but mixed evidence exists regarding its ability to reduce the severity of the associated penile curvature significantly.

Surgical management is indicated when curvature and ED are both present.[74] The Nesbit procedure and its multiple subsequent variations shorten the tunica albuginea by shortening the longer aspect of the penis to establish equilibrium and remove curvature. The ideal candidate for this technique has some erectile function, adequate penile length, and an hourglass plaque or narrowing deformity. Associated complications include penile shortening, ED, penile hematoma, urethral injury, numbness of the glans penis, and phimosis. Other surgical procedures attempt to lengthen the tunica albuginea by reconstructing the shortened aspect of the penis to restore equilibrium with the

TABLE 9-1 Oral Medications in the Management of Peyronie's Disease

DRUG AND DOSAGE	ACTION	NURSING IMPLICATIONS
Vitamin E, 200-300 mg daily	Antioxidant	Acts as antithrombotic when administered at higher doses; advise patient to consult physician about discontinuing medication prior to elective surgery
Potassium aminobenzoate, 20 g/day for 12 wk	Action unknown; may inhibit fibrinogenesis, increase action of monoamine oxidase	Most common adverse effect is gastrointestinal upset; advise patient to take with meal or snack
Colchicine, 0.6-1.2 mg/day for 1 wk, then increase to 1.8-2.4 mg for 12 wk	Inhibits collagen secretion from fibroblasts	Diarrhea, gastrointestinal upset occur in one third; advise patient to take with meals or a snack; liver enzyme levels should be monitored during therapy
Tamoxifen, 20 mg bid		Most common adverse effect is gastrointestinal upset; advise patient to take with meal or snack; alopecia occasionally occurs, reassure patient condition is transient
Acetyl-L-carnitine, 2 g/day	Action unknown; may act as antioxidant, restore phospholipid composition of mitochondria, inhibit apoptosis	May provide better pain control than tamoxifen; further research is needed to elucidate efficacy and identify any adverse side effects

longer aspect. These procedures are indicated for patients with severe curvature (Figure 9-8, C).

Finally, a penile prosthesis may be implanted into patients with severe Peyronie's disease and ED who do not respond to more conservative treatment options. Penile length may be restored by incising or excising the plaque, and a malleable or inflatable device can be implanted. See earlier for a more detailed discussion of nursing management for the patient undergoing implantation of a penile prosthesis.

PRIAPISM

Priapism is a painful and prolonged erection caused by abnormally high arterial perfusion of the cavernous bodies or incomplete drainage of venous blood from the cavernous bodies. The risk of ED following an episode of priapism is approximately 50%.[31] Episodes that persist beyond 4 to 6 hours typically indicate ischemia and represent a medical emergency; nonischemic priapism is less common and tends to be painless.[1,39,80] Priapism can present as an acute episode, and it may recur when caused or influenced by a chronic underlying disease or disorder. *Stuttering priapism* is the term used for prolonged and painful erections that resolve without medical intervention; these episodes are characteristic of men with sickle cell anemia. Table 9-2 outlines factors associated with an increased risk of priapism.[1,81-84]

The pathophysiology of priapism is not completely understood; it varies according to the underlying cause. Stasis or pooling of blood causes damage or destruction of the endothelium and necrosis in low-flow (ischemic) priapism, although unregulated blood inflow, often associated with trauma, neurologic disease, and fistula formation between arterial inflow and venous outflow, are common characteristics of high-flow (nonischemic) priapism.

Assessment

Priapism is usually diagnosed based on a history of a prolonged, usually painful, erection, combined with physical examination of the penis.[39] The cavernosal bodies will be fully to partly rigid and the penis may be dusky because of underlying ischemia. Unlike normal erections, the glans penis and corpus spongiosum are rarely involved. A blood sample is obtained to screen for hemoglobin S if sickle cell anemia is possible and previously undiagnosed and to rule out leukemia. Cavernous blood is obtained for blood gas analysis

to differentiate ischemic from high-flow priapism. If this test does not yield clear results, radionuclide scanning or dynamic infusion cavernosometry may be performed to establish the diagnosis.

Nursing Management

Because low-flow priapism is associated with ischemia and ultimately, necrosis and irreversible tissue damage, the goal of medical and nursing care is to reverse the erection rapidly and re-establish blood flow to compromised tissues.[39] A 21-gauge butterfly needle may be inserted into the corporal body to aspirate pooled blood. This maneuver is combined with intracavernosal injection of a vasoconstricting agent, such as phenylephrine or terbutaline. Alternatively, methylene blue, an inhibitor of guanylate cyclase, may be injected to reverse the effects of nitric oxide and induce tumescence.[85,86] Priapism associated with sickle cell anemia also may require interventions designed to reverse the underlying sickling process; these include hydration, oxygenation, and alkalinization. High-flow priapism may be prevented by early application of an ice pack. However, many patients will require embolization of the internal pudendal artery.

Following successful reversal of priapism, the underlying cause is explored and treated to reduce the risk of recurrence. The patient is taught to recognize the signs and symptoms of recurrence and the need to seek treatment promptly to minimize permanent damage or fibrosis of the cavernosal bodies. The patient is also advised of the risk for subsequent ED and told that other treatment can be pursued if this complication develops.

REPRODUCTIVE FUNCTION DISORDERS

Infertility, sometimes labeled subfertility, describes a wide variety of disorders that compromise the ability to fertilize a viable ovum and establish a successful pregnancy. Advances in technology and reproductive biology, however, have greatly increased our understanding of the factors that lead to fertility problems and enhanced the range and efficacy of treatment options.

MALE FACTOR INFERTILITY

Infertility may be caused by disorders affecting the male partner, female partner, or both. When infertility

TABLE 9-2 Causes of Priapism[1,81,82-84]

ASSOCIATED FACTOR	USUAL TYPE OF PRIAPISM	MECHANISM
Sickle cell anemia (affects 8% of African Americans)	Ischemic (low flow), stuttering, frequently recurs	Sludging of blood; leads to ED when seen in adults
Intracavernous injection for erectile dysfunction (ED); usually seen with psychogenic or neurogenic erections	Ischemic, acute	Hypersensitivity or higher dose of vasodilating drug causes prolonged erection and poor emptying via venous channels
Oral drugs–antidepressants (trazodone, fluoxetine, sertraline, lithium), tranquilizers (mesoridazine, perphenazine), antipsychotics (chlorpromazine), α-adrenergic blockers (prazosin, very rare with doxazosin, terazosin, tamsulosin), anticoagulants (warfarin, heparin) Illicit drugs (cocaine) Hormones (gonadotropin-releasing hormone)	Ischemic, acute	Varies; drugs may increase arterial flow to cavernosal sinusoids; enhanced firing of cavernosal nerves; many drug actions remain unknown
Neurologic disorders—spinal cord injury, disk disease, cauda equina syndrome, spinal anesthesia	Ischemic or nonischemic (high flow), frequently recurs	Abnormal release of neurotransmitters promoting erection or interfering with detumescence
Cancer—leukemia, prostate cancer, renal cell carcinoma, melanoma	Ischemic, sometimes recurs	Mechanical blockage of venous outflow or secondary via stasis of blood within corporal bodies
Total parenteral nutrition—when administered with 20% fat emulsion	Ischemic, stuttering	Unknown; higher density fat emulsion may adversely affect coagulability of blood, promote adverse cellular changes in blood, or cause fat embolus
Trauma—laceration of cavernous artery or its branches; blunt trauma to perineum	Arterial laceration—ischemic; blunt trauma—nonischemic	Laceration—unregulated leakage and pooling of blood in cavernosal sinusoids; blunt trauma—vasodilation with nocturnal erections leading to rupture of damaged arteries and unregulated high flow into corporal bodies
Hemodialysis	Ischemic	Hemoconcentration, hypovolemia causes sludging and stasis of blood within cavernosal sinusoids

involves the male partner, it is referred to as male factor infertility.

Definition and Epidemiology

The likelihood of a couple successfully conceiving is approximately 20% to 25% each month, with a cumulative chance of 75% within 6 months and about 90% within 1 year.[87] Fertilization usually occurs within 6 days of ovulation and the likelihood of conception peaks at approximately 24 years of age in men and women. Infertility is typically defined as the inability to conceive after 1 year of

TABLE 9-3 Modifiable Factors Associated with Male Factor Infertility[88,89]

FACTOR	MECHANISM AND NURSING IMPLICATIONS
Smoking	Increases serum prolactin and estradiol levels; smoking cessation postulated to have immediate beneficial effects for both partners
Alcohol consumption	Chronic alcoholism associated with testicular atrophy but moderate alcohol consumption not associated with impaired spermatogenesis
Psychological distress	Possible negative impact of semen quality; support and reassurance may improve fertility potential
Extreme physical exertion	Extreme exercise (e.g., running more than 100 miles/wk) may have detrimental effect but normal exercise regimen encouraged
Testicular hyperthermia	Continuous exposure to high environmental temperatures associated with reduced semen quality; underwear type does *not* significantly influence testicular temperature but sauna or hot tub use should be curtailed when attempting to conceive
Nutrition	Obesity adversely affects testosterone, estradiol levels; vitamin A deficiency may impair spermatogenesis; weight loss, vitamin supplementation based on recommended daily allowances may be recommended but magnitude of benefit from these interventions unknown
Occupational or environmental toxins, lead, ethylene glycol, mercury vapor, excessive heat, military radar, radiation, carbon disulfide	Diminish sperm count, associated endocrine function, sperm morphology
Prescription, over-the-counter, or illicit drugs; anabolic steroids; cimetidine; cyclosporine; phenothiazine; ketoconazole; sulfasalazine; spironolactone; valproic acid; allopurinol; calcium channel blockers; colchicine; nitrofurantoin; minocycline; marijuana; cocaine	Impair associated endocrine function, semen quality (including sperm count and morphology), fertilization potential; modification of prescription or over-the-counter drug regimens, immediate discontinuance of all illicit drugs maximize semen quality and fertility potential
Chemotherapy (multiple agents)	Impairs semen quality for 6-12 mo or permanently; administration of luteinizing hormone-releasing hormone during treatment may preserve fertility potential in some men
Herbal agents, echinacea, St. John's wort	Diminishes sperm count; should be discontinued to determine effect on fertility potential

intercourse, or when the couple complains of infertility and requests assistance from healthcare providers.[88] Approximately 20% of cases are attributable to male factors alone and 30% involve both male and female factors. Thus, approximately 50% of all cases of infertility involve male factors.

A number of disorders predispose to infertility. Among these, lifestyle factors are of particular interest to the urologic nurse because they are potentially modifiable and their alleviation or removal is likely to improve the likelihood of successful conception.[88,89] Table 9-3 summarizes common modifiable elements associated with male factor infertility. A number of medical, surgical or constitutional factors must also be addressed when managing the infertile couple with male factor infertility. (Table 9-4).

Assessment

Infertility is initally assessed with a careful history.[88] It begins with a review of sexual practices, including the duration of unprotected or anticipatory sexual intercourse and current sexual techniques. Questions about current techniques focus on behaviors that may reduce the likelihood of conception, including the use of potentially spermicidal lubricants, excessively frequent or infrequent intercourse, previous birth control methods, and timing of intercourse with respect to the occurrence of ovulation. Modifiable risk factors are carefully explored, as well as congenital, medical, and surgical conditions affecting fertility potential. The use of any prescription, over-the-counter, and illicit drugs should be explored in a manner that ensures patient confidentiality, avoids moral judgments, and provides factual information about the relationship between specific substances and fertility potential. Further queries should explore possible female factors, including previous infertility

evaluation involving the female partner or the patient. Both partners should be asked about children from relationships with previous sexual partners.

The physical examination begins with inspection of the man's body habitus, paying special attention to secondary male characteristics, hair distribution, and breast size. The genital examination includes testicular dimensions (length and width) using a goniometer and examination of the spermatic cord, specifically assessing for the presence of the vas deferens and varicocele (Figure 9-9).

Laboratory testing begins with collection of an adequate sample for a semen analysis. Two to three specimens are typically required, following abstinence

TABLE 9-4 Medical, Surgical, and Congenital Factors Associated with Male Factor Infertility[88]

FACTOR	FEATURES
Congenital and developmental factors	Cryptorchidism, anomalies of gender differentiation, urinary tract anomalies, central nervous system anomalies, cystic fibrosis, Kartagener's syndrome (immotile cilia syndrome), Young's syndrome (epididymal obstruction and frequent respiratory infections), Kallmann's syndrome (hypogonadotropic hypogonadism and anosmia [absence of sense of smell]), delayed onset of puberty, varicocele
Medical history	Recent febrile illness (within 1-3 mo), urinary tract infections, sexually transmitted diseases, testicular cancer, tuberculosis, viral orchitis, diabetes mellitus, gynecomastia, epididymitis, orchitis, renal insufficiency, hypothyroidism, perineal or testicular trauma, retrograde ejaculation
Surgical history	Orchiopexy (bilateral versus unilateral and age); varicocelectomy; herniorrhaphy; transurethral resection of prostate; transurethral incision of bladder neck; Y-V plasty of bladder; retroperitoneal surgery; other pelvic, inguinal or scrotal surgeries

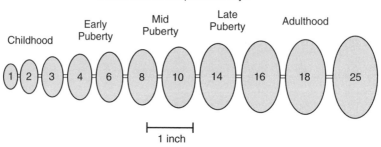

Fig. 9-9 A Prader orchidometer has 12 testicular models varying in size from 1 ml to 25 ml. Normal testicular volume should be approximately 20 ml with a maximum length of at least 4 cm.

from sexual activity for 2 to 3 days. The specimen should be collected within 1 hour of analysis in a clean but not necessarily sterile container that is completely devoid of spermicidal materials. The urologic nurse should advise the patient that the specimen can be obtained via masturbation, the preferred technique, or collected in a special nonspermicidal condom. The patient is also counseled against prolonged abstinence prior to specimen collection because the results of such a specimen are likely to be misleading. Table 9-5 outlines the minimal parameters of a normal semen analysis. Other analytical studies may be performed, such as a strict morphologic analysis and assays for white blood cells, antisperm antibodies, and various biochemical constituents of the semen. The semen analysis guides further evaluation and management. Additional testing may include endocrine testing, transrectal ultrasonography for ejaculatory duct obstruction, color Doppler ultrasonography for small varicoceles, venography for testicular venous reflux, vasography, sperm penetration assay, mucus migration testing, hemizonal assays, and hypo-osmotic swelling testing to differentiate immotile from dead sperm.

In some cases, a single causative disorder is identified, although other cases may have several contributing factors or no obvious predominant factor.

Table 9-6 outlines common identifiable causes of infertility.

Nursing Management

Management of the infertile couple requires coordination of efforts between both partners and often involves physicians who provide care to the female partner. Patient education should be carried out in close consultation with the urologist, the gynecologist, and the couple. Basic counseling often includes information about the usual chances of conception over 1, 6, and 12 months and intercourse timing with respect to ovulation. Couples should be advised to avoid using lubricants or to limit their use to products free from spermicidal substances. The couple may be advised that intercourse on an every other day basis, paying special attention to timing with regard to ovulation and specific physician advice, will help increase the chances of successful conception.

Modifiable risk factors should be addressed initially (see Table 9-3) although they may be combined with more invasive interventions, depending on the results of the semen analysis. Table 9-7 outlines medical treatment options directed at underlying causes of male infertility.

Surgery. Several surgical options may be performed to enhance fertility potential in the male. Varicocele repair requires ligation of the internal spermatic vein to reduce excessive venous flow. A varicocele is defined as dilated (varicose) veins in the scrotum, typically affecting the more dependent

TABLE 9-5 Semen Analysis: Minimal Standards of Adequacy

PROCEDURES	PARAMETER
On at least two occasions	Ejaculate volume = 1.5-5.0 ml
	Sperm density >20,000,000/ml or 50-60 $\times$ 10^6 total sperm
	Motility >0%
	Forward progression: = 2+ (on a scale of 0-4)
	Morphology (routine) >60% normal
Additional testing	No significant sperm agglutination
	No significant agglutination
	No significant pyospermia
	No hyperviscosity or inadequate liquefaction

Modified from Lipshultz LI, Howards SS (eds): Infertility in the Male, 3rd edition. St Louis: Mosby, 1996.

TABLE 9-6 Factors Closely Associated with Male Factor Infertility

FACTOR	FREQUENCY (%)
Varicocele	42
Idiopathic	23
Obstruction within reproductive tract	14
Cryptorchidism	3
Immunologic	1
Ejaculatory dysfunction	1
Drugs, irradiation	1
Sexual dysfunction	<1
Genetic congenital disorder	<1

Modified from Lipshultz LI, Howards SS (eds): Infertility in the Male, 3rd edition. St Louis: Mosby, 1996.

TABLE 9-7 Treatment Options Designed to Improve Reproductive Function

UNDERLYING DISORDER	INTERVENTION
Hypogonadotropic hypogonadism	Exogenous replacement of testosterone, human chorionic gonadotropin (hCG), with or without gonadotropin-releasing hormone as indicated
Hyperprolactinemia	Bromocriptine or cabergoline (long-acting dopaminergic agonist)
Congenital adrenal hyperplasia (CAH)	Corticosteroid treatment only if CAH is linked with infertility
Hypothyroidism	Synthroid supplementation
Anabolic steroid abuse	Discontinue all exogenous steroids, supplement with hCG for 12 wk
Pyospermia	Antimicrobial treatment following evaluation for source of infection and likely pathogen
Antisperm antibodies	Prednisone for 4 wk
Retrograde ejaculation	α-Adrenergic agonist (e.g., ephedrine or imipramine)
Idiopathic oligospermia	Clomiphene citrate, tamoxifen, hCG (with or without human menopausal gonadotropin), testolactone, gonadotropin-releasing hormone, kallikrein, pentoxifylline, carnitine, various antioxidants
Varicocele	Varicocelectomy

(left) testis. Clinically apparent varicoceles, in particular, are associated with compromised fertility potential,[90] which improves following their repair.[91] Varicocelectomy may be approached using an inguinal, scrotal, or retroperitoneal incision, laparoscopy, or via percutaneous venography. Postoperative nursing management includes use of a scrotal support to minimize discomfort although upright and avoidance of heavy lifting for 1 to 2 weeks following the procedure. Men are advised that scrotal bruising and modest swelling are anticipated, but increased swelling or pain after the first 24 to 48 postoperative hours, fever, or inability to urinate requires prompt intervention.

Vasovasostomy (anastomosis of the vas deferens) or epididymovasostomy (attachment of the vas deferens to the epididymis) may be performed to reverse vasectomy or correct ductal obstruction.[88,92] The procedure is performed in an outpatient surgery setting with microscopic equipment to visualize the small and delicate anatomy of the vas deferens and epididymis. Because of advances in reproductive medicine, men are now offered the option of sperm cryopreservation at the time of microsurgical reconstruction. Cryopreservation harvests and preserves motile sperm from the testicular end of the vas deferens or epididymis for intracytoplasmic sperm injection at a later date, if indicated.

Several techniques are used to retrieve sperm from subfertile men. Microsurgical sperm aspiration uses an operating microscope to harvest sperm from the epididymis via a small scrotal incision. Alternatively, sperm may be extracted by a needle using a percutaneous approach. Testicular sperm extraction requires an open testicular biopsy to harvest sperm or percutaneous aspiration using a fine needle. As anticipated, the maturity of the harvested sperm is inversely related to the retrieval location; sperm harvested from the testis are less mature than sperm harvested from the distal epididymis. Fortunately, with the advent of intracytoplasmic sperm injection (ICSI), the likelihood that these immature sperm cells can be used for fertilization and creation of a viable pregnancy has improved dramatically.

Intracytoplasmic Sperm Injection. ICSI has revolutionized management of the infertile male.[88] Specifically, it allows men to become genetic fathers whose options prior to ICSI were limited to adoption or donor insemination. The procedure unites harvested oocytes obtained from ovarian follicles via in vitro fertilization (IVF) with a single sperm cell obtained from ejaculate, the epididymis, or the testis using the techniques described above (Figure 9-10). The single sperm cell is injected through the zona pellucida and oolemma of the oocyte that has been transiently immobilized in a droplet of oil-based medium. During the injection, the oocyte is aspirated and injected to provoke activation and increase the likelihood of fertility. In addition, the tail of the sperm is crushed between the micropipette and

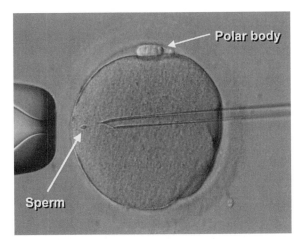

Fig. 9-10 Intracytoplasmic sperm injection (ICSI): A single sperm cell is injected through the zona pellucida of an oocyte. (From Wein AJ, Kavoussi LR, Novick AC, Partin AW, Peters CA (eds): Campbell-Walsh Urology, 9th edition. Philadelphia-Saunders, 2007.)

Petri dish to immobilize and activate it, further increasing the likelihood of fertilization. Success rates for ICSI range from 32% to 65% and appear to be highest in centers with extensive experience with the procedure.

In addition to educating the couple about the procedure, the urologic nurse should provide factual information about the cost of the procedure, insurance reimbursement, and risks associated with ICSI. As with many reproductive technologies, such as IVF, ICSI is relatively costly ($7000 to $12,000 in the United States) and may not be covered by medical insurance.[88] In addition, ICSI, similar to IVF, is associated with an increased likelihood of twin or multiple-fetus pregnancy of 38% or higher.[93] The possibility of genetic defects when a single immature sperm cell is selected and used to fertilize an ovum, as compared with the potential millions of sperm cells competing to fertilize the ovum with spontaneous pregnancy, is also a concern. Some studies have found a slightly increased rate of spontaneous abortions, but malformations in live births were similar to those observed in non–ICSI-assisted IVF, ranging from 1.7% to 1.8%.[93-95]

Adjunctive Therapies. Sperm may be obtained from selected men using procedures other than ICSI. For example, men with profoundly altered penile sensation because of spinal cord injury or other paralyzing neurologic disorders affecting cervical or high thoracic spinal segments may undergo vibratory stimulation to initiate an ejaculatory response. Vibratory stimulation is delivered via a handheld electric or battery-driven device applied to the dorsum of the glans penis and then to the frenulum and penoscrotal areas. Men with retrograde ejaculation caused by paralyzing spinal cord lesions or retroperitoneal lymph node dissection may undergo electroejaculation stimulation. This requires placement of a probe in the rectum that delivers an electric current, which stimulates the sympathetic efferents to produce an ejaculatory response. However, because the ejaculate is expressed in a retrograde rather than antegrade manner, the bladder must be prepared by drainage of urine prior to the procedure and a broth with a pH and nutrients favoring sperm survival is infused. Sperm are then concentrated in a pellet for IVF or intrauterine insemination.

SUMMARY

Revolutions have occurred in erectile and reproductive dysfunction, forever changing how patients are cared for and the indications for intervention. Unfortunately, positive attitudes toward sexual function are slow to evolve, often frustrating affected men, their partners, and their urologic care providers. In addition to playing a central role in providing services to the men and women seeking care for erectile and reproductive dysfunction, urologic nurses are in a key position to educate the public at large about the prevalence of these disorders, their importance to quality of life, and novel solutions for their treatment.

REFERENCES

1. Lue TF: Physiology of penile erection and pathophysiology of erectile dysfunction. In Wein AJ, Kavoussi LR, Novick AC, Partin AW, Peters CA (eds): Campbell-Walsh Urology, 9th edition. Philadelphia: Saunders, 2007; pp 718-49.
2. Walz J, Perrotte P, Suardi N, Hutterer G, Jeldres C, Bénard F, et al: Baseline prevalence of erectile dysfunction in a prostate cancer screening population. Journal of Sexual Medicne, 2008; 5(2):428-35.
3. NIH Consensus Development Panel on Impotence: NIH Consensus Conference. Impotence. Journal of the American Medical Association, 1993; 270(1):83-90.
4. Lewis JH, Rosen R, Goldstein I: Consensus Panel on Health Care Clinician Management of Erectile Dysfunction. Erectile dysfunction. American Journal of Nursing, 2003; 103(10):48-58.
5. Droupy S: Epidemiology and pathophysiology of erectile dysfunction. Annales d'Urologie, 2005; 39:71-84.
6. Sasayama S, Ishii N, Ishikura F, Kamijima G, Ogawa S, Kanmatsuse K, et al: Men's health study: epidemiology of erectile dysfunction and cardiovascular disease. Circulation Journal, 2003; 67:656-9.

7. Braun M, Wassmer G, Klotz T, Reifenrath B, Mathers M, Engelmann U: Epidemiology of erectile dysfunction: results of the 'Cologne Male Survey.' International Journal of Impotence Research, 2000; 12(6):305-11.

8. Martin-Morales A, Sanchez-Cruz JJ, Saenz de Tejada I, Rodriguez-Vela L, Jimenez-Cruz JF, Burgos-Rodriguez R: Prevalence and independent risk factors for erectile dysfunction in Spain: results of the Epidemiologia de la Disfuncion Erectil Masculina Study. Journal of Urology, 2001; 166(2):569-75.

9. Chew KK, Stuckey B, Bremner A, Earle C, Jamrozik K: Male erectile dysfunction: Its prevalence in Western Australia. Journal of Sexual Medicine, 2008; 5(1):60-9.

10. Masters WH, Johnson V: Human Sexual Response. Boston: Little-Brown, 1970.

11. McVary K: Lower urinary tract symptoms and sexual dysfunction: epidemiology and pathophysiology. BJU International, 2006; 97(Supplement 2):23-8.

12. Giuliano F., Rampin O: Alpha receptors in the central nervous system and its effects on erection. Journal of Andrology, 1999; 20:683-7.

13. Beutel ME, Weidner W, Brahler E: Epidemiology of sexual dysfunction in the male population. Andrologia, 2006; 38:115-21.

14. Rosen R, Altwein J, Boyle P, Kirby RS, Lukacs B, Meuleman E, O'Leary MP, Puppo P, Robertson, Giuliano F: Lower urinary tract symptoms and male sexual dysfunction: the multinational survey of the aging male (MSAM-7). European Urology, 2003; 44(6):637-49.

15. Kloner RA, Mullin SH, Shook T, Matthews R, Mayeda G, Burnstein S, et al: Erectile dysfunction in the cardiac patient: how common and how should we treat?. Journal of Urology, 2003; 170(Supplement):S46-50.

16. Roth A, Kalter-Leibovici O, Kerbis Y, Tenenbaum-Koren E, Chen J, Sobol T, Raz I: Prevalence and risk factors for erectile dysfunction in men with diabetes, hypertension, or both diseases: a community survey among 1,412 Israeli men. Clinical Cardiology, 2003; 26(1):25-30.

17. Bacon CG, Mittleman MA, Kawachi I, Giovannucci E, Glasser DB, Rimm EB: A prospective study of risk factors for erectile dysfunction. Journal of Urology, 2006; 176:217-21.

18. Sasaki K, Yoshimura N, Chancellor MB: Implications of diabetes mellitus in urology. Urologic Clinics of North America, 2003; 30(1):1-12.

19. Costabile RA: Optimizing treatment differences for diabetes mellitus–induced erectile dysfunction. Journal of Urology, 2003; 170(Supplement):S35-S39.

20. Darby E, Anawalt BD: Male hypogonadism: an update on diagnosis and treatment. Treatments in Endocrinology, 2005; 4:293-309.

21. Tweed MJ, Roland JM: Haemochromatosis as an endocrine cause of subfertility. British Medical Journal, 1998; 316:915-6.

22. Bellinghieri G, Savica V, Santoro D: Vascular erectile dysfunction in chronic renal failure. Seminars in Nephrology, 2006; 26:42-5.

23. Korplainen JT, Nieminen P, Myllyla VV: Sexual functioning among stroke patients and their spouses. Stroke, 1999; 30:715-9.

24. Brunner DW, Calvano T: The sexual impact of cancer and cancer treatments in men. Nursing Cinics of North America, 2007; 42(4):555-80.

25. Blanker MH, Bohnen AM, Groeneveld FP, Bernsen RM, Prins A, Thomas S, Bosch JL: Correlates for erectile and ejaculatory dysfunction in older Dutch men: a community-based study. Journal of the American Geriatrics Society, 2001; 49:436-42.

26. Simsek I, Asian G, Akarsu M., Koseoglu H, Esen A: Assessment of sexual function in patients with chronic liver disease. International Journal of Impotence Research, 2005; 17:343-5.

27. Rabkin JG, Wagner GJ, Rabkin R: The vicious cycling: bicycling related urogenital disorders. European Urology, 2005; 47:141-7.

28. Leibovitch I, Mor Y: Impotence and nerve entrapment in long distance amateur cyclists. Acta Neurologica Scandinavica, 1997; 95:233-40.

29. Shenfeld OZ, Gofrit ON, Gdor Y, Landau I, Katz R, Pode D: The role of sildenafil in the treatment of erectile dysfunction in patients with pelvic fracture urethral disruption. Journal of Urology, 2004; 172:2350-2.

30. Greenfield JM, Levine LA: Where we stand with medical therapy for Peyronie's disease. Contemporary Urology, 2005; 17:15-6.

31. Burnett AL, Bivalacqua TJ, Champion HC, Musicki B: Long-term oral phosphodiesterase 5 inhibitor therapy alleviates recurrent priapism. Journal of Urology, 2006; 67:1043-8.

32. Keene LC, Davies PH: Drug-related erectile dysfunction. Adverse Drug Reactions and Toxicological Reviews, 1999; 18(1):5-24.

33. Sikka SC: Drug, environment and chemical exposures in the realm of sexuality. In Hellstrom WJG (ed): Handbook of Sexual Dysfunction. San Francisco: American Society of Andrology, 1999; pp 27-34.

34. Nandipati KC, Raina R, Agarwal A, Zippe CD: Erectile dysfunction following radical retropubic prostatectomy: epidemiology, pathophysiology and pharmacological management. Drugs and Aging, 2006; 23:101-17.

35. Jayne DG, Brown JM, Thorpe H, Walker J, Quirke P, Guillou PJ: Bladder and sexual function following resection for rectal cancer in a randomized clinical trial of laparoscopic versus open technique. British Journal of Surgery, 2005; 92:1124-32.

36. Zippe C, Nandipati K, Agarwal A, Raina R: Sexual dysfunction after pelvic surgery. International Journal of Impotence Research, 2006; 18:1-18.

37. Fischer ME, Vitek ME, Hedeker D, Henderson WG, Jacobsen JG, Goldberg J: A twin study of erectile dysfunction. Archives of Internal Medicine, 2004; 164(2):165-8.

38. Rosen RC: Psychogenic erectile dysfunction. Classification and management. Urologic Clinics of North America, 2001; 28:269-278.

39. Lue TF, Broderick GA. Evaluation and nonsurgical management of erectile dysfunction and premature ejaculation. In Wein AJ, Kavoussi LR, Novick AC, Partin AW, Peters CA (eds): Campbell-Walsh Urology, 9th edition. Philadelphia: Saunders, 2007; pp 750-87.

40. Lewis JH: Acting as a primary care provider for patients with erectile dysfunction. Clinician Reviews, 2001; 11(Supplement):20-4.

41. Dean J, Rubio-Aurioles E, McCabe M, Eardley I, Speakman M, Buvat J, et al: Integrating partners into erectile dysfunction treatment: Improving the sexual experience for the couple. International Journal of Clinical Practice, 2008; 62(1):127-33.

42. Kirby RS: Basic assessment of the patient with erectile dsfunction. In Carson CC, Kirby RS, Goldstein I (eds): Textbook of Erectile Dysfunction. Oxford, UK: Isis Medical Media Ltd, 1999; pp 195-205.

43. Rosen RC, Riley A, Wagner G, Osterloh IH, Kirkpatrick J, Mishra A: The International Index of Erectile Function (IIEF): a multidimensional scale for assessment of erectile dysfunction. Urology, 1997; 49(6):822-30.

44. Mykletun A, Dahl AA, O'Leary MP, Fossa SD: Assessment of male sexual function by the Brief Sexual Function Inventory. BJU International, 2006; 97:316-23.

45. Donatucci CF, Lue TF: The combined intracavernous injection and stimulation test: diagnostic accuracy. Journal of Urology, 1992; 148:61-2.

46. Lue TF: Erectile dysfunction. New England Journal of Medicine, 2000; 342:1802-13.

47. Derby CA, Mohr BA, Goldstein I, Feldman HA, Johannes CB, McKinlay JB: Modifiable risk factors and erectile dysfunction: can lifestyle changes modify risk? Urology, 2000; 56:302-6.

48. Schwarzer U, Sommer F, Klotz T, Cremer C, Engelmann U: Cycling and penile oxygen pressure: the type of saddle matters. European Urology, 2002; 41(2):139-43.

49. Marceau L, Kleinman K, Goldstein I, McKinlay J: Does bicycling contribute to the risk of erectile dysfunction? Results from the Massachusetts Male Aging Study (MMAS). International Journal of Impotence Research, 2001; 13(5):298-302.

50. Dorey G, Feneley RC, Speakman MJ, Robinson JP, Paterson J: Pelvic floor muscle exercises and manometric biofeedback for erectile dysfunction and postmicturition dribble: three case studies.

Journal of Wound, Ostomy, and Continence Nursing, 2003; 30(1):44-52.

51. Ballard DJ: Treatment of erectile dysfunction: can pelvic muscle exercises improve sexual function? Journal of Wound, Ostomy, and Continence Nursing, 1997; 24(5):255-64.

52. Dutta TC, Eid JF: Vacuum constriction devices for erectile dysfunction: a long-term, prospective study of patients with mild, moderate, and severe dysfunction. Urology, 1999; 54(5):891-3.

53. Chen J, Mabjeesh NJ, Greenstein A: Sildenafil versus the vacuum erection device: patient preference. Journal of Urology, 2001; 166(5):1779-81.

54. Bratton RL, Cassidy HD; Vacuum erection device use in elderly men: a possible severe complication. Journal of the American Board of Family Practice, 2002; 5(6):501-2.

55. Ganem JP, Lucey DT, Janosko EO, Carson CC: Unusual complications of the vacuum erection device. Urology, 1998; 51(4):627-31.

56. Heaton JP, Morales A: Endocrine causes of impotence (nondiabetes). Urologic Clinics of North America, 2003; 30(1):73-81.

57. Kuhnert B, Byrne M, Simoni M, Kopke W, Gerss J, Lemmnitz G, et al: Testosterone substitution with a new transdermal hypoalcoholic gel applied to scrotal or non-scrotal skin: a multicentre trial. European Journal of Endocrinology, 2005; 153:317-26.

58. Cooper CS, Perry PJ, Sparks AE, MacIndoe JH, Yates WR, Williams RD: Effect of exogenous testosterone on prostate volume, serum and semen prostate-specific antigen levels in healthy young men. Journal of Urology, 1998; 159(2):441-3.

59. Carrier S: Pharmacology of phosphodiesterase 5 inhibitors. Canadian Journal of Urology, 2003; 10(Supplement 1):12-6.

60. Ernst E, Pittler MH: Yohimbine for erectile dysfunction: a systematic review and meta-analysis of randomized clinical trials. Journal of Urology, 1998; 159(2):433-6.

61. Vogt HJ, Brandl P, Kockott G, Schmitz JR, Wiegand MH, Schadrack J, Gierend M: Double-blind, placebo-controlled safety and efficacy trial with yohimbine hydrochloride in the treatment of nonorganic erectile dysfunction. International Journal of Impotence Research, 1997; 9(3):155-61.

62. Reid K, Surridge DH, Morales A, Condra M, Harris C, Owen J, Fenemore J: Double-blind trial of yohimbine in treatment of psychogenic impotence. Lancet, 1987; 2(8556):421-3.

63. Allard J, Giuliano F: Central nervous system agents in the treatment of erectile dysfunction: how do they work? Current Urology Reports, 2001; 2(6):488-94.

64. Enzlin P, Vanderschueren D, Bonte L, Vanderborght W, Declercq G, Demyttenaere K: Trazodone: a double-blind, placebo-controlled, randomized study of its effects in patients with erectile dysfunction without major organic findings. International Journal of Impotence Research, 2000; 12(4):223-8.

65. Hellstrom WJ, Bennett AH, Gesundheit N, Kaiser FE, Lue TF, Padma-Nathan H, Peterson CA, Tam PY, Todd LK, Varady JC, Place VA: A double-blind, placebo-controlled evaluation of the erectile response to transurethral alprostadil. Urology, 1996; 48(6):851-6.

66. Montorsi F, Salonia A, Deho' F, Cestari A, Guazzoni G, Rigatti P, Stief C: Pharmacological management of erectile dysfunction. BJU International, 2003; 91(5):446-54.

67. Richter S, Vardi Y, Ringel A, Shalev M, Nissenkorn I: Intracavernous injections: still the gold standard for treatment of erectile dysfunction in elderly men. International Journal of Impotence Research, 2001; 13(3):172-5.

68. Gregoire I: Pharmacologic erection program: an alternative solution for the man with erectile dysfunction. Urologic Nursing, 1995; 15(1):10-3.

69. Carson CC: Penile prostheses: are they still relevant? BJU International, 2003; 91(3):176-7.

70. Anastasiadis AG, Wilson SK, Burchardt M, Shabsigh R: Long-term outcomes of inflatable penile implants: reliability, patient satisfaction and complication management. Current Opinion in Urology, 2001; 11(6):619-23.

71. Montague DK: Prosthetic surgery for erectile dysfunction. In Wein AJ, Kavoussi LR, Novick AC, Partin AW, Peters CA (eds): Campbell-Walsh Urology, 9th edition. Philadelphia: Saunders, 2007; pp 788-801.

72. Quallich SA, Ohl DA: Penile prosthesis: patient teaching and perioperative care. Urologic Nursing, 2002; 22(2):81-90.

73. Mulcahy JJ: Long-term experience with salvage of infected penile implants. Journal of Urology, 2000; 163(2):481-2.

74. Gholami SS, Gonzalez-Cadavid NF, Lin CS, Rajfer J, Lue TF: Peyronie's disease: a review. Journal of Urology, 2003; 169:1234-41.

75. Schiavino D, Sasso F, Nucera E, Alcini E, Gulino G, Milani A, Patriarca G: Immunologic findings in Peyronie's disease: a controlled study. Urology, 1997; 50(5):764-8.

76. Biagiotti G, Cavallini G: Acetyl-L-carnitine vs tamoxifen in the oral therapy of Peyronie's disease: a preliminary report. BJU International, 2001; 88(1):83-7.

77. Dang G, Matern R, Bivalacqua TJ, Sikka S, Hellstrom WJ: Intralesional interferon-alpha-2B injections for the treatment of Peyronie's disease. Southern Medical Journal, 2004; 97(1):42-6.

78. Di Stasi SM, Giannantoni A, Stephen RL, Capelli G, Giurioli A, Jannini EA, Vespasiani G: A prospective, randomized study using transdermal electromotive administration of verapamil and dexamethasone for Peyronie's disease. Journal of Urology, 2004; 171(4):1605-8.

79. Hauck EW, Mueller UO, Bschleipfer T, Schmelz HU, Diemer T, Weidner W: Extracorporeal shock wave therapy for Peyronie's disease: exploratory meta-analysis of clinical trials. Journal of Urology, 2004; 171(2 Pt 1):740-5.

80. Keoghane SR, Sullivan ME., Miller MA: The etiology, pathogenesis and management of priapism. BJU International, 2002; 90(2):149-54.

81. Burnett AL: Pathophysiology of priapism: dysregulatory erection physiology thesis. Journal of Urology, 2003; 170(1):26-34.

82. Dodds PR, Batter SJ, Serels SR: Priapism following ingestion of tamsulosin. Journal of Urology, 2003; 169(6):2302.

83. Avisrror MU, Fernandez IA, Sanchez AS, Garcia-Pando AC, Arias LM, del Pozo JG: Doxazosin and priapism. Journal of Urology, 2000; 163(1):238.

84. Vaidyanathan S, Soni BM, Singh G, Sett P, Krishnan KR: Prolonged penile erection association with terazosin in a cervical spinal cord injury patient. Spinal Cord, 1998; 36(11):805.

85. deHoll JD, Shin PA, Angle JF, Steers WD: Alternative approaches to the management of priapism. International Journal of Impotence Research, 1998; 10(1):11-4.

86. Steers WD, Selby JB Jr: Use of methylene blue and selective embolization of the pudendal artery for high flow priapism refractory to medical and surgical treatments. Journal of Urology, 1991; 146(5):1361-3.

87. Spira A: Epidemiology of human reproduction. Human Reproduction, 1986; 1(2):111-5.

88. Kim ED, Lipshultz LI, Howards SS: Male infertility. In Gillenwater JY, Grayhack JT, Howards SS, Mitchell ME (eds): Adult and Pediatric Urology, 4th edition. Philadelphia: Lippincott Williams & Wilkins, 2002; pp 1683-757.

89. Sharpe RM: Lifestyle and environmental contribution to male infertility. British Medical Bulletin, 2000; 56(3):630-42.

90. Onozawa M, Endo F, Suetomi T, Takeshima H, Akaza H: Clinical study of varicocele: statistical analysis and the results of long-term follow-up. International Journal of Urology, 2002; 9(8):455-61.

91. Perimenis P, Markou S, Gyftopoulos K, Athanasopoulos A, Barbalias G: Effect of subinguinal varicocelectomy on sperm parameters and pregnancy rate: a two-group study. European Urology, 2001; 39(3):322-5.

92. Schroeder-Printzen I, Diemer T, Weidner W: Vasovasostomy. Urologia Internationalis, 2003; 70(2):101-7.

93. SART Registry: Assisted reproductive technology in the United States: 1996 results generated from the American Society for

Reproductive Medicine/Society For Assisted Reproductive Technology Registry. Fertility and Sterility, 1999; 71(5):798-807.

94. Simpson JL, Lamb DJ: Genetic effects of intracytoplasmic sperm injection. Seminars in Reproductive Medicine, 2001; 19(3):239-339.

95. Nudell DM, Lipshultz LI: Is intracytoplasmic sperm injection safe? Current status and future concerns. Current Urology Reports, 2001; 2(6):423-31.

96. Goldstein I, Lue TF, Padma-Nathan H, Rosen RC, Steers WD, Wicker PA: Oral sildenafil in the treatment of erectile dysfunction. Sildenafil Study Group. New England Journal of Medicine, 1998; 338(20):1397-404.

97. Donatucci C, Taylor T, Thibonnier M, Bangerter K, Gittleman M, Casey R, Vardenafil Study Group: Vardenafil improves patient satisfaction with erection hardness, orgasmic function, and overall sexual experience, although improving quality of life in men with erectile dysfunction. Journal of Sexual Medicine, 2004; 1:185-92.

98. Buvat J, van Ahlen H, Schmitt H, Chan M, Kuepfer C, Varanese L: Efficacy and safety of two dosing regimens of tadalafil and patterns of sexual activity in men with diabetes mellitus and erectile dysfunction: scheduled use vs. on-demand regimen evaluation (SURE) study in 14 European countries. Journal of Sexual Medicine, 2006; 3:512-20.

CHAPTER 10

Genitourinary Trauma

Trauma is defined as a significant injury or shock to the body, as from violence or an accident.[1] From a clinical perspective, genitourinary trauma typically includes unintentional injury or surgical misadventure. This chapter will review nursing management of renal, ureter, bladder, urethra, penis, scrotum, and testis trauma.

Traumatic injury is a persistent and significant public health issue throughout the world and across the life span. Millions of persons in Canada and the United States sustain significant injuries each year. Unintentional injury is the leading cause of death among persons aged 1 to 44 years and is the third leading cause of death in adults aged 45 to 54 years.[2] In the United States, injury-attributable medical costs in 2000 exceeded $117 billion. The psychosocial costs are even higher; trauma negatively affects the patient, family, and friends, particularly when the injury is associated with intentional violence. Trauma often leads to prolonged or permanent disability, sometimes so severe that it renders the person unable to work and generate income.[3] Serious injuries affect multiple organ systems and approximately 10% involve the genitourinary system.[4,5]

Because genitourinary injury usually occurs within the larger context of a multiple-system trauma, urologic management comprises one component of a team approach that first addresses more immediately life-threatening injuries involving the respiratory, cardiovascular, and neurologic systems. The initial evaluation and management often begin before the person enters an emergency department. Emergency medical personnel may make initial contact with the victim at the scene of the accident and initiate evaluation and basic management at the accident scene and during transport to an emergency department. Immediate management is characterized by the ABCDE mnemonic:

A. Establish an airway and protect the cervical spine.
B. Maintain or establish breathing.
C. Control blood loss and restore circulating blood volume.
D. Address disability or neurologic status.
E. Manage the environment, including maintenance of the victim's temperature and reversal of a state of undress.[6]

Because urologic trauma is often subtle and rarely poses the immediate threat to life associated with thoracic, abdominal, or head injury, it may be overlooked during the critical first hours following a multisystem injury. Urinary system injury should be suspected whenever gross or microscopic hematuria occurs.[7] Although it seems logical to assume that gross hematuria indicates more serious injury than microscopic hematuria, several studies have demonstrated that microscopic hematuria, particularly when associated with a systolic blood pressure lower than 90 mm Hg, is often associated with significant renal trauma affecting both the parenchyma and vascular structures.[8,9] In many cases, urologic trauma is first suspected when attempting to place an indwelling catheter.[4] This simple action should prompt a simple but essential maxim for assessing and managing urinary system trauma—proceed in a retrograde fashion when evaluating the urinary tract for injury. Specifically, urologic and emergency personnel should proceed with evaluation of the urethra and move in a stepwise and retrograde fashion from the lower to upper urinary tract and, ultimately, the kidneys.

RENAL INJURIES

The kidneys are the most commonly injured organ in the genitourinary system, with renal injuries occurring in 1.4% to 3.0% of all trauma cases.[5,10] Renal injuries vary widely in severity, ranging from self-limiting contusions to lacerations of the kidney involving the renal parenchyma, collecting system, or hilum. The American Association for the Surgery of Trauma has proposed a classification system with

277

five grades, based on the extent of damage to the renal parenchyma, collecting system, and hilum (Table 10-1), and this has been validated as an instrument to guide therapy.[11] This grading system is also applied to the results of an abdominal computed tomography (CT) scan, helping physicians make accurate and rapid decisions about surgical intervention when severe trauma necessitates nephrectomy or urgent repair. A review of a database containing more than 523,000 patients hospitalized for trauma between 1997 and 1998 has revealed that 1.2% had a renal injury.[12] Most (64%) were renal contusions (grade I), 26% had lacerations (grades II and III), and 4% had associated vascular injuries (grades IV and V).

Etiology and Pathophysiology

As noted in Chapter 2, the kidney is protected against trauma by its fascial coverings, perinephric fat, and adjacent structures, including the abdominal muscles, diaphragm, quadratus lumborum muscles, and overlying ribs. Collectively, these structures create a shock absorber effect designed to preserve the integrity of the renal parenchyma, hilum, and vessels despite

TABLE 10-1 American Association for the Surgery of Trauma Organ Injury Grading Schema for Renal Injuries[5]

GRADE	DESCRIPTION
I	Contusion associated with normal imaging studies and gross or microscopic hematuria
II	Perineal hematoma confined to retroperitoneum or laceration that extends less than 1 cm into renal cortex; not associated with extravasation
III	Laceration that extends more than 1 cm into renal cortex; not associated with extravasation or rupture of collecting system
IV	Laceration extends through cortex, medulla, and involes collecting system; may be associated with renal artery or vein injury but hemorrhage is contained
V	Shattered kidney or avulsion of renal hilum causing devascularization of the kidney

blunt force trauma to the abdomen or flank. Renal injury occurs when these protective elements are compromised by significant blunt force or penetrating trauma.

Blunt force is the most common cause of renal trauma, accounting for 90% to 95% of all such injuries in rural settings and 80% in urban settings.[5] Blunt force trauma to the upper abdomen is most likely to injure the kidney when it is associated with rapid deceleration, overwhelming the shock absorber function inherent to the kidneys. Common causes of blunt trauma include motor vehicle accidents (MVAs), sports injuries (football, hockey), a blow to the belly or flank, or a fall. In children, the most common cause of blunt trauma is as a pedestrian struck by a car or a bicycle accident[13,14]; for adults, the most common cause is an MVA. Although most blunt trauma results in contusion of the kidney, vascular injuries may occur in severe cases, when deceleration velocities cause shear and tearing of vessels.

Children carry a particularly high risk for renal trauma associated with blunt (or penetrating) abdominal trauma because of the comparatively large size of the kidney, the proportion that rests below the rib cage, the softness of the ribs, and the thinner, less well developed abdominal muscles. This risk is exacerbated by the presence of a congenital anomaly of the kidney, resulting in hydronephrosis, or ectopia bypassing the normal protective mechanisms of the ribs, spine, and adjacent organs.[15] In addition, children tend to release significant amounts of catecholamines in response to trauma.[7] As a result, blood pressure is unlikely to drop until as much as 50% of blood volume is lost, rendering the diagnosis "hemodynamic stability" less meaningful in children as compared with adults.

Penetrating injuries are usually caused by a gunshot or stab wound. Soft damage created by a gunshot wound of the kidney is profoundly influenced by the velocity of the bullet.[7] Bullets traveling at higher velocity create larger cavities, resulting in more tissue damage. Rifles and assault weapons tend to project bullets at higher velocities, whereas handguns generally propel projectiles at lower velocities. Cavitation and vaporization also influence soft tissue damage, but it must be remembered that additional, and sometimes extensive, trauma may arise from fragmentation of the bullet or use of ammunition specifically designed to maximize tissue destruction.

The extent of trauma resulting from a stab wound is influenced by the length and width of the weapon, depth of penetration, presence of any twisting after the body is penetrated, and patient's hemodynamic stability.[16] Stab wounds resulting in renal trauma generally occur in the abdomen, anterior chest, posterior chest, or occasionally the flank. They are typically associated with wounds affecting adjacent organs, often including penetration of the bowels, with fecal contamination of the abdomen.

Clinical Manifestations

As noted earlier, hematuria is the most common clinical manifestation indicating urinary system injury. Nevertheless, the presence of hematuria, or its magnitude, does not always indicate the extent of underlying injury. Patients with significant renal injuries may only have microscopic hematuria, whereas others with grade 1 hematomas may have grossly visible blood in the urine.[17] Other common

findings include diffuse abdominal tenderness with ecchymosis or contusion of the flank, with associated tenderness. Marked rigidity of the abdomen may indicate bowel injury and blood in the retroperitoneum. Retroperitoneal bleeding can also cause ileus, nausea, and vomiting. A palpable abdominal mass may occur, indicating a rapidly expanding retroperitoneal hematoma and impending shock. All trauma patients should be observed closely for signs and symptoms of shock and high-volume blood loss.

Diagnosis and Staging

Management of renal injuries is based on a staging system (Figure 10-1). The history focuses on the nature of the injury, location, magnitude and type of force leading to injury, and indications of deceleration force. The physical examination includes careful inspection of the abdomen and flank for symmetry and ecchymosis, abrasions, and signs of any penetrating trauma.[18] Ecchymosis over the posterior 11th or

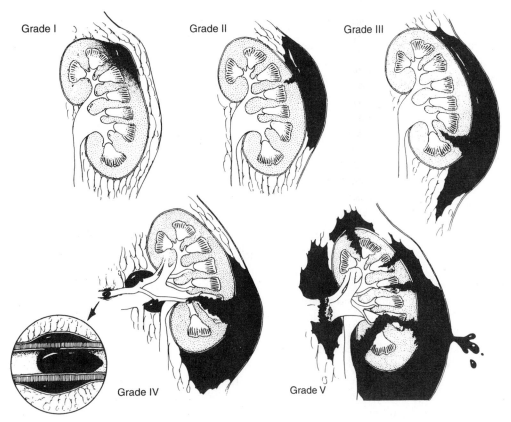

Fig. 10-1 American Association of the Surgery of Trauma Organ Injury Severity Scale for the Kidney. (From Walsh P, Retik A, Vaughen E, Wein A, et al: Campbell's Urology, 8th edition. Philadelphia, Saunders, 2002; p. 3709.)

12th rib, called Grey Turner sign, usually indicates renal trauma, but it does not develop rapidly. Gentle palpation of the abdominal flank and lower rib cage is completed, assessing for symmetry, masses, or pain. The history and physical examination may raise the suspicion of renal injury, but laboratory testing is required to confirm this suspicion, particularly when faced with blunt force trauma.

The initial laboratory study is a urinalysis. A finding of gross or microscopic hematuria indicates a strong suspicion of renal trauma, particularly when urethral and bladder trauma have been excluded. The ideal urine specimen is obtained as soon as possible after injury, because later specimens are likely to be significantly diluted because of parenteral fluid replacement.[7] A sample for serum hematocrit determination is drawn whenever hematuria is detected, or when hemodynamic instability (defined as a systolic blood pressure lower than 90 mm Hg) occurs, to assess the magnitude of blood loss. The hematocrit may be normal when initially measured, but serial measurement may reveal a steady or precipitous decline if significant blood loss occurs.

Imaging studies are indicated whenever an adult patient with blunt abdominal trauma is found to have gross hematuria or a patient with microscopic hematuria is found to be hemodynamically unstable.[7] Imaging studies are also indicated whenever a penetrating wound enters the trunk, regardless of the severity of associated hematuria. In contrast, hemodynamically stable adults with microscopic hematuria have an extremely low risk of significant renal trauma (less than 0.016%)[19] and do not require imaging studies.

Because children are at higher risk than adults for renal injury, and they exhibit hemodynamic instability only after severe blood loss, the indications for imaging differ. Unlike adults, obtaining an appropriate renal imaging study in a child with blunt or penetrating renal trauma and microscopic hematuria can be justified. Imaging every child with abdominal trauma and gross hematuria is mandatory, regardless of evidence of hemodynamic instability.[7]

Imaging studies are used to stage renal injuries and evaluate urinary system function. The patient with a severe injury mandating urgent surgery may undergo one-shot excretory urography. This study is selected because it is performed on the operative table and requires very little time. Unfortunately, it is relatively inaccurate for staging renal injuries and further imaging studies may be required if renal surgery is not imminent.

A contrast-enhanced or spiral CT scan is preferred in the hemodynamically stable patient because it allows more accurate staging of renal injuries.[20] Patients with grades III to V renal lacerations will also require a repeat CT scan in 2 to 4 days to identify any delayed complications.[21] Arteriography is useful for staging renal injuries and for diagnosing vascular trauma. Historically, arteriography was considered the gold standard for staging renal trauma, but it has now been replaced by abdominal CT. Current indications for arteriography are nonvisualization of a kidney on intravenous pyelography following blunt force trauma or when CT is unavailable. The major causes of nonvisualization are total pedicle avulsion, arterial thrombosis, severe contusion causing vascular spasm, and absence of a kidney (e.g., previous nephrectomy or congenital absence). Ultrasound is not recommended for the initial evaluation of renal trauma because of its poor sensitivity when assessing for parenchymal lacerations.[22]

Early Complications

Hemorrhage is the most common early complication seen following renal injury.[5] Rapid exsanguination may occur in patients with higher grade injuries, leading to hypovolemic shock and death unless promptly reversed. The nurse should carefully observe any patient with renal trauma for signs and symptoms of significant blood loss including vital signs—pulse, respirations, and blood pressure—serum hematocrit, oxygen saturation, restlessness, anxiety, and mental acuity.

Later Complications

Prolonged low-volume blood loss occurs in some patients with renal trauma. Persistent hematuria, combined with a slowly declining serum hematocrit value, indicates a slow hemorrhage that may require subsequent imaging studies, selective embolization, or surgery. Long-term complications associated with renal injury include urinoma, hydronephrosis, arteriovenous fistula, and renal vascular hypertension. A urinoma is a collection of extravasated urine formed when the anatomic integrity of the urinary system is compromised. It may result in abscess formation, sepsis, hydronephrosis, or perinephric fibrosis and ureteropelvic junction obstruction. Signs of a perinephric abscess are abdominal tenderness, flank pain, and fever above 38.3° C. The incidence of hypertension following renal injury has not been adequately studied; estimates vary from 0% to 9.4% in children.[23-26] Even less is known about the long-term risk for hypertension in adults; existing studies have shown that the risk is quite small during the initial months following renal injury, but long-term data are lacking. Several factors may contribute to this risk, including renovascular injury with subsequent renal artery stenosis, parenchymal damage with subsequent atrophy, or post-traumatic arteriovenous fistula causing local ischemia and activation of the renin-angiotensin system.[7]

Nursing Management

As noted earlier, urologic management of the patient with a renal injury and multiple trauma occurs in an emergency care setting and must be coordinated with urgent patient needs, as reflected in the ABCDE mnemonic (see earlier). Figure 10-2 provides an algorithm for managing renal injuries based on the American Association for the Surgery of Trauma Classification System.[5]

Observation. Conservative management, defined as observation while the body is allowed to heal, is preferred whenever feasible. Indications for observation include patients who have sustained blunt force trauma, have lower grade injuries, and remain hemodynamically stable (systolic blood pressure higher than 90 mm Hg).[27,28] In addition, selected patients with more severe injury may be managed conservatively following blunt renal trauma. Observation also comprises first-line management in children, but they require particularly close monitoring because they may remain normotensive for extended periods in the presence of major injury.[29] From a nursing perspective, observation is more than watchful waiting. Instead, it provides multiple opportunities for education and self-monitoring as well as counseling about the importance of adherence to formal follow-up with the urologist. The patient and family are taught to monitor the urine for signs of gross hematuria or for changes in urine color or character if gross hematuria is seen at the time of injury. The patient is also advised to drink adequate fluids to meet daily needs and to consume a diet with an adequate protein and vitamin intake needed to

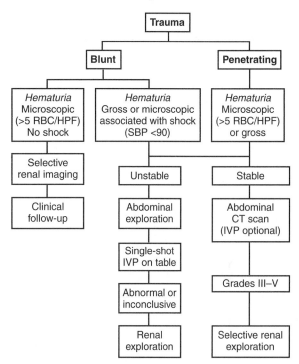

Fig. 10-2 Flow chart for adult renal injuries. *CT*, computed tomography; *HPF*, high-powered field; *IVP*, intravenous pyelography; *RBC*, red blood cell count; *SBP*, systolic blood pressure. (From Welsh P, Retik A, Vaughen E, Wein A, et al: Campbell's Urology, 8th edition. Philadelphia-Saunders, 2002; p. 3711.)

promote wound healing. The urologic nurse should consult with the urologist concerning parameters of bedrest and scheduled return to activities. Although recommendations vary, patients are generally counseled to remain in bed, except for meals and trips to the toilet, for 1 week. After this period, the patient may resume light ambulation and nonstrenuous activity. However, the patient should avoid strenuous activity for approximately 1 month, depending on the grade of the injury and clinician's judgment.

Surgery. Indications for surgery in the patient with blunt renal trauma are largely based on anecdotal experience and vary significantly among trauma centers.[5] Renal injuries caused by blunt trauma must be managed surgically when associated with an expanding or pulsatile hematoma or signs and symptoms of hemodynamic instability and impending shock. Lower grade injuries also may be managed surgically, particularly if the patient is hemodynamically unstable or if long-term renal function is likely to be impaired unless aggressive management is undertaken. Less well-accepted indications for surgery include evidence of urinary extravasation, nonviable renal parenchyma, or incomplete staging, combined with suspicion of vascular trauma or urinary extravasation. As an alternative to immediate surgery, the patient with urinary extravasation may be managed by insertion of a ureteral stent or percutaneous drainage.[29,30] If the urinoma does not resolve within about 5 days, or if a urinoma leads to a perinephric abscess, surgery is indicated.

Unlike blunt trauma, most penetrating renal injuries (70%) require surgical exploration.[5] The goal of surgery is to repair damage to the vascular or collecting system while maximizing preservation of renal parenchyma. When organ preservation is not feasible, a nephrectomy is performed to control blood loss or remove a no longer viable kidney.

Postoperative nursing management is similar to that for any significant abdominal procedure. The patient will have a nasogastric tube in place to rest the bowel and an indwelling catheter. Parenteral antimicrobial therapy may be maintained to prevent infection following a penetrating wound. Effluent from surgical drains should be monitored for character and volume. The volume of drainage may be particularly high in the patient with renal trauma; the effluent should be intraperitoneal fluid and not urine. The creatinine level of the drain effluent may be measured if urinary extravasation is suspected. The patient is also closely monitored for persistent bleeding. The operative wound, abdomen, and flank are monitored for signs of hemorrhage, as is the serum hematocrit and hemoglobin. The indwelling catheter is monitored for the presence of blood or clots and for patency. Grossly visible blood and clots are anticipated when the patient initially returns from surgery, but the urine should return to a yellowish or pink-tinged color within approximately 24 hours.

Following hospital discharge, the patient is educated about the importance of a follow-up imaging study, usually performed 3 months postoperatively. This imaging study is used to detect potential complications such as early-onset renal artery stenosis, urinary calculi, hydronephrosis, arteriovenous fistula, or chronic pyelonephritis with parenchymal scarring.[5] The long-term follow-up also includes imaging studies to ensure adequate renal function and

monitoring of blood pressure. Routine blood pressure monitoring should persist for at least 2 decades following injury because of several case reports of renovascular hypertension 15 years following renal injury.[31]

URETERAL INJURIES

Even when compared with other structures within the genitourinary system, ureteral injuries are rare.[7] The small caliber of the ureters, their location within the abdominal cavity, and their flexible connections to the upper and lower urinary tract contribute to the low likelihood of injury as a direct result of violence. Although rare, ureteral injuries are clinically significant and often lead to urinary obstruction, hydronephrosis, extravasation of urine, fistula formation, infection, or retroperitoneal fibrosis. Therefore, prompt diagnosis and effective management are necessary to restore urinary tract integrity and prevent serious secondary complications.

Etiology and Pathophysiology

The most common cause of ureteral trauma is unintentional injury during surgery, sometimes called surgical misadventure.[32] It occurs in about 1% of all pelvic surgeries.[7] The incidence in hysterectomy, the most commonly performed pelvic surgery in North America, is approximately 1.7%, particularly when surgery was complicated by pelvic organ prolapse.[33] The risk is greatest in patients with extensive bulky tumors, previous pelvic radiotherapy, pelvic inflammatory disorders, endometriosis, or devascularization after extensive lymph node dissection. The most common mode of injury is inadvertent ligation. Most injuries are recognized at the time of their occurrence, but some remain undetected until secondary complications occur, such as urinoma, sepsis, or obstruction and hydronephrosis. Other invasive procedures associated with ureteral injury include electrosurgical or laser-assisted ablation of endometriosis and inadvertent disruption during ureteroscopy.[7]

Because of their location within the abdominal cavity, more than 95% of cases of ureteral trauma associated with violence are caused by a penetrating wound, such as that produced by a gunshot or knife.[34] Blunt trauma is a rare cause; it may result from hyperextension of the spine or as one component of high-grade renal trauma.[21]

Clinical Manifestations

In contrast to other injuries of the urinary tract, hematuria is absent in 25% to 45% of cases.[35-37] Fever, flank, or lower quadrant pain may occur soon after the injury. If the patient is discharged without diagnosis of ureteric injury, the patient will likely present to the physician or emergency room within 10 days, symptomatic, and with a fistula, often accompanied by a watery discharge from the wound or vagina, or hematuria. Extravasation of urine leads to paralytic ileus, nausea, and vomiting.

Diagnosis

Diagnosis of a ureteral injury occurs in one of two distinctive clinical settings—during or following a surgical procedure or in the context of a multisystem trauma. Most intraoperative ureteral injuries are detected during the same procedure.[38] Nevertheless, imaging studies such as intravenous urography or contrast-enhanced CT scan are usually performed for patients with ureteral injuries caused by surgery or unintentional trauma to define the location and nature of the injury and its impact on urinary tract function better (see Table 10-2).[3] A dimercaptosuccinic acid (DMSA) radionuclide scan may be obtained to assess renal function after surgical correction. Assessment of a fistula may require analysis of effluent for creatinine (the urine creatinine level is higher than the serum creatinine level) and IV injection of 10 ml of indigo carmine, which will cause the discharge will appear blue.

Nursing Management

Symptoms of ureteral injury usually manifest by postinjury days 7 to 10 and require prompt treatment. Percutaneous nephrostomy, nephrostomy tube, or ureteral stenting is used to reestablish urine elimination. Small injuries may be allowed to heal spontaneously, but more extensive injuries may require surgical repair. If surgical repair is indicated, ureteral integrity may be reestablished by an end-to-side or end-to-end anastomosis, called a ureteroureterostomy. More severe tissue loss may require ureteral reimplantation with mobilization of a psoas hitch to minimize tension on the anastomosis, transureteroureterostomy, autotransplantation, or ureteral replacement with bowel or appendix.[29]

Conservative management of a ureteral injury necessitates long-term placement of a ureteral stent.

If a fistula is involved, a ureteral stent will remain in place for at least 6 weeks and it may require as long as 6 months before adequate healing occurs. The patient is counseled that a ureteral stent sometimes produces lower urinary tract symptoms, including urgency, urge incontinence or feelings of incomplete bladder emptying, or hematuria. Adequate fluid intake, antimuscarinic medications, and avoidance of bladder irritants will alleviate these symptoms. Refer to Chapter 7 for a description of the nursing management of a long-term nephrostomy tube. In addition to general management principles, the patient with a ureteral injury should be taught to irrigate the tube. This is particularly important because irrigation clears debris from the lumen of the tube and may avoid a trip to the emergency department. The significance of adherence with follow-up appointments and serial imaging studies to assess healing progress is emphasized.

Refer to Chapter 11 for a detailed description of postoperative management of ureteral surgery. In addition to these general principles, the patient is counseled that a return to full physical activity will require approximately 4 to 6 weeks, depending on the extent of the injury and the urologist's judgment. Patients are also taught to self-monitor for signs of urinary tract infection, obstruction, and urinary stone formation.

BLADDER INJURIES

Because of its location deep within the bony pelvis, bladder injuries caused by blunt or penetrating trauma represent less than 2% of all abdominal injuries requiring surgery.[39] As a result, associated injuries are typically extensive and the mortality rate varies from 12% to 22%.[39-41]

Similar to what can happen with the ureters, surgical misadventure represents a common cause of bladder injury.[42] Iatrogenic injury is an uncommon complication of urologic, gynecologic, and general surgical procedures, including especially hysterectomy, open or laparoscopic, and herniorrhaphy. Tension-free vaginal tape (TVT) is associated with a 10% incidence of bladder perforation.[43] Endoscopic evaluation of the bladder at the time of gynecologic or urologic procedures is routine in some centers and may detect unsuspected bladder injury.[44] Bladder lacerations can also occur during a cesarean section or vaginal delivery. Immediate recognition and treatment of iatrogenic injury with an indwelling catheter lead to rapid healing.

Etiology and Pathophysiology

Penetrating trauma is the most common cause of bladder injury associated with violence, most commonly following a gunshot wound.[7] Blunt force leading to pelvic fracture may cause extensive injury to the lower urinary tract, including the bladder. Blunt force trauma is usually associated with a MVA, fall, crush injury, or high-impact blow to the abdomen (Figure 10-3). The risk for bladder injury is greatest when blunt force trauma leads to pelvic fracture. Approximately 15% of all pelvic fractures result in injury to the bladder or urethra,[45] and more than 80% of all bladder injuries are associated with a pelvic fracture, usually involving one or both pelvic arches.[39] Children are at greater risk for bladder injury associated with blunt force trauma because the organ is found in a higher abdominal position

above the pubis and directly behind the poorly developed rectus abdominis muscle.[29] A full bladder is postulated to be at particular risk for decelerating injury when the person is subjected to blunt force trauma. The American Association for Surgery of Trauma (AAST) has developed an injury severity schema for assessing and managing bladder injury associated with blunt force trauma.[46]

Clinical Manifestations

Between 90% and 95% of patients with a bladder injury will have gross hematuria caused by penetrating trauma, piercing injury from a knife wound or gunshot, or bladder wall contusion.[42] Suprapubic pain and bruising are common, but these are often masked by the discomfort associated with a pelvic fracture or other injury. When a bladder injury is not immediately recognized, patients may develop additional signs, including inability to urinate, absence of bowel sounds, fever, peritoneal irritation,

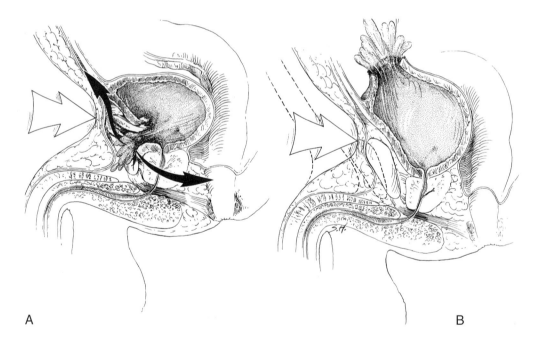

A

B

Fig. 10-3 Pathophysiology of bladder injury associated with blunt force trauma. **A,** Extraperitoneal injuries are usually associated with pelvic fracture when deceleration or shearing forces rupture the bladder base. Additional damage may occur when fragments tear the lower bladder or its base. **B,** Intraperitoneal injury occurs when blunt force is applied directly to the bladder; the risk for this type of injury is greatest when such force is applied to a distended (full) bladder. Rupture usually occurs near the dome, resulting in disruption of the peritoneum and intraperitoneal urine extravasation. (From Gearhart JP, Rink RC, Mouriquand PED (eds): Pediatric Urology. Philadelphia: Saunders, 2001; p 936.)

and elevated blood urea nitrogen level. The presence of these signs often indicates a higher grade bladder injury involving the intraperitoneal space.[42] Delayed detection of an intraperitoneal injury eventually leads to ascites, with abdominal distention. Prolonged extravasation also may lead to referred pain to the shoulder when the diaphragm is irritated or it may result in respiratory distress when extravasation is extensive.

Diagnosis

Because 10% to 29% of bladder injuries are associated with urethral injury or rupture,[7] the physical examination begins with inspection of the urethra for signs of blood. A urinalysis is performed whenever possible to identify the presence of hematuria.[47] Any patient suffering from multiple trauma with hematuria, particularly if the patient is hemodynamically unstable, and anyone who has a pelvic fracture should be investigated for bladder trauma.[48] If blood is detected at the urethral meatus, evaluation begins with retrograde urethrography or cystourethroscopy before a catheter is inserted and additional evaluations are begun. In addition to the signs and symptoms noted earlier, a rectal examination is completed that may reveal indistinct landmarks if a significant pelvic hematoma is present. Intraperitoneal rupture also may produce increased blood urea nitrogen creatinine, and potassium levels and low levels of serum sodium; abnormal laboratory findings are not characteristic of patients with an extraperitoneal bladder rupture, but these findings may be clinically masked in the patient with multiple trauma. Retrograde urethrography (RUG) may be followed by cystography or CT scanning, depending on the extent of injuries and the suspicion level for renal injury.[49] However, even RUG is avoided if a ruptured urethra is suspected. Although each of these studies may reveal bladder rupture, it should be emphasized that both have limited sensitivity and specificity for the diagnosis of a bladder rupture. The accuracy of diagnosis is maximized by obtaining cystographic images in anteroposterior, oblique, and lateral views, with the bladder distended with sufficient volume to ensure that clots or omentum do not temporarily seal a small disruption in its integrity.[42] A plain abdominal film of the kidney, ureter, and bladder also may be obtained. It is useful in the diagnosis of pelvic fractures and may demonstrate a generalized haziness throughout the lower abdomen because of

extravasation of blood or urine into the peritoneum. Table 10-2 outlines the AAST taxonomy for staging bladder injuries associated with blunt force trauma.

Nursing Management

A low-stage bladder injury (contusion) is usually managed by an indwelling catheter until hematuria resolves, usually within 10 to 14 days. A superficial laceration is managed similarly, but may require a longer period of catheterization to ensure adequate healing. Follow-up imaging is obtained before catheter removal to ensure adequate healing and to confirm that the patient is able to urinate normally following catheterization.[29] Figure 10-4 is an algorithm for assessing and managing patients with pelvic fractures and suspected lower urinary tract injury.

Extraperitoneal bladder rupture is usually managed by urethral catheterization until the injury heals, in approximately 10 days. Clots may require irrigation or surgical removal. If the patient has a fractured pelvis, mobilization can occur when the pubic ramus is stable; if the pelvic fracture is unstable, external fixation will cause a prolonged recovery. Postoperative care will include careful assessment for bleeding because, during bladder repair, disruption of pelvic hematomas will cause significant bleeding from pelvic veins.

High-stage bladder injuries involving intraperitoneal rupture require open surgical repair. Postoperatively, the patient will have a urethral or suprapubic catheter in place for 7 to 10 days.

TABLE 10-2 American Association for the Surgery of Trauma Taxonomy for Bladder Injury Associated With Blunt Force Trauma[5]

GRADE	CLINICAL CHARACTERISTICS
I	Bladder contusion with hematoma or partial thickness laceration
II	Extraperitoneal laceration of the bladder less than 2 cm in depth
III	Extraperitoneal laceration more than 2 cm in depth or intraperitoneal laceration less than 2 cm
IV	Intraperitoneal laceration greater than 2 cm in depth
V	Intraperitoneal or extraperitoneal laceration that extends into bladder neck, trigone, or ureteral orifice

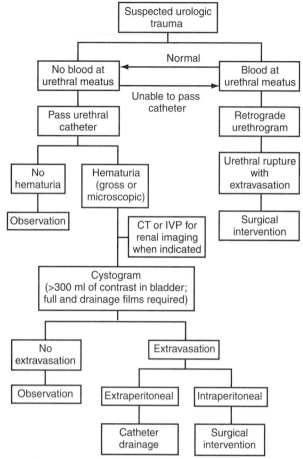

Fig. 10-4 Algorithm for evaluation and treatment of pelvic fracture and suspected lower urinary tract injury. *CT,* computed tomography; *IVP,* intravenous pyelography. (From Walsh PC, Retik AB, Vaughan ED, Wein AJ (eds): *Campbell's Urology,* 8th edition. Philadelphia: Saunders, 2002; p 3722.)

The volume and character of urine output and patency of the urinary drainage system are monitored hourly immediately after surgery. A follow-up cystogram is obtained prior to catheter removal to ensure wound healing and efficient urine evacuation with micturition. Long-term complications include calculus formation around a suture if any aspect piece protrudes into the bladder.

URETHRAL INJURIES

Location of Injury

Anterior Urethra. In the male patient, urethral injuries are classified according to their location.[42]

TABLE 10-3 Taxonomy for Urethral Injury in Men[43]

TYPE	CLINICAL CHARACTERISTICS
I	Posterior urethra stretched by shearing forces, but no rupture occurs
II	Partial or complete rupture above level of urogenital diaphragm, which remains intact
III	Partial or complete rupture, with rupture of urogenital diaphragm
IV	Bladder neck injury with extension into posterior urethra
V	Partial or complete anterior urethral injury

Anterior urethral injuries are usually associated with blunt trauma to the perineum, such as a straddle injury. The bulbar urethra is the most vulnerable; trauma typically occurs when the urethra is crushed against the pelvic bone. Although uncommon, anterior urethral injuries also may be associated with sexual activity or genital self-mutilation.[50] Iatrogenic urethral injury may occur with urethral instrumentation, accidental avulsion of a catheter through the urethra while the retention balloon remains inflated, or inflation of the catheter in the bulbous urethra.

Posterior Urethra. Almost all posterior urethral injuries are caused by a straddle injury, when blunt force trauma causes shear to the bladder base, prostate, and their fascial connections acting against the membranous urethra, the portion of the posterior urethra that lies beneath the apex of the bladder and contains the muscle fibers of the rhabdosphincter. The most common cause is MVA (90%); other etiologies include falls, crushing injuries, and sports injuries. Although only 10% to 15% of pelvic fractures result in urethral injury, almost all result in complete disruption of the posterior urethra. This risk is greatly increased in symphysis and inferior rami fractures combined with injury to the sacroiliac joint.[51] Table 10-3 outlines a classification schema for posterior urethral injuries.

Injuries in Certain Populations

Women. Because of its short length, mobility, and location behind the osseous pubis, urethral injuries associated with violence or trauma are rare in women as compared with men. Even when the bony pelvis is fractured, the incidence of associated urethral injury is 0% to 6%.[47] Vaginal injury will also occur and vaginal bleeding may be present. Women with a urethral injury have a high risk of permanent urinary incontinence. In addition, iatrogenic urethral injuries may occur with instrumentation or during surgical procedures. The diagnosis and management of urethral injury in association with vaginal delivery occur in an obstetric setting[29] and are beyond the scope of this chapter.

Children. Although boys are less likely to experience urethral trauma than adult men,[52] girls are at significantly higher risk than adult women.[47] The increased risk for urethral injury observed in girls younger than 17 years may be attributable to incomplete ossification of the bony pelvis or the more intraabdominal location of the lower urinary tract. Similar to adults, most are associated with an MVA, particularly when the accident has caused a pelvic bone fracture.

Clinical Manifestations

All patients with pelvic fracture or trauma to the perineum are suspected of sustaining a urethral injury until proven otherwise. Men with a urethral injury usually present with blood at the meatus, gross hematuria, significant pain on voiding, or inability to void. They also may have swelling of the penis, scrotum, or perineum. In addition to hematuria or urethrorrhagia, women may experience vaginal bleeding and laceration or an inability to void. Urethral injury associated with urine extravasation may produce labial edema or urine loss through the vagina.

Diagnosis

The presence of blood at the urethral meatus should serve as a strong warning against attempting urethral catheterization until urethral injury has been excluded. Physical examination is likely to reveal suprapubic tenderness, perineal hematoma, or a pelvic fracture in some patients, regardless of gender. Rectal examination of men with posterior urethral injuries may reveal a prostate that is displaced superiorly, often called a high-riding prostate. In women, vaginal bleeding, labial edema, or urine leaking through the vagina may be seen if urine extravasation and fistula occur.

RUG will show partial or complete extravasation at the prostatomembranous junction, depending on whether the injury is incomplete or complete. In women, excretory urography, voiding cystourethrography (VCUG), antegrade cystourethroscopy through a suprapubic tract, or vaginoscopy may be done to determine the size and location of the urethral injury.[53]

Nursing Management

Urethral contusion may be managed conservatively. If the patient can void without pain or bleeding, intervention is limited to pain control and perineal support. If the patient is unable to void, short-term urethral catheterization will be necessary until edema resolves. In patients who are hemodynamically unstable, a suprapubic catheter may be placed until a more detailed evaluation of potential urethra trauma can be undertaken. Depending on the extent of the injury, a suprapubic catheter may remain in place for a prolonged period, sometimes for 3 months or longer.[42] Those with type I injuries or partial disruptions typically heal spontaneously and the suprapubic tube can be removed within 2 to 3 weeks. More severe injuries associated with complete disruption require surgical reconstruction. Although there are no clear data on whether delayed reconstruction reduces the incidence of complications in men with posterior urethral injury,[54] it appears that delay does not significantly affect outcome and allows the patient to stabilize before undergoing reconstructive surgery.

Preoperative preparation will include cystography and urethrography to identify the length and location of the injury, typically immediately posterior to the pubic bone. Repair is usually a single-stage procedure, through a perineal or perineoabdominal approach, with the injured, strictured area (1 to 2 cm) fully excised and with a tension-free end-to-end anastomosis of the bulbous urethra to the prostatic apex.[55] Grafts from buccal tissue have achieved a high success rate, with a low incidence of stricture development.[56] Suprapubic and urethral catheters are left in place for approximately 4 weeks. Usual postoperative care is instituted, with early ambulation, oral intake once bowel sounds are heard, and bowel management with stool softeners. Patients should be instructed to avoid straining during a bowel movement because it may place undue stress on the anastomosis. Patients with a history of constipation may require anticipatory management with stool softeners during the immediate postoperative period. Patients should also be counseled to notify the urologic nurse or physician if they are experiencing bladder spasms because this also may place undue stress against the healing anastomosis site. Pharmacotherapy with an antimuscarinic or anticholinergic drug is indicated when bladder spasms occur.

Approximately 1 month after surgical repair, the urethral catheter is removed and a cystogram is obtained via the suprapubic catheter. If no extravasation occurs, the suprapubic catheter can be removed. If extravasation occurs, the suprapubic tube is left in place and serial repeat cystography is performed until urethral integrity is restored. Because patients with urethral injury are at risk for stricture formation at the anastomotic site, the urology nurse should teach the patient to recognize signs and symptoms of obstruction, including diminution of the force of the urinary stream, hesitancy, straining to void, frequency, and feeling of incomplete emptying. A transient period of in and out catheterization may be required to maintain urethral patency in some patients. Internal urethrotomy is a last resort because of the high risk of urinary incontinence following this procedure.

Complications

Several significant complications are associated with posterior urethral injuries, including urethral stricture, urinary incontinence and associated lower urinary tract symptoms, psychological distress, and erectile dysfunction (ED) in men. The risk of urethral stricture is significant in anterior and posterior urethral injuries (45% to 83%), even if the injury is managed by primary surgical repair.[57] The risk of urinary incontinence in men and boys is greatest when the posterior urethra is injured and the injury is associated with a pelvic fracture; this risk is particularly high in women and girls, because any injury is likely to involve the urethral sphincter mechanism.[7,58,59] ED affects as many as 72% of adult men and 18% of boys with posterior urethral injuries and pelvic fractures.[59,60] ED is typically attributable to local neurologic dysfunction, although 28% may have an identifiable vascular defect as well.[60] Given the prevalence of urinary incontinence, ED, and urethral stricture disease following urethral injury, it is not surprising that these patients are at high risk for psychological distress. Nevertheless,

several studies have found that these injuries are associated with more than just an impaired health-related quality of life. Instead, significant psychiatric disorders have been seen in both children and young adults, including dysthymia and major depression, social phobias, post-traumatic stress disorder, and separation anxiety in children.[59,61]

INJURIES OF THE EXTERNAL GENITALIA

In addition to their role in managing urinary system trauma, urologic nurses are frequently involved in the diagnosis and treatment of injuries affecting the male external genitalia. This chapter provides a brief overview of the management of penile, scrotal, and testicular injuries. In addition to these unintentional injuries, the reader should review Clinical Highlights for Advanced and Expert Practice: Female Genital Mutilation, for a description of intentional female genital mutilation, currently still being performed in many areas of the world.[62-64]

Penile Injuries

Various injuries may compromise the anatomy of the penis. Penile amputation usually occurs in the context of genital self-mutilation; patients who engage in this behavior tend to be psychotic at the time of injury, have suicidal ideation, and are at high risk of repeated self-injury.[65] Treatment focuses on recovery of the organ, surgical reattachment using microsurgical techniques, and psychiatric evaluation and management to treat underlying psychopathology.

A penile fracture describes injury to the tunica albuginea during vigorous sexual intercourse. It occurs when the penis slips out of the vagina and rams against the pubis during a deep thrust or when the penis is unintentionally thrust into an unforgiving surface; 38% are associated with urethral injuries.[5] Clinical manifestations include acute penile pain and hematoma. Conservative management is theoretically possible but surgical treatment is recommended because it reduces recovery time, hospital stay, and the risk of subsequent penile deformity. Various other factors may cause soft tissue injury to the penis, including human and animal bites, improper use of constriction bands, industrial accidents, and misadventure with common household devices, such as vacuum cleaners. Management is based on the severity of the wound, the potential

Clinical Highlights for Advanced and Expert Practice: Female Genital Mutilation

The term *female genital mutilation* is used to describe the practice of surgical removal of part or all of the female genitalia.[63] The procedure is typically performed by a traditional—not medically trained—practitioner. The procedure lasts about 20 minutes and may be performed with a razor blade, knife, cut glass, sharpened rocks, scissors, or fingernails.[65] Instruments are typically used without cleaning and the procedure is usually performed without anesthesia. Approximately 85% of these procedures are performed in Africa and involve removal of the clitoral hood, or clitoridectomy. The most extensive procedure, called infibulation, involves clitoridectomy and excision of the labia minora, followed by excision of the labia majora, which are then stitched together to cover the vaginal orifice. The age at which such procedures may be performed varies widely; it is most commonly performed between the ages of 4 and 10 years, but may be performed as early as 7 days after birth, at the time of marriage, during a first pregnancy, or during labor.

Female genital mutilation is associated with a number of significant physical and psychosocial complications.[64,65] Immediate complications include hemorrhage from the internal pudendal or dorsal artery damage, urethral or bladder injury, and acute urinary retention. Lack of cleanliness predisposes women and girls to urinary tract infection and death resulting from septic shock. Other reported complications include impaired wound healing, predisposing women to recurring urinary tract infection, keloid scar formation, chronic abscess formation, chronic vaginitis, vaginal stenosis, dysmenorrhea, and vesicovaginal or rectovaginal fistula. Psychological complications include post-traumatic stress disorder, depression, and severe sexual dysfunction. Although reconstructive surgery can be used to reverse existing genital and urethral injuries associated with this practice, the only truly effective strategy is immediate discontinuance of its practice on a global basis.[64]

for associated infection, and the presence of additional wounds or injuries. Among neonates, bleeding after circumcision is the most common penile injury, usually managed with pressure dressing, antibiotic ointment, and possibly suturing. Hair strangulation of the penile shaft of the neonate from a stray hair in the diaper has also been reported. In the older child, the usual penile injuries are trauma from a raised toilet seat falling and trapping a little boy's genitalia between the seat and the toilet bowl or a zipper injury in which the foreskin is trapped.

Scrotal Injury

Blunt trauma from fighting or sports is the most frequent cause of scrotal injury. Hematoma and ecchymosis are the usual signs of blunt injury and will resolve without intervention, although the injury is acutely painful and is often accompanied by lower abdominal pain and even nausea and vomiting. It is critical to ensure that the testis has not been injured along with the scrotum. Acute compression of the scrotum against the pubic bone can cause significant injury to the testicle, epididymis, and urethra or avulsion of the scrotal vessels.[29] Ultrasound should be routinely performed on any scrotal or testicular injury. If testicular rupture has occurred, even with immediate treatment, the risk of atrophy and reduced function is high.[66]

Avulsion of the Scrotal Skin

This injury usually occurs from a machinery accident and places the patient at risk for a contaminated wound. Thus, irrigation, débridement, and antibiotic therapy are mandatory. Treatment will involve primary or delayed closure of the wound, depending on the extent of injury and wound contamination. If injury is extensive, scrotal flaps may be necessary for skin grafting. Postoperative care will involve meticulous wound care and assessment of healing.

Blunt Trauma to Testicle

Blunt injury can cause contusion, intratesticular bleeding, or tunica albuginea rupture. Scrotal ultrasound may differentiate between minor testicular contusion and rupture of the testicle but the sensitivity of ultrasound is low and, if rupture is suspected, surgical exploration is indicated.[67] Rupture requires immediate exploration and repair.[68]

SUMMARY

Successful urologic management of patients with trauma typically occurs in the context of the emergency department. Initial interventions are directed at life-threatening trauma summarized earlier by the ABCDE mnemonic. During this period of emergent care, urologic issues are often managed by temporizing techniques, such as insertion of a suprapubic catheter or limited imaging studies to exclude severe urinary system trauma. However, once the patient is stabilized, it is essential that the urinary and reproductive systems undergo proper evaluation and treatment to restore anatomic and functional integrity to the genitourinary system.

REFERENCES

1. Soanes C, Stevenson A: Oxford Dictionary of English, 2nd edition. Oxford: Oxford University Press, 2003.
2. Centers for Disease Control and Prevention: Injury Fact Book: 2006. Retrieved February 13, 2008 from http://www.cdc.gov/ncipc/fact_book/InjuryBook2006.pdf
3. Gin-Shaw SL, Jorden RC: Multiple trauma. In Marx JA (ed): Rosen's Emergency Medicine, 5th edition. St Louis: Mosby, 2002; pp 242-55.
4. Schneider RE: Genitourinary system. In Marx JA (ed): Rosen's Emergency Medicine, 5th edition. St Louis: Mosby, 2002; pp 437-55.
5. McAninch JW, Santucci RA: Renal injuries. In Gillenwater JY, Grayhack JT, Howards SS, Mitchell ME (eds): Adult and Pediatric Urology, 4th edition. Philadelphia: Lippincott, Williams & Wilkins, 2002; pp 479-506.
6. American College of Surgeons Committee on Trauma: Advanced Trauma Life Support for Doctors. Chicago: American College of Surgeons, 1997.
7. McAninch JW, Santucci R: Renal and ureteral trauma. In Wein AJ, Kavoussi LR, Novick AC, Partin AW, Peters CA (eds): Campbell-Walsh Urology, 9th edition. Philadelphia: Saunders, 2007; pp 1274-92.
8. Nicolaisen GS, McAninch JW, Marshall GA, Bluth RF Jr, Carroll PR: Renal trauma: re-evaluation of the indications for radiographic assessment. Journal of Urology, 1985; 133(2):183-7.
9. Mee SL, McAninch JW: Indications for radiographic assessment in suspected renal trauma. Urologic Clinics of North America, 1989; 16(2):187-92.
10. Wright JL, Nathens AB, Rivara FP, Wessells H: Renal and extrarenal predictors of nephrectomy from the national trauma databank. Journal of Urology, 2006; 175(3):970-5.
11. Santucci RA, McAninch JW, Safir M, Mario LA, Service S, Segal MR: Validation of the American Association for the Surgery of Trauma organ injury severity scale for the kidney. J Trauma, 2001; 50:195-200.
12. Wessells H, Suh D, Porter JR, Rivara F, MacKenzie EJ, Jurkovich GJ, Nathens AB: Renal injury and operative management in the United States: results of a population-based study. Journal of Trauma, Injury, Infection and Critical Care, 2003; 54(3):423-30.
13. Durbin DR, Elliott M, Arbogast KB, Anderko RL, Winston FK: The effect of seating position on risk of injury for children in side impact collisions. Annual Proceedings/Association for the Advancement of Automotive Medicine. Association for the Advancement of Automotive Medicine 2001; 45:61-72.
14. Gerstenbluth RE, Spirnak JP, Elder JS: Sports participation and high-grade renal injuries in children. Journal of Urology, 2002; 168:2575-8.
15. Stylianos S: Outcome from pediatric solid organ injury: role of standardized care guidelines. Current Opinion in Pediatrics, 2005; 17:402-6.
16. Armenakas NA, Duckett CP, McAninch JW: Indications for non-operative management of renal stab wounds. Journal of Urology, 1999; 161(3):768-71.
17. McAninch JW: Injuries to the genitourinary tract. In Tanagho EA, McAninch JW (eds): Smith's General Urology, 16th edition. New York: Lange Medical Books/McGraw-Hill, 2004; pp 291-310.
18. Cassabaum VD, Bourg PW: The ins and outs of renal trauma: early identification of renal injury in the ED is critical. AJN, American Journal of Nursing, 2002; Supplement:4-7, 25-7.
19. Miller KS, McAninch JW: Radiographic assessment of renal trauma: our 15-year experience. Journal of Urology, 1995; 154(2 Pt 1): 352-5.
20. Smith JK, Kenney PJ: Imaging of renal trauma. Radiology Clinics of North America, 2003; 41:1019-35.
21. Blankenship JC, Gavant ML, Cox CE, Chauhan RD, Gingrich JR: Importance of delayed imaging for blunt renal trauma. World Journal of Surgery, 2001; 25:1561-4.
22. McGahan JP, Richards JR, Jones CD, Gerscovich EO: Use of ultrasonography in the patient with acute renal trauma. Journal of Ultrasound Medicine, 1999; 18:207-13.
23. Nance ML, Lutz N, Carr MC, Canning DA, Stafford PW: Blunt renal injuries in children can be managed nonoperatively: outcome in a consecutive series of patients. Journal of Trauma, 2004; 57(3):474-8.
24. Margenthaler JA, Weber TR, Keller MS: Blunt renal trauma in children: experience with conservative management at a pediatric trauma center. J Trauma, 2002; 52:928-32.
25. Smith EM, Elder JS, Spirnak JP, et al: Major blunt renal trauma in the pediatric population: is a nonoperative approach indicated?. Journal of Urology, 1993; 149:546-8.
26. Russell RS, Gomelsky A, McMahon DR, Andrews D, Nasrallah PF: Management of grade IV renal injury in children. Journal of Urology, 2001; 166:1049-50.
27. Velmahos GC, Toutouzas KG, Radin R, Chan L, Demetriades D: Nonoperative treatment of blunt injury to solid abdominal organs: a prospective study. Archives of Surgery, 2003; 138(8):844-51.
28. Toutouzas KG, Karaiskakis M, Kaminski A, Velmahos GC: Nonoperative management of blunt renal trauma: a prospective study. American Surgeon, 2002; 68:1097-1103.
29. Peppas DS: Pediatric urologic emergencies. In Gearhart JP (ed): Pediatric Urology. Totawa, NJ: Humana Press, 2003; pp 17-50.
30. Moudouni SM, Patard JJ, Manunta A, Guiraud P, Guille F, Lobel B: A conservative approach to major blunt renal lacerations with urinary extravasation and devitalized renal segments. British Journal of Urology International, 2001; 87:290-4.
31. Jakse G, Putz A, Gassner I, Zechmann W: Early surgery in the management of pediatric blunt renal trauma. Journal of Urology, 1984; 131:920-4.
32. Ghali AM, El Malik EM, Ibrahim AI, Ismail G, Rashid M: Ureteric injuries: diagnosis, management, and outcome. Journal of Trauma, 1999; 46(1):150-8.
33. Vakili B, Chesson RR, Kyle BL, Shobeiri SA, Echols KT, Gist R, Zheng YT, Nolan TE: The incidence of urinary tract injury during hysterectomy: a prospective analysis based on universal cystoscopy. American Journal of Obstetrics and Gynecology, 2005; 192(5):1599-1604.
34. Elliott SP, McAninch JW: Ureteral injuries from external violence: the 25-year experience at San Francisco General Hospital. Journal of Urology, 2003; 170(4 Pt 1):1213-6.
35. Presti JC, Carroll PR, McAninch JW: Ureteral and renal pelvic injuries from external trauma: diagnosis and management. Journal of Trauma, 1989; 29:370-4.
36. Palmer LS, Rosenbaum RR, Gershbaum MD, Kreutzer ER: Penetrating ureteral trauma at an urban trauma center. 10-year experience. Urology, 1999; 54:34-6.
37. Brandes SB, Chelsey MJ, Buckman RF, Hanno PM: Ureteral injuries from penetrating trauma. Journal of Trauma, 1994; 36:766-9.
38. Hammontree LN, Wade BK, Passman CM, Prieto JC, Burns JR, Kolettis PN: Ureteral injuries: Recent trends in etiologies, treatment, and outcomes. Journal of Pelvic Medicine and Surgery, 2005; 11(3):129-36.

39. Hsieh CH, Chen RJ, Fang JF, Lin BC, Hsu YP, Kao JL, et al: Diagnosis and management of bladder injury by trauma surgeons. American Journal of Surgery, 2002; 184(2):143-7.

40. Corriere JN Jr, Sandler CM: Management of the ruptured bladder: seven years of experience with 111 cases. Journal of Trauma, 1986; 26(9):830-3.

41. Cass AS: Diagnostic studies in bladder rupture. Indications and techniques. Urologic Clinics of North America, 1989; 16(2):267-73.

42. Corriere JN Jr: Trauma to the lower urinary tract. In Gillenwater JY, Grayhack JT, Hoards SS, Mitchell ME (eds): Adult and Pediatric Urology, 4th edition. Philadelphia: Lippincott, Williams & Wilkins, 2002; pp 507-30.

43. Barry C, Lim YN, Muller R, Hitchins S, Corstiaans A, Foote A, et al: A multi-centre, randomized clinical control trial comparing the retropubic (RP) approach versus the transobturator approach (TO) for tension-free, suburethral sling treatment of urodynamic stress incontinence: The TORP study. International Urogynecology Journal and Pelvic Floor Dysfunction, 2008; 19(2):171-8.

44. Kwon CH, Golberg RP, Koduri S, Sand PK: The use of introperative cystoscopy in major vaginal and urogynecologic surgeries. American Journal of Obstetrics and Gynecology, 2002; 187:1466-72.

45. Demetriades D, Karaiskakis M, Toutouzas K, Alo K, Velmahos G, Chan L: Pelvic fractures: epidemiology and predictors of associated abdominal injuries and outcomes. Journal of American College of Surgeons, 2002; 195:1-10.

46. Moore EE, Cogbill TH, Jurkovich GJ, McAninch JW, Champion HR, Gennarelli TA, Malangoni MA, Shackford SR, Trafton PG: Organ injury scaling. III: chest wall, abdominal vascular, ureter, bladder, and urethra. Journal of Trauma, 1992; 33(3):337-9.

47. Hartanto VH, Nitti VW: Recent advances in management of female lower urinary tract trauma. Current Opinions in Urology, 2003; 13:279-84.

48. Iverson AJ, Morey AF: Radiographic evaluation of suspected bladder rupture following blunt trauma: critical review. World Journal of Surgery, 2001; 25:1588-91.

49. Morey AF, Iverson AJ, Swan A, Harmon WJ, Spore SS, Bhayani S, et al: Bladder rupture after blunt trauma: guidelines for diagnostic imaging. Journal of Trauma, 2001; 51:683-6.

50. Catalano G, Catalano MC, Carroll KM: Repetitive male genital self-mutilation: a case report and discussion of possible risk factors. Journal of Sex and Marital Therapy, 2002; 28(1):27-37.

51. Aihara R, Blansfield JS, Millham FH, LaMorte WW, Hirsch EF: Fracture locations influence the likelihood of rectal and lower urinary tract injuries in patients sustaining pelvic fractures. Journal of Trauma, 2002; 52:205-8.

52. Holland AJA, Cohen RC, McKertich KMF, Cass TD: Urethral trauma in children. Pediatric Surgery International, 2001; 17:58-61.

53. Podesta ML, Jordan GH: Pelvic fracture urethral injuries in girls. Journal of Urology, 2001; 165:1660-5.

54. Ku JH, Jeon YS, Kim ME, Lee NK, Park YH: Comparison of long-term results according to the primary mode of management and type of injury for posterior urethral injuries. Urologia Internationalis, 2002; 69:227-32.

55. Koraitim MM: Failed posterior urethroplasty: lessons learned. Urology, 2003; 62:719-22.

56. Pansadoro V, Emiliozzi P, Gaffi M, Scarpone P, DePaula F, Pizzo M: Buccal mucosa urethroplasty in the treatment of bulbar urethral strictures. Urology, 2003; 61:1008-10.

57. Asci R, Sarikaya S, Buyukalpelli R, Saylik A, Yilmaz AF, Yildiz S: Voiding and sexual dysfunctions after pelvic fracture urethral injuries treated with either initial cystostomy and delayed urethroplasty or immediate primary urethral realignment. Scandinavian Journal of Urology and Nephrology, 1999; 33(4):228-33.

58. Dorairajan LN, Gupta H, Kumar S: Pelvic fracture-associated urethral injuries in girls: experience with primary repair. British Journal of Urology International, 2004; 94(1):134-6.

59. Onen A, Ozturk H, Kaya M, Otcu S: Long-term outcome of posterior urethral rupture in boys: a comparison of different surgical modalities. Urology, 2005; 65(6):1202-7.

60. Shenfeld OZ, Kiselgorf D, Gorfit ON, Verstandig AG, Landau EH, Pode D: The incidence and causes of erectile dyfunction after pelvic fracture associated with posterior urethral disruption. Journal of Urology, 2003; 169(6):2173-6.

61. Subasi M, Arslan H, Necmioglu S., Onen A, Ozen S, Kaya M: Long-term outcomes of conservatively treated pediatric pelvic fractures. Injury, 2004; 35(8):772-81.

62. Toubia NF, Sharief EH: Female genital mutilation: have we made progress? International Journal of Gynecology and Obstetrics, 2003; 82(3):251-61.

63. Cook RJ, Dickens BM, Fathalla MF: Female genital cutting (mutilation/circumcision): ethical and legal dimensions. International Journal of Gynecology and Obstetrics, 2002; 79:281-7.

64. Kelly E, Hillard PJ: Female genital mutilation. Current Opinion in Obstetrics and Gynecology, 2005; 17(5):490-4.

65. Romilly CS, Isaac MT: Male genital self-mutilation. British Journal of Hospital Medicin, 1996; 55:427-31.

66. Cross JJ, Berman LH, Elliott PG, Irving S: Scrotal trauma: a cause of testicular atrophy. Clinicial Radiology, 1999; 54:317-20.

67. Corrales JG, Corbel L, Cipolla B, Staerman F, Darnault P, Guille F, et al: Accuracy of ultrasound in diagnosis of rupture after blunt testicular trauma. Journal of Urology, 1993; 150:1834-6.

68. Mulhall JP, Gabram SG, Jacobs LM: Emergency management of blunt testicular trauma. Academic Emergency Medicine, 1995; 2:639-43.

CHAPTER

11

Surgical Procedures

....

PRINCIPLES OF CARE FOR ALL SURGICAL PATIENTS
....

Surgery is a unique experience and every person will react differently to the stressors it produces. Although surgical procedures are commonplace for the urologic nurse, we must remain sensitive to the fears and concerns that all patients experience when undergoing an operative procedure. Although many patients draw on multiple resources when coping with the anxiety associated with a surgical procedure, others are reluctant to voice their fears to a physician or family members. The urologic nurse can play an essential role in helping these patients express and cope with their fears. Even when a patient has acknowledged anxiety related to a surgical procedure, the related stress can compromise physiologic and psychosocial function and negatively influence recovery. Box 11-1 lists common fears expressed by patients undergoing urologic surgery. In addition to providing factzual information about a surgical procedure and the anticipated course of recovery, preoperative teaching provides an opportunity to confront and allay related anxieties and fears. All preoperative and postoperative patient teaching should include procedural, sensory, and behavioral content and materials (Box 11-2). In addition, teaching should be presented in an oral, written, and/or audiovisual format; it should be frequently reviewed and altered to reflect current institutional policies and practice and the patient's cognitive abilities and learning style.[1]

Preoperative assessment focusing on surgical and anesthesia risk is a critical component of urologic nursing (Table 11-1). The urologic nurse traditionally has worked under the direct supervision of the urologist and in close consultation with the patient's primary care provider and anesthetist to ensure preoperative assessment. Although each one continues to play an essential role in preoperative assessment, an advanced practice nurse is increasingly likely to complete the preoperative evaluation and ensure clearance from

anesthesia. Refer to Clinical Highlights for Expert and Advanced Practice: Completing a Preoperative Assessment for a detailed description of this critical component of surgical practice.

SURGERY OF THE KIDNEY
....

Urologic practice incorporates various surgical manipulations involving one or both kidneys. The most extensive of these is the radical nephrectomy, which is the principal treatment option for renal cell carcinoma. A detailed discussion of the pre- and postoperative management of the patients undergoing radical nephrectomy is presented. This discussion is followed by more concise reviews of other common urologic surgeries involving the kidneys. Although each of these procedures differs from the radical surgery procedure in important ways, essential principles of preoperative and postoperative management are similar to those described for radical nephrectomy.

Radical Nephrectomy

Radical nephrectomy is the surgical removal of the kidney, ipsilateral adrenal gland, and Gerota's fascia.[2] An open or laparoscopic approach may be selected, depending on the urologist's training and preference, the size of the tumor, and its stage. Laparoscopic procedures are typically reserved for stage I and II tumors that are 10 cm or smaller in size. A number of criteria also enter into the decision to submit a patient to any laparoscopic procedure (Table 11-2, see p. 296). A standard laparoscopic approach can be used for radical nephrectomy, but the hand-assisted technique has gained widespread use because of shorter operative times, avoidance of the need for specimen morcellation, and better control of the operative field.[3] The hand-assisted technique typically requires placement of two or three ports and a small incision in the periumbilical area over McBurney's point (about 5 cm to the left of the

BOX 11-1 Fears Related to Surgery
• •

General
Fear of the unknown
Loss of control
Loss of love from significant others
Threat to sexuality

Specific
Diagnosis of malignancy
Anesthesia
Dying
Pain
Disfigurement
Permanent limitations

BOX 11-2 Preoperative Teaching Content for the Urologic Patient
• •

Procedural
• Informed consent
• Preoperative screening and clearance for anesthesia (laboratory and diagnostic tests, preoperative history, physical assessment)
• Preoperative routines (shower, skin preparation, vital signs, clothing, personal belongings)
• NPO status
• Transfer to surgical suite and postanesthesia care routines, including dressings, intravenous fluids and medications, indwelling urethral catheters, stents or other drains, incision
• Pain control
• Postoperative routines (coughing, deep breathing, leg exercises, antiembolism stockings, ambulation, diet, discharge date, home care needs)

Sensory
• Needle insertion
• Medication effects—drowsiness, dry mouth, amnesia, dizziness
• Operating room environment
• Pain
• Sensations associated with catheters, IV, nasogastric tube

Behavioral
• Demonstration and explanation of exercise routines (coughing and deep breathing, leg exercises)
• Transfer techniques, splinting of incision, ambulation

right anterior superior iliac spine), allowing for insertion of a single hand, although the classic technique requires a third port (Figure 11-1, see p. 296).

An open surgical approach can be used for all stages of nephrectomy, but it is the only approach currently feasible for bulkier or higher grade tumors, particularly when they extend into the inferior vena cava.[2] An anterior subcostal, thoracoabdominal, midline, or flank incision is created to gain access to the renal fossa (Figure 11-2, see p. 297). The surgeon ensures early control of the renal pedicle in preparation for removing Gerota's fascia and its contents (kidney and ipsilateral adrenal gland). Large tumors may invade the vena cava and extend as far as the atrium. In these cases, the patient may require cardiopulmonary bypass and hypothermia to remove the entire mass safely.

Complications. Serious complications associated with laparoscopic radical nephrectomy include vascular injury, fatal gas embolism, hypercarbia, and postoperative pneumothorax.[4] Minor vascular injuries may be managed with blood transfusion, but significant lacerations of major blood vessels require the surgeon to convert from a laparoscopic to an open procedure to ensure rapid reversal of blood loss.[3] Other complications include cardiac arrhythmia, abdominal infection, ventral hernia, ascites, back spasm, shortness of breath, and crepitus related to creation of a pneumoperitoneum. Patients also may experience retention or urinary tract infection associated with manipulation of the urinary tract and transient ileus when the bowel is manipulated.

The complexity of the surgery and the proximity of the kidney to major blood vessels account for the relatively high incidence of complications (up to 20%) seen with open radical nephrectomy.[2] Intraoperative hemorrhage may occur if the inferior vena cava (IVC) or its tributaries are injured. Undetected lacerations of the IVC rarely occur during surgery, and they lead to oozing or frank bleeding postoperatively. Laceration of the liver or gastric tissue also may occur. Other potential complications include pancreatic fistula, pleural injury, particularly if a thoracoabdominal or modified flank incision has been used, postoperative atelectasis caused by operative positioning, wound infection, urinary tract obstruction, transient renal insufficiency, and incisional hernia, particularly with a flank incision. The patient is also at risk for the

TABLE 11-1 History and Physical Examination Components

BODY SYSTEM	CRITICAL COMPONENTS OF PREOPERATIVE ASSESSMENT	SPECIAL CONSIDERATIONS FOR PATIENT UNDERGOING SURGERY
Cardiovascular	Blood pressure, pulse rate, evaluation of heart sounds on auscultation, recent 12-lead electrocardiogram, any history of cardiovascular disease and current treatment, results of laboratory tests (complete blood count, hematocrit and hemoglobin), coagulation factors and use of prescription, over-the-counter, or herbal products that alter these factors, peripheral circulation determined by assessment of peripheral pulses, capillary refill or more sophisticated testing as indicated	Positive history of MI within 6 mo of anticipated surgery, congestive heart failure with jugular venous distention or S3 gallop significantly increase risk for myocardial events during surgery or immediate postoperative period; hypertension also increases risk for cardiovascular complications, particularly if associated with coronary artery disease
Respiratory	Respiratory rate, lung sounds, history of smoking, history of respiratory disease including COPD, emphysema, recent X-ray of chest, ability to cough and deep breathe, oxygen saturation (Sao_2) of peripheral blood	Increased risk of atelectasis in older adults because of diminished ciliary action in lungs, reduced respiratory excursion, cough reflex, and stiffer rib cage, risk of pulmonary or cardiovascular complications highest for persons who have smoked cigarettes for 20 yr or longer
Renal	Serum creatinine and BUN levels, obtain or review more sophisticated tests for renal function (creatinine clearance, radionuclide tests) as indicated, current hydration, urine elimination patterns, evaluate for signs and symptoms of renal insufficiency, including fluid and electrolyte imbalance, anemia, serum pH	Glomerular filtration rate diminishes with aging, wound healing impaired in patients with renal insufficiency, renal failure increases risk for postoperative mortality
Integumentary	Integrity of skin, including presence of acute or chronic wounds related to previous surgery, pressure, vascular or neuropathic etiology, previous scars, rashes, cutaneous infections	Older adults (particularly the very old, age 80 yr or older) have thinner stratum corneum, reduced elasticity of skin, increased risk for pressure ulceration or moisture-related skin damage (incontinence-associated dermatitis) during or following surgery
Musculoskeletal	Strength, mobility, dexterity, range of motion of neck and shoulders, history of musculoskeletal diseases, including arthritides	Older adults at increased risk for arthritides, impaired mobility following surgery
Neurologic	Special senses, with particular attention for corrective eyeglasses, hearing aids that require special management during and following surgery, mental acuity, understanding of surgical procedure and anticipated course of recovery, history of stroke, neurologic disease or lesions, including disk problems	Older adults at increased risk for acute dementia or confusion; patients with paralyzing spinal cord lesions at increased risk for multiple complications, including pressure injury and atelectasis
Gastrointestinal	Electrolytes, nutritional status (determine serum albumin and prealbumin levels if indicated), dentition and presence of false teeth, fecal elimination patterns	Patients undergoing manipulation of gastrointestinal tract at risk for prolonged ileus; extensive use of opioid analgesics during immediate postoperative period increases this risk; incorporation of bowel into urinary tract reconstruction increases risk for metabolic acidosis, malabsorption, chronic or recurring diarrhea.

BUN, Blood urea nitrogen; *COPD,* chronic obstructive pulmonary disease; *MI,* myocardial infarction.

Advanced practice nurses function in various roles within the specialty of urology. One of the most rapidly expanding roles for nurse practitioners in particular is preoperative preparation of patients undergoing a surgical procedure. Nurse practitioners are uniquely qualified to fulfill this role because of their holistic approach to patient care and their ability to identify factors that lie beyond the urinary system and determine how these factors may affect anesthesia, surgery, or recuperation. This clinical highlight outlines the essential components for preparing a patient for urologic surgery.

History and Physical Examination

A health history and physical examination is completed prior to any surgical procedure. Both the history and physical examination must be comprehensive and focus on physical or psychosocial factors likely to influence a patient's response to the stressors of undergoing surgery, anesthesia, the procedure itself, or the anticipated recovery. Assessment begins with a general inspection that incorporates skin color, height and weight, body habitus, grooming and clothing, mobility (ability to ambulate, gait, sitting or rising from a chair or examination table), cognitive status (orientation, mental acuity, knowledge and comprehension of upcoming surgery), and the presence of family or significant others. The vital signs are measured, including temperature, blood pressure, pulse, and respirations. Although each assessment must be individualized, the health history and physical examination should cover the areas noted in Table 11-1.

Metabolic Status

For the patient undergoing urologic surgery, evaluation of the metabolic status focuses on renal, hepatic, and adrenal function and nutrition. Assessment of hepatic function includes measurement of liver enzyme and albumin levels and coagulation factors. Patients with compromised hepatic function may require special preparation for surgery, including transfusion with fresh frozen plasma or administration of vitamin K. Those with cirrhosis may require boosting of nutritional status, limiting sodium intake, and administration of a diuretic to reduce ascites. In addition to the evaluation of renal function discussed above, patients with renal insufficiency may have underlying fluid and electrolyte disorders that must be corrected prior to surgery.

Several adrenal hormone levels, including catecholamines and glucocorticoids, are elevated during and immediately following anesthesia and surgery. Persons with potentially compromised adrenal function, such as those on chronic corticosteroids, may experience an acute and life-threatening insufficiency of steroids when the body is challenged by the physical demands of anesthesia and surgery. The urologist and anesthesiologist are informed of the patient's status, and stress level corticosteroids such as Decadron (dexamethasone sodium phosphate) or Solu-Cortef (hydrocortisone sodium succinate) are administered during and immediately following surgery. In contrast, patients with a pheochromocytoma experience overproduction of the adrenal medullary hormones epinephrine and norepinephrine. Clinical manifestations of a pheochromocytoma include palpitations, sweating, headaches, and difficulty sleeping. However, within the context of surgery, the most important manifestation is labile swings in blood pressure that significantly raise the overall mortality risk. Therefore, any suspicion of a pheochromocytoma indicates the need for a complete evaluation and endocrine consultation before surgery is undertaken, as well as suppressive drugs administered during and immediately following surgery.

Nutrition

The basal metabolic rate is defined as the average caloric requirement for the resting human. The physical and psychosocial demands of anesthesia and surgery raise the basal metabolic demands of the body, resulting in increased caloric needs, despite a decrease in physical activity. During routine, elective surgery, this increase is approximately 10% but it may be as high as 25% during trauma surgery complicated by multiple bone fractures, or much higher in the patient with severe burns. Nutritional requirements may be further challenged when the patient banks blood for autotransfusion following surgery. Because of these challenges, the nurse practitioner should work with the patient, urologist, anesthesiologist, and family to ensure that nutritional deficits are resolved prior to surgery and that postoperative nutritional intake is adequate to meet the needs of the transient increase in basal metabolism and wound healing.

TABLE 11-2 Patient Selection for a Laparoscopic Surgical Procedure

CLINICAL CONDITION	IMPACT ON LAPAROSCOPIC APPROACH
Uncorrected coagulopathy, massive hemoperitoneum, abdominal wall infection, peritonitis, suspected malignant ascites	Absolute contraindications for laparoscopic approach because of high risk for uncontrolled hemorrhage, spread of abdominal or peritoneal infection, bowel injury in case of malignant ascites
Morbid obesity	Renders entire procedure more technically difficult, increases risk for postoperative complications (however, these risks have not been found to be greater than those seen with open procedures)
Multiple prior surgical procedures or pelvic fibrosis	Increases difficulty establishing an adequate gas retroperitoneum; risk for CO_2 leakage may lead to inflammation and fibrosis in patient with artificial hip prosthesis
Organomegaly	Increased risk of damage to enlarged organ; difficulty when establishing pneumoperitoneum
Diaphragmatic hernia	Increased risk for leakage of CO_2 from mediastinum increases risk for pneumopericardium
Umbilical hernia	Absolute contraindication for using the umbilicus as site for establishing CO_2 pneumoperitoneum
Ileal or aortic aneurysm	Access to abdomen must be obtained at safe distance from any aneurysm; accessory trocars must be inserted under strict endoscopic control to avoid risk of catastrophic laceration of aneurysm
Pregnancy	Access to abdomen must be obtained at safe distance from gravid uterus, which becomes progressively difficult as pregnancy progresses; prolonged pneumoperitoneum must be avoided because of increased risk for maternal hypercarbia and acidosis, with subsequent fetal distress

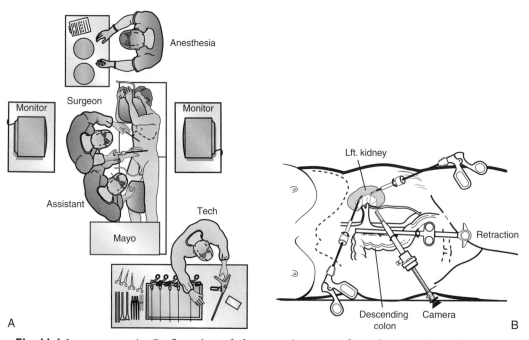

Fig. 11-1 Laparoscopy. **A,** Configuration of the operating room for a laparoscopic nephrectomy. **B,** Trocar position for laparoscopic nephrectomy. (From Wein AJ, Kavoussi LR, Novick AC, Partin AW, Peters CA [eds]: Campbell-Walsh Urology, 9th edition. Philadelphia: Saunders, 2007; p 1763; Walsh PC, Retik AB, Wein AJ, Vaughan ED (eds): Campbell's Urology, 8th edition. Philadelphia: Saunders, 2002; p 3657.)

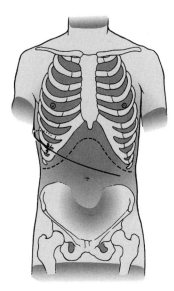

Fig. 11-2 Common incisions used for open radical nephrectomy. Thoracoabdominal or subcostal. (From Wein AJ, Kavoussi LR, Novick AC, Partin (eds): Campbell-Walsh Urology, 9th edition. Philadelphia, Saunders, 2007; p 1176.)

systemic complications common to all major surgical procedures, such as pulmonary complications, deep vein thrombosis, pulmonary embolus, and pneumonia. Transient ileus is also seen with open procedures, particularly when extensive bowel manipulation is required.

Preparation for surgery. Preparation for radical nephrectomy is profoundly influenced by the decision to approach the procedure via a laparoscopic or open technique. Laparoscopic procedures avoid the large incisions required for open surgery, but they require insufflation of the abdomen with carbon dioxide (CO_2) or another gas and significant anesthesia time, and may require conversion to an open procedure if significant hemorrhage occurs. In contrast, open procedures may require less anesthesia time, but they rely on a significant incision in the abdomen or flank and a subsequent increase in recovery time.

Laparoscopic radical nephrectomy. The patient is informed that two or three small incisions will be made in the abdomen or flank and a larger (2-inch) incision will be created to the left or right anterior superior iliac spine if a hand-assisted technique is used. Bowel preparation is required, including a clear liquid diet and bisacodyl (Dulcolax) tablets or suppository the day before surgery. A more aggressive preparation, including GoLYTELY and an antibiotic,

may be required for selected patients or when the procedure is complicated by fibrosis because of multiple prior procedures or radiation therapy. Counseling about potential complications, including the risk for bleeding and potential for conversion to an open procedure, is provided and the patient is advised to bank blood based on institutional policy.

Open surgery. The patient is advised that the procedure may cause significant blood loss, necessitating the need for transfusion and blood banking based on institutional policy. Frail or older patients should be counseled about increasing the amount of dietary iron and protein when banking blood and preparing for radical nephrectomy. Preoperative bowel preparation is required, using a combination of a clear liquid diet and bisacodyl preparation, GoLYTELY, or a sodium phosphate (Fleet Phospho-Soda) enema.

Postoperative care. Postoperative care is also influenced by the surgical approach. Although laparoscopic procedures avoid a surgical incision and reduce postoperative recovery times in certain patients, each technique carries a risk of shared or unique complications that are most likely to be prevented or reversed by prompt identification and intervention.

Laparoscopic radical nephrectomy. Several complications unique to laparoscopic nephrectomy may affect the procedure and subsequent postoperative recovery period.[5] A gas embolism may occur if the Veress needle, used to create the pneumoperitoneum, unknowingly pierces an organ and insufflation proceeds. This complication is usually identified and managed in the operative setting. Hypercarbia may occur, especially in patients with chronic obstructive pulmonary disease (COPD), leading to respiratory and metabolic distress. To prevent this complication, the urologist may create a pneumoperitoneum using an alternative gas, such as helium. A pneumomediastinum or pneumopericardium may occur, compromising cardiovascular function. It is usually detected during surgery and corrected at that time, although it is occasionally diagnosed during the immediate postanesthesia recovery period. Mechanical bowel injuries are typically detected and managed intraoperatively, but undetected injuries occasionally occur and produce signs and symptoms of peritonitis during the early postoperative recovery period. An electrosurgical bowel injury is rarely detected during the procedure itself. Instead, it usually manifests as fever, nausea, and signs of peritonitis about

3 to 7 days following surgery. Minor bowel injuries can be managed conservatively by the administration of antibiotics and an elemental diet, although surgical repair may be required when more extensive injury creates tissue necrosis.

Pain following a laparoscopic radical nephrectomy is significant but comparatively less than that experienced by patients who undergo an open procedure. This pain can be roughly divided into two manifestations, localized and diffuse. Early intense pain occurring during the immediate postoperative period localized to a single port incision and accompanied by nausea and signs of an ileus may indicate herniation of bowel through the site, although localized pain occurring several days following the procedure is more likely to be associated with a wound infection. Diffuse abdominal discomfort associated with a fever raises a suspicion of peritonitis. Diffuse abdominal pain occurring during the early postoperative period also may indicate irritation from the pneumoperitoneum, release of noxious material during laparoscopy, or bowel injury. The discomfort produced by a pneumoperitoneum is transient because the CO_2, will be absorbed rapidly, usually within 24 to 48 hours. In contrast, persistent pain is more likely to indicate bowel injury or infection. The initial management of postlaparoscopic pain focuses on identifying its probable cause and treating its underlying pathophysiology, complemented by appropriate analgesic medications and nonpharmacologic comfort interventions.

Open nephrectomy. Postoperative care of the patient undergoing an open radical nephrectomy follows the principles followed for all major surgery, including routine use of compression stockings and early mobilization to prevent deep vein thrombosis, and routine monitoring of vital signs, relevant laboratory findings, fluid intake, and urine output. However, several issues are particularly relevant to the postoperative recovery of the patient undergoing a radical nephrectomy. They include (1) compromised pulmonary function; (2) pain; (3) wound healing; (4) altered gastrointestinal function; and (5) altered urine elimination.

Because of the location, size, and nature of the incision, patients undergoing radical nephrectomy are at high risk for atelectasis and pneumonia. Therefore, breath sounds are routinely monitored and active deep breathing and coughing exercises are augmented with the use of an incentive spirometer. Patients with a flank incision will return from surgery with a chest tube and they should be carefully monitored for signs and symptoms of a pneumothorax.

Postoperative pain can be significant following open radical nephrectomy. Incisional pain is managed by splinting the abdomen and flank during pulmonary toilet, careful positioning in the bed or chair, and analgesic management. An epidural or patient-controlled analgesia (PCA) pump is used to manage initial postoperative pain, followed by oral opioid or nonsteroidal analgesics, when feasible. Routine assessment of the postoperative wound provides important information about the progress of wound healing and the cause of underlying pain. For example, a sudden increase in incisional pain may indicate a wound infection or an accumulation of fluid or blood in the wound. Superficial infections may be managed by removal of skin sutures or staples to allow drainage and subsequent healing, but more serious infections require systemic antibiotics. Similarly, although a mild collection of serous wound fluid may not require immediate intervention, a buildup of blood or purulent materials requires more aggressive evaluation and intervention.

Because radical nephrectomy requires manipulation of the bowel, a nasogastric tube will be placed during the initial postoperative period. Oral feeding occurs only after the return of bowel function, typically within the first week following surgery. Early ambulation and avoidance of excessive opioid analgesics promote an early return of bowel function.

Urine drainage is managed by an indwelling catheter and urine output is regularly monitored for volume and urine character. The urologic nurse closely monitors the catheter for excessive bleeding and for passage of clots in particular, which may block urinary drainage. Transient renal insufficiency may occur because of venous thrombus formation caused by a vena caval thrombus or following surgical ligation of a renal vein.[6] Renal insufficiency is typically transient, but it may necessitate hemodialysis.

Patient teaching highlights. Patients are advised to avoid lifting, straining, and prolonged automobile rides until cleared by their surgeon. Teach the patient to consume adequate fluids and to use a mild laxative and/or stool softener when needed to ensure a soft formed stool and avoid the straining associated with constipation. Over-the-counter medications, high-dose vitamin E, and other products known to thin the blood should be avoided during the first 4 to 6 weeks following surgery unless specifically cleared by a physician. Patients are counseled to contact their urologist or urologic nurse if they experience gross hematuria, gross bleeding from the incision, fever, signs of a wound infection, or nausea and vomiting. Box 11-2 summarizes general information related to postoperative patient teaching.

Partial Nephrectomy

Partial nephrectomy is the surgical removal of a tumor from the kidney while preserving as much of that kidney's parenchyma as possible.[6] It is also indicated for benign lesions such as atrophic pyelonephritis in a duplicated renal system, caliceal diverticulum complicated by infection or stones, renovascular hypertension caused by stenosis of a branch of the renal artery, trauma to a single renal pole or segment, and resection of a benign tumor, such as an angiomyolipoma or oncocytoma. The procedure is frequently described as nephron sparing because it avoids removal of the entire kidney. Candidates for partial nephrectomy include those with a solitary kidney, bilateral renal tumors for whom radical nephrectomy would render the person anephric and in need of immediate dialysis, compromised function of the opposite kidney, or a diagnosis such as diabetes, likely to compromise renal function in the future. The ideal candidate for partial nephrectomy has a small (less than 4 cm) tumor that is well localized and contained within the cortex.

Similar to radical nephrectomy, laparoscopic or open approaches are feasible alternatives for partial nephrectomy.[7] Laparoscopic partial nephrectomy typically uses a transperitoneal or retroperitoneal approach and three ports to gain access to and manipulate the kidney. In addition, a ureteroscope is passed to visualize the renal pelvis. Because the goals of partial laparoscopic nephrectomy include removal of the kidney and simultaneous sparing of normal nephrons, minimization of ischemic damage is of paramount importance. Ischemic damage to the renal parenchyma is limited by hypothermic techniques, such as packing the kidney with finely shaved ice, thus limiting the period of warm ischemia, when renal perfusion is compromised and hypothermia is not present, to 30 minutes.

Various open surgical techniques may be used to accomplish partial nephrectomy, including simple enucleation, wedge resection, polar segmental nephrectomy, and transverse resection. Each of these approaches dictates that the surgeon gain early vascular control, thus limiting parenchymal ischemia, followed by excision of the tumor and repair of residual parenchyma. When applied to carefully selected patients with small, well-contained tumors, partial nephrectomy provides 5-year cancer-free survival rates of 87% to 90%.[6]

Simple Nephrectomy

Simple nephrectomy requires removal of the entire kidney, but does not involve the en bloc resection required for radical surgery. Indications include renovascular hypertension, extensive parenchymal damage caused by pyelonephritis, congenital dysplasia, cystic disease, reflux nephropathy, and nephrosclerosis. An open or laparoscopic approach may be used to complete a simple nephrectomy. Techniques used for these procedures are similar to those used for radical surgery.

Donor Nephrectomy

Unlike simple nephrectomy, a donor nephrectomy seeks to remove an otherwise healthy kidney for the purpose of transplantation into a patient with chronic renal failure.[8] Traditionally, donor nephrectomy was performed using an open surgical technique via a flank incision. The renal vessels are clamped as close to the aorta and vena cava as possible in anticipation of reestablishing vascular access in the transplant recipient. The ureter is cut, leaving adequate length to attach it to the recipient's bladder, typically in a refluxing manner. After removal, the kidney and ureter are placed in an iced saline solution and flushed with a cooled preservation fluid until venous effluent is clear and the kidney discolored. Complication rates vary from 4% to 8%.[6] Common postoperative complications include wound infection, chronic wound pain, incisional hernia, and pneumothorax.

Laparoscopic donor nephrectomy using a transperitoneal approach is a potential alternative to open surgery. After insufflation of the abdomen with CO_2, four or five trocars are introduced and a small suprapubic incision created to allow ureteral amputation. Potential advantages of the laparoscopic procedure include reduced blood loss, less postoperative pain, shorter length of hospital stay, and a more rapid return to work. Disadvantages include longer anesthesia and operating times, longer renal ischemia times, and shorter renal vessels. Operative and warm ischemia times are reduced by a hand-assisted approach, but this approach necessitates an additional small incision.

Cryotherapy of the Kidney

From a surgical perspective, cryotherapy is defined as the application of extreme cold for the purpose of tissue ablation. Renal cryotherapy is undergoing investigation for its efficacy in the management of small, localized renal tumors (smaller than 4 cm).[9] Access to the tumor may be gained laparoscopically, percutaneously, or via open incision. Cryoprobes are then placed intraoperatively using ultrasonic guidance and the tumor is ablated (Figure 11-3). Potential advantages of cryotherapy include reduction of renal ischemia and minimization of hospital length of stay, about 3 to 4 days for open techniques and 1 to 2 days for laparoscopic procedures. Complications associated with renal cryotherapy are similar to those encountered with partial nephrectomy and include bleeding and injury of adjacent organs caused by inadvertent contact with a cryoprobe. Further investigation is needed to determine what role, if any, cryotherapy will ultimately play in the surgical management of renal cell carcinoma.

SURGERY OF THE RENAL PELVIS AND URETERS

With the advent of endourology, the need for open surgical repair of the ureter in adults has been largely replaced by endoscopic, laparoscopic, or extracorporeal techniques. Nevertheless, pyeloplasty, open repair of a ureteral stricture or trauma, surgical anastomosis of one ureter to the other, or reimplantation of one or both ureters into the bladder (ureteroneocystostomy) is required in some adult patients. Chapter 7 provides a detailed discussion of endourologic management of the patient with urinary calculi and Chapter 18 reviews the surgical management of patients undergoing surgery of the ureter and renal pelvis.

SURGERY OF THE LOWER URINARY TRACT

A number of surgical procedures are indicated for the management of lower urinary tract disorders. This section will review surgical procedures used to manage lower urinary tract malignancies, including transurethral resection of bladder tumors and radical cystectomy, and selected procedures used to manage urinary incontinence.

Surgical Management of Bladder Cancer

As noted in Chapter 8, treatment options for bladder cancer are based on the tumor stage. Superficial disease, stages T1 and T2, is typically managed by resection and intravesical chemotherapy, although invasive tumors, stage T3 and higher, require more aggressive treatment, often including radical cystectomy.

Transurethral Resection of Bladder Tumors. Transurethral resection of bladder tumors (TURBT) is indicated for localized bladder cancer. The procedure is usually performed using a 24- or 25F resectoscope and rigid outer sheath, up to 30F. The resectoscope houses a malleable wire loop connected to an electrosurgical unit whose current can be manipulated to cut or coagulate. The urologist's ability to visualize the bladder and resect tumors, and to differentiate these from normal urothelium, may be enhanced by the use of a photosensitizing agent that fluoresces when exposed to a certain wavelength of light. An appropriate irrigant for TURBT, such as 1.5% glycine and sterile water, is infused throughout the procedure and all tissues are collected and preserved for pathologic analysis. Following resection, a careful bimanual pelvic or rectal examination is done to assess for residual mass or tumor that is adherent to the pelvic side wall, because fixed tumors have a poor prognosis.[10]

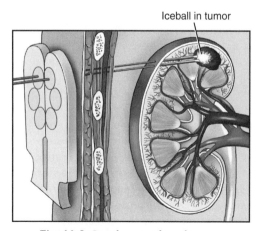

Iceball in tumor

Fig. 11-3 Cryotherapy of renal tumor.

Alternatives to traditional transurethral resection include fulguration of very small, superficial lesions using a Bugbee electrode or thermal destruction via laser energy. Laser energy is useful in the management of papillary lower urinary tract tumors because it destroys tissue and provides excellent vascular coagulation. The most commonly used laser light sources for resecting bladder tumors are neodymium YAG (yttrium-aluminum-garnet), argon, or KTP (potassium–titanyl phosphate). Limitations to laser treatment include the inability to retain a tissue specimen for pathologic analysis and lack of efficacy for carcinoma in situ. In addition, extensive training and education are imperative for all operative personnel when laser energy is used to manage lower urinary tract tumors.

Complications. Complications associated with TURBT include those associated with all endoscopic procedures involving the lower urinary tract, including urinary tract infection in 7% to 13% of cases.[11,12] Over 90% of patients who have TURBT and/or intravesical chemotherapy will experience lower urinary symptoms such as voiding frequency, urgency, and dysuria. In addition, transurethral resection of urothelial tumors carries small but significant risks for perforation of the bladder wall, severe hematuria, and vesicoureteral reflux or distal ureteral injury.[13-15]

Complications associated with the use of laser energy for fulguration include optic or cutaneous injuries to operating room personnel.[16] Patient-related complications include thermal laser injury to the patient's bladder, urethral or ureteral stricture, bladder perforation, undetected coagulation necrosis, and thermal damage to adjacent structures, such as the bowel.

Preparation for surgery. Preparation incorporates principles for any lower urinary tract endoscopic procedure (see the discussion of cystourethroscopy in Chapter 4). Patients with low-grade tumors are advised that the principal goal of resection or laser fulguration is to destroy all visible malignant tumors, but resection may be limited if higher grade (invasive) tumors are found that indicate the need for radical cystectomy. Although the procedure remains investigational in the United States, Canadian patients with carcinoma in situ may be counseled concerning treatment with a photodynamic sensitizing agent such as porfimer (Photofrin PDT) prior to transurethral resection to improve the surgeon's ability to identify and ablate malignant tissue.[10] In addition to instruction about transurethral surgery and its anticipated course of recovery, teaching also incorporates basic information about the anticipated type of energy used for tumor resection, the role of tissue collection and pathologic analysis, and the critical importance of scheduled follow-up appointments and ongoing cancer surveillance.

Postoperative care. Bothersome, irritative lower urinary tract symptoms are usually managed conservatively by adequate fluid intake, avoidance of bladder irritants such as caffeine or alcohol, and administration of urinary analgesics or antimuscarinics as directed. Patients can be advised that these symptoms are likely to peak by the third day following the procedure and then subside. Bladder spasms, experienced as intermittent cramping discomfort, are also more likely to respond to a urinary analgesic or antimuscarinic agent as compared with an opioid analgesic. Bladder irrigation to control bleeding may be required for up to 24 hours if extensive resection was undertaken. Hematuria is usually transient and mild, but the nurse should carefully monitor the patient for high-volume blood loss manifested as bright red blood in the urine and passage of blood clots.

Patient teaching highlights. Teach the patient the signs and symptoms of hematuria or urinary obstruction. Warn them that mild dysuria and hematuria may occur for a few days after tumor resection but it should gradually resolve. In addition to the interventions described for managing bothersome lower urinary tract symptoms, the patient can be counseled that as many as three warm sitz baths each day may relieve discomfort. Patients are also advised that urinary tract analgesics or antimuscarinics should be taken as prescribed rather than as needed because their actions are not the same as those of opioid or nonsteroidal analgesics. Although rare, patients should also be taught to contact the urologist or urologic nurse immediately if they experience signs and symptoms of peritonitis, indicating infection associated with bladder rupture or coagulation necrosis.

Radical Cystectomy. Radical cystectomy remains the primary treatment strategy for controlling locally invasive bladder cancer (Table 11-3).[17,18] It requires removal of the bladder, perivesical fat, overlying peritoneum, and pelvic lymph nodes. In women, it includes the uterus and a portion of the anterior

TABLE 11-3 Management of Invasive Bladder Tumors

CYSTECTOMY	RECURRENT SUPERFICIAL STAGE T2 DISEASE
Surgery + chemotherapy	Locally advanced (T3b, T4a)
Chemotherapy (± surgery)	T4b, N-positive, possibly for select M-positive

TABLE 11-4 Urinary Diversions

TYPE	DIVERSION
Noncontinent	Conduit—ileal, colonic; cutaneous ureterostomy, percutaneous nephrostomy
Continent	Nonorthotopic—use small and/or large-bowel Indiana pouch, colon with terminal ileum, Kock pouch
	Orthotopic—more complicated, improved body image; Studer pouch, hemi-Kock pouch

vagina; in men, the prostate and seminal vesicles. The bladder is approached via a lower midline abdominal incision and a gap is developed between the bladder and pubic bones (space of Retzius). The peritoneal cavity is entered and explored to ensure the absence of metastatic masses, and a pelvic lymphadenectomy is completed. The bladder vessels are ligated and the bladder removed, using a nerve-sparing technique whenever possible. A urethrectomy may be performed in men and the vagina reconstructed in women. In patients with negative nodal involvement the 5- and 10-year recurrence rates after radical cystectomy are 8% and 14%, and 32% and 34%, respectively, even when nodal metastases are present.[18]

After the bladder is safely removed, attention is then directed to diversion or reconstruction of the lower urinary tract to create a low-pressure escape route for urine (ileal or intestinal conduit), an ectopic storage reservoir for urine that can be emptied by intermittent catheterization (continent urinary diversion), or a reconstructed reservoir connected to the trigone and urethra (orthotopic neobladder). This chapter will review multiple options for managing urinary elimination following radical or simple cystectomy. Detailed discussions or pre- and postoperative management will focus on the most common type of incontinent urinary diversion, the ileal conduit, several common continent urinary diversions, and the orthotopic neobladder in detail.

Partial Cystectomy. Partial cystectomy is the surgical removal of a portion of the bladder wall, followed by reconstruction of the remaining bladder. Indications for the procedure are limited to cases in which bladder cancer is confined to one portion of the bladder wall that is sufficiently removed from the bladder base so that an organ-sparing procedure is feasible. However, the relatively small proportion of patients who qualify for the procedure, and higher

cancer recurrence rates when compared with those of radical cystectomy, severely limit the clinical role for this procedure.[19]

Simple Cystectomy. A simple cystectomy is the surgical removal of the bladder without the en bloc resection of adjacent structures essential to radical cystectomy.[17] Indications for simple cystectomy include neurogenic bladder dysfunction associated with upper urinary tract distress, refractory radiation or chemotherapy-induced cystitis, locally invasive prostate cancer that extends into the bladder base, pyocystis in a defunctionalized (previously diverted) lower urinary tract, severe urethral trauma, and severe interstitial cystitis that has proven refractory to all other reasonable treatment options.

Ureteral Diversions. Ureteral diversion is reserved for patients who are poor candidates for any other type of diversion (Table 11-4).[20] The surgery involves bringing the ureters through a small incision in the abdominal wall and creating a budded stoma. The result is an incontinent diversion that must be drained by an ostomy pouch. Significant disadvantages associated with the ureterostomy include the technical challenge of creating an adequately budded stoma in a good location on the abdomen and a high incidence of stomal stenosis.

Urinary Conduits. The Bricker ileal conduit is the most commonly performed conduit type diversion (Figure 11-4). It is constructed from a small segment of ileum that is isolated from the fecal stream and attached to the ureters; it allows free urine drainage via a stoma brought through the abdominal wall. A 10- to 12-cm segment of ileum that is at least 12 to 15 cm away from the ileocecal valve is selected for the procedure. The ileum near the

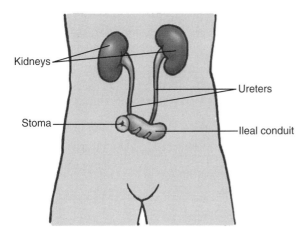

Kidneys

Ureters

Stoma

Ileal conduit

Fig. 11-4 Ileal conduit. The conduit is constructed from comparatively short segment of ileum isolated from the fecal stream. One end is closed and the other used to create a bedded stoma brought through the abdominal wall. The ureters are implanted into the conduit in a refluxing manner. (From Black JM, Hawks JH [eds]: Medical-Surgical Nursing, 7th edition. Philadelphia: Saunders, 2005; p 873.)

valve is avoided because of its critical role in vitamin B_{12} metabolism. Surgery is combined with a simple or radical cystectomy.

The procedure begins with location and resection of the ileum, along with its blood supply and mesentery. The remaining bowel is then rejoined to ensure integrity of the fecal stream. The proximal end of the conduit is closed and its distal end is brought through a small opening in the abdominal wall and formed into a budded stoma. The ureters are implanted into the segment in a refluxing manner. The urostomy does not store urine; instead, it acts as a conduit for rapid urine expulsion into an ostomy bag that fits around the abdominal stoma and is regularly emptied to ensure unimpeded urine efflux.

Alternatively, colonic segments can be used to construct a conduit.[21] A colonic conduit offers potential advantages when compared with the ileal conduit, including a more robust blood supply and proximity to the right lower quadrant of the abdomen, the most common location for an abdominal stoma. The large lumen of the colonic conduit results in a wide-mouthed stoma at lower risk for stenosis or obstruction, and its thicker wall allows the surgeon to create an antirefluxing ureteral implantation when desired. Multiple segments of colon have been incorporated into conduits, but the proximal sigmoid is generally used. In the context of

managing bladder cancer, colonic conduits are generally reserved for patients with extensive pelvic irradiation affecting the terminal ileum.

Complications. The most common complications involve the abdominal stoma; they include stomal stenosis, bowel necrosis, parastomal herniations, and stomal retraction or prolapse.[20] Obstruction or fistula may occur at the level of the ureterointestinal anastomosis, particularly if the patient has scant omentum, limiting the ability to move the intestinal segment easily from the intestinal tract to the abdominal wall. Bacteriuria of the diverted urinary tracts is a common finding during the early postoperative period; although bacteriuria is typically asymptomatic and does not require treatment, it does reflect a significant long-term risk for pyelonephritis.[22] Early complications related to the reanastomosed fecal stream include prolonged ileus or (rarely) anastomotic leak. Diarrhea may occur but is usually attributable to bile salt malabsorption and changes in bowel flora caused by antibiotic use.

Long-term complications include chronic bacteriuria, sometimes interspersed with episodes of pyelonephritis. Long-term deteriorations in renal function may be attributable to reflux associated with chronic bacteriuria and recurring pyelonephritis, obstruction from a stone, anastomotic stricture, or stomal stenosis. The incidence of long-term renal damage varies from 10% to 28% of adults with a long-term ileal conduit.[23,24] Urinary calculi occur in 5% to 20% of patients with ileal conduits.[23,25] The potential for cancer developing when the fecal stream is exposed to the presence of urine was originally observed in patients undergoing ureterosigmoidostomy, but it is very rare in patients undergoing an ileal conduit, in which the fecal and urinary streams remain strictly isolated.[26]

Preparation for surgery. Preoperative counseling about the procedure and the nature of the ostomy helps the patient begin the prolonged journey toward integrating this significant change in body habitus and elimination function into his or her existing body image. A visit with a volunteer from an ostomy patient support group is invaluable for many patients, although the optimal timing of a visit varies from patient to patient. Stoma marking by a wound, ostomy, continence (WOC; enterostomal) nurse prior to surgery is critical because it reduces the risk of postoperative complications while maximizing success with pouching.[27] Preoperative bowel preparation usually consists of a 1- or 2-day regimen comprising a low-residue diet, mechanical cleansing with GoLYTELY, sodium phosphate enemas, and neomycin or an equivalent antibiotic.

Postoperative care. Principles of postoperative management are consistent with those for any major abdominal procedure requiring extensive manipulation of the bowel. In addition to adherence to these principles, the urologic nurse will focus care on several issues specific to the patient undergoing cystectomy and ileal conduit creation: (1) altered urine elimination; (2) wound healing and initial stoma maturation; (3) alterations in fecal elimination; and (4) changes in body image.

The patient will arrive from the postanesthesia care unit with ureteral stents and an indwelling catheter or closed suction drain in the remaining urethra or suprapubic area. The ureteral stents may differ in length or color, allowing rapid differentiation of right versus left. It is important to maintain drainage of all tubes and stents and to use straps or binders to ensure that no drainage tube is subjected to excessive traction or accidentally dislodged, particularly during dressing pouch changes. Drainage into the ostomy pouch is regularly monitored for amount, color, and consistency. The urine will initially be pinkish, but it should not be bright red or characterized by passage of significant clots. It will be cloudy and is expected to contain significant amounts of mucus following the integration of the small or large bowel into the urinary stream. Ureteral stents and drainage tubes are usually removed 5 to 7 days following surgery.

The stoma is expected to undergo changes in appearance and size during the early postoperative period (Table 11-5). The urologic nurse should work closely with the patient, family, and WOC nurse to ensure that the patient and at least one significant other is able to change the ostomy pouch and assess the stoma and peristomal skin.

Because the procedure involves bowel reconstruction, the patient will have a nasogastric tube and orders to remain NPO until bowel function returns. With the return of bowel function, many patients will experience diarrhea because of bile salt malabsorption or antibiotic use. If diarrhea is severe, stool culture for *Clostridium difficile* should be performed and the patient treated accordingly. Conservative management, including bulking agents and adequate fluid intake, is encouraged otherwise. Of note, the patient should be advised to avoid taking medications that suppress motility during recovery from a procedure that involved bowel manipulation. Patients can also be reassured that diarrhea typically subsides within 4 to 6 weeks.

Creation of an ostomy, particularly in the context of a cancer diagnosis, exerts a profoundly negative influence on body image and perceived quality of life. During the immediate postoperative period, professional nurses will manage pouch changes for the patient, although it is essential that the patient and at least one significant other learn to change the pouch as soon as possible, particularly given ever-shortening hospital stays. Whether changing an ostomy pouch or teaching the patient and significant others to change the pouch, the nurse must maintain a compassionate and caring attitude and avoid all behaviors that imply aversion or distaste with any step of the procedure. In addition, the nurse should openly acknowledge the difficulty most patients experience when adjusting to an ostomy and maintain a nonjudgmental and supportive attitude as each patient struggles to cope with and accept this profound change in body image.

TABLE 11-5 Postoperative Stoma Assessment

ASSESSMENT CRITERIA	CHARACTERISTICS
Stoma type	Inspection, abdominal location, operative report
Stoma viability	Color and turgor (moist, beefy red, pale pink, taut, shiny, translucent)
Stoma height (degree of protrusion)	Flush with skin, moderately protruding, or long; ideal height = 2.5 cm
Abdominal location	Right or left side, upper or lower quadrant; description of peristomal contours, proximity of stoma to waistline, skin folds, incisions, bony prominences
Stoma size	Measure with disposable stoma-measuring guide, at stomal base
Effluent	Measure amount, note consistency, measure pH
Peristomal skin	Monitor color, integrity (rashes, ulcerations, erythema, blister formation)

Patient teaching highlights. Teaching and support of the patient who has undergone a cystectomy is an ongoing process. Patients and family should be advised that a period of grieving and adjustment to the changing body is normal, while simultaneously providing information and resources designed to assist the patient to cope with changes at the cognitive, psychomotor, and emotional levels. Table 11-6 summarizes teaching highlights that focus on practical matters related to the activities of daily living. In addition, patient teaching focuses on the need for follow-up with a WOC nurse and urologic care providers. Many patients also benefit from participation in a support group. The United Ostomy Association has chapters throughout North America designed to provide networking and support for adults and children living with an ostomy.

Continent Urinary Diversions. All continent urinary diversions, sometimes called cutaneous urinary pouches, contain two essential components; one is a urinary reservoir connected to the ureters, and the other is a continent catheterizable stoma. They are usually fashioned from isolated segments of the bowel, although the fundus of the stomach has been used in one type.

The Kock pouch combines a proximal nipple mechanism made from approximately 17 cm of bowel, a urinary reservoir constructed from approximately 78 cm of ileum, and a distal nipple constructed from an additional 17 cm of small bowel (Figure 11-5). Continence is achieved by intussuscepting a segment of small bowel that is attached to the abdominal wall to form a budded stoma. A segment is constructed in a similar manner

TABLE 11-6 Teaching Highlights for the Patient with New Ileal Conduit and Ostomy

ACTIVITY	TEACHING HIGHLIGHT
Pouch changes	Details of pouch changes usually taught by WOC nurse; urologic nurse should help patient obtain adequate supplies for initial use and identify medical supply or retail source for ongoing supply needs; patients also advised to bring extra supplies in case leakage occurs while away from home
ADLs	Patients reassured that they should be able to resume all (or almost all) ADLs; counsel patient anxious about resumption of ADLs to begin with activities they feel most comfortable with, practice activities in supportive setting before attempting in less controlled situation (e.g., person who fears swimming may wish to wear pouch in bathtub filled with water before bathing at beach or in a pool)
Bathing and showering	Patients can bathe with pouch on or off; ileal conduit will continue to produce urine while pouch is off, so most prefer to shower
Clothing styles	Little or no change in clothing style necessary; snug-fitting underclothing flattens urine in pouch, may provide better contour than loose-fit styles; men may generally need to wear shirts that do not tuck in at waist if stoma is located directly above belt line

ADLs, Activities of daily living; *WOC,* wound, ostomy, continence.

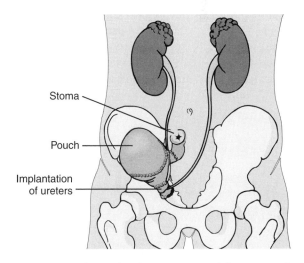

Fig. 11-5 Kock pouch. This is constructed from approximately 133 cm of small bowel reconstructed to form a low-pressure urinary reservoir, continent and catheterizable stoma, and nonrefluxing mechanism for ureteral implantation. (From Lewis SL, Heitkemper MM, Dirksen SR, O'Brien PG, Bucher L [eds]: Medical Surgical Nursing, 6th edition. St Louis: Mosby, 2007; p 1190.)

and is used to form a nonrefluxing mechanism to attach the ureters to the reservoir. The reservoir is constructed from the largest segment of ileum; it is detubularized and formed into a spherical pouch designed to avoid the powerful bolus contractions observed in normal bowel.

Alternatively, another type, such as the Indiana pouch, incorporates one or more segments of the right colon with a segment of distal ileum to construct a catheterizable continent urinary diversion. An Indiana pouch is made by incorporating an isolated and detubularized segment of the ileum and ascending colon to construct a urinary reservoir (Figure 11-6). The ureters are then implanted into the side of the reservoir and a special nipple and valve constructed to attach the reservoir to the skin. The ureters may be implanted in a refluxing or nonrefluxing manner, depending on the surgeon's clinical experience and judgment. The anti-incontinence mechanism incorporates the ileocecal valve, which is reinforced by infolding the bowel wall and creating a budded stoma placed within the abdominal wall. A number of alternatives, including the Florida, Miami, Penn, and Mainz pouches, have been described over the past several decades. The reader is referred to a urologic surgery text for a detailed discussion of each of these procedures.

Mitrofanoff Procedure. Because of long-term problems associated with maintaining a continent stoma using stapled, intussuscepted, or surgically reconstructed bowel loops, Mitrofanoff has described an alternative continent mechanism that incorporates the appendix.[28,29] A continent stoma is constructed using a small-caliber tubular organ, such as the appendix or a ureteral segment, with sufficient length to extend from the reservoir to the abdominal wall or umbilicus to form a small stoma (Figure 11-7). An antirefluxing connection is then established within the urinary reservoir and a submucosal tunnel constructed using a flap valve mechanism. Alternatively, the stoma can be placed at the umbilicus, providing a more cosmetic effect with the abdominal wall. This procedure has gained popularity because it maintains continence in approximately 98% of patients,[29] has a straighter lumen between the stoma and reservoir, and produces less mucus than continent stomas constructed from bowel.

Complications. Metabolic complications may be encountered whenever any bowel segment is incorporated into the urinary tract, but the risk is greatest with continent cutaneous or orthotopic pouches constructed from larger segments of bowel as compared with the ileal conduit. Hypokalemia, hypomagnesemia, and hyperammonemia contribute to metabolic acidosis in 10% to 50% of patients with continent cutaneous diversions.[30-32] Blood urea nitrogen and creatinine levels also tend to rise, and some patients may develop constitutional symptoms, including fatigue, anorexia, weight loss, and polydipsia.

Metabolic acidosis may occur whenever urine is regularly stored in a reservoir made of bowel. Although the bladder's urothelium forms an effective barrier against the reabsorption of fluid or salts from urine, intestinal reservoirs secrete and reabsorb

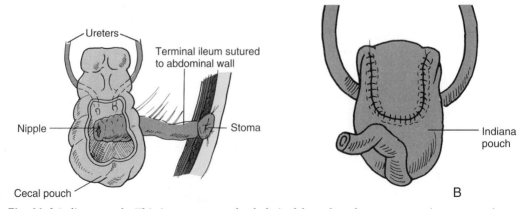

Fig. 11-6 Indiana pouch. This incorporates a detubularized large bowel to create a urinary reservoir. (From Black JM, Hawks JH [eds]: Medical-Surgical Nursing, 8th edition. Philadelphia: Saunders, 2009; p 741.)

various ions and water, including sodium ions; these are exchanged for hydrogen ions and bicarbonate, which is exchanged for chloride. In addition, ileal or intestinal reservoirs reabsorb ammonium ions, resulting in a rise in serum urea and creatinine levels. Unless this condition is corrected, the patient may experience significant bone demineralization and related complications.[33] Malabsorption of fat-soluble vitamins, including B_{12}, may occur, particularly if extensive segments of ileum are incorporated into the diversion. However, because the liver is able to store significant supplies of this vitamin, vitamin B_{12} loss may not become clinically apparent until 2 to 5 years after the procedure.

Other potential complications include the formation of urinary calculi.[32] The risk of forming an obstructive stone is affected by the type of diversion (Table 11-7) as is the composition of the stone. Although calculi typically form in the upper urinary tracts in the ileal or intestinal conduit, they often form in the reservoir in the orthotopic or cutaneous continent diversion. Pouch perforation affects up to 9% of patients, parastomal herniations in 4% to 5%, and stomal stenosis associated with difficult catheterization occurs in 20% to 50%. Urinary incontinence rates in cutaneous urinary diversions range from 0% to 20%. Nighttime urine loss is more common than

daytime incontinence, possibly because of increased urine volumes in a reservoir constructed from bowel as compared with bladder lined with urothelium. Asymptomatic bacteriuria occurs in up to 80% of patients. It may lead to bothersome symptoms related to inflammation of the urinary reservoir in some, and febrile urinary tract infections occur in approximately 2%.

Preparation for surgery. Physical preparation for a continent urinary diversion is similar to that for an ileal conduit, including the need for extensive bowel cleansing. Preoperative educational needs vary based on the type and extent of the planned surgical

TABLE 11-7 Incidence of Urinary Calculi in Urinary Diversions[32,34,35]

DIVERSION TYPE	REPORTED INCIDENCE OF URINARY CALCULI (%)
Ileal conduit	9
Intestinal conduit	11
Kock pouch	26-28
Indiana pouch	0-13
Mainz pouch	9
Ileal neobladder	3
Kock neobladder	4

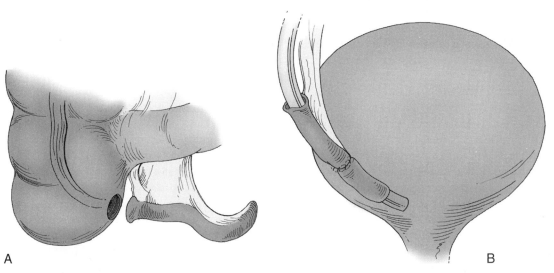

Fig. 11-7 Mitrofanoff procedure. **A,** The Mitrofanoff continent stoma is created from the appendix or an isolated segment of ureter. **B,** The narrow-lumen tube is connected to the urinary reservoir or urinary bladder and brought to the abdominal wall or umbilicus to create an easily catheterizable stoma. (From Wein AJ, Kavoussi LR, Novick AC, Partin AW, Peters CA [eds]: Campbell-Walsh Urology, 9th edition. Philadelphia: Saunders, 2007; p 3694.)

procedure. For the patient with cancer, preoperative educational counseling must reinforce flexibility regarding the procedure that will ultimately be performed, because the ability to complete a continent urinary diversion or neobladder may be altered based on intraoperative findings. Counseling also includes teaching about self-care practices, including intermittent catheterization, the anticipated number and type of postoperative drains, and the need for a temporary nasogastric tube. Stoma site selection must be completed by the WOC nurse.

Postoperative care. Postoperative management incorporates the principles and major issues discussed for the patient undergoing construction of an ileal conduit. In addition to those issues, several management challenges are more specific to cutaneous continent urinary diversions.[33-35] Although ureteral stents are used for both types of diversion, their location will vary, depending on the surgeon's preference and diversion type. Stents may terminate in the urinary reservoir, or they may protrude from a separate stab wound within the abdominal wall or the cutaneous stoma. A suprapubic catheter is often placed in the urinary reservoir via a small stab wound in the abdomen. A second catheter is typically inserted through the stoma to facilitate drainage of urine not flushed by the stents. A Jackson-Pratt drain in the lower pelvic cavity and an indwelling catheter inserted through the urethra facilitate drainage of pelvic fluid accumulation. Use of a Velcro-type catheter holder will help stabilize drainage tubes and prevent unintentional dislodgment.

Adequate decompression of the urinary reservoir is critical because the patient is at risk for urinary extravasation until the suture lines completely heal. Early signs of urinary or fecal leakage from anastomosis include an increased abdominal girth, fever, and drainage through the incision or around tubes or drains. Fecal anastomotic leaks are uncommon, but they will lead to peritonitis and require prompt surgical repair. Clinical manifestations include fever, abdominal pain, rigidity, and absence of bowel sounds.

Similar to the ileal conduit, all catheters, stents, and drainage containers should be labeled and a closed gravity drainage system for each device maintained. The use of separate drainage systems is promoted because it minimizes the risk of infection and allows easy evaluation of the volume and character of drainage from each tube.

Assessment of urine clarity and character must integrate knowledge of the anticipated outcomes when bowel is incorporated into the urinary tract. The urinary reservoir will initially produce large volumes of mucus, causing the urine to appear cloudy and turbid. In addition, it will be light red to pink during the first several days following surgery. In contrast to these anticipated findings, bright red blood or clots in the urine must be reported promptly, because they may indicate a loss of anastomotic integrity or infection causing the hematuria.

All tubes must be regularly monitored to ensure patency. Unimpeded flow is encouraged by positioning the drainage bag below the level of the kidneys to maximize the effect of gravity and by gentle irrigation as directed to prevent occlusion from mucus or small clots within drainage tubes. A Penrose drain is typically present and its drainage also must be monitored for volume and character. Drainage is expected to be high volume during the immediate postoperative period and may require transient containment via an ostomy appliance. However, the volume of drainage should diminish quickly.

Patient teaching highlights. In contrast to a urinary conduit, the cutaneous pouch is emptied by intermittent catheterization.[36] This necessity of ongoing intermittent catheterization was introduced during the preoperative period, and it is critical to ensure that the patient and at least one family member or significant other can perform the procedure by the time the continuous drainage tubes are discontinued, approximately 4 to 6 weeks postoperatively. The importance of regular and effective evacuation of the pouch is emphasized, and the patient is warned that allowing the pouch to become overdistended increases the difficulty when catheterizing the continent stoma and may increase the risk for spontaneous perforation. The patient must also be provided with a Medic-Alert bracelet that specifies continent urinary diversion. This is critical because it alerts health care professionals to seek immediate urologic consultation if the patient becomes incapacitated and unable to participate actively in ensuring urinary elimination from a cutaneous continent urinary diversion.

The patient is taught to self-monitor for signs and symptoms of pouch inflammation (pouchitis), including cramping pain at the diversion site, acute onset of urinary incontinence, hematuria, and fever. The patient is further counseled that malodorous or cloudy urine without other symptoms does not indicate pouchitis and should be managed by an increase in fluid volume and/or adjustment in the types of fluids consumed.

The patient is advised that the diversion will continue to produce mucus, although the volume typically subsides over time. Instruction should include various interventions to ensure regular evacuation of mucus from the reservoir and counseling that failure to remove mucus adequately will increase the risk for problems with intermittent catheterization because of mucus blockage and stones in the reservoir. Interventions that reduce mucus include daily irrigation, consumption of an adequate daily fluid volume, and consumption of mucolytic nutritional products, such as cranberry or blueberry products.

Patients are also advised that systemic alkalization is usually required to offset metabolic acidosis. The diet is altered to restrict chloride intake. Sodium bicarbonate or potassium citrate–citric acid (Polycitra-K) may be administered to supplement the body's store of these buffering substances. In addition, weight-dependent doses of chlorpromazine (Thorazine) or nicotinic acid may be used to reduce production of cyclic adenosine monophosphate (cAMP)–dependent acids from the urinary reservoir.[37,38]

Patients whose diversion surgeries sacrifice the ileocecal valve are advised that they may experience changes in the resorptive potential of the small bowel and reduced intestinal transit time, creating a greater risk for diarrhea and problems absorbing fat-soluble vitamins, including B_{12}, A, D, E, and K. The malabsorption of bile acid salts also increases the synthesis of bile acids, and patients are taught signs and symptoms of cholelithiasis and steatorrhea—passage of frothy malodorous stool with a high fat content.

Orthotopic Neobladder. An orthotopic neobladder involves reconstructing a bowel that is attached to the trigone (Figure 11-8, *A*). From a strictly technical perspective, the neobladder represents an ideal procedure because it preserves the patient's ability to evacuate urine via the native urethra. Even when compared with cutaneous continent urinary diversions, it avoids the need for an ostomy and ongoing intermittent catheterization. Because of these advantages, the proportion of patients

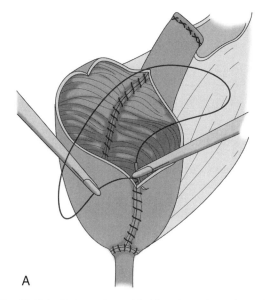

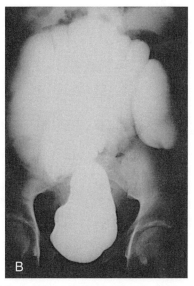

Fig. 11-8 A, Orthotopic neobladder. An orthotopic neobladder attaches a urinary reservoir constructed of large or small bowel to the trigone and urethra to recreate more normal voiding and avoid an abdominal stoma. **B,** Orthotopic neobladder with volvulus. Gross distension of orthotic right colon bladder because of urinary retention and patient inability to adhere to an intermittent catheterization regimen. (From Wein AJ, Kavoussi LR, Novick AC, Partin AW, Peters CA [eds]: Campbell-Walsh Urology, 9th edition. Philadelphia: Saunders, 2007; pp 2548, 2551.)

undergoing radical cystectomy for bladder cancer with simultaneous construction of an orthotopic neobladder now varies between 50% and 90% in most major medical centers in North America.[39] Nevertheless, these advantages must be carefully weighed against limitations of the procedure, including urinary incontinence (particularly at night), potential for residual malignancy within the trigone or urethra, and the need for substantial abdominal straining to evacuate urine from the neobladder adequately.[40] Therefore, patients must be carefully counseled and screened prior to the procedure. Absolute contraindications for orthotopic diversion are mental or physical disability, inability to adhere to the bladder catheterization protocol, elevated creatinine level, irritable bowel disease, carcinoma of the prostate or urethra, or tumor invasion into the prostate or bladder neck (Figure 11-8, *B*). Other contraindications are pelvic irradiation, carcinoma in situ (CIS), and recurrent urethral stricture.

For the patient with cancer, radical cystectomy is modified to preserve the trigone, bladder neck, and entire urethra. A number of procedures have been described; Table 11-8 outlines the major characteristics of common neobladder procedures in men and associated nighttime continence rates. Because of differences in urethral anatomy and length, special considerations apply when constructing an orthotopic neobladder in a woman. They include (1) ensuring adequate volume reservoir to maximize continence potential; (2) avoidance of mucosal folds near the bladder outlet to prevent obstruction; (3) placement of an omental segment between the neobladder and vagina or use of some other maneuver to avoid any kinking of the reservoir and obstruction or fistula formation; (4) preventing enterocele or rectocele by reinforcing the endopelvic fascia at the pouch of Douglas; and (5) carefully preserving the endopelvic fascial supports of the bladder.[21]

Complications. Certain complications are similar to those seen with continent diversions, including nocturnal incontinence, urinary calculi (particularly in the neobladder), and all the metabolic complications associated with isolation of a large segment of bowel from the gastrointestinal tract. Additional

TABLE 11-8 Alternative Procedures for Constructing an Orthotopic Neobladder[21]

NAME	DESCRIPTION	NIGHTTIME CONTINENCE RATES (%)
Camey	60 cm of ileum isolated from fecal stream, detubularized, reconstructed to form a U-shaped neobladder; ureters implanted in nonrefluxing manner	60
Studer	60 cm of ileum found at least 25 cm proximal to ileocecal valve isolated from fecal stream, detubularized, reconstructed to form approximately spherical structure; ureters implanted in refluxing manner using technique similar to that for ileal conduit	74
Hautmann	60-80 cm of distal ileum isolated from fecal stream, detubularized, reconstructed to form M-shaped reservoir; ureters implanted using nonrefluxing technique	85
Mainz	10-15 cm of cecum and 20-25 cm of associated ileum isolated from fecal stream and detubularized, sacrificing ileocecal valve, and combined large- and small-bowel segment reconstructed to form W-shaped neobladder; ureters are implanted in tunneled manner that resists reflux	75
Le Bag	20 cm of cecum and ascending colon isolated from fecal stream, along with approximately equal length of terminal ileum; entire segment detubularized and folded to form elongated sphere; ureters reimplanted using technique similar to that used for colonic conduits	54
UCLA	10-15 cm of cecum and 30 cm of terminal ileum isolated from fecal stream; all but 10 cm of ileum detubularized and reconstructed to form elongated spherical neobladder similar to Le Bag technique; ureters implanted in a refluxing manner using technique described for ileal conduit procedure	32

complications include incomplete emptying of the neobladder, sometimes called hypercontinence, and ureteral obstruction.[41] Table 11-9 summarizes common complications associated with orthotopic neobladders.

Preparation for surgery. Preoperative evaluation and preparation are similar to those described for cutaneous urinary diversions. However, routine intermittent catheterization is performed only once daily for a period of 2 to 3 months after surgery.[41] Catheterization is continued only if the patient has copious mucus production or is unable to empty the bladder effectively using a combination of voiding and straining. Patients are also advised that effective bladder emptying will require a combination of pelvic floor muscle relaxation, contraction of the muscular component of the neobladder, and straining to maximize urine evacuation.

Postoperative care. The main issues related to postoperative management are consistent with those discussed for continent cutaneous urinary diversions, including maintenance of urine flow and monitoring of volume or character of effluent from all tubes and drains, prompt recovery of bowel function, wound

healing, and pain management. However, unlike cutaneous urinary diversions, the patient must be taught to differentiate neobladder function from that of the native bladder and provided with strategies to ensure adequate bladder evacuation and prevent calculus formation.

Patient teaching highlights. Because the neobladder is constructed from detubularized small and/or large bowel, micturition represents a combination of smooth muscle contraction within the reservoir wall, elevation of abdominal pressure by straining, and relaxation of the pelvic floor muscles. Therefore, patients are taught to identify, isolate, rapidly contract, and maximally relax the pelvic floor muscles during micturition. They are taught to supplement spontaneous voiding with abdominal straining while maintaining pelvic floor muscle relaxation to evacuate urine from the neobladder further. Voiding efficiency is also maximized by avoidance of overdistention; therefore, patients are advised to void when the bladder feels full or to urinate by the clock (every 3 to 4 hours).[42,43]

Augmentation Cystoplasty. Augmentation cystoplasty incorporates a segment of the gastrointestinal tract into the bladder to augment bladder capacity, increase bladder wall compliance, and diminish or abolish overactive detrusor contractions. The most common indication is hostile neurogenic bladder dysfunction, characterized by a reduced bladder capacity, low bladder wall compliance, and obstruction of the bladder outlet. Other indications include intractable detrusor overactivity, refractory to all forms of conservative or pharmacologic management, particularly when complicated by incomplete bladder emptying requiring intermittent catheterization. A detailed discussion of augmentation cystoplasty is provided in Chapter 18.

Procedures for Stress Urinary Incontinence

To date, there are more than 150 procedures and numerous variations of these for the treatment of urinary incontinence in women.[44] This remarkably large number indicates an ongoing search for the ideal procedure. Surgical treatment for stress urinary incontinence has been divided into six main categories: (1) anterior colporrhaphy; (2) needle urethropexies; (3) abdominal or laparoscopic retropubic urethropexies; (4) suburethral sling procedures; (5) suburethral injections (bulking agents); and

TABLE 11-9 Common Complications in Patients with Orthotopic Neobladders

TYPE OF NEOBLADDER	COMPLICATION	INCIDENCE (%)
Ileal	Diurnal urinary incontinence	7
	Nighttime urinary incontinence	31
	Incomplete emptying, requiring IC	14
	Ureteral obstruction	10
Colonic	Diurnal urinary incontinence	12
	Nighttime urinary incontinence	30
	Incomplete emptying, requiring IC	11
	Ureteral obstruction	12

IC, Intermittent catheterization.

(6) artificial urinary sphincter.[45] Each of the procedures is designed to address the underlying cause of the incontinence—urethral hypermobility, intrinsic sphincter incompetence, or both—and none are indicated for overactive bladder dysfunction (urge incontinence) in the absence of stress incontinence. This chapter will include detailed discussions of only the most commonly performed procedures.

Anterior Colporrhaphy. Anterior colporrhaphy requires an anterior vaginal wall incision, dissection to expose the proximal two thirds of the urethra, and placement of one or two Kelly sutures to elevate the position of the bladder base and proximal urethra. However, the percentage of women who remained continent after anterior colporrhaphy is low (about 37%), and it is no longer widely used for managing stress urinary incontinence.[46,47]

Needle Urethropexy. Needle urethropexy procedures are designed to restore continence by restoring the bladder base and proximal urethra to an abdominal position. Modern procedures are based on a technique originally described by Pereyra in 1959[48] and modified throughout the past 4 decades.[49] The original procedure avoided the extensive retropubic dissection required for retropubic urethropexy procedures popular in the 1950s by passing sutures through a small suprapubic skin incision using a special cannula, with a stylet inserted through a hollow shaft. Significant modifications of this procedure were promulgated by Stamey and colleagues.[49] However, systematic literature review has revealed that continence rates at 4 years or more after surgery are approximately 67%, significantly less than the 83% to 84% continence rates found for suburethral slings or retropubic suspensions.[50] As a result, these procedures are no longer widely performed for the management of stress incontinence in women.

Retropubic Urethropexy. Once considered first-line surgical management of stress incontinence by many surgeons, retropubic suspension procedures represent one of several options for women whose incontinence is judged to be caused primarily by hypermobility of the urethra and bladder base in the absence of significant urethral sphincter incompetence, a condition that is also called intrinsic sphincter deficiency (Figure 11-9).[51] Multiple techniques for retropubic urethropexy have been described, but the most commonly performed are the Burch colposuspension

and paravaginal fascial repair. Regardless of technique, retropubic urethropexy seeks to restore continence by returning the bladder base and proximal urethra to an abdominal position.

Historically, the Marshall-Marchetti-Krantz (MMK) procedure was the most commonly performed retropubic procedure, but it fell from widespread use during the late 1970s and early 1980s. It regained some popularity when the technique was adapted for laparoscopy, but it was ultimately supplanted by the laparoscopic Burch colposuspension, based on technical considerations. The MMK requires placement of suspensory sutures through the ostium of the pubic symphysis to elevate the bladder base anteriorly. Its durability, expressed as the proportion of patients who remain continent, at 10 years is approximately 64%.[52]

The paravaginal fascial repair reattaches the vaginal sulcus and overlying endopelvic (pubocervical) fascia to the pelvic side wall and arcus tendineus fasciae pelvis, sometimes referred to as the white line based on its appearance during surgery (Figure 11-9, *D*). It can be performed using an open vaginal or abdominal approach, or laparoscopically.[53] The durability of the paravaginal repair has not been widely studied. One randomized trial that enrolled 36 subjects has found that 61% of patients who underwent paravaginal repair remain continent at 3 years as compared with 100% of those who underwent the Burch colposuspension.[54]

The Burch colposuspension raises the bladder base by attaching sutures passed through the vaginal wall and into Cooper's ligament rather than the ostium of the pubic symphysis. Unlike other retropubic procedures, the colposuspension also provides some compression at the level of the proximal urethra (Figure 11-9, *A-C*). At the dawn of the twenty-first century, the Burch colposuspension is the most commonly performed retropubic suspension. Its popularity is partially based on a solid 5-year durability of approximately 82%[47] and a low incidence of associated complications.[55]

Complications. All retropubic urethropexies share the potential for complications associated with any abdominopelvic surgery, including atelectasis and pneumonia, wound infection or dehiscence, abscess formation, and venous thrombosis or embolism. However, the most common complications of these procedures are transient obstructed voiding

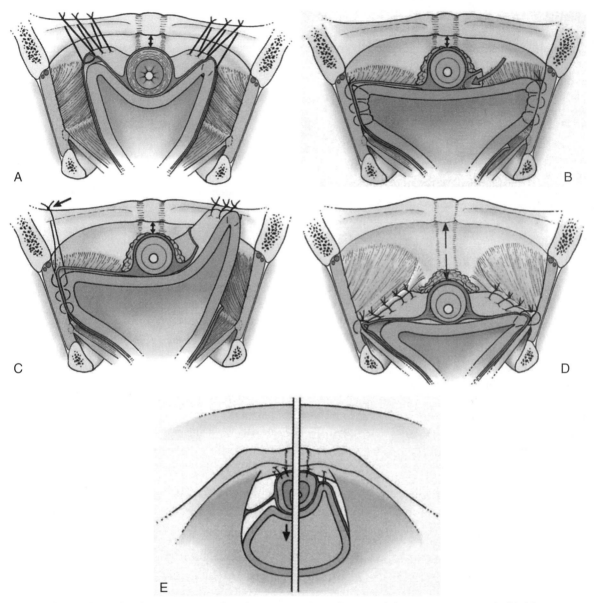

Fig. 11-9 Burch colposuspension. This places sutures through Cooper's ligament to support the bladder base and urethra. **A,** Coronal view. **B,** Coronal view, vagino-obturator shelf procedure. **C,** Coronal view, vagino-obturator shelf procedure on the *left*, augmented by stitching to the iliopectineal line and a Burch procedure on the *right*. **D,** Coronal view, paravaginal repair. **E,** Sutures in a Marshall-Marchetti-Krantz procedure and their proximity to the urethra. (From Wein AJ, Kavoussi LR, Novick AC, Partin AW, Peters CA [eds]: Campbell-Walsh Urology, 9th edition. Philadelphia: Saunders, 2007; p 2171.)

or urinary retention, usually caused by postoperative inflammation of the bladder base, urethra, and adjacent structures. Persisting obstructive voiding problems may be caused by overcorrection of the urethral axis or denervation during dissection. Persistent or recurring urinary incontinence may be caused by denervation leading to intrinsic sphincter deficiency, or de novo or persistent detrusor overactivity leading to overactive bladder syndrome.[56] Uncommon but significant complications include injury to the bladder, ureter, or urethra.

In addition to these conditions, each of the procedures is associated with unique complications arising from the particular surgical technique used to restore continence. For example, osteitis pubis is a persistent and painful inflammation of the ostium of the symphysis pubis and pubic bones. It occurs in approximately 1% to 3% of patients undergoing MMK. [44,57] Similarly, as many as 10% of patients undergoing a Burch colposuspension may develop postoperative pelvic organ prolapse, prompting the incorporation of several modifications of the surgical procedure to reduce this risk. [58]

Preparation for surgery. The nurse should inform the patient that an indwelling or suprapubic catheter will be in place for 24 hours to approximately 5 days postoperatively. [59] Suprapubic catheters may be clamped to allow the bladder to fill and provide an opportunity to attempt voiding. Once a pattern of voiding is reestablished, the patient may be asked to measure postvoid residual volumes in preparation for discontinuing the suprapubic catheter when the volume remains below a certain point (often 50 to 75 ml). Alternatively, patients may be taught intermittent catheterization (IC) preoperatively. This strategy avoids the necessity of leaving a catheter in place, but postoperative edema and pain make IC a less comfortable option for most patients.

Preoperative counseling should include the possibility of urinary retention following surgery. In addition, women with urge incontinence, overactive bladder syndrome, or urodynamically documented detrusor overactivity should be counseled that these symptoms may not be relieved by the surgery. Nevertheless, patients should be reassured that these symptoms are expected to respond to behavioral or pharmacologic treatments.

Postoperative care. In addition to general postoperative management principles for any patient undergoing an abdominopelvic procedure, the following issues must be addressed when caring for the patient recuperating from a retropubic urethropexy: (1) altered urine elimination, (2) pain, and (3) wound healing.

The patient typically returns from surgery with a suprapubic catheter. The catheter is monitored for patency and the urine output observed for volume and character. Pink-tinged urine is anticipated, but the urologist should be informed promptly if the urine is bright red or the drainage bag is filled with blood clots. The catheter typically remains in place for 1 to 5 days following surgery and the patient must be carefully monitored to ensure that effective micturition occurs. If a suprapubic catheter remains in place, the patient is taught to clamp the tube until an urge to void is perceived or a period of 3 to 4 hours elapses without the urge to urinate. The patient is advised to urinate into a graduated container, such as a voiding hat, without straining, and then to unclamp the catheter and measure the postvoid residual volume. The maneuver should be repeated approximately once every 24 hours as directed until the postvoid residual remains at or below acceptable threshold values for 2 to 3 days.

Management of pain begins with an informed assessment to determine the likely cause. Incisional pain tends to be dull, penetrating, and continuous, and the pain associated with bladder spasm is perceived as sharp, cramplike, and intermittent. Moderate to moderately severe incisional pain is anticipated during the first several days following surgery, but a sudden increase in incisional pain may indicate a wound infection or extravasation of urine. Bladder spasms may or may not occur, but their presence should prompt the urologic nurse to evaluate the patient carefully for catheter blockage or a urinary tract infection. Incisional pain is managed by an appropriate analgesic, although the discomfort of bladder spasms can be relieved by an antimuscarinic, such as oxybutynin or tolterodine, or a combination agent, such as belladonna and opium suppositories. Avoidance of bladder irritants while consuming adequate clear fluids will reduce the risk for and severity of bladder spasms.

A suction drain may be placed in the retropubic space to drain oozing from the paravaginal veins. The volume and character of drainage should be carefully monitored and passage of high-volume bloody drainage or urine reported to the physician immediately. Drainage tubes are typically removed between 1 and 3 days postoperatively, depending on the amount of drainage.

Patient teaching highlights. Emphasis is placed on teaching the patient that wound healing requires time and strict adherence to activity restrictions. The nurse should consult with the urologist concerning activity restrictions, which usually require the patient to avoid lifting any object heavier than 10 pounds or sexual intercourse for a period of 4 to 6 weeks following surgery. The patient is also taught to self-monitor for signs and symptoms of urinary retention and urinary tract infection. The patient can also be taught behavioral interventions designed to promote voiding, including consumption of a mild bladder irritant, such as a cup of caffeinated coffee or tea, followed by attempts to relax the pelvic floor muscles and urinate while standing in a warm shower or sitting in a tub of warm water. Patients who are discharged from hospital with a suprapubic catheter in place are advised to continue clamping and unclamping the catheter as directed by their physician, measure voided and residual urine volumes, and record and report data to their physician. In some cases, IC may be taught or preoperative teaching reinforced at the time of hospital discharge.

Patients are also counseled about the possibility of de novo or persistent overactive bladder dysfunction. Many will require considerable nursing support for assistance in dealing with this frustrating postoperative complication. Bladder retraining, fluid adjustment, and antimuscarinic therapy may assist in ameliorating the symptoms (see Chapter 7). Patients can be advised that these symptoms may subside over time; however, it is important to avoid establishing this as an anticipated outcome of a surgical procedure designed to relieve stress rather than urge urinary incontinence.

Suburethral Slings. A suburethral sling refers to any strip of material placed (tunneled) underneath the urethra. Suburethral slings are designed to restore continence by elevating and stabilizing the hypermobile urethra and by compressing the middle third of the urethra when the woman assumes an upright (sitting or standing) position.

A number of materials may be used to create suburethral slings. Commonly used autologous materials include fascia harvested from fascia surrounding the rectus abdominis or fascia lata or from the vaginal wall. Cadaveric fascia harvested from the rectus abdominis or fascia lata or fascia from animal sources also may be used. These alternatives avoid the morbidity associated with harvesting autologous fascia, but they have not proved as durable as autologous or synthetic materials.[60]

The surgery is typically performed through suprapubic and vaginal incisions; an additional incision may be necessary to harvest autologous fascia from an area other than the rectus. The fascia is placed suburethrally and careful attention given to avoid placing any tension against the urethra. Avoiding tension during sling placement is critical, because the change from a supine position during the operative procedure to a standing or sitting position will provide adequate compression of the urethra during bladder filling and storage while circumventing obstruction of urinary outflow during micturition.

Particularly among urologists, suburethral slings have emerged as the preferred surgical technique for managing stress incontinence associated with intrinsic sphincter deficiency, bladder base descent, or a combination of these factors.[45] Fascial slings have proved durable, with 88% of women retaining continence at a mean follow-up of 51 months in one study.[46] Unfortunately, patients with mixed incontinence experience somewhat less favorable outcomes than those with stress incontinence alone, but urge incontinence is likely to resolve in up to 74% of cases and only 7% will experience de novo detrusor overactivity.[61,62]

Synthetic Slings. A number of synthetic materials have been used to create suburethral slings, including Gore-Tex, Prolene, and Marlex. However, two synthetic slings have emerged in recent years that have risen to prominence because of their ease of insertion and initial efficacy. Based on a survey of 530 surgeons belonging to the International Urogynecological Association, the most commonly used synthetic sling material for management of stress or mixed urinary incontinence is tension-free vaginal tape (68%), followed by transobturator tape (13%).[63] Nevertheless, the choice of synthetic materials continues to advance rapidly, and the preferences reflected in this survey may change as urologists and urogynecologists gain more experience with these materials and as the evidence base for their use evolves.

Transvaginal tape. Tension-free transvaginal tape (TVT) is constructed from a polypropylene mesh. It is designed to provoke a tissue response resulting in collagen deposition that coalesces into a scar; this acts as a urethral support mechanism for the pubourethral ligaments.[64] However, the true mechanism of its action when implanted into the suburethral area is not completely understood.

The TVT procedure can be performed on an outpatient basis. The patient is placed in a lithotomy position and the procedure is performed under general or spinal (epidural) anesthesia, or under local anesthesia with hydrodistention of the space of Retzius.[65] A vaginal incision and blunt dissection are completed, producing a space lateral to the urethra, which becomes the starting position for each of the TVT sling needles. Two abdominal incisions, approximately 2 to 3 cm from midline and above the pubic symphysis, are made for the intended exit points of the needles. Through a vaginal incision, the TVT needle is inserted through the periurethral fascia, into the space of Retzius, and upward until the needle comes through the abdominal incisions. Cystoscopy may be done to confirm the position of the needle and inspect the bladder and bladder neck for perforations or injury. The TVT tapes are then pulled through the tissues and placed on the abdomen and the tension adjusted with the patient coughing or straining; then the plastic sheath is removed and cut. A small dressing may be applied over the two abdominal incisions (Figure 11-10).

In a multicenter randomized trial comparing TVT with retropubic colposuspension, results were similar for cure (66% versus 57%). More women in the TVT group had a bladder injury but more women in the colposuspension group were unable to void postprocedure.[66] One author has described an inside-out technique designed to reduce urethral injury.[67] Long-term outcomes with TVT, including continence rates, are not yet known.

Transobturator tape. Transobturator tape (TOT) is constructed of a nonwoven, nonelastic polypropylene with a 15-mm-wide central silicone-coated zone placed in a tension-free manner beneath the middle of the urethra, extending from one obturator foramen to the other.[68,69] Similar to TVE, TOT is performed under general, spinal, or local anesthesia, and may be combined with other pelvic procedures, such as hysterectomy or prolapse surgery, when indicated. Short-term results (less than 5 postoperative years) reveal cure or significant improvement in stress urinary incontinence (UI) in 87.5% to 96% of women, and significant improvement or resolution of urge urinary incontinence in as many in 80%.[67,70,71] A single study comparing TOT and TVT found no significant differences when short-term continence rates were compared in a group of 102

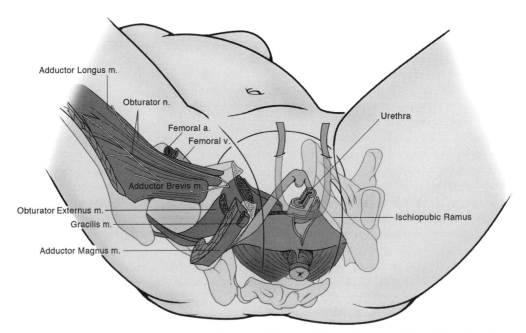

Fig. 11-10 Suburethral sling. Autologous fascia can be harvested from the rectus abdominis or fascia lata, or vaginal wall. It is then fashioned into a sling that is placed underneath the proximal urethra to provide both support and compression. Care is taken to avoid any tension when placing the sling. (From Wein AJ, Kavoussi LR, Novick AC, Partin AW, Peters CA [eds]: Campbell-Walsh Urology, 9th edition. Philadelphia: Saunders, 2007; p 2253.)

patients. Complications of TOT surgery are comparable to those of TVT and include hematoma, urinary retention, de novo urgency and detrusor overactivity, and the potential for urethral injury when the tape is placed. Like the TVT, long-term outcomes, including continence rates, are not known (Figure 11-11).

Complications. Similar to the retropubic urethropexies, the most common complication of the use of suburethral slings is transient urinary retention. Persistent or de novo detrusor overactivity or urge incontinence may develop in up to 25% of cases.[72] However, unlike the retropubic procedures, suburethral slings carry a risk for erosion of the sling, with a reported incidence varying from less than 1% to 23%.[73] Multiple materials have been associated with sling erosion, including autologous fascia, synthetic materials, and cadaveric fascia.[74] Hemorrhagic complications occur in 1% to 2% of cases; the most common is retropubic hematoma, with rare reported cases of major vessel injury and serious bleeding. Prolonged pain may occur after sling placement; it is usually localized to the surgical wound, but occasionally presents as periosteal pain.

Complications associated with synthetic material slings are generally similar to those associated with autologous or heterologous fascia. A perioperative complication unique to the TVT procedure is bladder perforation by the trocar, which occurs in up to 23% of cases.[75] To address these potential but rare complications, alternative methods of trocar placement have been proposed, such as antegrade placement (SPARC sling system, American Medical Systems, Minnetonka, Minn). Severe sphincter incompetence may occur if the scarring caused by placement of the tape fixes the bladder neck or proximal urethra in an open position.

Preparation for surgery. Patients undergoing pubovaginal sling procedures are advised that the surgery will require a brief hospital admission, usually about 2 to 3 days. In contrast, TVT and TOT placement are typically completed on an outpatient basis. Patients are counseled that a urethral catheter will be left in place following surgery; they are advised of the possibility that the catheter may require reinsertion or a finite period of catheterization may be necessary if they are unable to urinate successfully when the catheter is removed initially.

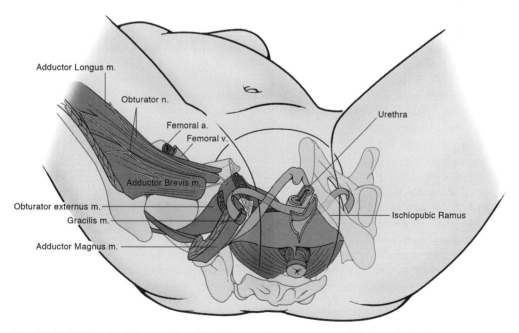

Fig. 11-11 Midurethral sling as placed by the transobturator approach (any technique). (From Wein AJ, Kavoussi LR, Novick AC, Partin AW, Peters CA [eds]: Campbell-Walsh Urology, 9th edition. Philadelphia: Saunders, 2007; p 2268.)

Postoperative care. Principles for postoperative management following a pubovaginal suburethral sling are similar to those used for patients undergoing a retropubic urethropexy. Important issues related to postoperative management following placement of a suburethral sling include the following: (1) altered urine elimination and risk for retention; (2) wound healing; and (3) pain. Urinary drainage typically occurs through an indwelling urethral catheter and urine output is monitored for volume and character. The catheter is generally removed within 5 to 7 days and the patient undergoes a trial of voiding. Patients are advised that the surgery is expected to alter the urinary stream and that special care should be taken to ensure efficient bladder evacuation. Helpful strategies include scheduled voiding, usually every 2 to 3 hours during the early postoperative period, double voiding (urinating, sitting on the toilet for a few minutes, and then urinating a second time), and voluntary pelvic floor muscle relaxation in preparation for voiding.

Patients undergoing a pubovaginal sling procedure will have a small midline incision in the suprapubic area and a vaginal incision. Perineal drainage is usually blood-tinged or spotty because of light bleeding, but significant bleeding must be promptly reported to the surgeon. Regular assessment for wound healing includes monitoring for signs and symptoms of infection, as well as indications of sling erosion. Signs and symptoms of sling erosion include persisting pain, bothersome urinary urgency combined with difficulty urinating, and a bloody, purulent, or malodorous perineal discharge.

Pain management begins with identification of its probable source and management of both the symptom and underlying cause, when feasible. Incisional pain (described earlier) may be managed by opioid analgesics during the immediate postoperative period. A warm sitz bath will also reduce perineal discomfort. Bladder spasm is managed by ensuring adequate fluid intake, avoidance of bladder irritants such as caffeine, and antimicrobial therapy if a urinary tract infection is present.

Patient teaching highlights. Similar to the retropubic urethropexy, teaching emphasizes strict avoidance of heavy lifting, straining, sexual intercourse, or other activities likely to interfere with postoperative wound healing. The patient is taught to self-monitor for urinary retention, urinary tract infection, and sling erosion. Patients who experience episodes of urinary retention may be taught to self-catheterize to avoid bladder overdistention. They can also be reassured that the likelihood of urinary retention greatly diminishes after the first 4 to 6 weeks following surgery. Patients are also gently introduced to the possibility of de novo detrusor overactivity and counseled that this condition, if it occurs, does not imply failure of the surgical procedure and can be managed with a combination of behavioral and pharmacologic interventions.

Suburethral Bulking Agents. Suburethral bulking agents were described for women with urinary incontinence as early as 1938.[76] The procedure is done under local anesthetic on an outpatient basis. A cystoscope is used to inject the bulking agent under the urethral mucosa, or a small suprapubic cystostomy is developed for the purpose of antegrade injection. The goal of injection is to restore coaptation of the urethral lumen, thus increasing more efficient urethral compression during physical activity. However, because the implant does not increase urethral closure forces, it does not obstruct voiding. Ideal patients include those who are poor surgical candidates and have incontinence caused by sphincter incompetence. Current bulking agents for men and women are glutaraldehyde cross-linked collagen, silicone microimplants suspended in a Plasdone hydrogel (Macroplastique, Uroloplasty, Minneapolis), pyrolytic carbon-coated zirconium oxide beads (Durasphere, Advanced UroScience, St Paul, Minn), or autologous fat. The short-term results have shown a high rate of continence, but repeated injections are typically required within 2 to 3 years for most agents.[77] The long-term results for autologous fat are even lower, from 10% to 50%.[78] Figure 11-12 shows the technique used for injection of periurethral bulking agents.

Complications. The most likely complication is transient urinary obstruction, urinary tract infection, hematuria, or de novo urgency. In addition, some patients will demonstrate hypersensitivity to the bulking agent.

Preparation for surgery. Patients are counseled about the need for repeated injections over time. Those undergoing injection of GAX collagen are given a skin test 1 month before injection. A small amount of collagen is injected subdermally into the arm and evaluated over a period of 72 hours. The patient is taught to observe the injection site

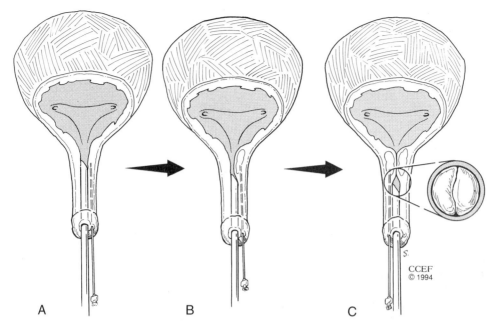

Fig. 11-12 Multiple bulking agents, including bovine collagen, polytef paste, and silicone beads, may be injected suburethrally to improve urethral sphincter competence without compromising the ability to empty the bladder via micturition. **A,** The procedure is done under cystoscopic guidance. **B,** A special needle is passed through a working port of the cystoscope and the urethral bulking agent injected underneath the urethral mucosa. **C,** Adequate volume is injected to coapt (close) the urethral walls. (From Walsh PC, Retik AB, Wein AJ, Vaughan ED [eds]: Campbell's Urology, 8th edition. Philadelphia: Saunders, 2002; p 1177.)

for redness, itching, induration, or swelling over a 72-hour period. Any reactions should be evaluated by a health care professional at 72 hours. Absence of a reaction indicates a very high likelihood that the patient will tolerate the collagen well. However, a small minority of patients will experience hypersensitivity following collagen injection, despite a negative skin sensitivity test. The patient is further advised that the procedure is typically completed on an outpatient basis and counseled about a small risk for transient urinary retention.

Postoperative care. Instruct the patient about the signs and symptoms of urinary tract infection and urinary retention. Some physicians recommend that the patient be instructed in IC. The patient should be seen for a postvoid residual 24 to 48 hours postinjection and for assessment of improvement. If continence is not restored, further injections may be offered, approximately 7 to 10 days apart.

Artificial Urinary Sphincter. An artificial urinary sphincter (AUS) is a urologic prosthetic device with three principal components—an abdominal reservoir, periurethral cuff, and pump mechanism.

The device is operated by baffling fluid through a tubing network connecting the cuff and abdominal reservoir (Figure 11-13, *A*). When activated, the cuff is filled with a small volume of fluid that surrounds the urethra and raises closure pressure. Immediately prior to micturition, the patient compresses a small pump placed in the scrotum or underneath loose skin of the labia majora, shunting water from the cuff to the abdominal reservoir. This provides a 1- to 2-minute period of time, allowing the patient to urinate without obstruction. In addition, the prosthesis contains a palpable button that deactivates the AUS by baffling water to the abdominal reservoir, thus leaving the urethral cuff in a persistently open (deflated) state.

The AUS provides an alternative for the patient with severe sphincter incompetence. It can be placed in women or men, but the greatest experience has been in men (Figure 11-13, *B*). The most common indication is moderate to severe stress urinary incontinence in men following radical prostatectomy, although it also may be implanted following any transurethral or open procedure that results in damage to the urethral sphincter mechanism. Although the likelihood of total continence is comparatively low (most patients continue to require one pad daily), the magnitude of improvement and patient satisfaction is quite high, even in men with a history of radiation therapy.[79,80] Specifically, the proportion of men who achieve total continence is about 27%, and the proportion of men who achieve significantly improved continence is about 87%.

For women, an AUS may be implanted when severe stress urinary incontinence persists, despite multiple prior surgeries. In one long-term follow-up study of women who had received an AUS, the reoperation rate was over 40%, even though 81% remained socially continent.[81] However, no woman who had undergone pelvic radiotherapy achieved continence when the AUS was implanted.

The AUS is also used for patients with sphincter incompetence caused by congenital or acquired neurologic disorders, such as myelodysplasia or low spinal cord injury. In one study that followed patients who had an AUS implanted during childhood, 92% remained socially continent, with follow-up periods of up to 22 years.[82] A small percentage of children undergoing implantation of an AUS void spontaneously, but most rely on intermittent catheterization to ensure regular bladder evacuation. Findings of reoperation, urethral erosion, and infection were similar to those of other studies.

The surgery is performed under very strict aseptic technique to reduce the risk of implant colonization.[83,84] The individually sized cuff is placed near the bladder neck or bulbous urethra in men and near the bladder neck in women. A balloon that regulates the pressure exerted by the periurethral cuff is placed in the prevesical space in the abdomen. The choice of balloon size and the amount of pressure to be exerted on the urethra are influenced by the size of the cuff and characteristics of the urethral tissue. It is important to remember that the higher the cuff pressure, the greater the likelihood of effective urethral closure but also the higher the risk of urethral ischemia or erosion. The pump mechanism of the artificial sphincter is placed in the scrotum in men or underneath the labia in women.

Complications. Infection of the device, usually by *Staphylococcus epidermidis*, is thought to occur during implantation.[83,84] Unfortunately, once infected, most prostheses cannot be salvaged and must be explanted. Reimplantation can be pursued within 3 to 6 months. Mechanical problems, such as kinking of tubes, device leakage, or pump malformation caused by

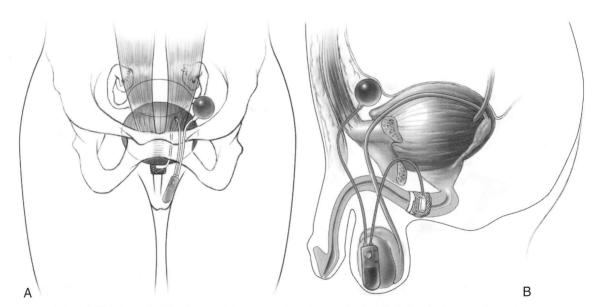

A   B

Fig. 11-13 The artificial urinary sphincter consists of a urethral cuff, abdominal reservoir, and pump device used to baffle water from the cuff to the reservoir. **A,** Artificial sphincter in a female. **B,** Artificial sphincter in a male. (From Walsh PC, Retik AB, Wein AJ, Vaughan ED [eds]: Campbell's Urology, 8th edition. Philadelphia: Saunders, 2002; pp 1188, 1191.)

air lock, blood, or crystals from the contrast material used to fill the device, result in a 7% to 8% surgical revision rate. Urethral erosion is an uncommon complication but urethral atrophy associated with recurring stress urinary incontinence affects 3% to 9% of patients within about 5 years.[83,84]

Preparation for surgery. Teaching concerning the purpose, appearance, and function of the prosthesis is reinforced, including the probable location of the activation device and the need for a brief hospital stay, about 1 to 3 days. The urologic nurse should work closely with the patient and surgeon to ensure that the patient has adequate dexterity and sensation to operate the AUS following implantation and deactivate the device if necessary. Patients should be counseled that, while the device is expected to reduce urine loss significantly, many find they will continue to use approximately one pad daily, even after implantation.

Prevention of device infection begins with documentation of sterile urine within 2 weeks of surgery and aggressive treatment of bacteriuria.[85] The patient is instructed to shower the night before and morning of surgery with chlorhexidine; the shave preparation is performed immediately before surgery and only in the operating suite. A limited bowel preparation may be administered and broad-spectrum antibiotics given immediately before the procedure.

Postoperative care. Parenteral antibiotics are usually administered until hospital discharge, and the oral antibiotics are given for an additional 7 to 10 days. The patient will have an indwelling catheter for approximately 1 week postprocedurally and urine output monitored for volume and character. Care is taken to avoid traction against the catheter and analgesics are administered as needed for pain.

The AUS will remain deactivated for approximately 6 to 8 weeks postoperatively to reduce the risk for urethral erosion and promote optimal wound healing.[84] During this period, the patient can be instructed to place gentle downward traction on the prosthesis to ensure that healing and subsequent scar formation do not cause upward migration, which would render the pump mechanism difficult to locate and manipulate.

Patient teaching highlights. Patients are advised to avoid heavy lifting and sexual intercourse for 6 to 8 weeks.[85] Long car trips should be avoided, if possible; if a trip is necessary, the patient is advised to make frequent stops, leave the car, and take a short walk about every 45 minutes.

The patient is counseled that long-term survival of the AUS relies on avoidance of infection, regular device use, and avoidance of needless lower urinary tract trauma. The patient is given a Medic-Alert bracelet or card informing care providers for the AUS and alerting them to the need for urologic consultation before urethral catheterization. Patients are also counseled about the need for prophylactic antibiotic therapy before certain invasive tests are carried out.

SURGERY OF THE PROSTATE

Prostate surgery is probably the most common intervention undertaken in urologic practice. Transurethral, open, or laparoscopic techniques may be completed to manage benign prostatic hyperplasia and localized prostate cancer.

Transurethral Resection of the Prostate

Transurethral resection of the prostate (TURP) is surgical resection of the prostate gland under endoscopic control. Thorough cystoscopic examination using a rigid cystoscopic system is completed prior to TURP. The surgeon then inserts a 24F or 25F resectoscope containing a malleable wire loop connected to an electrosurgical unit (Figure 11-14).

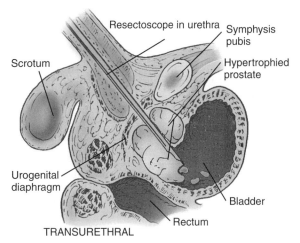

TRANSURETHRAL

Fig. 11-14 Transurethral resection of the prostate (TURP). This uses a malleable wire loop connected to an electrosurgical unit. Tissue resection is achieved by gently pulling the electrically active resecting loop toward the resectoscope. (From Black JM, Hawks JH [eds]: Medical-Surgical Nursing, 8th edition. Philadelphia: Saunders, 2009; p 1021.)

Tissue resection is achieved by gently pulling the resecting loop toward the resectoscope itself, with the urologist taking care to avoid the verumontanum or ureteral orifices to prevent stress urinary incontinence or vesicoureteral reflux. The area of resection varies with each patient but typically includes the bladder neck and prostatic fossa. A glycine or sorbitol solution is irrigated through the resectoscope during the procedure, removing blood and tissue from the operative field. The solution also allows electrocauterization of the prostatic vascular bed without injury to the adjacent tissue.

The traditional resectoscope system uses an electrical current that is modified for cutting or coagulation, but a newer system has been developed that is designed to decrease blood loss.[86] The coagulating intermittent cutting (CIC) device uses a constant voltage pulse current with controlled pulse intervals to reduce bleeding. Transurethral resection with a VaporTrode is another alternative to the traditional resection loop. The VaporTrode uses a higher than usual electrocautery power setting, and substitutes a ball or grooved ball to vaporize prostatic tissue and provide instantaneous cauterization.[87]

Despite a growing variety of minimally invasive alternatives, TURP remains the gold standard procedure for relief of the lower urinary tract symptoms associated with benign prostatic hyperplasia, including hesitancy, straining, intermittent stream, incomplete emptying and urinary retention, nocturia, urinary frequency, and bothersome urgency.

Preparation for surgery. Teaching reinforces the differentiation between transurethral and open surgery. Patients are advised that a brief hospital stay will be necessary, and that an indwelling catheter as well as continuous bladder irrigation are required during the immediate postoperative period. The patient is advised that the catheter will be placed under gentle traction to prevent excessive bleeding from the prostate. Nevertheless, he is counseled that mild hematuria is expected for a period of 4 to 6 weeks following TURP.

Postoperative care. The patient will return from surgery with a three-way bladder irrigation system that must remain patent at all times (Figure 11-15). Patency is ensured by maintaining continuous flow of irrigation solution, regular emptying of the drainage bag when it is no more than two thirds full, and ongoing monitoring of the catheter for patency.

Urine output is monitored every 1 to 2 hours for signs of excessive bleeding. Although a red-tinged fluid is anticipated in the drainage bag, the patient should not have bright red fluid or be passing bright red clots. Urine volume is calculated by subtracting the amount of irrigation fluid instilled from the total amount of fluid in the drainage. A large urine drainage bag, 2 L, designed for bladder irrigation is necessary. The nurse also maintains gentle traction on the indwelling catheter. Specifically, the patient will return to the floor with a three-way indwelling catheter taped to the leg using minimal tension (traction). The nurse maintains traction by ensuring

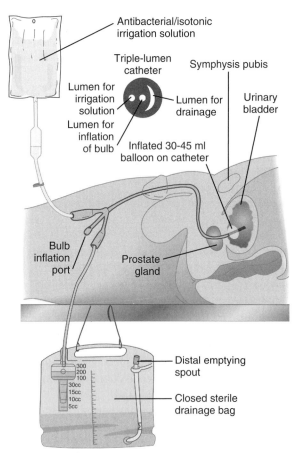

Fig. 11-15 Continuous irrigation of the bladder. This is done via a three-way indwelling catheter, which allows simultaneous infusion and drainage of an irrigating solution (normal saline) through the bladder. Rapid infusion flushes blood or debris from the bladder vesicle and prevents catheter blockage from blood clots or other debris. (From Black JM, Hawks JH [eds]: Medical-Surgical Nursing, 8th edition. Philadelphia: Saunders, 2008; p 1023.)

that the catheter remains in this position until irrigation is discontinued and bleeding has stopped. Traction is critical because it acts as a tamponade, preventing excessive bleeding from the newly resected tissue. The catheter may be irrigated with saline to evacuate large blood clots and prevent urinary retention, if necessary, but the nurse should only carry out this procedure in immediate and direct consultation with the urologist.

Pain after transurethral resection may be associated with trauma to the prostatic urethra or bladder spasms. Maintenance of a patent irrigation system, administration of opioid analgesics for pain arising from surgical resection, and administration of anticholinergics such as oxybutynin or belladonna and opium suppositories are typically effective.

Because of the positioning necessary to perform a TURP, patients are at high risk for deep vein thrombosis (DVT). Therefore, patients undergoing TURP should be fitted for compression stockings before the procedure and wear these garments during the immediate postoperative period. Raising the foot of the bed postoperatively 20 to 30 degrees promotes venous return from the lower extremity and may further reduce the risk for DVT. Teaching and reminding the patient to perform passive leg exercises until he is out of bed is also strongly recommended.

TUR syndrome. TUR syndrome is an uncommon consequence of TURP caused by excessive absorption of irrigation fluid through the prostatic veins.[88] The pathophysiology is only partly understood, but dilutional hyponatremia probably plays a central role. Clinical manifestations include mental confusion, bradycardia, hypotension or hypertension, nausea, vomiting, and visual disturbances. Risk factors include patients with very large prostates and total resection times longer than 90 minutes. Additional factors are liver disease, significant muscular atrophy, and bladder calculi.

Furosemide can be given immediately postoperatively to patients judged to be at high risk. In addition, the risk is reduced by the use of iso-osmotic solutions such as mannitol, glycine, or sorbitol during TURP. The height of the irrigating bag during the procedure can also influence absorption and it is recommended that the bag be placed just above the level of the pubis to reduce the intravesical pressure. Following the procedure, each patient is carefully monitored for signs and symptoms of hyponatremia. The physician is informed immediately if TUR syndrome is suspected because it can rapidly progress to fatal arrhythmias or myocardial infarction unless it is managed aggressively.

Patient teaching highlights. The patient is advised that hematuria may persist or clear and recur over the first 4 to 6 weeks postoperatively. The patient should be reassured that lightly tinged urine and the passage of dark red flecks or very small clots reflect wound healing, and that small scabs will be shed as the prostatic urethra heals. In contrast, the patient is advised to contact a urologist or urologic nurse promptly if he passes large, bright red clots or persistent bright red urine. Mild hematuria may be relieved by drinking water or clear liquids and temporarily limiting physical activity. Education also includes information about the potential for urinary retention. If unable to void, the patient can be taught strategies to encourage urination, but he also must be cautioned to contact the urologist promptly or seek immediate assistance if retention persists.

Patients are advised to avoid lifting objects that weigh more than 10 pounds for the first 2 weeks following TURP and to avoid long car trips, if possible. If a long trip is necessary, frequent stops (about every 45 minutes) are recommended. The patient is counseled to avoid sexual intercourse based on the urologist's recommendation and is further advised that orgasm is not expected to produce a visible expulsion of semen, as it did before the procedure. Instead, the patient is counseled that he will experience a perception of orgasm that may be subjectively different from that experienced preoperatively, and that seminal elements will pass harmlessly into the bladder and be expelled with his next urination.

Constipation should be avoided using a combination of fluid intake and dietary or prescriptive stool softeners. Straining to defecate should be avoided because of the potential to interfere with wound healing. Although rare, stress urinary incontinence may occur following TURP. Patients may be counseled that performance of pelvic floor muscle exercises may reduce or prevent stress uinary incontinence following TURP.[89]

Minimally Invasive Therapies

A number of minimally invasive alternatives to TURP have been developed over the last several decades.[90] They are indicated for men who do not wish or are unfit to undergo more invasive procedures, or who have not responded to medical management. This section will review the most common of these procedures, including transurethral microwave thermotherapy (TUMT), transurethral needle ablation (TUNA), water-induced thermotherapy (WIT), high-energy focused ultrasound (HIFU), and interstitial laser ablation. A common feature of these techniques is the use of an energy source to produce coagulation tissue necrosis. This procedure tends to minimize blood loss but prostatic tissue may be destroyed in the process, removing the opportunity for subsequent pathologic analysis for possible malignancy.

Transurethral Microwave Thermotherapy.

TUMT uses microwave energy to ablate prostatic tissues approximately 6 to 7 mm from a heat source located within a triple-lumen urethral catheter.[91] A cooling system circulates water within the catheter applicator, protecting adjacent tissues from thermal damage; also, a fiberoptic thermosensor monitors treatment temperature, ensuring that temperature in the target tissue is sufficiently high to ablate obstructive tissue. A rectal probe is also inserted, which monitors rectal temperatures during the procedure. Surface cooling of the urethra extends the depth of heating (up to 80° C). Cooling is important because it reduces discomfort during and following TUMT and preserves urethral integrity. A number of studies have examined the efficacy of TUMT and found significant improvements in bothersome lower urinary tract symptoms and reduction in obstruction severity, as assessed by urodynamic testing.[92] In contrast, one study failed to show any improvement in urodynamically measured obstruction magnitude, but this result has been attributed to the use of relatively low energy levels during a comparatively early phase of microwave thermotherapy.[93]

Similar to other studies, studies comparing TUMT with TURP have tended to demonstrate a smaller reduction in obstruction, a smaller magnitude of symptomatic relief, and less durable results with microwave thermotherapy.[92] Nevertheless, these results must be carefully weighed against the advantages of TUMT and other minimally invasive therapies for benign prostatic hyperplasia, such as avoidance of hospitalization, reduced bleeding and associated morbidity, and reductions in cost.

Transurethral Needle Ablation.

TUNA uses low-level radiofrequency, about 490 kHz, delivered via 12- to 22-mm needle electrodes to heat obstructive prostatic tissue to 110° C.[94,95] Needle electrodes are placed in the region intended for ablation, ensuring preservation of adjacent tissues, especially the urethra and rectum. The TUNA catheter is advanced under direct vision, but the position of the needle tips is visualized via transrectal ultrasound. Treatment requires 30 to 45 minutes, resulting in the creation of four distinctive areas of tissue destruction. Urethral and intraprostatic sensors monitor temperatures and a slow constant drip of saline keeps urethral temperatures below 43° C.

Several studies have examined long-term data from TUNA. Zlotta and colleagues[96] evaluated 188 consecutive cases managed by TUNA for a mean follow-up of 63 months. Durable reductions in the magnitude of obstruction, lower urinary tract symptom scores (using the international prostate symptom score [IPSS]), and peak urinary flow rates were achieved by TUNA. However, 21% required additional treatments, including pharmacotherapy (6%), a second TUNA procedure (4%), and open or transurethral prostate surgery (11%). Hill and co-workers[97] compared TUNA and TURP in a 5-year randomized clinical trial. Following randomization to either TUNA or TURP, subjects underwent annual follow-up, including lower urinary tract symptom score (IPSS), uroflowmetry, postvoid residual urinary volume measurement, and quantification of prostate size. They found that both TUNA and TURP produce durable reductions in bothersome symptoms, combined with durable increases in urinary flow rates. In addition, they noted that no patients who underwent TUNA experienced retrograde ejaculation, as compared with 41% of those undergoing TURP. Although changes from baseline were measured for each modality across five annual follow-up evaluations, no statistical comparisons were made between them to determine differences in the magnitude of reductions achieved by each.

Because of its ability to produce local denervation while avoiding the morbidity of more invasive procedures, such as transurethral incision of the prostate or bladder neck, TUNA has been investigated to determine its effect on men with chronic pelvic pain syndrome. In a pilot study of 27 subjects, 21 were randomly assigned to undergo TUNA and 6 underwent sham therapy (cystoscopy alone).[98] Although both groups experienced a transient increase in maximum urinary flow rate, the change was statistically significant in the TUNA group and not the sham group. In addition, patients undergoing TUNA experienced statistically significant pain relief and 72% had persistent relief at 12-month follow-up. Nevertheless, differences in the TUNA group were not statistically different when compared with those experienced by the sham group. Although these results are encouraging, further study is needed before it is possible to determine what role, if any, TUNA may play for the management of men with chronic pelvic pain syndrome.

Water Infusion Thermotherapy. WIT uses conductive heating produced by circulating high-temperature water (60° to 70° C) to heat and destroy obstructive prostatic tissue.[99] Treatment is delivered via an 18F 50-ml balloon urethral catheter and lasts for approximately 45 minutes; patients are usually able to tolerate the procedure with topical (intraurethral) anesthesia alone. The catheter is thermally insulated to protect adjacent tissues, especially the striated urethral sphincter. After insertion and positioning, the treatment balloon is inflated and the catheter is withdrawn to appose the positioning balloon snugly against the bladder neck, thereby placing the treatment balloon in the prostatic urethra.

Because of the procedure's relative novelty, long-term data about its safety and efficacy are not available. In a shorter term study of 125 patients from eight centers, treatment failures were reported as 6% after 1 year, 10% at 2 years, and 11% at 3 years.[100] In another study of 29 frail older men with chronic indwelling catheters associated with benign prostatic hyperplasia, 73% were able to void spontaneously and no longer required catheterization.[101]

High-Intensity Focused Ultrasound. HIFU uses focused high-energy ultrasound pulses to heat and destroy the prostatic adenoma.[102,103] A theoretical advantage of HIFU over the other minimally invasive procedures is the absence of any significant temperature increase or damage to tissue along the path of the ultrasound beam. Before HIFU is commenced, imaging ultrasound is used to identify the obstructive prostatic adenoma. This is followed by alternating pulses between high-energy and ablative pulses or low-energy pulses. The result is heating targeted tissue to 80° to 100° C. An indwelling catheter is

inserted in the bladder to enhance the ultrasound effect. Targeted tissue undergoes almost instantaneous coagulative necrosis caused by high local temperatures. To maintain a constant baseline temperature lower than 37° C in the transrectal probe, a semiautomatic cooling process is applied throughout the procedure.

Despite these potential advantages, a study comparing TURP to four minimally invasive therapies showed a smaller magnitude in symptom improvement as compared with TURP,[93] and another study of 98 men showed poor long-term durability, with 44% requiring additional treatment (TURP) within 5 years of HIFU.[103]

HIFU has also been advocated for the treatment of selected localized prostate cancers, with potentially promising initial results.[104,105] Patients have achieved a negative postoperative prostate biopsy and no elevation of prostate-specific antigen (PSA) level at successive intervals. However, the incidence of side effects may be relatively high, and include prolonged indwelling catheterization, rectal fistula in 5%, and erectile dysfunction (ED) in 30%. Long-term follow-up studies must be completed before the efficacy of HIFU for the management of localized prostate cancer can be determined.

Laser Ablation. The use of laser energy emerged in 1992 as urologists searched for minimally invasive alternatives to TURP with comparable efficacy in the relief of obstruction and associated lower urinary tract symptoms.[106] However, the cost of equipment, need for specialized training to operate equipment, time needed to achieve adequate vaporization, and postprocedural requirements such as the need for prolonged indwelling catheterization led to a decline in its popularity. Nevertheless, recent advanced have led to a resurgence of interest in two types of laser energy, holmium and KTP.

Holmium laser energy is used for multiple urologic procedures, including lithotripsy, prostatectomy, and bladder neck incision.[107-109] Holmium is a rare element found in gadolinite, a black mineral containing yttrium, iron, cerium, iron, and holmium. When applied to laser prostatectomy, holmium laser energy is directed to prostatic tissue using an end-firing laser fiber incorporated into a specially designed continuous flow resectoscope. The laser can be used to resect comparatively large sections of prostate tissue, which are then reduced into smaller pieces before removal.

More recently, an enucleation system has been developed that uses holmium laser energy. It allows resection of intact prostatic lobes that are passed into the bladder and then divided into smaller pieces prior to removal via a continuous drainage resectoscope.[108-110] Holmium laser energy offers several advantages when compared with older laser energy sources. It rapidly creates a large cavity in the prostate comparable to the cavities created by traditional TURP. As a result, it can be used for prostate glands weighing 125 g or more.[111] It also provides simultaneous and effective anticoagulation of resected tissue planes, minimizing blood loss and the need for transfusion,[110] as well as the risk for TUR syndrome associated with traditional TURP.[112] Because blood loss and the risk of dilutional hyponatremia are minimized, patients undergoing holmium laser prostatectomy tend to have less need for irrigation and reduced hospital stays.

Holmium laser prostatectomy or enucleation may be performed under general or spinal anesthesia. It has been shown to reduce the magnitude of bladder obstruction associated with benign prostatic hyperplasia, improve urinary flow rates, reduce postvoid residual volumes, and alleviate associated lower urinary tract symptoms.[108-112] Long-term outcomes of the procedure are not yet known.

Photoselective prostate vaporization has also emerged as a more effective alternative to older techniques of laser prostatectomy.[106] Sometimes called green light laser prostatectomy, photoselective prostate vaporization uses a high-energy KTP energy source. The wavelength of the KTP laser is avidly absorbed by oxyhemoglobin, so that it penetrates only 1 to 2 mm of prostate tissue. This allows the urologist to confine tissue necrosis to a smaller area, thus avoiding the adverse side effects associated with excessive tissue coagulation. Laser energy is delivered using a side-firing laser fiber introduced via a resectoscope designed for the procedure. The procedure may be performed under spinal or general anesthesia. Photoselective prostate prostatectomy has been found to reduce the magnitude of bladder obstruction associated with benign prostatic hyperplasia, improve urinary flow rates, reduce postvoid residual volume, and alleviate associated lower urinary tract symptoms.[106,113,114] Long-term outcomes following photoselective vaporization of the prostate are not yet known; one study found that urinary flow rates,

postvoid residual volumes, smaller prostate volumes, and lower IPSS scores persisted for 1 year in a group of 240 patients.[115]

Complications. The principal clinical advantages of minimally invasive procedures are fewer complications. Nevertheless, complications do occur, and they include urinary tract infection, prolonged or excessive dysuria, epididymitis, prolonged or severe hematuria, transient impotence, transient urinary urge incontinence, urethral pain, proctitis, transient urinary retention, and urethral stricture. Patients undergoing HIFU also may experience hematospermia.

Preparation for surgery. A prophylactic fluoroquinolone antibiotic is usually given 24 hours before the procedure and continued 7 to 14 days postprocedure. Obtaining a lower urinary tract symptom score such as the IPSS is recommended to establish a baseline for comparison following treatment. Transurethral rectal ultrasound may be done to determine prostate size, and biopsies will be obtained if a suspicion of prostate cancer exists. Cystoscopy may be performed to determine prostatic urethral length or rule out other abnormalities, such as stricture or bladder mass. Most urologists recommend that patients have no food or drink 8 hours prior to the procedure and that they eliminate alcohol, caffeine, and cigarettes at least 48 hours preprocedure. Generally, acetylsalicylic acid is stopped 7 days and nonsteroidal anti-inflammatory drugs (NSAIDs) and warfarin 3 days preprocedure, in consultation with the cardiology service. A limited bowel preparation (cleansing enema) may also be administered the night prior to the procedure. Even though these procedures are usually performed on an outpatient basis, patients are advised that they must arrange for transportation home following treatment.

In some cases, oral or intravenous sedation or a local prostatic or perineal block can be given for discomfort or anxiety. In addition, 2% lidocaine is usually instilled into the urethra prior to catheter insertion; this is usually the only pain control necessary for patients undergoing WIT. One center has recommended catheterizing the patient while in the Trendelenburg position with a 14- or 16F catheter and instilling 60 ml of chilled 2% lidocaine.[94] The catheter is then slowly withdrawn as the lidocaine is instilled. This is immediately followed by 10 ml of intraurethral lidocaine instillation, held in place with a penile clamp for 20 minutes.

Postoperative care and patient teaching highlights. Because these procedures are usually performed on an outpatient basis, the primary focus of postprocedural care is education for self-management and recognition of complications. The teaching plan for minimally invasive procedures must be individualized based on the specific procedure; the setting in which it occurs; the use of systemic, regional, or topical anesthesia; and comorbid conditions.

The nurse should explain to the patient that an indwelling catheter will remain in place for a variable amount of time, often 2 to 7 days, until swelling and edema are resolved, depending on the procedure, volume of tissue resected, and other factors. Consumption of a robust daily volume of fluids, usually 2 to 3 L, is encouraged to ensure passage of necrotic materials and to prevent occlusion of the catheter. Blood clots and small pieces of dark red brown necrotic tissue will appear in the catheter bag and in the voided urine for 7 to 30 days. Patients should be taught to differentiate the passage of small flecks of necrotic materials and old blood from active or excessive bleeding.

Patients are also counseled about irritative lower urinary tract symptoms—frequent urination, bothersome urgency, dysuria, and nocturia—that typically occur following minimally invasive procedures. These symptoms are expected to persist for several days after catheter removal until edema and inflammation subside. Two procedures, HIFU and laser vaporization, are particularly likely to produce bothersome lower urinary tract symptoms.

Relatively few restrictions are required after a minimally invasive procedure. Nevertheless, patients should be counseled that vigorous activities such as running, jogging, or digging should be avoided for several weeks to allow the ablated area to heal completely.

TREATMENT OF PROSTATE CANCER

Multiple treatment options have proved effective for the management of early-stage, localized prostate cancer. This section will review the nursing management of open surgery (radical prostatectomy) and cryotherapy. Refer to Chapter 8 for a detailed discussion of the nursing management of the patient undergoing brachytherapy.

Radical Prostatectomy

Radical prostatectomy is removal of the prostate and seminal vesicles. It is accompanied by pelvic lymphadenectomy in selected cases. A number of approaches have been used for the procedure, including open, laparoscopic, and robot-assisted laparoscopic surgery.

Radical Retropubic Prostatectomy. Originally described in 1947, radical retropubic prostatectomy was favored by many surgeons because it allowed an anatomic approach technically feasible for accomplishing the primary goal of surgery, complete resection of malignant tissue (Figure 11-16).[116] Application of the procedure was initially hampered by difficulties with bleeding and postoperative complications, such as ED and urinary incontinence. It gained widespread popularity in the 1990s because of increased understanding of the neurovascular bundles, allowing surgeons to improve their ability to control bleeding during the procedure dramatically and to reduce the incidence and/or severity of specific postoperative complications, including ED and urinary incontinence.

The patient is placed in a supine position and an incision is created in the midline of the lower abdomen, extending from the umbilicus to the pubis. The prostate is released from the endopelvic fascia and dorsal vein complex and the urethra is separated from the lateral and posterior portions of the membranous urethra.

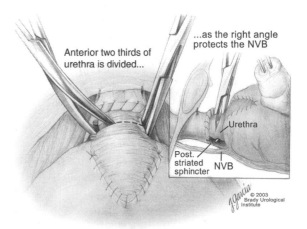

Fig. 11-16 Open radical retropubic prostatectomy. (From Wein AJ, Kavoussi LR, Novick AC, Partin AW, Peters CA [eds]: Campbell-Walsh Urology, 9th edition. Philadelphia: Saunders, 2007; p 2964.)

The proximal urethra is also transected and the prostate and seminal vesicles removed. Depending on the extent of local invasion, one or both neurovascular bundles are preserved, a maneuver that reduces the risk for ED and urinary incontinence. In addition, the bladder neck also may be preserved in an effort to increase the likelihood for maintaining continence.[117] An indwelling catheter is placed, the urethra reanastomosed. and the incision closed.

Complications. The most common complications following any radical prostatectomy are urinary incontinence and ED.[116,118] Multiple factors have been examined for their influence on the likelihood of these negative outcomes and several modifiable factors, such as preservation of the neurovascular bundles, surgeon's experience with the procedure, and bladder neck preservation, have been shown to exert some influence. Uncommon complications include stricture of the urethrovesical anastomosis, delayed bleeding, deep vein thrombosis, and pulmonary embolism.[119] One review of 15 cases has reported inguinal hernias in 21% of patients who underwent both prostatectomy and pelvic lymph node dissection.[120]

Preparation for surgery. Patients are instructed about the need for bowel preparation to reduce the risk of fecal contamination if the prostate adheres to the bowel and a bowel nick occurs. Preparation varies but usually incorporates a cleansing enema, magnesium citrate solution, suppositories, or bisacodyl tablets. Compression stockings are applied immediately prior to surgery to reduce the risk of DVT. The patient is given instruction about blood banking—storing autologous blood—as described in the preparation for radical nephrectomy (see earlier). The patient is advised that he will have an indwelling catheter following surgery that is expected to remain in place for approximately 7 to 21 days. Teaching the management of an indwelling catheter should begin prior to surgery and is reinforced during the early postoperative period. Five randomized trials have been conducted regarding the benefit of preoperative pelvic floor muscle exercises; one of these showed benefit in return to continence but overall the evidence remains weak about the effect.[121,122] What is known is that men benefit greatly from the support and encouragement when they participate in pelvic floor therapy preoperatively or postoperatively.

Postoperative care. Principles of postoperative management are the same for any patients undergoing abdominopelvic surgery. Specific issues related to open radical retropubic prostatectomy include (1) altered urine elimination, (2) pain management, (3) wound healing, and (4) prevention of DVT.

The hospital stay is typically brief, usually about 2 to 4 days. The patient will have an indwelling urethral catheter in place following surgery. Urine output is monitored closely for the first several days. Reddish to pink-colored urine is expected during the immediate postoperative period, but this should convert to a yellow hue by 1 to 2 days postoperatively. Frank bleeding or passage of clots should not occur and requires immediate management. If clots or blockage of the catheter is suspected, the nurse should promptly contact the urologist but avoid irrigation of the catheter, because this action might compromise delicate anastomoses at the bladder neck. The patient starts on a clear liquid diet when bowel sounds are heard, usually on the first postoperative day, and progresses to solid foods as tolerated.

Promotion of wound healing focuses on the incision and urethral anastomosis. A Penrose or Jackson-Pratt drain will drain the wound. Effluent from the drain is assessed for volume and character; serous drainage that is tinged with blood is expected, but passage of urine or bright red blood with clots must be reported promptly to the physician. Drains are removed when they cease to produce significant volumes of effluent, usually on postoperative day 3 or 4. Meticulous care is taken to ensure that traction is not placed against the catheter, particularly because the retention balloon is located near the newly created and healing urethral anastomosis. In addition, patients are counseled that they must not strain to defecate during the immediate postoperative period because this maneuver could place undue force against the newly created urethral anastomosis.

Compression stockings and anticoagulant therapy to reduce the risk of DVT are generally maintained over the first 1 to 2 postoperative days or until the patient is walking, particularly if a perineal approach is used requiring intraoperative positioning in an exaggerated dorsal lithotomy position.

Parenteral opioid analgesics are typically used to manage initial postoperative pain and an antiemetic may be administered if nausea occurs. Analgesics should be combined with nonpharmacologic pain reduction interventions such as (1) positioning the patient so that pressure on the incision is avoided;

(2) splinting the incision during pulmonary toilet; and (3) prevention of constipation, which exacerbates pressure and discomfort. Patients also may experience painful bladder spasms. They should be treated with an antimuscarinic agent such as tolterodine, oxybutynin, or opium or belladonna suppositories, rather than opioid analgesics.

Patient teaching highlights. Almost all men can be counseled that they will be discharged home with an indwelling catheter in place. The patient and family should be instructed about the indwelling catheter, including routine monitoring for blockage and excessive bleeding. The patient is advised that the catheter will be removed between 7 and 21 days postsurgery (average, about 14 days).[123,124]

While the catheter remains in place, the patient is counseled that particular care must be taken to avoid traction against the newly created urethral anastomosis. Specifically, the catheter must be secured in a manner that avoids traction against the anastomotic site, such as that provided by use of a Velcro-based catheter strap. Constipation also must be avoided. A soft diet, walking, and stool softeners are used to nsure passage of soft, formed stools. However, the patient and family also must be taught that enemas and suppositories should be avoided because of the risk of inadvertent trauma to the surgical site.

Preoperative instruction focuses on the anticipated changes in genitourinary function, such as urinary incontinence and ED after the catheter is first removed. Basic principles of pelvic floor muscle rehabilitation may be taught by the urologic nurse, including strategies to identify, contract, and relax the pelvic floor muscles and the concept of a graded muscle exercise routine. The patient can be reassured that continence typically improves dramatically over the initial days to weeks following catheter removal, and then gradually over the first year following surgery.[125] Patients can also be reassured that more aggressive treatment for the 10% to 15% who experience persistent incontinence is available.

Although thoughts about the risk of ED are often sublimated in favor of more basic concerns during the immediate postoperative period, these concerns almost always resurface as recovery progresses and initial fears and anxieties subside. The nurse can assist the patient and partner by bringing up the topic of sexual function in an objective and compassionate manner. Some evidence supports early treatment of ED using alprostadil (Caverject), or a phosphodiesterase type 5 inhibitor such as sildenafil, vardenafil, or tadalafil may enhance the efficacy of erectile function,[126] and many patients will be placed on one of these medications during the early postoperative period. The urologic nurse often plays a critical role in adherence to preventive treatment by reinforcing the purpose of the therapy; this is combined with ongoing education about additional options for managing this significant but often underappreciated aspect of prostate cancer treatment.

Laparoscopic and Robotic-Assisted Radical Retropubic Prostatectomy. Laparoscopic techniques also may be used to perform a radical retropubic prostatectomy. Techniques for laparoscopic prostatectomy have been championed by urologists in France,[127] North America,[128] and Germany.[129] Preparation for surgery is similar to that for open surgery, with the exception of bowel preparation, which is not routinely performed. Three small incisions are created for trocars and a Veress needle is inserted at the umbilicus to insufflate the abdomen with CO_2 or another gas if indicated. After inspecting the abdomen for trocar injury, pelvic lymphadenectomy is performed before the prostatectomy when indicated. Laparoscopic instruments are then used to free the prostate from the endopelvic fascia, transect the urethra, remove the prostate and seminal vesicles, and reanastomose the urethra. Similar to the open procedure, preservation of one or both neurovascular bundles is undertaken whenever feasible.

The advantages and disadvantages associated with laparoscopic versus open radical retropubic prostatectomy are similar to those for any laparoscopic procedure. Advantages include avoidance of a midline incision, with reductions in postoperative recovery time and pain. Disadvantages include the risk for conversion to an open procedure, risk for significant bowel injury, increased time under anesthesia, a higher positive margin rate as compared with published reports of open surgery, and higher direct cost.[130] Development of the experience and skill needed to complete a laparoscopic procedure efficiently and effectively requires significant dedication, leading some researchers to conclude that these procedures should be limited to dedicated centers.[131]

Robotic-assisted retropubic radical prostatectomy offers several technical advantages to laparoscopic techniques, including a three-dimensional vision system and an articulated robotic arm that mimics the wrist movement of the surgeon while extending the operator's ability to rotate the arm to a degree not allowed by the human wrist.[132] These features allow the surgeon to perform fine dissections in narrow areas such as the male pelvis while maintaining excellent visualization of critical anatomic structures. In addition, robotic-assisted techniques are more intuitively similar to open techniques than many classic laparoscopic maneuvers, which may help lower the steep learning curve observed with traditional laparoscopy. Although clinical experience with robotic-assisted prostatectomy remains limited, systematic literature reviews of initial results have demonstrated that this technique diminishes intraoperative blood loss (200 ml) and the need for subsequent transfusion, maintains higher serum hematocrit level at discharge, reduces hospital stay (by 1or 2 days), and optimizes recovery time.[133,134] Pathologic analysis has revealed positive margin rates, indicating residual tumor cells despite surgery, comparable to those

for open or laparoscopic radical prostatectomy. Costs remain higher for robotic-assisted radical prostatectomy, however, primarily because of equipment costs and maintenance.[133] In studies to date, the incidence of urinary incontinence and ED has been described as "comparable" to that of open or laparoscopic radical prostatectomy.[135]

Robotic-assisted prostatectomy is typically performed through small abdominal incisions comparable to those used for laparoscopic prostatectomy.[135] The time required for the procedure varies based on the characteristics of the patient and tumor, as well as the experience of the surgeon. However, robotic-assisted prostatectomy is intuitively more similar to open surgical techniques and an average time of 3 hours is reasonable when the procedure is performed by an experienced surgeon. The surgeon is seated at a console and manipulates robotic arms that are inserted into the patient using laparoscopic ports (Figure 11-17, *A*). A first assistant, often an

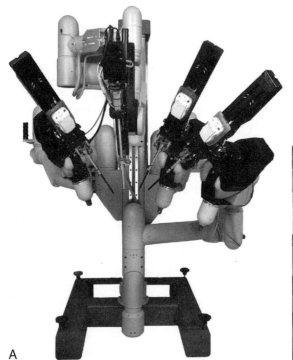

A

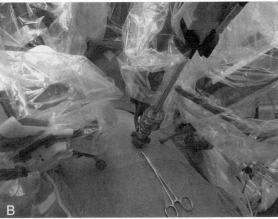

B

Fig. 11-17 A, Robotic-assisted laparoscopic radical prostatectomy. This combines a three-dimensional vision system and articulated robotic arm that mimics wrist movement while extending the operator's ability to rotate the arm to a degree not allowed normally (Courtesy of Intuitive Surgical, Sunnyville, CA). **B,** Trocar placement for laparoscopic radical prostatectomy. (From Wein AJ, Kavoussi LR, Novick AC, Partin AW, Peters CA [eds]: Campbell-Walsh Urology, 9th edition. Philadelphia: Saunders, 2007; pp 2988, 2989.)

advanced practice nurse or physician's assistant, passes and cuts suture materials and provides suction and retraction as indicated. Five to six laparoscopic ports are typically placed, including a camera port above the umbilicus, three working ports in the abdominopelvic region for the robotic arms, and one or two ports for the first assistant [135,136] (Figure 11-17, *B*). Similar to laparoscopic procedures, a pneumoperitoneum is maintained during the procedure using CO_2 or another gas. Prostatectomy is accomplished using a transperitoneal or extraperitoneal approach with the patient in lithotomy position with steep Trendelenburg (Figure 11-18).

Open Radical Perineal Prostatectomy. Radical perineal prostatectomy is an open surgical procedure and is an alternative to the retropubic approach. The patient is placed in an exaggerated lithotomy position with the legs elevated in stirrups and pressure points padded to prevent intraoperative pressure ulcerations. A slightly curvilinear incision is made from one midischial tuberosity to the other, about 1.5 cm above the anus. The prostate is freed from its endopelvic attachments and the urethra is transected at the level of the bladder neck and above the membranous urethra, where the rhabdosphincter is located. Pelvic lymphadenectomy cannot be simultaneously performed through the same incision; most patients who are considered to need this surgery undergo laparoscopic lymphadenectomy.

Potential advantages of radical perineal prostatectomy when compared with the retropubic approach include better visualization of the prostate when the patient is placed in an exaggerated lithotomy position and good ability to preserve the neurovascular bundles, when feasible. [137] When compared with the retropubic approach, patients undergoing perineal prostatectomy require less analgesia, ambulate and return to oral intake earlier than those managed by a retropubic procedure, and tend to have shorter hospital stays. Potential disadvantages include the inability to perform a simultaneous lymphadenectomy and a potential for rectal sphincter damage. [138-140]

Controversy exists as to whether the perineal technique provides the anatomic approach thought to afford the critical cancer control provided with the retropubic approach. Comparison studies between the two procedures have yielded mixed results, but the perineal approach tends to have comparable outcomes in terms of negative margins and long-term cancer control, slightly better continence rates, comparable rates of ED, and higher rates of postoperative rectal sphincter laceration with associated fecal incontinence (1% to 11%). [125,137]

Cryotherapy

Cryotherapy is the use of hypothermia (tissue freezing) to destroy tissue. In a urologic context, cryotherapy involves the delivery of extreme cold temperatures via a rectal probe to destroy localized prostate cancer. [141] Although cooling tissues to temperatures lower than $0°$ C causes crystallization of the extracellular fluid and cellular distress, cells

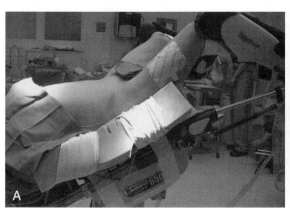 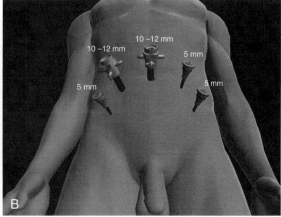

Fig. 11-18 Patient position for laparoscopic radical prostatectomy. (From Wein AJ, Kavoussi LR, Novick AC, Partin AW, Peters CA [eds]: Campbell-Walsh Urology, 9th edition. Philadelphia: Saunders, 2007; p 2988.)

cooled to temperatures of $-40°$ C or lower are completely destroyed. At least three cryosurgical devices are sold in North America. One uses liquid nitrogen that evaporates at the tip of the probe, causing cooling, another uses ultracooled liquid nitrogen compressed and cooled to $-206°$ C, and another uses liquid argon to achieve freezing. In 1993, Onik and colleagues[142] first reported the currently used technique of percutaneous transperineal ultrasound–guided cryoablation for localized prostate cancer. Treatment is most successful for lower grade, highly localized tumors and has fewer irritative and obstructive voiding symptoms than does brachytherapy.[143]

The procedure is performed under general or regional anesthesia. The patient is placed in a lithotomy position, a urethral catheter is inserted, the bladder is filled with saline to displace perineal structures from the treatment area, and a urethral warmer is placed. Up to 30 cryotherapy probes are placed in the prostate under transrectal ultrasonic guidance and a probe may be placed in the seminal vesicle if indicated. Two freeze cycles are performed to maximize malignant tissue destruction and the probes removed. The urethral warmer is left in place until thawing is completed. It is subsequently withdrawn and replaced with an indwelling catheter.

Complications. Long-term complications are related to the freezing of vulnerable surrounding tissue, such as the urethra, striated urethral sphincter, pelvic muscles, rectum, and ureters.[141-142] Impotence (almost 100%), incontinence (as high as 70%), tissue sloughing, and pelvic pain are all potential problems about which the patient should be informed prior to the procedure. Tissue sloughing may occur 3 to 8 weeks after the procedure, which can place the patient at risk for irritated and obstructed voiding and pyuria. Patient teaching must include the signs and symptoms of obstruction and urinary tract infection. Some men complain of pelvic and rectal pain; others may describe penile numbness caused by nerve injury.

Cryotherapy is not recommended for patients who have undergone previous radiation therapy. The incidence of rectourethral fistula and total incontinence after cryosurgery was 0.33% for patients who had not received radiation, but 8.7% for those patients who had been treated previously with radiation.[141,143]

Preparation for surgery. Because multiple probe placements are required, the patient should be counseled that all prescription medications, over-the-counter products, and herbal preparations with anticoagulant properties must be discontinued 3 to 7 days prior to the procedure based on institutional policies or physician's order. The patient is taught to self-administer a mechanical bowel preparation. It usually consists of oral magnesium citrate taken 1 day before the procedure at varying intervals plus a clear fluid diet, and a sodium phosphate enema on the day of the procedure.[144]

Postoperative care. The patient is expected to return home the same day. He is informed that he will have an indwelling catheter for approximately 3 weeks following cryotherapy. The patient is counseled that he is expected to pass sloughed tissue and debris and some blood, leading to light red or pink-tinged urine. However, passage of large volumes of bright red blood or clots is not expected and should provoke a prompt call to the urologist or urologic nurse. The patient is also taught to monitor the catheter and drainage bag for patency and to alert the urologic team if he experiences signs or symptoms of a urinary tract infection. After the catheter is removed, the patient is advised that he is likely to experience lower urinary tract symptoms, including voiding frequency, and possibly urgency and urinary leakage. Symptoms are expected to be transient, but the urologist or if urologic nurse should be informed if he is unable to urinate or if irritative lower urinary tract symptoms persist. A 6-month follow-up visit is typically scheduled that will include a reevaluation of lower urinary tract symptoms and examination of the prostate gland. The prostate gland is expected to be small and fibrotic; lower urinary tract symptoms experienced when the catheter was first removed should have subsided or disappeared. The IPSS provides a useful measure of urinary symptoms after cryotherapy. Bothersome lower urinary tract symptoms, including stress or urge incontinence, should be addressed at this time.[144]

Patient teaching highlights. In addition to catheter management, patients are educated that pelvic and rectal pain or penile numbness may occur but are expected to subside with time. Men are also counseled that the serum PSA level is expected to surge postbrachytherapy. The urologist or advanced practice nurse will review the complications of ED and urinary incontinence. In the case of ED, it is very important preoperatively that patients understand that this is likely to be permanent and difficult to treat.

SURGERY OF THE SCROTUM AND TESTES

A number of urologic conditions affecting the scrotum and testes may be managed by surgical intervention. This section will discuss three of the most common scrotal procedures in the adult: (1) bilateral orchiectomy for the management of advanced-stage prostate cancer; (2) radical orchiectomy for testicular cancer; and (3) vasectomy for voluntary sterilization. Refer to Chapter 18 for a discussion of scrotal and testicular procedures commonly performed in children.

Bilateral Orchiectomy

Bilateral orchiectomy is the surgical removal of both testes for the purpose of reducing the serum testosterone levels.[145] It is indicated for androgen blockade in men with advanced-stage prostate cancer and it remains the gold standard against which more novel treatments are compared. Nevertheless, its success must be carefully weighed against the psychological distress associated with its performance.[146] The procedure is usually performed on an outpatient basis, using local anesthesia (1% lidocaine or 0.5% bupivacaine). Various approaches may be used, including midline or transverse scrotal incisions. The skin, underlying dartos muscle, and fascial coverings (tunics) are incised until the parietal layer of the tunica vaginalis is reached. The testes and distal spermatic cord are removed, along with the epididymis. A prosthetic device can be implanted if the patient desires.

Complications. Serious complications are uncommon following bilateral orchiectomy. Sudden androgen deprivation is associated with a number of adverse side effects including hot flushes, which may be bothersome for some men.[147] Other adverse effects associated with androgen deprivation are osteoporosis, loss of lean muscle mass, depression, and mood swings.

Preparation for surgery. Because of advances in the last decade, particularly the advent of androgenic blocking agents and luteinizing hormone–releasing hormone (LH-RH) analogues, and the psychological distress associated with bilateral orchiectomy, comparatively few men undergo the procedure. It is critical that the nurse ensure that the patient understands the surgery, comprehends that it is irreversible, and is aware of available medical alternatives. The patient can be counseled that bilateral orchiectomy is expected to provide a 95% reduction in the serum testosterone level. However, the urologic nurse must also reinforce counseling that this procedure will not prevent the emergence of androgen-resistant prostate cancer. Nevertheless, patents can be reassured that effective androgen deprivation is anticipated to provide 5 years of cancer control for most men.

Postoperative care. Patients are instructed to wear a scrotal support to prevent excessive swelling and to check the surgical incision for signs and symptoms of bleeding or infection. Bacitracin ointment may be applied to the incision as directed, and the patient is advised to avoid lifting objects weighing more than 10 pounds for 3 to 4 weeks. Patients should increase their activity in a graded fashion, typically starting with a 5- to 10-minute walk, increasing to 30 minutes over the next 30 days.

Patient teaching highlights. Postoperative instruction focuses on the need for ongoing monitoring of prostate cancer and management of adverse effects of androgen deprivation. Chapter 8 provides a detailed description of the nursing management of hot flushes following surgical or medical androgen deprivation. See the following discussion of radical orchiectomy for care instructions following orchiectomy.

Radical Orchiectomy

A radical orchiectomy is the removal of one or both testes and high ligation of the spermatic cord, at the level of the internal ring. It is used to treat localized testicular cancer and assists with grading and staging of the tumor. The procedure is performed using general, spinal, or local anesthesia, with the patient supine. A 5- to 7-cm inguinal incision is made approximately 2 cm above the pubic tubercle. The incision may be extended onto the upper scrotum to facilitate removal of large tumors. Dissection extends to the level of the internal inguinal ring, with preservation of the ilioinguinal nerve. The spermatic cord, vas deferens, affected testis, and surrounding tunics are all removed. A testicular prosthesis may be inserted at the same time as the radical orchiectomy. Compressive dressings and scrotal support are used to minimize postoperative edema.

Complications. The most common complication is postoperative bleeding, which may occasionally result in a scrotal or retroperitoneal hematoma. Infection is rare. Scrotal edema is common and patients may be more comfortable with an athletic support. Support of the scrotum while the patient is in bed and intermittent use of ice packs, no more than 20 minutes at a time, will help with discomfort and swelling.

Preparation for surgery. Men with testicular cancer are usually young, between the ages of 15 and 35 years, and healthy, with few comorbid conditions. They should be counseled about banking sperm prior to treatment and should have a spouse or partner involved with this discussion whenever feasible. Support and encouragement to express concerns about body image and sexuality should begin preoperatively and continue throughout recovery.

Postoperative care. Postoperative care is similar to that for bilateral orchiectomy, but additional interventions may be necessary because of the more extensive dissection associated with radical orchiectomy and the need for spinal, regional, or general anesthesia. Particular care should be taken when monitoring the operative site for bleeding and the patient should be firmly counseled against attempts to increase activity before adequate wound healing can occur. Most importantly, the patient and his family will require support and open communication about pathology reports and further treatment of the testicular tumor.

Patient teaching highlights. The urologic nurse should provide opportunities for the patient to express feelings of anxiety and fear related to the suspicion of cancer and its treatment. The patient should be informed that testicular cancer and its treatment will impair sperm production, but that many men regain fertility following treatment. For cosmetic purposes, many men choose to have a testicular prosthesis placed. All male patients should be encouraged to do monthly testicular self-examination, and men with testicular cancer are especially counseled to examine the remaining (contralateral) testicle because of the increased risk for malignancy. The patient with testicular cancer is also advised about the importance of regularly attending follow-up appointments, particularly because late relapses can occur.[148]

Vasectomy

Vasectomy is the most commonly performed urologic surgery in the United States. It is used by almost 7% of couples in the United States and approximately 500,000 vasectomies are performed annually.[149] Evidence has suggested that vasectomy is equally popular in Canada, where the number of men undergoing the procedure increased by 39% during the 1980s, although the number of women undergoing tubal ligation declined by 28%.[150]

The procedure is performed on an outpatient basis using local anesthesia (Figure 11-19).[149] Initially, the right vas deferens is located in the hemiscrotum and brought just underneath the surface of the skin using the thumb, middle finger, and index finger. Lidocaine is injected to serve as a nerve block and the left vas deferens is located and anesthetized using similar maneuvers. Following mobilization, each vas deferens is held in place with a towel clip, fingers, or needle. A small 1-cm incision is typically made to expose each vas and a small segment incised and sent for tissue analysis. The segment may be clipped or cauterized or fascia interposed to prevent recannulization.[151] The incisions may be sutured or left open to reduce swelling and hematoma, depending on the surgeon's preference.

Several alternative or complementary maneuvers have been promulgated to reduce the pain associated with vasectomy or to reduce postoperative complications, such as scrotal hematoma. A no-scalpel approach gains access to the vas deferens through a tiny puncture hole in the scrotum rather than via the two small incisions created during traditional vasectomy.[152] Success of the procedure is greatly enhanced if it is performed in a warm room and efforts are made to relax the patient and scrotum. Advantages of the procedure include lower risks for postoperative infection, hematoma, and pain. A potential disadvantage is the need for greater training and skill. However, given adequate training, the procedure is quicker than traditional vasectomy.[149] The effectiveness of the no-scalpel technique versus traditional surgery has been evaluated in a randomized trial involving 1429 men seeking vasectomy; no difference in fertility outcomes was noted, but men randomized for the no-scalpel approach were found to have less pain and resumed intercourse sooner than those treated by the traditional approach.[153] A percutaneous vasectomy technique has also been described[154] using a ring lamp and blunt needle, and attempts have been made to incorporate laser energy or high-frequency ultrasound. Further research is required before the efficacy of percutaneous techniques can be clearly established. Several attempts have been made to develop reversible vasectomy procedures, but none has proved successful.

Complications. Hematoma and infection are the most common complications associated with vasectomy; their incidence varies from 1% to as high as

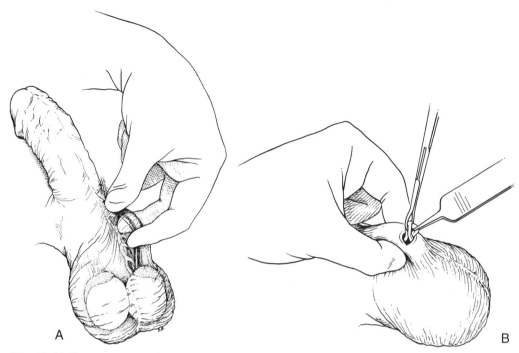

Fig. 11-19 Vasectomy. **A,** Each vas deferens is identified via palpation. **B,** Both vasa are clipped, cauterized, and/or fascia interposed to prevent recannulization. (From Walsh PC, Retik AB, Wein AJ, Vaughan ED [eds]: Campbell's Urology, 8th edition. Philadelphia: Saunders, 2002; p 1542.)

38%.[149] The incidence of both complications is reduced when performed by a highly experienced surgeon. Sperm granulomas occur in 10% to 30%, and a proportion of affected men may experience associated pain. Uncommon complications, affecting less than 1%, include chronic orchialgia and recannulization.[155]

Much attention and controversy have arisen from several studies that revealed a statistically significant correlation between vasectomy and long-term risk for prostate cancer[156,157] or cardiovascular disease.[158] Such observations have led to widespread speculation about a possible causal link between vasectomy and the risk for prostate cancer or heart attack, leading to evidence of some changes in urologic practice with regard to patient teaching and counseling about vasectomy.[159] However, several large and well-designed epidemiologic studies have found no evidence linking vasectomy with an increased risk for cardiovascular disease or prostate cancer.[158,160-162]

Preparation for surgery. A shave preparation of the scrotum is completed, and men are advised that injection of local anesthesia will occur underneath the scrotal skin. Some urologists recommend administering an anxiolytic such as diazepam to relax the patient and scrotum and minimize scrotal hematoma following the procedure.[149] Although reversal of a vasectomy is possible, men are counseled that the procedure should be considered permanent. Patients are further advised that no technique, short of resection of the entire vas deferens, is 100% effective for sterilization, and follow-up semen analyses are essential before resuming unprotected sexual intercourse.

Postoperative care. Men are taught to self-monitor the scrotum and small incisions. The incisions may be left open and fluff gauze dressings are placed in a snug-fitting athletic supporter following surgery. Dressings may be changed daily or every other day until the incisions heal. The open wounds are expected to seal themselves within about 4 days or less, and patients are advised to contact the urologist or urologic nurse if the wounds have not healed within this time frame or if significant drainage occurs.

Ice packs may be applied intermittently to the scrotal area for about 36 hours to reduce discomfort and swelling. An opioid analgesic will be used during the immediate postoperative period, but NSAIDs are usually adequate after the first 2 to 3 days.

Patient teaching highlights. Men are advised that they should avoid lifting heavy objects, such as those weighing more than 10 to 40 pounds, and to refrain from sexual activity for 1 to 2 weeks. The patient is advised that he can shower 36 hours after vasectomy, but should avoid scrubbing the scrotal skin. In addition to education about wound care and potential complications, patient teaching focuses on critical steps to ensure successful sterilization. Men undergoing vasectomy should be advised that follow-up semen analysis is critical to ensure the absence of sperm in the semen. This counseling is especially important because one retrospective study of 551 men who underwent vasectomy has found that 42% did not adhere to recommended follow-up schedules.[163] Advice about the optimal schedule for follow-up varies. Based on the urologist's judgment and clinical experience, men may be asked to provide a specimen as soon as 1 month following the procedure and not before the man has ejaculated at least 20 times to clear any residual sperm from the reproductive tract. Some patients will have absence of any sperm on this first sample, but many others will have a low number of sperm (often 1 or 2 sperm cells per high-powered field) that persists for a period of weeks to months. To ensure azoospermia following vasectomy, it is generally recommended that men have at least two specimens that are free from sperm when analyzed. When two specimens are found to be sperm-free, the chances of later recannulization and pregnancy are very low (0.6%).[164] Nevertheless, low sperm counts may persist for as long as 6 to 12 months, resulting in considerable frustration for the affected patient or couple. In contrast, if sperm counts rise during follow-up monitoring, recannulization is suspected and additional evaluation is warranted before the surgery can be considered successful.

SUMMARY

From the medical perspective, urology is a surgical specialty, and preoperative and postoperative management remain a central focus of urologic nursing practice. However, in contrast to the latter half of the twentieth century, management has increasingly moved from the inpatient unit in the acute care facility to the clinic, office, or ambulatory surgery center. As a result, urologic nursing management has shifted from providing direct care to teaching the patient and family to provide care in her or his home environment.

REFERENCES

1. Fagermone MS, Hamilton G: Preparing patients for urological surgery. International Journal of Nursing Studies, 2003; 40:281-90.
2. Hinman F Jr: Atlas of Urologic Surgery, 2nd edition. Philadelphia: Saunders, 1998.
3. Nelson CP, Wolf S: Comparison of hand-assisted versus standard laparoscopic radical nephrectomy for suspected renal cell carcinoma. Journal of Urology, 2002; 167(5):1989-94.
4. Eichel L, McDougall EM, Clayman RV: Basics of laparoscopic urologic surgery. In Wein AJ, Kavoussi LR, Novick AC, Partin AW, Peters CA (eds): Campbell-Walsh Urology, 9th edition. Philadelphia: Saunders, 2007; pp 171-220.
5. Manohar T, Desai M, Desai M: Laparoscopic nephrectomy for benign and inflammatory conditions. Journal of Endourology, 2007; 21(11):1323-8.
6. Novick AC: Open surgery of the kidney. In Wein AJ, Kavoussi LR, Novick AC, Partin AW, Peters CA (eds): Campbell-Walsh Urology. 9th edition. Philadelphia: Saunders, 2007; pp 1686-758.
7. Kaouk JH, Gill IS: Laparoscopic partial nephrectomy: a new horizon. Current Opinion in Urology, 2003; 13:215-9.
8. Lind MY, Ijzermans JNM, Bonjer HJ: Open vs laparoscopic donor nephrectomy in renal transplantation. International, 2002; 89:262-8.
9. Lowry PS, Nakada SY: Renal cryotherapy: 2003 clinical status. Current Opinion in Urology, 2003; 13:193-7.
10. Jones JS, Campbell SC: Non–muscle-invasive bladder cancer (Ta, T1, and CIS). In Wein AJ, Kavoussi LR, Novick AC, Partin AW, Peters CA (eds): Campbell-Walsh Urology, 9th edition. Philadelphia: Saunders, 2007; pp 2447-67.
11. Appell RA, Flynn JT, Paris AM, Blandy JP: Occult bacterial colonization of bladder tumors. Journal of Urology, 1980; 124(3):345-6.
12. Lytton B: Urinary infection in cystoscopy. British Medical Journal, 1961; 5251:547-9.
13. Pansadoro A, Franco G, Laurenti C, Pansadoro V: Conservative treatment of intraperitoneal bladder perforation during transurethral resection of bladder tumor. Urology, 2002; 60(4):682-4.
14. Kawakami M, Ishikawa M, Kontani K, Iijima K, Kobayashi S, Nishizawa O: Flexible video cystoscope with built-in high-frequency cauterizing element for transurethral resection of bladder tumor. International Journal of Urology, 2001; 8(12):713-4.
15. Chepurov AK, Nemenova AA: The complications of transurethral resection of the bladder for tumor. Urologiia i Nefrologiia, 1996; 2:21-3.
16. Kabalin JN: Complications of lasers in urologic surgery. In Taneja SS, Smith RB, Ehrlich R (eds): Complications of Urologic Surgery, 3rd edition. Philadelphia: Saunders, 2001; pp 257-67.
17. Nieh PT, Marshall FF: Surgery of bladder cancer. In Wein AJ, Kavoussi LR, Novick AC, Partin AW, Peters CA (eds): Campbell-Walsh Urology, 9th edition. Philadelphia: Saunders, 2007; pp 2479-2505.
18. Schoenberg MD, Gonzalgo ML: Management of invasive and metastatic bladder cancer. In Wein AJ, Kavoussi LR, Novick AC, Partin AW, Peters CA (eds): Campbell-Walsh Urology. 9th edition. Philadelphia: Saunders, 2007; pp 2468-78.
19. Montie JE: Against bladder sparing: surgery. Journal of Urology, 1999; 162(2):452-7.
20. Tomaselli N, McGinnis DE: Urinary diversions: surgical management. In Colwell JS, Goldberg MT, Carmel JE (eds): Fecal and Urinary Diversions: Management Principles. St Louis: Mosby, 2003; pp 184-204.
21. Michel K, deKernion JB: Urinary diversions and continent reservoirs. In Gillenwater JY, Grayhack JT, Howards SS, Mitchell ME

(eds): Adult and Pediatric Urology, 4th edition. Philadelphia: Lippincott, Williams & Wilkins, 2002; pp 1362-1400.

22. Link RE, Lerner SP: Rebuilding the lower urinary tract after cystectomy: a road map for patient selection and counseling. Seminars in Urology, 2001; 19(1):24-36.

23. Schmidt JD, Hawtrey CE, Flocks RH, Culp DA: Complications, results and problems of ileal conduit diversions. Journal of Urology, 1973; 109(2):210-6.

24. Yang WJ, Cho KS, Rha KH, et al: Long-term effects of ileal conduit urinary diversion on upper urinary tract in bladder cancer. Urology, 2006; 68(2):324-7.

25. Sullivan JW, Grabstald H, Whitmore WF Jr: Complications of ureteroileal conduit with radical cystectomy: review of 336 cases. Journal of Urology, 1980; 124(6):797-801.

26. Ide H, Kikuchi E, Shinoda K, Mukai M, Murai M: Carcinoma in situ developing in an ileal neobladder. Urology, 2007; 69(3):576.e9-11.

27. Bass EM, Del Pino A, Tan A, Pearl RK, Orsay CP, Abcarian H: Does preoperative stoma marking and education by the enterostomal therapist affect outcome? Diseases of the Colon and Rectum, 1997; 40(4):440-2.

28. Mitrofanoff P: Trans-appendicular continent cystostomy in the management of the neurogenic bladder. Chirurgie Pediatrique, 1980; 21(4):297-305.

29. Reidmiller H, Gerharz EW: Continent catheterizable reservoir made from colon. In Graham SD, Keane TE, Glenn JF (eds): Glenn's Urologic Surgery, 6th edition. Philadelphia: Lippincott Williams & Wilkins, 2004; pp 677-688.

30. Klimaszewski AD: Prospective study of metabolic abnormalities in patient with Kock pouch urinary diversion. Journal of Urology, 1989; 33:85-8.

31. Okada Y, Hamaguvhi A, Kageyama S, et al: Postoperative complications of self-catheterizable continent urinary diversions (Kock, Indiana and appendicial Mainz) and patient care. Acta Urologica Japonica, 1995; 41(11):947-52.

32. Wiesner C, Pahernik S, Stein R, et al: Long-term follow-up of submucosal tunnel and serosa-lined extramural tunnel ureter implantation in ileao caecal continent cutaneous urinary diversion (Mainz pouch I). British Journal of Urology International, 2007; 100(3):633-7.

33. Gray M, Cluff D, Johnson VY, Dixon L, Wasson D: Urinary diversions: perspectives on nursing care. Perspectives, 2000; 2:1-8.

34. Madersbacher S, Schmidt J, Eberle JM, Thoeny HC, Burkhard F, Hochreiter W, Studer UE: Long-term outcome of ileal conduit diversion. Journal of Urology, 2003; 169(3):985-90.

35. Turk TM, Koleski FC, Albala DM: Incidence of urolithiasis in cystectomy patients after intestinal conduit or continent urinary diversion. World Journal of Urology, 1999; 17(5):305-7.

36. Hautmann RE, Paiss T, de Petriconi R: The ileal neobladder in women: 9 years of experience with 18 patients. Journal of Urology, 1996; 155:76-81.

37. Koch MO, McDougal WS: Nicotinic acid: treatment for the hyperchloremic acidosis following urinary diversion through intestinal segments. Journal of Urology, 1985; 134(1):162-4.

38. Koch MO, McDougal WS: Chlorpromazine: adjuvant therapy for the metabolic derangements created by urinary diversion through the intestinal segments. Journal of Urology, 1985; 134(1):165-9.

39. Hautmann RE: Urinary diversion: ileal conduit to neobladder. Journal of Urology, 2003; 169(3):834-42.

40. Stein R, Fichtner J, Thuroff JW: Urinary diversion and reconstruction. Current Opinion in Urology, 2000; 10(5):391-5.

41. Carrion R, Arap S, Corcione G, Ferreyra U, Neyra Argote G, Cantor A, Seigne J, Lockhart J; Confederation of American Urology: A multi-institutional study of orthotopic neobladders: functional results in men and women. British Journal of Urology International, 2004; 93(6):803-6.

42. Gotoh K, Yamanaka N, Shimogaki H, et al: A urodynamic study on neobladder function. Japanese Journal of Urology, 1998; 89(12):939-48.

43. Park JM, Montie JE: Mechanisms of incontinence and retention after orthotopic neobladder diversion. Urology, 1998; 51(4):601-9.

44. Stoffel JT, Bresette JF, Smith JJ: Retropubic surgery for urinary incontinence. Urologic Clinics of North America, 2002; 29(3):585-96.

45. Walters MD, Daneshgari F: Surgical management of stress urinary incontinence. Clinical Obstetrics and Gynecology, 2004; 47(1):93-103.

46. Bergman A, Elia G: Three surgical procedures for genuine stress incontinence. Five-year follow-up of a randomized prospective study. American Journal of Obstetrics and Gynecology, 1976; 173(1):66-71.

47. Agarwala N, Liu CY: Minimally invasive management of urinary incontinence. Current Opinion Obstetrics Gynecology, 2002; 14:429-33.

48. Peryera AJ: A simplified surgical procedure for the correction of stress incontinence in women. Western Journal of Surgery, 1959; 67:223-6.

49. Bodell DM, Leach GE: Needle suspensions for female incontinence. Urologic Clinics of North America, 2002; 29(3):575-84.

50. Glazener CMA, Cooper K: Bladder neck needle suspension for urinary incontinence in women. Cochrane Database of Systematic Reviews, 2002; (2):CD003636.

51. Chapple CR. Retropubic suspension surgery for incontinence in women. In Wein AJ, Kavoussi LR, Novick AC, Partin AW, Peters CA (eds): Campbell-Walsh Urology, 9th edition. Philadelphia: Saunders, 2007; pp 2168-86.

52. Demirci F, Yildirim U, Demirci E, Ayas S, Arioglu P, Kuyumcuoglu U: Ten-year results of Marshall Marchetti Krantz and anterior colporrhaphy procedures. Australian and New Zealand Journal of Obstetrics and Gynecology, 2002; 42(5):513-4.

53. Nguyen JK: Current concepts in the diagnosis and surgical repair of anterior vaginal prolapse caused by paravaginal defects. Obstetrical and Gynecological Survey, 2001; 56(4):239-46.

54. Colombo M, Milani R, Vitobello D, Maggioni A: A randomized comparison of Burch colposuspension and abdominal paravaginal defect repair for female stress urinary incontinence. American Journal of Obstetrics and Gynecology, 1996; 175(1):78-84.

55. Kenton K, Oldham L, Brubaker L: Open Burch urethropexy has a low rate of perioperative complications. American Journal of Obstetrics and Gynecology, 2002; 187(1):107-10.

56. Paik JS, Cho MC, Oh SJ, Kim SW, Ku JH: Factors influencing the outcome of mid urethral sling procedures for female urinary incontinence. Journal of Urology, 2007; 178(3 Pt 1):985-9.

57. Kammerer-Doak DN, Cornella JL, Magrina JF, Stanhope CR, Smilack J: Osteitis pubis after Marshall-Marchetti-Krantz urethropexy: a pubic osteomyelitis. American Journal of Obstetrics and Gynecology, 1998; 179(3 Pt 1):586-90.

58. Langer R, Lipshitz Y, Halperin R, Pansky M, Bukovsky I, Sherman D: Prevention of genital prolapse following Burch colposuspension: comparison between two surgical procedures. International Urogynecology Journal, 2003; 14(1):13-6.

59. Leach GE, Dmochowski RR, Appell RA, Blaivas JG, Hadley HR, Luber KM, et al: Female stress urinary incontinence clinical guidelines panel summary report on surgical management of female stress urinary incontinence. Journal of Urology, 1997; 158:875-80.

60. Carbone JM, Kavaler E, Hu JC, Raz S: Pubovaginal sling using cadaveric fascia and bone anchors: disappointing early results. Journal of Urology, 2001; 165:1605-11.

61. Haab F, Trockman BA, Zimmern PE, Leach GEl: Results of pubovaginal sling for the treatment of intrinsic sphincteric deficiency determined by questionnaire analysis. Journal of Urology, 1997; 158:1738-41.

62. Morgan TO Jr, Westney OL, McGuire EJ: Pubovaginal sling: 4-year outcome analysis and quality of life assessment. Journal of Urology, 2000; 163:1845-8.

63. Jha S, Arunkalaivanan AS, Davis J: Surgical management of stress urinary incontinence: a questionnaire-based survey. European Urology, 2005; 47(5):648-52.

64. Falconer C, Ekman-Ordeberg G, Malmstrom A, Ulmsten U: Clinical outcome and changes in connective tissue metabolism after intravaginal slingplasty in stress incontinent women. International Urogynecology Journal of Pelvic Floor Dysfunction, 1996; 7:133.

65. Sander P, Lose G: Surgical options in the treatment of stress urinary incontinence in women. Minerva Ginelologia, 2007; 59(6):619-27.

66. Ward K, Hilton P; United Kingdom and Ireland Tension-free Vaginal Tape Trial Group: Prospective multicenter randomized trial of tension-free vaginal tape and colposuspension as primary treatment for stress incontinence. British Medical Journal, 2002; 325(7355):67-74.

67. Costa P, Delmas V: Trans-obturator-tape procedure—"inside out or outside in": current concepts and evidence base. Current Opinion in Urology, 2004; 14(6):313-15.

68. Delorme E: Transobturator urethral suspension: mini-invasive procedure in the treatment of stress urinary incontinence in women. Progres en Urologie, 2001; 11(6):1306-13.

69. Delorme E, Droupy S, de Tayrac R, Delmas V: Transobturator tape (Uratape). A new minimally invasive method in the treatment of urinary incontinence in women. Progres en Urologie, 2003; 13(4):656-9.

70. Costa P, Grise P, Droupy S, Monneins F, Assenmacher C, Ballanger P, Hermieu JF, Delmas V, Boccon-Gibod L, Ortuno C: Surgical treatment of female stress urinary incontinence with a trans-obturator-tape (T.O.T.) Uratape: short-term results of a prospective multicentric study. European Urology, 2004; 46(1):102-7.

71. Tamussino K, Hanzal E, Kölle D, et al: Transobturator tapes for stress urinary incontinence: Results of the Austrian registry. American Journal of Obstetrics and Gynecology, 2007; 197(6):634e1-5.

72. Schrepferman CG, Griebling TL, Nygaard IE, Kreder KJ: Resolution of urge symptoms following sling cystourethropexy. Journal of Urology, 2000; 164:1628-31.

73. Aundsen CL, Flynn BJ, Webster GD: Urethral erosion after synthetic and nonsynthetic pubovaginal slings: differences in management and continence outcome. Journal of Urology, 2003; 170:134-7.

74. Boublil V, Ciofu C, Traxer O, Sebe P, Haab F: Complications of urethral sling procedures. Current Opinion in Obstetrics and Gynecology, 2002; 14(5):515-20.

75. Rodriquez L, Blander DS, Raz S: New millennium, new slings. Current Urology Reports, 2001; 2:399-406.

76. Karram M: Surgical correction of genuine stress incontinence secondary to intrinsic urethral sphincter dysfunction. In Walters MD, Karram MM (eds): Clinical Urogynecology. St Louis: Mosby, 1993; pp 210-24.

77. Wilson TS, LeMack GE, Zimmern PE: Management of intrinsic sphincteric deficiency in women. Journal of Urology, 2003; 169:1662-9.

78. Dmochowski RR, Appell RA: Injectable agents in the treatment of stress incontinence in women: where are we now?. Urology, 2000; 56(6 Supp. 1):32-41.

79. Dalkin BL, Wessells H, Cui H: A national survey of urinary and health-related quality of life outcomes in men with an artificial urinary sphincter for post-radical prostatectomy incontinence. Journal of Urology, 2003; 169:237-9.

80. Gomha MA, Boone TB: Artificial sphincter for post prostatectomy incontinence in men who had prior radiotherapy: a risk and outcome analysis. Journal of Urology, 2002; 167:591-6.

81. Thomas K, Venn SN, Mundy AR: Outcome of the artificial urinary sphincter in female patients. Journal of Urology, 2002; 167:1720-2.

82. Herndon CD, Rink RC, Shaw MB, Simmons GR, Cain MP, Kaefer M, et al: The Indiana experience with artificial urinary sphincters in children and young adults. Journal of Urology, 2003; 169:650-4.

83. Venn SN, Greenwell TJ, Mundy AR: The long-term outcome of artificial urinary sphincters. Journal of Urology, 2000; 164(3 Pt 1):702-7.

84. Tse V, Stone AR: Incontinence after prostatectomy: the artificial urinary sphincter. British Journal of Urology International, 2003; 92(9):886-9.

85. Quallich SA, Ohl DA: Artificial urinary sphincter, part II: patient teaching and perioperative care. Urologic Nursing, 2003; 23(4):269-77.

86. Littlejohn JO Jr, Ghafar MA, Kang YM, Kaplan SA: Transurethral resection of the prostate: the new old standard. Current Opinion in Urology, 2002; 12(1):19-23.

87. Gray M, Allensworth D: Electrovaporization of the prostate: initial experiences and nursing management. Urologic Nursing, 1999; 19(1):25-32.

88. Chambers A: Transurethral resection syndrome—it does not have to be a mystery. AORN Journal, 2002; 75(1):156-70.

89. Porru D, Campus G, Caria A, Madeddu G, Cucchi A, Rovereto B, Scarpa RM, Pili P, Usai E: Impact of early pelvic floor rehabilitation after transurethral resection of the prostate. Neurourology and Urodynamics, 2001; 20:53-9.

90. Larson TR: Rationale and assessment of minimally invasive approaches to benign prostatic hyperplasia therapy. Urology, 2002; 59:12-6.

91. Djavan B, Seitz C, Ghawidel K, Basharkhad A, Bursa B, Hruby S: High-energy transurethral microwave thermotherapy in patients with acute urinary retention caused by benign prostatic hyperplasia. Urology, 1999; 54:18-22.

92. Zlotta AR, Djavan B: Minimally invasive therapies for benign prostatic hyperplasia in the new millennium: long-term data. Current Opinion in Urology, 2002; 12(1):7-14.

93. Ahmed M, Bell T, Lawrence WT, Ward JP, Watson GM: Transurethral microwave thermotherapy (Prostatron version 2.5) compared with transurethral resection of the prostate for the treatment of benign prostatic hyperplasia: a randomized, controlled, parallel study. British Journal of Urology, 1997; 79(2):181-5.

94. Parrott EK: TUNA of the prostate in an office setting: nursing implications. Urologic Nursing, 2003; 23:33-9.

95. Rosario DJ, Woo H, Potts KL, Cutinha PE, Hastie KJ, Chapple CR: Safety and efficacy of transurethral needle ablation of the prostate for symptomatic outlet obstruction. British Journal of Urology, 1997; 80(4):579-86.

96. Zlotta AR, Giannakopoulos X, Maehlum O, Ostrem T, Schulman CC: Long-term evaluation of transurethral needle ablation of the prostate (TUNA) for treatment of symptomatic benign prostate hyperplasia: clinical outcome up to five years from three centers. European Urology, 2003; 44:89-93.

97. Hill B, Belville W, Bruskewitz R, Issa M, Perez-Marrero R, Roehrborn C, Terris M, Naslund M: Transurethral needle ablation versus transurethral resection of the prostate for the treatment of symptomatic benign prostatic hyperplasia: 5-year results of a prospective, randomized, multicenter clinical trial. Journal of Urology, 2003; 171(6 Pt 1):2336-40.

98. Aaltomaa S, Ala-Opas M: The effect of transurethral needle ablation on symptoms of chronic pelvic pain syndrome—a pilot study. Scandinavian Journal of Urology and Nephrology, 2001; 35(2):127-31.

99. Mynderse LA, Larson TR: Transurethral hot water balloon thermotherapy for benign prostatic hypertrophy. Current Urology, 2003; 4:287-91.

100. Muschter R: Conductive heat: hot water–induced thermotherapy for ablation of prostatic tissue. Journal of Endourology, 2003; 17(8):609-16.

101. Breda G, Isgro A: Treatment of benign prostatic hyperplasia with water-induced thermotherapy: experience of a single institution. Journal of Endourology, 2002; 16(2):123-6.

102. Schatzl G, Madersbacher S, Djavan B, Lang T, Marberger M: Two-year results of transurethral resection of the prostate versus four 'less invasive' treatment options. European Urology, 2000; 37(6):695-701.

103. Madersbacher S, Schatzl G, Djavan B, Stulnig T, Marberger M: Long-term outcome of transrectal high-intensity focused

ultrasound therapy for benign prostatic hyperplasia. European Urology, 2000; 37(6):687-94.

104. Murat FJ, Poissonnier L, Pasticier G, Gelet A: High-intensity focused ultrasound (HIFU) for prostate cancer. Cancer Control, 2007; 14(3):244-9.

105. Uchida T, Sanghvi NT, Gardner TA, Koch MO, Ishii D, Minei S, et al: Transrectal high-intensity ultrasound for treatment of patients with stage T1b-2N0M0 localized prostate cancer: a preliminary report. Urology, 2002; 59:394-8.

106. Te AE, Malloy TR, Stein BS, Ulchaker JC, Nseyo UO, Hai MA, Malek RS: Photoselective vaporization of the prostate for the treatment of benign prostatic hyperplasia: 12-month results from the first United States multicenter prospective trial. Journal of Urology, 2004; 172(4 Pt 1):1404-8.

107. Maheshwari PN, Shah HN: In-situ holmium laser lithotripsy for impacted urethral calculi. Journal of Endourology, 2005; 19(8):1009-11.

108. Gupta N, Sivaramakrishna, Kumar R, Dogra PN, Seth A: Comparison of standard transurethral resection, transurethral vapour resection and holmium laser enucleation of the prostate for managing benign prostatic hyperplasia of >40 g. British Journal of Urology International, 2006; 97(1):85-9.

109. Aho TF, Gilling PJ, Kennett KM, Westenberg AM, Fraundorfer MR, Frampton CM: Holmium laser bladder neck incision versus holmium enucleation of the prostate as outpatient procedures for prostates less than 40 grams: a randomized trial. Journal of Urology, 2005; 174(1):210-4.

110. Elzayat EA, Habib EI, Elhilali MM: Holmium laser enucleation of the prostate: a size-independent new "gold standard." Urology, 2005; 66(Suppl 5):108-13.

111. Matlaga BR, Kim SC, Kuo RL, Watkins SL, Lingeman JE: Holmium laser enucleation of the prostate for prostates of >125 mL. British Journal of Urology International, 2006; 97(1):81-4.

112. Shah HN, Kausik V, Hegde S, Shah JN, Bansal MB: Evaluation of fluid absorption during holmium laser enucleation of prostate by breath ethanol technique. Journal of Urology, 2006; 175(2):537-40.

113. Bachmann A, Schurch L, Ruszat R, Wyler SF, Seifert HH, Muller A, Lehmann K, Sulser T: Photoselective vaporization (PVP) versus transurethral resection of the prostate (TURP): a prospective bi-centre study of perioperative morbidity and early functional outcome. European Urology, 2005; 48(6):965-72.

114. Bachmann A, Ruszat R, Wyler S, Reich O, Seifert HH, Muller A, Sulser T: Photoselective vaporization of the prostate: the Basel experience after 108 procedures. European Urology, 2005; 47(6):798-804.

115. Sarica K, Alkan E, Luleci H, Tasci AI: Photoselective vaporization of the enlarged prostate with KTP laser: long-term results in 240 patients. Journal of EndoUrology, 2005; 19(10):1199-1202.

116. Han M, Partin AW: Retropubic and suprapubic open prostatectomy. In Wein AJ, Kavoussi LR, Novick AC, Partin AW, Peters CA (eds): Campbell-Walsh Urology, 9th edition. Philadelphia: Saunders, 2007; pp 2845-53.

117. Selli C, De Antoni P, Moro U, Macchiarella A, Giannarini G, Crisci A: Role of bladder neck preservation in urinary continence following radical retropubic prostatectomy. Scandinavian Journal of Urology and Nephrology, 2004; 38(1):32-7.

118. Maffezzini M, Seveso M, Taverna G, Giusti G, Benetti A, Graziotti P: Evaluation of complications and results in a contemporary series of 300 consecutive radical retropubic prostatectomies with the anatomic approach at a single institution. Urology, 2003; 61(5):982-6.

119. Lepor H, Kaci L: Contemporary evaluation of operative parameters and complications related to open radical retropubic prostatectomy. Urology, 2003; 62(4):702-6.

120. Ichioka K, Yoshimura K, Utsunomiya N, Ueda N, Matsui Y, Terai A, Arai Y: High incidence of inguinal hernia after radical retropubic prostatectomy. Urology, 2004; 63(2):278-81.

121. Hunter KF, Moore KN. Glazener CMA: Conservative management for postprostatectomy urinary incontinence. Cochrane Database of Systematic Reviews, 1999; (4):CD001843.

122. Burgio KL, Goode PS, Urban DA, Umlauf MG, Locher JL, Bueschen A, Redden DT: Preoperative biofeedback assisted behavioral training to decrease post-prostatectomy incontinence: a randomized, controlled trial. Journal of Urology, 2006; 175(1):196-201.

123. Lepor H, Nieder AM, Fraiman MC: Early removal of urinary catheter after radical retropubic prostatectomy is both feasible and desirable. Urology, 2001; 58:425-9.

124. Scolieri MJ, Resnick MI: The technique of radical perineal prostatectomy. Urologic Clinics of North America, 2001; 28:521-33.

125. Gray M, Petroni GR, Theodorescu D: Urinary function following radical prostatectomy: a comparison of the retropubic and perineal approaches. Urology, 1999; 53:881-90.

126. Montorsi F, Guazzoni G, Strambi LF, Da Pozzo LF, Nava L, Barbieri L, et al: Recovery of spontaneous erectile function after nerve-sparing radical retropubic prostatectomy with and without early intracavernous injections of alprostadil: results of a prospective, randomized trial. Journal of Urology, 1997; 158:1408-10.

127. Guillonneau B, Vallancien G: Laparoscopic radical prostatectomy: the Montsouris technique. Journal of Urology, 2000; 163(6):1643-9.

128. Gill IS, Zippe CD: Laparoscopic radical prostatectomy: technique. Urologic Clinics of North America, 2001; 28(2):423-36.

129. Turk I, Deger S, Winkelmann B, Schonberger B, Loening SA: Laparoscopic radical prostatectomy. Technical aspects and experience with 125 cases. European Urology, 2001; 40(1):46-53.

130. Guillonneau B, Vallancien G: Laparoscopic radical prostatectomy: the Montsouris experience. Journal of Urology, 2000; 163(2):418-22.

131. Rassweiler J, Seemann O, Hatzinger M, Schulze M, Frede T: Technical evolution of laparoscopic radical prostatectomy after 450 cases. Journal of EndoUrology, 2003; 17(3):143-54.

132. Hemal AK, Manon M: Robotics in urology. Current Opinion in Urology, 2004; 14:89-93.

133. Tewari A, El-Hakim A, Leung RA: Robotic prostatectomy: a pooled analysis of published literature. Expert Review of Anticancer Therapy, 2006; 6(1):11-20.

134. Hu JC, Nelson RA, Wilson TG, Kawachi MH, Ramin SA, Lau C, Crocitto LE: Perioperative complications of laparoscopic and robotic-assisted laparoscopic radical prostatectomy. Journal of Urology, 2006; 175(2):541-6.

135. Jacobsen NE, Moore KN, Estey E, Voaklander D: Open versus laparoscopic radical prostatectomy: a prospective comparison of postoperative urinary incontinence rates. Journal of Urology, 2007; 177(2):615-619 http://www.ncbi.nlm.nih.gov/entrez/utils/fref.fcgi?itool=AbstractPlus-def&PrId=3048&uid=17222646&db=pubmed&url=http://linkinghub.elsevier.com/retrieve/pii/S0022-5347(06)02519-5

136. Van Appledorn S, Bouchier-Hayes D, Agarwal D, Costello AJ: Robotic laparoscopic radical prostatectomy: setup and procedural techniques after 150 cases. Urology, 2006; 67(2):364-7.

137. Melman A, Boczko J, Figueroa J, Leung AC: Critical surgical technique for radical perineal prostatectomy. Journal of Urology, 2004; 171(2):786-90.

138. Sullivan LD, Rabbani F: Should we reconsider the indications for ileo-obturator node dissection with localized prostate cancer? British Journal of Urology, 1995; 75:33-7.

139. Bluestein DL, Bostwick DG, Bergstralh EJ, Oesterling JE: Eliminating the need for bilateral pelvic lymphadenectomy in select patients with prostate cancer. Journal of Urology, 1994; 151:1315-20.

140. Narayan P, Fournier G, Gajendran V, Leidich R, Lo R, Wolf Jr JS, et al: Utility of preoperative serum prostate-specific antigen concentration and biopsy Gleason score in predicting risk of pelvic lymph node metastases in prostate cancer. Urology, 1994; 44:519-24.

141. Polascik TJ, Nosnik I, Mayes JM, Mouraviev V: Short-term cancer control after primary cryosurgical ablation for clinically localized

prostate cancer using third-generation cryotechnology. Urology, 2007; 70(1):117-21.

142. Onik GM, Cohen JK, Reyes GD, Rubinsky B, Chang Z, Baust J: Transrectal ultrasound-guided percutaneous radical cryosurgical ablation of the prostate. Cancer, 1993; 72:1291-9.

143. Hubosky SG, Fabrizio MD, Schellhammer PF, Barone BB, Tepera CM, Given RW: Single center experience with third-generation cryosurgery for management of organ-confined prostate cancer: Critical evaluation of short-term outcomes, complications, and patient quality of life. Journal of EndoUrology, 2007; 21(12): 1521-31.

144. Lam JS, Pisters LL, Belldegrun AS: Cryotherapy for prostate cancer. In Wein AJ, Kavoussi LR, Novick AC, Partin AW, Peters CA (eds): Campbell-Walsh Urology, 9th edition. Philadelphia: Saunders, 2007; pp 3032-52.

145. Kozlowski JM, Grayhack JT: Carcinoma of the prostate. In Gillenwater JY, Grayhack JT, Howards SS, Mitchell ME (eds): Adult and Pediatric Urology, 4th edition. Philadelphia: Lippincott Williams & Wilkins, 2002; pp 1417-1564.

146. Lucas MD, Strijdom SC, Berk M, Hart GA: Quality of life, sexual functioning and sex role identity after surgical orchidectomy in patients with prostatic cancer. Scandinavian Journal of Urology and Nephrology, 1995; 29(4):497-500.

147. Gomella LG. Contemporary use of hormonal therapy in prostate cancer: Managing complications and addressing quality-of-life issues. British Journal of Urology International, 2007; 99 Suppl 1:25-29; discussion 30.

148. Pottek TS, Dieckmann KP: Aftercare in testicular cancer is worthwhile. Recurrences are curable. Urologe, 2005; 44(9):1024-30.

149. Sandlow JI, Winfield HN, Goldstein M: Surgery of the scrotum and seminal vesicles. In Wein AJ, Kavoussi LR, Novick AC, Partin AW, Peters CA (eds): Campbell-Walsh Urology, 9th edition. Philadelphia: Saunders, 2007; pp 1098-1127.

150. Alderman PM, Gee EM: Sterilization: Canadian choices. CMAJ Canadian Medical Association Journal, 1989; 140(6):645-9.

151. Labrecque M, Nazerali H, Mondor M, Fortin V, Nasution M: Effectiveness and complications associated with 2 vasectomy techniques. Journal of Urology, 2002; 168(6):2495-8.

152. Li S: Ligation of vas deferens by clamping method under direct vision. Chinese Medical Journal, 1976; 4:213-4.

153. Sokal D, McMullen S, Gates D, Dominik R: A comparative study of the no-scalpel and standard incision approaches to vasectomy in 5 countries. Journal of Urology, 1999; 162(5):1621-25.

154. Li S: Percutaneous injection of vas deferens. Chinese Journal of Urology, 1980; 1:193-8.

155. Preston JM: Vasectomy: common medicolegal pitfalls. British Journal of Urology International, 2000; 86(3):339-43.

156. Emard JF, Drouin G, Thouez JP, Ghadirian P: Vasectomy and prostate cancer in Quebec, Canada. Health and Place, 2001; 7(2):131-9.

157. Mo ZN, Huang X, Zhang SC, Yang JR: Early and late long-term effects of vasectomy on serum testosterone, dihydrotestosterone, luteinizing hormone and follicle-stimulating hormone levels. Journal of Urology, 1995; 154(6):2065-9.

158. Goldacre MJ, Wotton CJ, Seagroatt V, Yeates D: Cancer and cardiovascular disease after vasectomy: an epidemiological database study. Fertility and Sterility, 2005; 84(5):1438-43.

159. Sandlow JI, Kreder KJ: A change in practice: current urologic practice in response to reports concerning vasectomy and prostate cancer. Fertility and Sterility, 1996; 66(2):281-4.

160. Dennis LK, Dawson DV, Resnick MI: Vasectomy and the risk of prostate cancer: a meta-analysis examining vasectomy status, age at vasectomy, and time since vasectomy. Prostate Cancer and Prostatic Diseases, 2002; 5(3):193-203.

161. Cox B, Sneyd MJ, Paul C, Delahunt B, Skegg DC: Vasectomy and risk of prostate cancer. Journal of the Amercian Medicall Association, 2002; 287(23):3110-5.

162. Chacko JA, Zafar MB, McCallum SW, Terris MK: Vasectomy and prostate cancer characteristics of patients referred for prostate biopsy. Journal of Urology, 2002; 168(4 Pt 1):1408-11.

163. Christensen RE, Maples DC Jr: Postvasectomy semen analysis: are men following up? Journal of the American Board of Family Practice, 2005; 18:44-7.

164. Haldar N, Cranston D, Turner E, MacKenzie I, Guillebaud J: How reliable is vasectomy? Long-term follow-up of vasectomised men. Lancet, 2000; 356:43-4.

165. Girard N: Preoperative assessment. Nurse Practitioner Forum, 1997; 8(4):140-6.

166. McDougal WS: Perioperative care. In Gillenwater JY, Grayhack JT, Howards SS, Mitchell ME (eds): Adult and Pediatric Urology, 4th edition. Philadelphia: Lippincott, Williams & Wilkins, 2002; pp 449-78.

CHAPTER 12

Congenital Anomalies of the Genitourinary System

The term *congenital anomaly* describes various defects affecting embryonic development.[1] Malformations are defects of organogenesis; they represent abnormal development of an organ caused by environmental or genetic factors. Deformities occur when mechanical factors remold the architecture of an organ. They are clinically relevant when they compromise function or further growth and development of the affected organ. A disruption such as a fistula affects a fully developed organ and can also be caused by environmental or genetic factors. Because of the complexities of embryogenesis, genitourinary system organs are frequently the sites of malformations, deformities, or disruptions. The overall incidence of urinary tract anomalies is approximately 5%. The kidneys are most commonly affected, accounting for 45% of these defects, the ureters account for 29%, the renal

vessels 12%, the urethra 5%, the bladder 4%, and fistulae 3%.[2]

Congenital anomalies are often encountered by urologic nurses caring for pediatric and adult patients. Although these defects influence urologic management, they may not comprise the primary complaint or disorder leading the individual to seek care. This chapter will review the causes and pathophysiology of anomalies affecting the urinary and reproductive systems, their diagnosis, and primary management or possible influence on other urologic procedures or disorders. Refer to the box, Clinical Highlights for Advanced and Expert Practice: Signs and Symptoms in the Neonate Indicating the Need for an Urgent Urologic Evaluation, for a review of urologic conditions encountered during newborn examination that represent a urologic emergency.

Clinical Highlights for Advanced and Expert Practice: Signs and Symptoms in the Neonate Indicating the Need for an Urgent Urologic Evaluation

Background
In addition to congenital defects, the urologic nurse or nurse practitioner is often queried about signs and symptoms seen in the neonate that may or may not indicate an underlying genitourinary disorder. This clinical highlights box will focus on physical signs or symptoms that indicate a possible urologic disorder demanding prompt assessment and urgent intervention.

Abdominal Mass
An abdominal mass is the most common finding on newborn examination indicating the need for prompt urologic evaluation. About 50% of all abdominal masses are of renal origin, 83% involve the genitourinary system, and only 17% originate in the gastrointestinal tract. Common urologic conditions leading to an abdominal mass include the following:
- Hydronephrosis
- Polycystic or multicystic kidney
- Renal vein thrombosis
- Bladder enlargement with ureterohydronephrosis caused by urethral valves in male neonates
- Solid tumor (uncommon)

Nonurologic explanations for abdominal mass include the following:
- Liver cyst
- Gastrointestinal system congenital anomalies
- Volvulus of the ileum

Continued

Clinical Highlights for Advanced and Expert Practice: Signs and Symptoms in the Neonate Indicating the Need for an Urgent Urologic Evaluation–cont'd

Evaluation
A kidney, ureter, and bladder (KUB) study is performed to define basic landmarks. Abdominal ultrasound is typically done first to define the size, architecture, and character of the mass. A radionuclide scan (DTPA or MAG3) is obtained if the mass is determined to be renal in origin; intravenous urography is not usually performed because of the neonate's inability to concentrate and excrete contrast media and the associated risk of nephrotoxicity (see Chapter 4). If hydronephrosis is diagnosed, a voiding cystourethrogram (VCUG) is obtained to diagnose bladder outlet obstruction or vesicoureteral reflux.

Nursing Management
The presence of any abnormality on neonatal physical examination causes intense anxiety in the entire family. The nurse can assist the parents by providing an explanation of each procedure and its purpose and by ensuring communication between the family and various specialty practice physicians involved in the neonate's care. In addition, parents can be provided with basic statistics concerning the possible causes of an abdominal mass in a neonate. This information is particularly reassuring to the parent who equates the presence of an abdominal mass with a malignancy in an adult.

Hematuria
Hematuria in the neonate is rare, but is a clinically sign that demands prompt evaluation. Renal vein thrombosis accounts for approximately 20% of all cases of hematuria; the second leading cause is renal artery thrombosis, either spontaneous or caused by umbilical artery catheter use. Unlike in the adult urologic patient, however, it is not commonly associated with a malignant tumor. Common causes of hematuria in the newborn include the following:
- Renal vein thrombosis
- Renal artery thrombosis
- Polycystic kidney disease
- Medullary sponge kidney
- Urinary calculus
- Obstruction of the urinary tract (particularly urethral polyps)

Nonurologic conditions associated with hematuria are particularly uncommon. Possible causes include the following:
- Adrenal hemorrhage
- Endocarditis
- Iatrogenic (e.g., associated with use of umbilical artery catheters)

Thrombosis of the renal vein or artery constitutes a true emergency that may threaten the life of the neonate, particularly if it affects both kidneys. It may be diagnosed on prenatal ultrasound or detected on newborn examination. Approximately 65% of cases occur during the first 2 weeks of life and 20% of all cases are bilateral. Risk factors include any disorder that predisposes the neonate to dehydration and thrombotic events, including polycythemia, trauma, infection, or dehydration caused by gestational or established diabetes mellitus in the mother.

Renal artery thrombosis usually occurs in neonates who require catheterization of the umbilical artery for monitoring purposes, particularly if the tip of the catheter is placed above spinal segment L1. Other risk factors include trauma during arterial catheterization, injection of hyperosmotic solutions via the catheter, sepsis, and infection.

Adrenal hemorrhage, a nonurologic cause of hematuria in the neonate, is a rare condition thought to arise from a sudden increase in inferior vena cava pressure that is transmitted to the adrenal veins, leading to intimal rupture and bleeding. Risk factors include prolonged labor and delivery, traumatic delivery, and resuscitation efforts in the infant with pulmonary compromise.

Evaluation
The infant with hematuria is rapidly assessed for breathing, cardiovascular function, and hydration status. Clinical manifestations associated with renal vein thrombosis include low blood pressure and signs of shock and sepsis. The kidney is enlarged and may be easily palpated; laboratory analysis of the serum will reveal anemia, thrombocytopenia, and azotemia. Urinalysis will reveal hematuria and proteinuria. Ultrasonography can be used to image the thrombosis as an enlargement of the contralateral kidney. Absent renal function of the affected kidney is revealed on a radionuclide study.

Clinical Highlights for Advanced and Expert Practice: Signs and Symptoms in the Neonate Indicating the Need for an Urgent Urologic Evaluation–cont'd

Renal artery stenosis produces edema and signs of congestive heart failure, often with ischemia of the lower extremities. Urinalysis reveals hematuria and proteinuria and blood studies demonstrate an elevated creatinine level. Unlike the child with renal vein thrombosis, the blood pressure remains elevated.

Adrenal hemorrhage causes severe blood loss, leading to unilateral or bilateral flank masses, pallor, and lethargy or hypovolemic shock. Unlike the gross hematuria characteristically seen with thrombosis of the renal veins or artery, adrenal hemorrhage usually produces microscopic hematuria only; ultrasonography is performed to confirm the diagnosis.

Nursing Management

When faced with a child with hematuria, the urologic nurse recommends immediate referral and urgent care. The acutely ill child with hematuria requires hospitalization and management of blood loss, dehydration, congestive heart failure, infection, and/or acute renal insufficiency. Heparin therapy is indicated for the management of renal vein thrombosis, typically administered over a period of 2 weeks. Renal artery thrombosis requires critical care to reverse hypertension, congestive heart failure, and renal ischemia; surgical revascularization is indicated in some cases. Alternatively, aggressive medical therapy using intraarterial thrombolytic agents is preferred for certain cases. Aggressive medical therapy is also indicated for the patient with adrenal hemorrhage, including blood transfusion and fluid support and antimicrobial therapy when indicated. Adrenal hemorrhage is usually self-limiting, but surgery is occasionally necessary when blood loss is severe and not adequately controlled by aggressive medical treatment.

Abnormal Micturition

Oliguria, anuria, or a dribbling urinary stream in the neonate may indicate a urologic emergency. The vast majority of neonates void within hours of their birth and a delay in micturition for more than 24 hours is a clear indication of inability to urinate or lack of urine production by the kidneys. Common causes of abnormal micturition in the neonate include the following:

- Bilateral renal agenesis (Potter's syndrome)
- Bilateral renal artery or renal vein thrombosis
- Urethral valves or polyps
- Adverse effect of magnesium sulfate or ritodrine administered to mother

Potter's syndrome causes anuria and leads to rapid death. Bilateral renal artery or vein thrombosis acutely compromises renal function, resulting in oliguria. Urethral valves or polyps cause bladder outlet obstruction. Polyps are more likely to be associated with hematuria than urethral valves. Medications such as magnesium sulfate or ritodrine exert an anticholinergic effect that may transiently compromise detrusor contraction strength, leading to bladder overdistention and absent or dribbling micturition, despite the presence of a large volume of urine in the bladder.

Evaluation

Physical examination may reveal the presence of an abdominal mass with hydronephrosis or distention of the bladder with urinary retention. Ultrasonography can identify or exclude hydronephrosis, the presence of a thrombosis in a major renal vessel, or bladder overdistention. Radionuclide studies may be indicated when renal function is compromised.

Nursing Management

Refer to discussions in this chapter on the management of bilateral renal agenesis, urethral valves, or polyps. The management of renal vein or artery thrombosis is discussed in this clinical highlights box. Transient urinary retention caused by a medication is managed by a temporary indwelling catheter. Parents are reassured that the catheter is expected to remain in place for only a brief period, until the effects of the medication subside.

Scrotal Mass

A firm scrotal mass is assumed to be torsion of the testes in the newborn until proven otherwise. Additional causes of a scrotal mass include the following:

- Teratoma
- Yolk sac tumors

Continued

Clinical Highlights for Advanced and Expert Practice: Signs and Symptoms in the Neonate Indicating the Need for an Urgent Urologic Evaluation–cont'd

- Gonadal stroma tumors
- Incarcerated inguinal hernia

Evaluation
Careful palpation and transillumination of the scrotum are completed to determine the likely origin of the mass and any connection to the inguinal canal.

Nursing Management
Urgent referral to a pediatric surgeon or pediatric urologist is indicated whenever a scrotal mass is detected in a neonate. Because of the risk of torsion, initial evaluation should occur within a matter of hours of discovery of the mass.

ANOMALIES OF THE KIDNEYS

Renal anomalies include defects of renal growth, position, and internal architecture. Defects of renal number include absence of one or both kidneys (agenesis) or accessory (supernumerary) kidneys.

Bilateral Renal Agenesis

Renal agenesis is defined as an absence of one or both kidneys; it is postulated to arise from an abnormal interaction between the metanephric cap and ureteric bud.[3,4] Bilateral renal agenesis (Potter's syndrome) occurs in approximately 1 in 4000 to 5000 births and is associated with characteristic facial and body features caused by oligohydramnios (paucity of amniotic fluid), renal insufficiency, and pulmonary hypoplasia. The causes of bilateral renal agenesis are unknown. At least some cases of Potter's syndrome are thought to arise from an obstructive uropathy occurring very early during embryogenesis and preventing development of either kidney.[5] As a result, amniotic fluid production is severely curtailed, leading to insufficient space within the uterus for normal embryogenesis. This causes facial deformities, pulmonary hypoplasia, and a low-birth-weight fetus. Additional factors associated with an increased risk of bilateral renal agenesis include administration of methimazole, a drug used to treat hyperthyroidism, during early pregnancy[6]; cystic adenomatoid malformation of the lung[7]; an autosomal dominant genetic defect seen in certain families[8]; esophageal atresia[9]; and maternal cocaine abuse.[10] Spontaneous preterm abortion is not unusual in patients with Potter's syndrome, and death occurs rapidly among those who survive to term, usually within 24 hours.

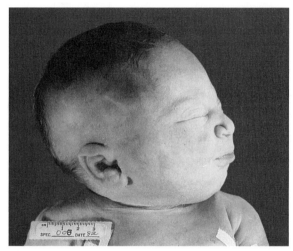

Fig. 12-1 Potter's facies, demonstrating flattening of the nose and low-set ears. (From Carlson B: Human Embryology and Developmental Biology, 3rd edition. St Louis: Mosby, 2005; p 403.)

Assessment. Potter's syndrome is usually diagnosed on prenatal ultrasound.[11,12] In addition to absence of the kidneys, oligohydramnios and pulmonary hypoplasia are characteristic of Potter's syndrome. Infants who are delivered have facial deformities that are caused by crowding in the oligohydramniotic uterine environment. These include flattening of the nose, low-set compressed ears, inner canthal skin folds, and thickened fingers (Figure 12-1).

Nursing Management. Because many fetuses with Potter's syndrome die in utero or rapidly following birth, urologic nurses do not commonly encounter this devastating congenital anomaly. Nursing care of a mother who gives birth to an infant with Potter's syndrome focuses on counseling about bilateral renal agenesis and anticipatory grieving.

Unilateral Renal Agenesis

Unilateral renal agenesis is more common than bilateral absence, occurring in approximately 1 in every 1000 to 1500 births.[4] Male infants are at a slightly higher risk compared with female infants (ratio, 1.8:1). Unilateral renal agenesis does not compromise growth and development, and it may be diagnosed only as an incidental finding. Although the term *unilateral agenesis* is defined as absence of a kidney, clinical experience reveals that many persons who appear to have absence of one kidney actually have a defect in renal development, causing multicystic renal dysplasia and hypoplasia. This distinction is important, particularly if the malformed kidney retains sufficient dysplastic parenchyma to contribute to hypertension or when it is susceptible to infection.

Fortunately for the infant with unilateral agenesis, the contralateral kidney is able to counterbalance the absence of its partner. This process, called compensatory hypertrophy, begins as early as week 22 of embryonic development. It is characterized by hyperplasia of the parenchyma, resulting in a larger kidney with functional abilities and reserve comparable to those of persons with paired kidneys.[13] Although the remaining kidney tends to be large and robust in function, it does not contain more nephrons than those found in a person with paired kidneys. Some research has suggested that a solitary kidney may be at greater risk for disease and mortality, but more recent data have shown that the life expectancy of those with a solitary kidney is no different than that of persons with paired kidneys.[4] Nevertheless, these persons do have an increased risk of proteinuria, hypertension, and renal insufficiency as compared with age-matched persons with paired kidneys.[14]

Assessment. Unilateral renal agenesis is typically identified during the routine evaluation of patients with defects of the external genitalia or an internal organ system or bothersome urologic symptoms, such as recurring urinary tract infections or intermittent flank pain. It may present as an incidental finding in a woman undergoing evaluation for menstrual difficulties or an abdominal mass. Multiple imaging studies can detect absence of a kidney, including intravenous pyelography (IVP), renal or abdominal ultrasound, abdominal computed tomography (CT), or magnetic resonance imaging (MRI).

Differentiation of unilateral agenesis from a small dysplastic or multicystic kidney relies on a radionuclide study capable of detecting functioning parenchyma, such as a ^{99m}Tc-mercaptoacetyltriglycine (MAG3) or diethylenetriaminepentaacetic acid (DTPA) study. The purpose of a radionuclide scan is to identify any residual parenchyma and its potential to cause hypertension, proteinuria, or urinary infection. It also allows the clinician to determine whether absence of the kidney in the retroperitoneal space coincides with the presence of a hypoplastic kidney in the pelvis. A radionuclide study is justified whenever unilateral renal agenesis is discovered in the course of an evaluation for urologic or nephrologic disorders, including assessment of genitourinary anomalies. A radionuclide study, or any further imaging, may not be indicated if agenesis is found on a CT or MRI scan in an adult patient without urologic symptoms or hypertension.

A diagnosis of unilateral renal agenesis in a child justifies further investigation to rule out additional congenital anomalies. Additional urinary system anomalies are found in up to 48% of patients with a solitary kidney.[15,16] The most common urinary defect is vesicoureteral reflux affecting the remaining kidney; other common anomalies include ureterovesical and ureteropelvic junction (UPJ) obstruction. Congenital anomalies affecting organs outside the urinary system occur in 25% of cases.[4] The cardiovascular, gastrointestinal, and skeletal systems are most commonly involved. Children with unilateral renal agenesis are also at increased risk for genital system anomalies. Girls are particularly susceptible and tend to have defects arising from incomplete or nonunion of the müllerian ducts, leading to defects of the vagina and uterus. Boys may have a cryptorchid testis, hypospadias, or defects of the vas deferens, seminal vesicles, or prostate.

Nursing Management. Unilateral renal agenesis is frequently encountered as an incidental finding in a patient with multisystem congenital defects or as part of a urologic disorder, such as vesicoureteral reflux or ureterovesical junction obstruction.[4] When encountered in a child, patient and family education includes an explanation of compensatory hypertrophy and reassurance that the remaining kidney is adequate for a normal life. Nevertheless, education must also include the significance of ensuring that the function of the remaining kidney is preserved. Several strategies have been advocated for the preservation of solitary kidney function. Restriction of contact sports seeks to minimize the risk of renal trauma associated with blunt force flank or abdominal injuries. A range of advice may be offered, including avoidance of all contact sports, engaging in sports only with padding designed to reduce blunt force trauma to the flank or abdomen, or no restrictions. However, because there is inadequate evidence to support or refute whether restricting contact sports is protective of a solitary kidney, the urologic nurse should consult with the physician and counsel families and patients accordingly. Physicians or surgeons caring for the patient should be informed that the individual has a solitary kidney, particularly when managing a situation such as obstruction, trauma, or infection affecting a solitary kidney. Although there is no evidence that a solitary kidney increases any risk of hypertension, patients should be screened for blood pressure on an annual basis. Elevation of the blood pressure should be followed with a functional imaging study (e.g., radionuclide scan) to identify a dysplastic or hypoplastic kidney if blood pressure is elevated in a child or young adult.

Although true agenesis does not require surgical intervention, a hypoplastic kidney may secrete enough renin to cause secondary hypertension or may act as a focus of infection. In either case, a nephrectomy may be needed to control secondary hypertension or prevent febrile infections. In addition, surgery may be required to repair associated urinary system anomalies, such as high vesicoureteral reflux or ureteral obstruction.[15]

Supernumerary Kidneys

A supernumerary kidney is characterized by one or more completely formed accessory kidneys with their own blood supply.[1,4,17] It is extremely rare, with fewer than 100 cases reported as of 1999.[17] The accessory kidney is usually ectopic and located in a caudal position—closer to the pelvis—with respect to the dominant paired kidneys. It may be drained by a separate ureter, but is often associated with a bifid ureter that also drains one of the dominant kidneys. The condition is often asymptomatic, but as many as

50% of patients will be hydronephrotic or develop calculi.[1,4] The cause of supernumerary kidneys is unknown, but it is postulated to arise from multiple ureteric buds interacting with a single metanephric cap or from multiple ureteric buds, each with its own metanephric cap.[18]

Assessment. A supernumerary kidney is diagnosed by abdominopelvic CT scanning, MRI, ultrasound, intravenous urography, or radionuclide scanning.[19] It may be associated with congenital defects such as horseshoe kidney or coarctation of the aorta,[20] but is most commonly discovered as an unexpected finding when evaluating an abdominal or pelvic mass.[21,22]

Nursing Management. The supernumerary kidney may be asymptomatic, but the nurse should educate the patient that ongoing monitoring (e.g., annual blood pressure measurement, urinalysis) is justified because of the risk for dysplasia or structural defects predisposing the individual to infection or secondary hypertension. In addition, given its association with other congenital anomalies, children should undergo evaluation for additional congenital anomalies.

Defects of the Renal Parenchyma

Abnormalities of the architecture of the renal parenchyma are called renal dysplasia.[23-25] From a histologic perspective, dysplastic kidneys are characterized by malformed and poorly differentiated cells, incomplete branching of the ureteral buds, and primitive tissue, such as cartilage. Nevertheless, because histologic diagnosis requires renal biopsy, the diagnosis is usually based on appearance on an imaging study combined with indirect clinical indicators, such as family history and measurements of renal function. The cause of renal dysplasia is thought to be similar to that associated with agenesis—abnormal interactions between the ureteric bud and metanephric cap lead to malformations in ureteral branching and nephron development. Alterations in the protein signal transduction agents responsible for normal nephrogenesis and renal development (see Chapter 1) can lead to an upregulation of cell growth and abnormally large kidneys, with multiple cysts (polycystic or multicystic dysplasia). In contrast, upregulation of other protein signal transduction agents can promote apoptosis (programmed cell death) characterized by a small kidney with undifferentiated metaplastic elements or involution of a kidney that was previously large and cystic during prenatal development or following birth. Maternal use of angiotensin-converting enzyme (ACE) inhibitors also leads to renal dysplasia, particularly when ingested during the second and third trimesters of pregnancy.[26]

Dysplasia is further classified as total or subtotal.[24] Total dysplasia involves both the renal cortex and medulla; it is almost always seen with ureteral atresia, absence of the ureter, and a small renal artery. It is the outcome of an early insult to parenchymal development and is typically associated with renal ectopia, defects affecting the contralateral upper urinary tract (80%), and anomalies of other organ systems. A kidney with total dysplasia may be hypoplastic or enlarged. It lacks adequate function to be visualized on intravenous urography, although a calcified shell may render the renal shadow visible to the trained eye. Subtotal dysplasia selectively affects the medulla or cortex, or is limited to a focal area within the kidney (segmental dysplasia). It is associated with less severe ureteral anomalies such as ureterocele, megaureter, prune-belly syndrome, and myelodysplasia. Kidneys with subtotal dysplasia retain more function than those with total dysplasia, and they will be visualized on a contrast-enhanced imaging study such as IVP or CT. Nevertheless, they are frequently associated with defects of the kidney.

Polycystic Kidney Disease

Renal cysts occur when proliferation of the renal epithelium leads to a diverticulum within the tubular wall.[25] Subsequent collection of fluid, from the glomerular filtrate or interstitial fluid, within the cyst can cause it to become large enough that is easily visualized on an imaging study such as a CT, sonography, or intervenous urography (Figure 12-2). A cyst becomes clinically relevant when it reduces or replaces enough functioning parenchyma to reduce renal function, or when it causes clinical symptoms such as flank or back pain. Renal cysts may occur as a genetic disorder, congenital anomaly, or acquired disorder; this chapter will focus on heritable or congenital cysts.

Polycystic kidney disease is a genetic disorder seen as two clinical syndromes—autosomal dominant (sometimes referred to as adult) and autosomal recessive (sometimes referred to as infantile).[27] Autosomal dominant polycystic kidney disease (ADPKD) is caused by a defect of at least one of

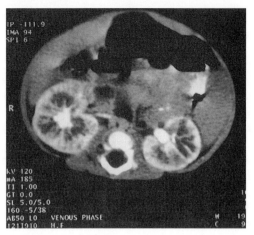

Fig. 12-2 Ultrasonography of a polycystic kidney demonstrates multiple cysts replacing both the parenchyma and distorting the pelvicalyceal system. (From Moore K, Persaud TVN: The Developing Human, 7th edition. Philadelphia: Saunders, 2003; p 301.)

three genes (polycystic kidney disease 1 [*PKD1*], *PKD2*, or *PKD3*).[25,28] Defects of the *PKD1* and *PKD2* genes account for over 95% of cases of ADPKD. The autosomal dominant form comprises approximately 90% of all cases of polycystic kidneys, affecting approximately 1 in 1000 live births.[27] During embryogenesis, the kidneys develop normally and continue to function normally during the first decade of life. However, around the age of 10 years, cysts begin to develop and proliferate. These cysts soon compromise and ultimately replace the normal parenchyma, causing renal failure, usually by the third to fourth decades of life. These cysts generally cause clinical symptoms, including abdominal mass with flank pain, microscopic or gross hematuria, urinary tract infection, and renal colic caused by obstructing blood clots. By the fifth decade of life, the renal parenchyma is sufficiently damaged that dialysis is usually necessary. In addition to these patients, some persons are being diagnosed with ADPKD on imaging studies, but renal insufficiency or symptoms may not develop until the seventh decade of life. Risk factors for early progression to end-stage renal disease include male gender, gravida 4 or higher in women, hematuria, and hypertension.[29]

ADPKD is also associated with extrarenal cyst formation. For example, about 50% of these patients will develop liver cysts, which are often moderate, but 15%

to 20% of those affected will have more severe and symptomatic hepatic disease requiring orthotopic liver transplantation.[30,31] Cysts also develop in the pancreas, lung, ovaries, esophagus, thyroid, uterus, subarachnoid space, and male reproductive organs, including the testes, prostate, epididymis, and prostate.[25] Pancreatic cysts are particularly common in persons older than 20 years (98.5%) but these rarely lead to pancreatitis.

Autosomal recessive polycystic kidney disease (ARPKD), sometimes called infantile polycystic kidneys, is comparatively uncommon, affecting only 1 in 20,000 live births.[32] The gene associated with ARPKD has been identified as *PKHD1* (polycystic kidney and hepatic disease gene 1); it is located on chromosome 6. In 30% to 50% of cases, renal enlargement occurs during embryonic development, leading to oligohydramnios and respiratory compromise at birth.[25,33,34] In a few cases, the kidneys are so large that they interfere with vaginal delivery. Congenital hepatic fibrosis is commonly associated with ARKPD because of defects in the ductal plate. Although renal and hepatic enlargement vary, approximately 75% of infants with ARPKD and congenital hepatic fibrosis develop enlarged palpable kidneys during infancy, and 50% will require renal transplantation for renal failure by age 20 years.[35]

Assessment. The most common clinical manifestations leading to the diagnosis of polycystic kidneys include enlarged (and often palpable) kidneys, enlargement of the liver, hypertension, urinary tract infection, hematuria, and flank pain. Patients with autosomal dominant polycystic kidneys tend to present with pain.[25] The pain of ADPKD usually predates the evolution of palpable kidneys; it is localized to the abdomen or flank and may radiate to the epigastric or suprapubic area. It is usually characterized as dull and appears to crescendo as cystic formation progresses, possibly caused by distention of the renal capsule or traction on the renal pedicle. It may be accompanied by episodes of acute pain, associated with rupture of a cyst. Hypertension is present in 60% of patients at diagnosis; it is usually mild to moderate and attributable to compression of blood vessels in the kidney, with subsequent activation of the renin-angiotensin system. Hypertension may be interrupted by transient periods of hypotension when a cyst ruptures, leading to an acute decompression of local vessels within the kidney.

Autosomal recessive polycystic kidneys may be diagnosed on prenatal ultrasound or during neonatal examination (see Clinical Highlights for Advanced and Expert Practice: Signs and Symptoms in the Neonate Indicating the Need for an Urgent Urologic Evaluation). Typical presenting features include bilateral enlarged, palpable kidneys, an enlarged liver, hypertension, urinary tract infection, and respiratory difficulties.[33] Growth retardation will be seen in 25%, particularly when renal function is impaired.

One or more imaging studies are completed to characterize the kidneys and liver. Ultrasound usually reveals large kidneys that retain their characteristic beanlike (reniform) structure, with greater than normal echogenicity because of multiple cysts.[36] The presence of a single cyst in a child raises the suspicion of ADPKD. Contrast-enhanced imaging studies, such as intravenous urography or a CT scan, typically reveal striations of the parenchyma and multiple fluid-filled cysts. Imaging of the liver demonstrates malformed and dilated bile ducts, periportal fibrosis, and varying numbers of hepatic cysts. Of note, the involvement of the kidney and liver in the disease process tends to be inversely proportional; children with more severely affected kidneys tend to have less hepatic involvement, whereas those with more profound liver involvement have fewer renal cysts.

Differentiating autosomal dominant from recessive polycystic kidney disease is often difficult and occasionally not possible.[34] When polycystic kidneys are diagnosed in a child or adult, both parents are asked to undergo abdominal ultrasound whenever feasible. If ultrasonography reveals renal cysts in one parent, ADPKD is diagnosed; however, if both parents are free from cysts, the likelihood of the disease is dramatically reduced to that of a spontaneous genetic mutation.

Alternative diagnostic possibilities include Meckel or Bardet-Biedl syndrome, congenital hepatic fibrosis, or other particularly unusual conditions. Diagnosis of the less common autosomal polycystic kidney disease is based on the presence of cysts involving the kidneys and/or liver, negative ultrasonography in both parents (who must be older than 30 years), and liver biopsy. Diagnosis of ADPKD is based on evaluation of gross or microscopic hematuria in 35% of cases.[25] Hematuria is related to cyst rupture, infection, or participation in sports or strenuous exercise. Genetic analysis can be used to diagnose ADPKD, but it is expensive and technically demanding, and requires testing of two related and affected individuals.

Nursing Management. Treatment of ADPKD is aimed at delaying end-stage renal disease and managing interim complications, including infection, hypertension, and pain. Renal function is regularly monitored by urinalysis and measurement of serum creatinine and blood urea nitrogen (BUN) levels. The patient is advised of risk factors for early development of renal failure, including male gender, multiple pregnancies, hematuria, and hypertension. Emphasis is placed on potentially mutable risk factors, including counseling women of childbearing years about the risk associated with more than three pregnancies and the associated risk of bearing children with ADPKD. Although treatment of hypertension has not been proved to reduce the risk in humans, data in animals suggest that treatment may slow progress to end-stage renal disease.[37] In addition, blood pressure control is important because it helps alleviate or prevent secondary cardiac complications, including left ventricular hypertrophy and congestive heart failure.[38] Limited evidence also exists showing that restriction of protein in the diet to 15 to 30 g/day, particularly when combined with intake of soy protein, may slow renal deterioration.[37] Patients also should be counseled that dietary supplementation with flax oil or fish oil, rich in α-linoleic acid, might slow renal deterioration and cyst formation, but there is insufficient evidence to prove or disprove any clinically significant benefit. In addition, patients may be counseled that the physician or nurse practitioner may prescribe a cholesterol-lowering agent that might slow renal deterioration and cyst development because of the drug's antiproliferative and antioxidant properties.

Although these strategies may slow renal deterioration, no treatment exists that will arrest the inevitable decline to end-stage renal disease experienced by most patients with ADPKD. Fortunately, the onset of renal failure occurs relatively late in life, with a median onset of 53 years in patients with a defect in *PKD1* and 70 years in those with a defect in *PKD2*.[25] Dialysis and renal transplantation are required when renal function falls to levels that are insufficient to maintain internal homeostasis.

Hemodialysis is a good alternative for these patients, partially because it has proved effective in lowering blood pressure and the risk of related cardiac complications. Renal transplantation is also effective for patients with ADPKD; the nurse can reassure the patient considering transplantation that there is no increased risk for developing cysts in a transplanted kidney. Nevertheless, it is important to note that special considerations exist when a living relative is undergoing consideration as a donor for a patient with ADPKD.

Goals of therapy for infants or young children with the autosomal recessive form are similar to those of other causes of renal insufficiency, including ADPKD.[35] Immediate treatment focusing on respiratory support in the neonatal period is required when cystic replacement of renal parenchyma has progressed significantly during embryogenesis. In children who survive the neonatal period with functioning kidneys, efforts to preserve renal function are instituted and renal function is routinely monitored. Growth and development are closely monitored, and a diet that ensures maximal growth while avoiding excessive protein intake is monitored in consultation with a nephrologist and nutritionist. Liver function also must be closely monitored, and portosystemic shunting is completed when fibrosis leads to symptomatic portal hypertension.

Urinary tract infection presents special challenges for the patient with polycystic kidney disease.[25] Unlike the unaffected person, the urine culture is often not revealing, depending on the location of the infection. Acute bacterial interstitial nephritis occurs in nonobstructed urinary tracts and is characterized by fever, dysuria, voiding frequency, and bothersome urinary urgency. These patients typically have a suggestive urinalysis and positive urine culture and respond rapidly to sensitivity-guided antimicrobial therapy. In contrast, children or adults with sterile urine, or those who fail to respond to several weeks of antibiotic therapy, may have a pyonephrosis (infection of a calyceal system that is obstructed by a stone, blood clot, or compressing cyst), pyocyst (infected cyst) or perinephric abscess (see Chapter 5). In this case, percutaneous or laparoscopic incision and drainage, open surgical drainage, or nephrectomy may be required to reverse infection. Treatment of urinary tract infections is further complicated in these patients because few drugs effectively penetrate renal cysts, particularly when infected with gram-negative organisms. Urinary tract instrumentation should be avoided whenever possible because of the risk of secondary infection. Other healthcare providers should be advised of this precaution, which carries a risk of symptomatic infection of approximately 43% and a small but significant risk of overwhelming infection and death.[39] Patients with polycystic kidney disease should be taught strategies to reduce the risk of community-acquired urinary tract infection, including good perineal hygiene, the possible benefit of regular consumption of cranberry juice or cranberry products,[40] and regular, complete bladder evacuation. The urologic nurse should consult with the physician or nurse practitioner concerning the possibility of intravaginal hormone replacement in postmenopausal women who are free from significant hepatic disease.[25]

Frequently for the patient with polycystic kidney disease, obstructing calculi, clots, or cysts may obstruct the urinary tract. Various endourologic techniques may be used to manage stones, obstructing clots, or persistent hematuria in polycystic kidneys, including extracorporeal shock wave lithotripsy, percutaneous nephrolithotomy, retrograde endoscopy, and stone manipulation.[41] Although particular care must be taken to prevent or manage infection, these interventions provide an attractive alternative to open surgical manipulation of the kidney or nephrectomy.

Multicystic Dysplastic Kidneys

Multicystic dysplasia of the kidney is among the most common causes of abdominal mass in the newborn (Figure 12-3). Unilateral dysplasia affects 1 in every 3000 to 5000 births and bilateral dysplasia affects 1 in every 10,000 births.[42] Unilateral multicystic dysplasia usually arises as a spontaneous malformation,[43] but bilateral involvement may be caused by an inherited or genetic defect. Patients with multicystic dysplasia are at very high risk for urinary tract obstruction; the affected kidney is typically, but not always, attached to an atretic—incompletely cannulated—ureter. Moreover, many features of dysplasia can be reproduced in the experimental animal model by obstructing a ureter.[44] The cause of multicystic dysplasia remains unclear, but there is some evidence that obstruction, teratogens, and genetic defects are likely to cause or contribute to this anomaly.

Like many defects of the urinary system, multicystic dysplasia may be associated with other anomalies.

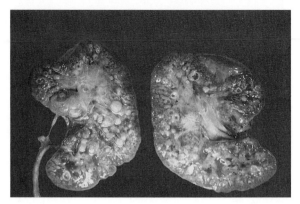

Fig. 12-3 Multicystic kidney is characterized by relatively large cysts that replace the renal parenchyma and distort the pelvicalyceal collecting system. (From Carlson B: Human Embryology and Developmental Biology, 3rd edition. St Louis: Mosby, 2005; p 405.)

In one series of 138 fetuses evaluated by ultrasonography, 66% with multicystic renal dysplasia were noted to have additional anomalies and it was further observed that 22% of affected fetuses did not survive pregnancy or the neonatal period.[45] Associated defects affect approximately 40% of children with multicystic dysplasia; these include vesicoureteral reflux or UPJ obstruction of the contralateral kidney, cystic defects affecting the ipsilateral testis in boys, and abnormalities of the bladder wall.[25]

Involution may occur in the multicystic dysplastic kidney, either during embryonic development or during early life.[46] The presence of an involuted multicystic kidney in the neonate or infant may be mistaken for renal agenesis (see earlier discussion). When children born with multicystic dysplasia are monitored with ultrasonography during infancy and early childhood, nearly 50% will experience some reduction in renal size and 23% of kidneys will become undetectable.[47] Accurate differentiation of an involuted, multicystic, dysplastic kidney from a congenitally absent kidney is clinically relevant because the scarred areas in the former contain renin-producing cells that are capable of activating the renin-angiotensin system, leading to secondary hypertension.[48]

Assessment. Multicystic dysplasia is often detected by prenatal ultrasound.[42-46] These contain multiple thin-walled cysts that do not communicate. The cysts are typically larger than those found in the polycystic kidney and individual cysts may be quite large.

Parenchyma is found between the cysts, but is often hypoechogenic, possibly suggesting adverse effects of dysplasia. The presence of an abdominal mass on a newborn examination also may provide the first clue to a multicystic dysplastic kidney. When detected by intravenous urography, the multicystic dysplastic kidney will be observed as an enlarged nonfunctioning kidney, usually with enlargement of the parenchyma of the contralateral kidney suggesting compensatory hypertrophy. Functional radionuclide studies provide more detailed information; when viewed on a DTPA radionuclide scan, less than 5% of these kidneys will demonstrate any activity.[49] However, when the dimercaptosuccinic acid (DMSA) radionuclide is injected, 15% will demonstrate some function, although this contributes very little to total renal function.[50]

Nursing Management. Differentiation of bilateral from unilateral multicystic dysplasia is critical to management. Children with bilateral multicystic dysplasia are at greater risk for end-stage renal disease, more likely to have a familial disorder causing the defects, and have a poorer prognosis when compared with children with unilateral disease.[42,44,45] Fetuses with bilateral multicystic kidneys are more likely to die before being carried to term and those who survive to birth are at greater risk for death because of a combination of renal failure and pulmonary hypoplasia. Peritoneal dialysis has been advocated as a routing intervention for children with significant bilateral multicystic dysplasia.[45] However, this option is associated with secondary complications, and the urologic nurse should coordinate discussions between the physician and parents when this treatment option is contemplated. Children with bilateral disease who survive to early childhood before end-stage renal disease occurs have a much better diagnosis because dialysis is technically easier and renal transplantation becomes possible once the child reaches 20 to 22 pounds (9 to 10 kg).

In addition to routine monitoring of pulmonary and renal function, the urologic nurse should consult with the physician concerning the need for chromosomal analysis. Screening ultrasonography of the parents and siblings also may be considered and the mother should be screened for diabetes mellitus, because its presence greatly increases the risk of bearing subsequent children with multicystic dysplasia.[51]

Patients with unilateral multicystic dysplasia are less likely to experience renal failure or pulmonary hypoplasia. Rather, they may remain asymptomatic, particularly if the contralateral kidney undergoes compensatory hypertrophy. However, nearly 50% of these children will have a risk of hypertension, justifying the need for routine annual blood pressure measurement. The proportion of patients with hypertension remains controversial, with estimates ranging from 0% to 20%.[25,45,52] Using ambulatory blood pressure monitoring, it was found that 20% of a group of 25 children with multicystic dysplasia had evidence of hypertension. Although the majority demonstrated elevated blood pressure during waking hours and while asleep, 40% had normal readings while awake but experienced elevated blood pressure while sleeping. Pharmacotherapy is indicated when hypertension-complicated dysplasia occurs to reduce the risk of renal failure and secondary cardiac complications. Highly selected children with multicystic dysplasia and hypertension may benefit from nephrectomy, but adults rarely achieve a significant reduction in blood pressure from nephrectomy alone.[25,52]

In addition to blood pressure monitoring, patients with multicystic dysplasia should undergo evaluation of the contralateral kidney, paying particular attention to the presence of obstruction or vesicoureteral reflux. Patients and parents should be advised of the significance of urinary tract infection with a solitary functioning kidney. In addition, the urologic nurse should advise the family that children with multicystic dysplasia have a 3- to 10-fold greater risk for Wilms' tumor. Although this risk is considered too small to justify prophylactic nephrectomy, ultrasonic monitoring should be completed every 3 months, up to age 8 years.[25]

Surgical therapy is rarely indicated for the patient with unilateral multicystic dysplasia. Possible indications for nephrectomy include hypertension in a child, pain (sometimes caused by massive enlargement of the kidney), and malignancy. A laparoscopic approach may be used to minimize the perioperative morbidity and pain associated with open nephrectomy.[53]

Defects in Renal Position. Because the kidneys must migrate from the pelvis to the retroperitoneum and rotate to a position parallel to the spinal column, defects of embryonic development may lead to malposition of the kidneys.[4] A malrotated kidney is typically seen on radiographic or ultrasonic imaging as being rotated on its vertical axis, so that the renal pelvis faces anteriorly. Malrotation does not typically cause clinically relevant dysfunction, but it may coexist with defects of the pelvicalyceal system, resulting in hydronephrosis and obstruction.[54]

Renal Ectopia. An ectopic kidney is found somewhere other than the retroperitoneum.[4] In some cases, the ectopic kidney is associated with a ureter and renal vessels that are normal in length, a condition called ptosis. However, an abnormality of renal migration during embryonic development can lead to a kidney located in the pelvis or lower abdomen. In this case, the ureters and renal vessels will also be shortened and the kidney will be malrotated. The most common form of renal ectopia involves one kidney that is located in the pelvis, called a pelvic kidney (Figure 12-4). Pelvic kidneys remain asymptomatic in about 50% of cases and are discovered as an incidental finding during an imaging study. Urologic symptoms leading to the discovery of a pelvic kidney include abdominal pain, abdominopelvic mass, and infection. Pelvic kidneys are more susceptible to stone formation than normally located kidneys and pain raises suspicion of urinary calculi. This increased risk may be caused by abnormal relationships and architecture in the pelvicaliceal system that predispose the kidney to urinary stasis.

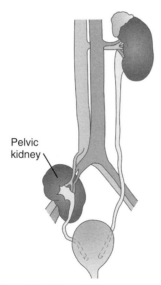

Pelvic kidney

Fig. 12-4 The pelvic kidney is the most common form of ectopia. (From Carlson B: *Human Embryology and Developmental Biology*, 3rd edition. St Louis: Mosby, 2005; p 404.)

Ureterohydronephrosis in the absence of obstruction is found in approximately 50% of pelvic kidneys, and angiography frequently reveals abnormalities of the renal vasculature. Similar to other renal anomalies, ectopia is associated with an increased risk for other urinary system defects, including vesicoureteral reflux, renal dysplasia, cryptorchidism, and hypospadias.[55]

The intrathoracic kidney is a rare form of renal ectopia characterized by a kidney located above the retroperitoneal space and within the thorax.[56] It may not require treatment, although it has been reported to be associated with other congenital anomalies, such as trisomy 21[57] and patent ductus arteriosus.[58,59]

Assessment. Renal ectopia is detected on an imaging study, although it may be palpated as a mass in the abdominopelvic region of the infant or small child. When ectopy is found in a child, careful examination of the contralateral kidney should be done because up to 85% of these patients will have a defect affecting the contralateral urinary tract. The child is also examined for anomalies of the reproductive tract and cardiac and skeletal systems, paying careful attention to exclude the most commonly associated defects, such as hypospadias, cryptorchidism, vaginal agenesis, and vertebral anomalies, known to affect 15% to 45% of children found to have renal ectopia.[4]

Even when discovered as an incidental finding in the older child or adult, ectopia has particular significance for the urologic nurse and urologist. Evaluation in this case includes the location of the kidney, characterization of the pelvicalyceal system, differentiation of obstructive from nonobstructive ureterohydronephrosis, and mapping of its vasculature. This evaluation is critical because it affects the approach and techniques used in multiple urologic procedures, including laparoscopic or open surgery,[60,61] lithotripsy,[62] and percutaneous endourologic procedures.[63]

Nursing Management. Ectopy per se does not require treatment, and the urologic nurse can reassure the patient and parents that the presence of this defect does not imply an imminent risk of renal failure in the otherwise healthy individual. Instead, urologic management focuses on identification of associated anomalies and prevention or treatment of complications. Parents of the child with renal ectopy are counseled to inform health care providers of the presence of an ectopic kidney, particularly if abdominal or pelvic surgery is considered. They are also taught that obstruction or infection of an ectopic kidney may produce atypical pain when compared with persons with normally located kidneys. This information is particularly useful if the patient experiences renal colic, which may be confused with a gastrointestinal disorder unless the physician is made aware of the presence of a pelvic kidney.

Because of their abnormal locations, ectopic kidneys present unusual technical challenges when urinary stones lead to obstruction and pain. Percutaneous nephrolithotomy is often elected over extracorporeal shock wave lithotripsy when positional defects are severe,[64] and patients or parents are counseled to seek care from a urologist with considerable training and experience in endourology, preferably including prior experience in managing those with renal ectopia.

Ectopia Complicated by Fusion Anomalies

Fusion anomalies occur when the metanephric caps merge to form a single organ. The most common, called the horseshoe kidney, involves only the lower poles of the kidneys. Less common forms are characterized by the crossing of one kidney to the contralateral side of the body; these anomalies are collectively called crossed renal ectopia with fusion (Figure 12-5).

Horseshoe Kidney. The most common form of fusion is the horseshoe kidney, which occurs in approximately 1 in every 400 births. It is characterized by a relatively thin isthmus of merged tissue, fusing the lower poles into a single organ resembling

a horseshoe (Figure 12-6). The horseshoe kidney is frequently lower than a normal kidney; anterior malrotation of the renal pelves and elongation of its lower poles also occur.[65] Additional congenital anomalies involving the genitourinary, skeletal, cardiovascular, and gastrointestinal systems are found in approximately one third of all patients with horseshoe kidneys, regardless of whether the kidney causes bothersome symptoms. Occasionally, the horseshoe kidney is dysplastic and associated with an increased risk of malignancy in later life, particularly Wilms' tumor,[66,67] renal carcinoid,[68,69] and transitional cell carcinoma of the renal pelvis.[70]

Assessment. The horseshoe kidney remains asymptomatic in many patients and is often discovered as an incidental finding on an imaging study. However, unlike many other congenital anomalies, the horseshoe kidney is not easily diagnosed by contrast-enhanced or ultrasonic imaging studies because of the small size of the isthmus connecting the kidneys.[4,65] The diagnosis is suspected when the pelves are malrotated so that the vertical axes of the renal bodies point downward, toward the lower spine. Prenatal ultrasound will reveal an abnormal renal-pelvic angle, measured between the long axis of the renal pelves on the axial view of the abdomen, but this angle is not routinely measured.[71] IVP will detect the isthmus, provided it contains functioning parenchyma capable of concentrating contrast media, or a radionuclide study such as the DTPA or MAG3 scan may be useful because it will identify the presence of functioning parenchyma in the isthmus of the kidney and differentiate clinically relevant obstruction of

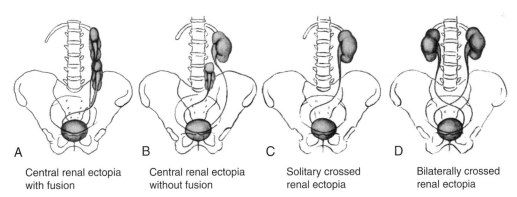

A	B	C	D
Central renal ectopia with fusion	Central renal ectopia without fusion	Solitary crossed renal ectopia	Bilaterally crossed renal ectopia

Fig. 12-5 Crossed renal ectopia with fusion. (From Walsh P, Retik AB, Vaughan ED, Wein AJ [eds]: Campbell's Urology, 8th edition. Philadelphia: Saunders, 2002; p 1899.)

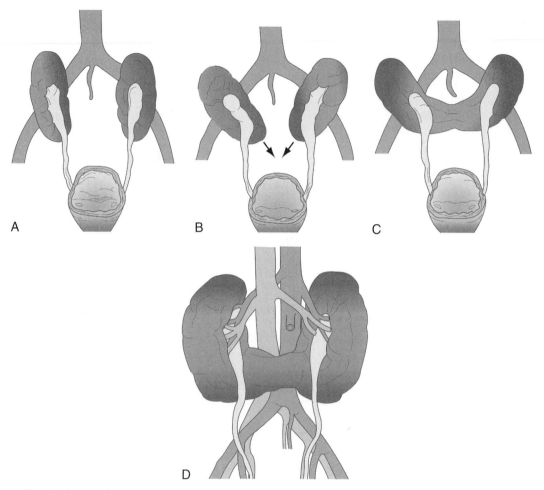

A   B   C

D

Fig. 12-6 Horseshoe kidney demonstrating the isthmus of tissue fusing the lower poles of the kidneys and malrotation of the renal pelves. (From Carlson B: *Human Embryology and Developmental Biology*, 3rd edition. St Louis: Mosby, 2005; p 405.)

the upper urinary tract from nonobstructive uretero-hydronephrosis. This distinction is often important, because 80% of all horseshoe kidneys are associated with dilation of the pelvicalyceal system and ureter, usually in the absence of significant obstruction. Alternatively, bothersome urologic disorders may lead to incidental diagnosis of a horseshoe kidney; the most common conditions include renal colic caused by urinary calculi, infection, and hematuria.

Nursing Management. Traditionally, surgery was often undertaken in patients with horseshoe kidneys in an attempt to relieve obstruction and improve drainage of the upper urinary tracts.[4] However, subsequent clinical experience has demonstrated that

separation of the isthmus does not change the clinical course in most patients so the practice has been abandoned.

Therefore, management of the horseshoe kidney has shifted to education, monitoring for complications, and adaptation of surgical, laparoscopic, or endoscopic procedures to the altered anatomy created by this congenital anomaly. When discovered in a child, the patient and family should be educated about the nature of the defect and the possibility of associated anomalies. When discovered in an adult or child, teaching includes information about the increased risk for stone formation and the signs and symptoms of renal colic. Families are also advised of a slight increase in the risk of Wilms' tumor, which requires routine monitoring by a physician, probably with ultrasonic imaging of the kidney. Similarly, adults with a horseshoe kidney are advised of a slight increase in the risk of renal carcinoid or transitional cell carcinoma of the upper urinary tract. Routine monitoring in this case should include routine urinalysis and further evaluation if unexplained hematuria occurs. Finally, patients should be counseled that adaptation of invasive techniques, including laparoscopic and endoscopic urologic procedures,[72] open surgery (e.g., transplantation[73]), and abdominal procedures (e.g., repair of abdominal aortic aneurysm[74]) might be necessary.

Crossed Renal Ectopy With Fusion. Crossed renal ectopia occurs when a developing metanephric cap crosses the midline.[4,74,75] In this case, both ureters develop and implant into the bladder, but the metanephric caps fuse into a single kidney that is to the right or left of the midline. Typically, the metanephric caps also fuse into a single renal parenchyma with two collection systems. Historically six types of renal ectopia have been described,[76] but the clinical relevance of this classification schema has not been demonstrated.[4] Crossed renal ectopia is uncommon, affecting approximately 1 in 2000 births. Malrotation of the kidney and nonobstructive hydronephrosis are common, but renal function is typically adequate. Nevertheless, abnormalities of ureteral position may lead to UPJ obstruction or vesicoureteric reflux. Evaluation and management are similar to those described for the horseshoe kidney.

ANOMALIES OF THE CALICES, RENAL PELVES, AND URETERS

Congenital anomalies can also affect the calices, renal pelvis, or ureters. Defects in the architecture of the collecting system typically produce obstruction or poor contractility because of abnormal development of the smooth muscle of the ureter. Defects in ureteral number present as complete or incomplete duplication of a ureter associated with a single or, rarely, supernumerary renal parenchyma.

Defects of the Calices

Dilation of one or more calices may be the result of an obstruction or nonobstructive process. For example, a calyceal diverticulum is a cystic dilation of the calyx that is not associated with an obstructive lesion.[4] It is

hypothesized to arise from abnormal development of one division of the ureteric bud. Calyceal diverticula are frequently asymptomatic and incidentally detected during an upper urinary tract imaging study. However, they are associated with urinary stasis and an increased risk of secondary urinary calculi.[77]

Megacalycosis is a term used to describe an enlarged calyx detected in the absence of obstruction.[78] It is typically detected during an evaluation for a childhood urinary tract infection, although it may be initially detected as an incidental finding in adults. Megacalycosis is associated with a transient delay in the recanalization of the upper ureter after the ureteral buds connect to the metanephros or abnormal development of the renal pyramids, with incomplete projection of the papillae into the calices. Congenital megacalycosis is a rare anomaly characterized by dilation of all the renal calices and hypoplasia of the renal pyramids in the absence of renal pelvic dilation or obstruction.[79,80] Renal function is normal in these patients, but there is an increased risk of urinary calculi.

Congenital obstruction of a calyx occurs as the result of an infundibular stenosis; it is often associated with multicystic or polycystic renal dysplasia, simple renal cysts, or megacalycosis.[81] Associated abnormalities of the ureter are rare, but the condition typically affects both kidneys (90%) and is associated with an increased risk of end-stage renal disease.[82] This risk arises from dysplasia or glomerulosclerosis, rather than being a direct result of the obstructed calyx.

Ureteropelvic Junction Obstruction

Ureteropelvic junction (UPJ) obstruction is defined as blockage of the tapered junction where the pelvic joins the tubular ureter. It is a relatively common defect, affecting as many as 1 in 500 births.[83] UPJ obstruction usually affects only one kidney, but from 10% to 40% will have bilateral defects. In 90% of cases, an intrinsic defect leads to obstruction[84] and the remaining 10% are attributable to extrinsic compression of the ureter[85] (Figure 12-7). The cause of intrinsic UPJ obstruction is unknown; it is hypothesized to arise from a defect in the tubular progress of the ureter itself, which is characterized by several phases of canalization and occlusion prior to formation of the mature urinary tract seen in the adult. Histologic analysis implicates inflammation

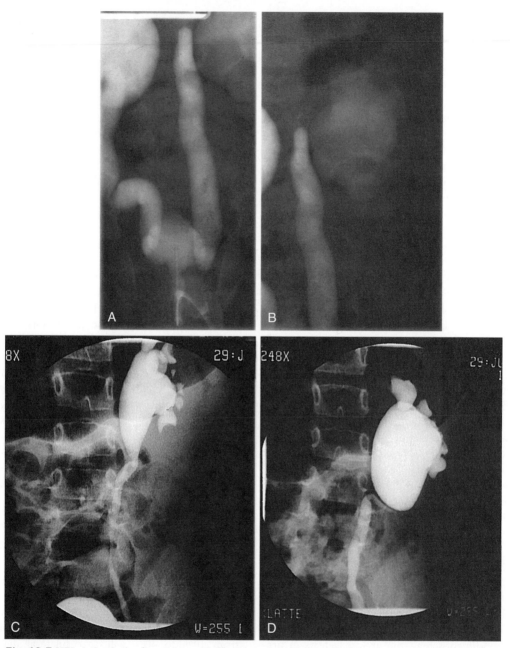

Fig. 12-7 UPJ. **A,** Intrinsic obstruction with fibrosis and narrowing of upper ureter. **B,** Extrinsic obstruction with ureteral kinking caused by crossing vessel. (From Walsh P, Retik AB, Vaughan ED, Wein AJ [eds]: Campbell's Urology, 8th edition. Philadelphia: Saunders, 2002; p 2074.)

and fibrosis of the pelvic and ureteral wall,[84] apoptosis of smooth muscle cells,[86] or defects of the smooth muscle myosin chains in the affected area.[87] Extrinsic cases are often attributed to crossing renal vessels, but a study of normal (unobstructed) ureteropelvic junctions has revealed crossing vessels in 19%[88] as compared with 13% of patients with UPJ obstruction.

Traditionally, UPJ obstruction was diagnosed only when it caused bothersome symptoms such as pain or hematuria, or led to complications such as a urinary calculus or infection.[4] However, with the rise of prenatal ultrasonography, urologists and urologic nurses frequently encounter infants with asymptomatic UPJ obstruction, and questions arise concerning the efficacy of preventive interventions, as well as their safety when compared with a watchful waiting strategy. UPJ obstruction is associated with an increased risk of vesicoureteral reflux affecting both the obstructed and contralateral kidneys; whether this represents a sequela of the embryonic defect leading to the UPJ defect is not known.

Assessment. The diagnosis of UPJ obstruction often is made on prenatal ultrasonic examination, and recent evidence has suggested that this trend leads to increased diagnosis of UPJ obstruction during the perinatal area and an increased likelihood of early surgical repair.[89] The indications for prenatal ultrasound continue to evolve, but they generally include the following: (1) discrepancies in expected fundal height for gestational age; (2) oligohydramnios (placental fluid volume less than 500 ml); (3) elevated level of serum alpha-fetoprotein; and (4) previous pregnancies associated with congenital anomalies.[90] The prenatal sonogram is typically performed at 16 to 20 weeks' gestation, after the pronephron and metanephron have regressed and the developing metanephric kidneys are beginning to assume some of the renal function necessary to sustain life. When a urinary system abnormality such as hydronephrosis is detected, further ultrasonic imaging is completed to assess fetal size and maturity, amniotic fluid volume, gender (which influences the possible causes of urinary tract obstruction), localization of the obstructing lesion (such as a UPJ obstruction), and its effect on fetal health and development. The severity of hydronephrosis is also graded and this is used to guide subsequent interventions (Table 12-1).

In cases of moderate to severe UPJ obstruction, grades 2 to 4, follow-up evaluation after birth is indicated. A renal ultrasound is completed at around age 3 to 5 days. Even if the ultrasound at this time is normal, a voiding cystourethrogram (VCUG) is obtained to determine the presence of vesicoureteral reflux. If both the VCUG and renal ultrasonogram are normal, one or more follow-up ultrasonograms are obtained to ensure that hydronephrosis does not recur. If the renal ultrasonogram is normal, but

TABLE 12-1 Hydronephrosis Grading System for Prenatal Ultrasonography[90]

GRADE	DESCRIPTION
0	Normal upper urinary tract
1	Mild dilation of renal pelvis, no caliectasis
2	Moderate dilation of renal pelvis and calices
3	Severe dilation of renal pelvis and calices, parenchyma remains normal
4	Severe dilation of renal pelvis and calices, renal parenchyma is thin

vesicoureteral reflux is diagnosed, the patient is managed as having primary reflux, and prophylactic antibiotic therapy is begun under the direction of the urologist. In addition, a radionuclide scan will be obtained to measure differential renal function, quantify the magnitude of obstruction, and identify whether surgical intervention may be indicated. Persistent hydronephrosis on the renal ultrasonogram obtained at age 3 to 5 days also indicates the need to obtain a VCUG to determine whether UPJ obstruction is complicated by vesicoureteral reflux.

Renal function is assessed in the child with moderate to severe hydronephrosis both prenatally and following birth. Prenatal assessment occurs under the direction of the obstetrician, but pediatric urology and nephrology also may play a role in this assessment. Prenatal assessment relies on multiple indirect assessments, including measurement of amniotic fluid volume (partly consisting of fetal urine) and of fetal urine electrolyte and protein levels. Measurements of the specific gravity of the fetal urine and the β_2-microglobulin or α_1-microglobulin level also may be done. Following birth, serum creatinine and blood urea nitrogen levels are combined with results of urinalysis and ultrasonic or radionuclide scans to assess renal function.

Nursing Management. The primary goals of management of patients with UPJ obstruction include preservation of renal function, prevention of infection, particularly when vesicoureteral reflux coexists with UPJ blockage, and control of pain. When moderate to severe hydronephrosis is found by prenatal ultrasound, the parents are counseled about the need for close prenatal monitoring, particularly if the condition is bilateral or evidence of oligohydramnios exists. The urologic nurse may be in contact with the parents of a fetus with hydronephrosis and suspected UPJ obstruction prior to birth. Counseling and education at this point include explanations that a postnatal ultrasonogram will be obtained during early life. The nurse should explain that the initial ultrasonogram is delayed until age 3 to 5 days to avoid the risk of a false-negative result produced by the mild dehydration and oliguria found during the first 24 to 38 hours following delivery. The parents are advised that this ultrasound also allows confirmation of persisting hydronephrosis, and that approximately 20% of neonates with prenatal hydronephrosis have no evidence of the condition when assessed at age 3 to 5 days. The optimum length of follow-up required for children with prenatal hydronephrosis and a normal ultrasound at birth, however, is unknown. Some have argued that a 3-month follow-up ultrasound is adequate,[90] but others have observed recurrence up to 22 months of age.[91] The urologic nurse should consult with the pediatric urologist when counseling parents about ongoing monitoring when the prenatal ultrasonogram shows hydronephrosis and the postnatal study is normal.

The parents are counseled that a VCUG is indicated because of the high risk for vesicoureteral reflux. Teaching should also include the need for early and ongoing assessment and the goals of treatment. Infants found to have vesicoureteral reflux will be placed on prophylactic antibiotics. Based on the age of the neonate, amoxicillin or trimethoprim may be selected. Education for the family of a neonate with UPJ obstruction and reflux includes teaching about renal growth during the first year of life and the importance of preventing and recognizing the signs and symptoms of a urinary infection, particularly in the infant who is unable to report dysuria or flank pain and who may not be able to mount a particularly impressive fever, even in the presence of pyelonephritis. The urologic nursing management of reflux management is discussed in detail later in this chapter.

When hydronephrosis persists on the initial ultrasonogram, parents are advised that a radionuclide study will be performed to assess differential renal function and obstruction severity. If differential renal function testing shows significant compromise of the affected kidney, early surgical intervention

is considered. Pyeloplasty is performed to relieve UPJ obstruction; it is typically approached using an open surgical technique.[92] Alternative techniques include laparoscopic, robotic-assisted laparoscopic, and endourologic approaches (see Chapter 11 for detailed descriptions of pyeloplasty techniques). If renal function is robust and obstruction is not severe, conservative treatment is typically preferred, regardless of the severity of the hydronephrosis. In this case, ongoing monitoring of renal function using ultrasound or radionuclide imaging techniques should be done. The urologic nurse should reinforce teaching concerning the need for routine follow-up in the child with UPJ obstruction, even when symptoms are absent and imaging study results are encouraging, because of the risk for recurrence.

Pain secondary to UPJ obstruction may be caused by passage of a stone or by rapid filling of the UPJ secondary to diuresis. This can occur in young adults following consumption of alcohol or in younger children following consumption of a particularly large volume of fluids over a brief period. Parents and patients are advised to ensure adequate overall fluid intake but avoid drinking large volumes of fluid in a short time to avoid flank pain and renal colic.

DEFECTS IN URETERAL NUMBER
Bifid Renal Pelvis

A duplicated renal pelvis is referred to as a bifid. It is characterized by two pelvicalyceal systems that join at the ureteropelvic junction.[91] A bifid renal pelvis is seen in as many as 40% of patients undergoing IVP for unrelated reasons. Even the earliest reports found no urinary system dysfunction unless associated with other congenital defects.[93] Therefore, it is considered a variant of normal.

Ureteral Duplication

In contrast to the kidneys, defects in ureteral number are described as duplication anomalies.[91] Duplications may be complete or incomplete; an incomplete duplication refers to partial replication of the ureter that drains into a single orifice at the bladder base (Figure 12-8). Incomplete duplication is also referred to as a bifid ureter. Complete duplication of the ureter refers to two separate ureters ending in two orifices (Figure 12-9). A complete duplication of the ureter frequently arises from a single kidney with a duplicated pelvicalyceal system. In this case, the upper pole ureter drains the upper most pelvicalyceal system of the kidney while the lower pole ureter drains the lower most pelvicalyceal system. The ureteral orifice that drains the upper pole is described as the upper pole orifice, regardless of its location in the bladder base. Similarly, the lower pole ureteral orifice describes the ureter draining the lower pole of the kidney, regardless of its relation to the corresponding upper pole ureter.

Duplication of the ureter occurs in approximately 1 in 125 births; about 40% involve both kidneys and 60% are limited to one side.[91] With incomplete duplication (a bifid ureter), a replicated upper segment terminates to a single orifice in the bladder, but a portion of its course is drained by two cannulized ureters.[94] A duplication that terminates at a relatively short distance below the renal pelvis is referred to as a Y defect and duplication that persists to the distal ureter is referred to as a V defect.[95] Evaluation of the segment where the duplication merges into a single ureter reveals a high incidence of fibrosis,

smooth muscle abnormality, and functional obstruction, including stricture in 24% of cases.[94] These defects lead to the stasis and infection often observed in patients with incomplete ureteral duplication.

Complete ureteral duplication is characterized by two distinctive ureters that typically drain a single kidney, with two distinctive pelvicalyceal systems.[96] The anatomic configuration of complete ureteral duplication follows the Weigert-Meyer law, which states that the upper pole ureter will terminate in an orifice medial to the lower pole ureter (see Figure 12-9).[36] Because of its medial position, it has a relatively long submucosal tunnel and rarely refluxes. In contrast, the lower pole ureter will terminate in a laterally placed orifice, which usually allows vesicoureteric reflux. Exceptions to this principle have been encountered, but are extremely rare.[97] Additional defects associated with complete ureteral duplication include ectopic ureterocele, ectopic insertion of a ureteral orifice, and UPJ obstruction. Despite the risk for associated anomalies, ureteral duplication is often discovered incidentally on an imaging study and found to have exerted no apparent deleterious effects on urinary system function.

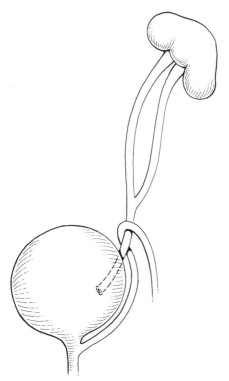

Fig. 12-8 Incomplete ureteral duplication (bifid ureter) draining into single ureteral orifice. (From Walsh P, Retik AB, Vaughan ED, Wein AJ [eds]: Campbell's Urology, 8th edition. Philadelphia: Saunders, 2002; p 2008.)

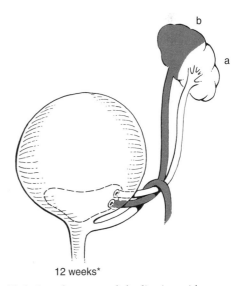

12 weeks*

Fig. 12-9 Complete ureteral duplication with two ureters demonstrates the Weigert-Meyer law. The lower pole ureter drains into the superiorly placed ureteral orifice and the inferiorly placed ureteral orifice drains the upper pole ureter. (From Walsh P, Retik AB, Vaughan ED, Wein AJ [eds]: Campbell's Urology, 8th edition. Philadelphia: Saunders, 2002; p 2012.)

In rare cases, three ureteral buds will develop, leading to ureteral triplication affecting one kidney.[98,99] The left kidney is affected most commonly, and the ureters typically drain through a single ureteral orifice. Urologic disorders associated with ureteral triplication include urinary tract infection, vesicoureteral reflux, and urinary calculi.

Assessment. Ureteral duplication is often discovered as an incidental finding during an imaging study such as a VCUG. This study is typically done as part of an evaluation following a urinary tract infection in an infant or child. Vesicoureteral reflux commonly occurs in the ureter draining the lower renal segment, because of its lateral (higher) location within the bladder base. When associated with reflux and urinary tract infection, a renal ultrasonogram or intravenous pyelogram is obtained to elucidate the anatomy of the affected and contralateral upper urinary tracts further. When invasive interventions are being considered, a radionuclide study may be performed to assess the function of each renal segment and to identify any obstruction.

Nursing Management. When discovered in the adult as an incidental finding, ureteral duplication may not require treatment or evaluation. Nevertheless, the urologic nurse should ensure that the patient understands both the name of the anomaly, and the related anatomy, a duplication of a ureter of one or both kidneys. This information is particularly helpful if the patient experiences pelvic trauma or will undergo urologic surgery in the future.

Ureteral duplication with vesicoureteral reflux requires immediate management. Low-grade reflux is managed conservatively with prophylactic antibiotic therapy and ongoing monitoring; higher grade reflux may require surgical intervention. Surgical intervention may be indicated if high-grade reflux is found or if reflux fails to resolve, despite a prolonged period of watchful waiting (see Chapter 14).

Ureterocele

Ureterocele is a cystic dilation of the distal ureter (Figure 12-10).[91] When the defect is contained entirely in the bladder, it is classified as an intravesical ureterocele. In contrast, one that is partly located in the bladder neck or urethra is referred to as an ectopic ureterocele. Ureteroceles are relatively uncommon; estimates of their incidence vary from 1 in 4000 to 12,000 live births. They tend to affect one ureter, but 10% are bilateral and 60% to 80% are

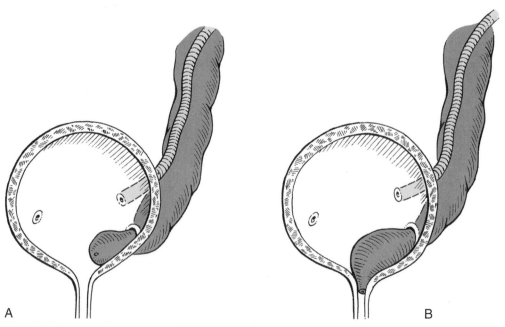

Fig. 12-10 Ureteroceles. **A,** Intravesical ureterocele is contained entirely within the bladder vesicle. **B,** Ectopic ureterocele extends into the proximal urethra. (From Walsh P, Retik AB, Vaughan ED, Wein AJ [eds]: Campbell's Urology, 8th edition. Philadelphia: Saunders, 2002; p 2009.)

ectopic. Approximately 80% of ectopic ureteroceles occur in patients with complete ureteral duplication.

Ureteroceles exert variable influence on urinary system function, depending on their size and location. Ureterocele size varies from barely visible on imaging studies to large dilations that occupy a significant portion of the bladder vesicle and obstruct the urinary outflow tract. Intravesical ureteroceles rarely obstruct the bladder outlet; they are typically diagnosed as an incidental finding during an imaging study. In contrast, ectopic ureteroceles tend to drain the upper pole of a duplicated pelvicalyceal system and 74% to 90% of these upper poles are damaged because of long-term obstruction. They are more likely to be associated with a urologic disorder such as a urinary tract infection, bladder outlet obstruction, hematuria. or urinary incontinence. The lower pole of a duplicated system associated with a ureterocele tends to be displaced downward, giving it the appearance of a drooping lily when imaged during IVP. Dilation of the ureter may be attributable to several causes, including vesicoureteral reflux and ureteral obstruction, or it may occur when neither reflux nor obstruction is present.

Assessment. Traditionally, ureteroceles were diagnosed on intravenous urography, but most are now detected during ultrasonography. When viewed during sonography, they appear as a well-defined cyst (dark hole) in the posterior aspect of the bladder base (Figure 12-11). When viewed during intravenous urography, the cystocele appears as a semicircular

defect resembling a spring onion or cobra's hood seen in the bladder base. When viewed during cystography, the ureterocele appears as a dark bubble or shadow, despite surrounding contrast (Figure 12-12). The evaluation of a ureterocele should include obtaining an imaging study of the upper urinary tracts, such as an intravenous urogram or ultrasonogram, and a VCUG. The VCUG is used to classify the ureterocele as intravesical or ectopic and to identify vesicoureteral reflux or obstruction of the bladder outlet. The risk of vesicoureteral reflux is relatively high; it occurs in 50% of lower pole ureters in ectopic ureteroceles associated with ureteral duplication and in 25% of contralateral ureters. Urethral obstruction is rare among intravesical ureteroceles, and uncommon among ureteroceles; nevertheless, it is the most common cause of urethral obstruction in girls.

Imaging of the upper urinary tract is completed to characterize the results of reflux and to define

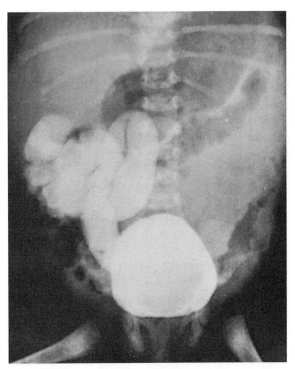

Fig. 12-12 Postvoiding film shows reflux to the lower right pole. The girl had bilateral ureteroceles, with the right one being a small ureterocele that was not demonstrated on the cystogram. (From Wein AJ, Kavoussi LR, Novick AC, Partin AW, Peters CA [eds]: Campbell-Walsh Urology, 9th edition. Philadelphia: Saunders-Elsevier, 2007, p 3401.)

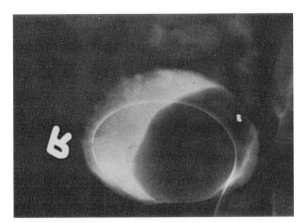

Fig. 12-11 Cystogram outlines a left ureterocele. (From Wein AJ, Kavoussi LR, Novick AC, Partin AW, Peters CA [eds]: Campbell-Walsh Urology, 9th edition. Philadelphia: Saunders-Elsevier, 2007; p 3401.)

anatomy when an ectopic ureterocele is associated with ureteral duplication. In selected cases, the urologist may perform cystoscopy to assess the orifice of the defect or as part of an endoscopic incision (unroofing) procedure.[91]

Nursing Management. The goals of ureterocele treatment include protection of urinary system function, relief of obstruction, maintenance (or restoration) of urinary continence, treatment of infection, and resolution of vesicoureteral reflux. A ureterocele may be diagnosed by prenatal ultrasound, during an imaging study for an unrelated health problem, or as the result of a urinary tract infection, hematuria, or urinary incontinence.

When diagnosed during prenatal ultrasonography, a decision must be made as to whether the infant should undergo invasive treatment designed to correct the defect, conservative treatment such as prophylactic antibiotics designed to reduce symptoms, or watchful waiting, with active surveillance and intervention only if symptoms or sequelae of obstruction occur. If the ureterocele is small, intravesicular, and not associated with hydronephrosis, watchful waiting may be recommended. Watchful waiting typically involves routine ultrasound at 3- to 6-month intervals for the first 2 years and at 6-month to 2-year intervals thereafter. In contrast, treatment of ectopic ureteroceles associated with ureteral duplication and hydroureteronephrosis may justify early treatment to reverse obstruction and reduce the risk of infection. Conservative treatment typically consists of postnatal evaluation with ultrasonography and obtaining a VCUG, as well as prophylactic antibiotic therapy if vesicoureteral reflux exists. Alternatively, if obstruction or hydronephrosis exists, more invasive therapy may be considered. Because of the infant's age and small size, some pediatric urologists advocate a minimally invasive approach, consisting of endoscopic incision (unroofing) of the cystocele or possibly endoscopic puncture using a laser. Others advocate open surgery, which may include ureteroneocystostomy or partial nephrectomy of an obstructed, poorly functioning renal segment. Longitudinal studies have provided no clear evidence favoring either approach. In one study of 52 patients with a mean follow-up of 8 years, conservative (nonsurgical) management of ectopic ureteroceles diagnosed prenatally showed that 27% experience no adverse effects.[100] Another

study compared 40 children with prenatally diagnosed ureteroceles managed with aggressive surgical intervention to 55 children whose ureteroceles were diagnosed when they were evaluated postnatally for a urinary tract infection.[101] In this study, prenatal diagnosis and early intervention decreased both the morbidity and rate of secondary procedures as compared with children whose ureteroceles were diagnosed and managed postnatally.

When a neonate with a prenatally diagnosed ureterocele is encountered, the urologic nurse should teach the parents about the signs and symptoms of urinary tract infection, regardless of the anticipated plan for managing the ureterocele. They are also taught to monitor the infant for difficulty voiding caused by partial blockage of the urethral outlet with micturition. If postnatal evaluation reveals vesicoureteral reflux, the infant is placed on prophylactic antibiotic therapy and the family is taught to administer the medication and monitor for side effects (see Chapter 14). The importance of ongoing monitoring of renal function using imaging studies is emphasized, and the possibility that a ureterocele may interfere with achievement of continence is gently introduced to the parents, particularly if the ureterocele is ectopic or large. The parents are also reassured that surgical reconstruction of an obstructing ureterocele can be undertaken if it proves obstructive or contributes to urinary incontinence.

The occurrence of a urinary tract infection is the most common reason for detection of a ureterocele in the older infant or child.[91] Initially, the urinary tract infection is treated, followed by institution of prophylactic antibiotics if vesicoureteral reflux is diagnosed. Invasive treatment of a ureterocele may be indicated, particularly if it is ectopic, associated with duplex ureters, or associated with vesicoureteral reflux or hydroureteronephrosis and obstruction.

A number of considerations influence the surgical approach in the child with a ureterocele, including the ureterocele type and size, the patient's age, presence of reflux or ureteral duplication, volume of functioning renal parenchyma, magnitude of ureteral dilation, and severity of obstruction. Three primary techniques are used for ureterocele repair—endoscopic decompression, sometimes called unroofing, open reconstruction of the ureterocele, often accompanied by ureteroneocystostomy, or partial ne-phrectomy of an obstructed and usually dysplastic renal segment.[91] More recently, a holmium laser has been used to puncture the wall of the ureterocele, producing rapid decompression with minimal bleed-ing.[102] For the child undergoing surgical repair of a ureterocele, the urologic nurse plays an essential role in teaching the patient and family about the antici-pated surgery, including preoperative and postoper-ative management. This also includes postoperative expectations concerning correction of vesicoureteral reflux. Clarifying these expectations is particularly important because certain procedures are expected to correct reflux, although endoscopic decompression may create reflux at the same time that it relieves obstruction.

Megaureter

The term *megaureter* is used to describe a dilated or wide ureter, regardless of its cause.[103] A number of classification schemes have been proposed to clarify this broad term; a functional system proposed in 1977[104] and still widely used today[91,103] will be used in this discussion (Table 12-2). Although the original schema also incorporated causes of secondary mega-ureter, this chapter will focus exclusively on congen-ital (primary) megaureter, postulated to arise from abnormal embryogenesis.

The epidemiology of megaureter is unknown; in one study of 185 neonates with urinary obstruction, 23% were found to have megaureter caused by an obstructive lesion near the ureterovesical junction.[104] In addition, it is known that the primary megaureter is four times more common in boys as compared with girls and affects only one ureter in 75% of cases. Dysplasia of the affected kidney is common and the contralateral kidney is dysplastic or hypoplas-tic in 10% to 15% of cases.[103]

Three principal causes can lead to an obstructed megaureter. In most cases, a short acontractile seg-ment of ureter exists just above the ureterovesical junction. Although this segment may have a lumen that is about the same diameter as a normal ureter, its low-compliant wall and inability to propagate a peri-staltic contraction render it functionally obstructed. The refluxing megaureter is caused by inadequate tunneling of the intravesical ureter through the blad-der wall to prevent reflux. It is sometimes associated

TABLE 12-2 Classification Schema for Primary Megaureter (Wide Ureter)

DESCRIPTION	CHARACTERISTICS
Obstructed	Congenital obstructive lesion caused by a dynamic segment at ureterovesical junction, ureteral valve, ureteral stricture
Refluxing	Ureteral dilation caused by congenital defect of ureterovesical junction resulting in vesicoureteral reflux
Nonrefluxing, unobstructed	Cause unknown; may represent resolved obstruction of ureter (obstruction followed by recannulation)

with an enlarged bladder and bilateral hydronephro-sis. The cause of the nonrefluxing unobstructed megaureter is unknown; possible causes include changes in urine production just prior to and imme-diately following birth and transient ureteral obstruc-tion that resolves with further maturation of the urinary system.[103]

Assessment. Like many urinary system defects, approximately 50% of cases are discovered on prena-tal ultrasound although the other half are detected during evaluation of microscopic hematuria, infec-tion, or a urinary calculus. When imaged on ultra-sound, the ureter may be traced from the renal pelvis to the bladder, a task that is not feasible when imag-ing a normal-sized ureter. Images of the kidney may reveal hydronephrosis and the bladder may be abnor-mally enlarged as well. On intravenous urography, the ureter will be massively dilated and tortuous, sim-ilar to the appearance of a loop of small bowel.

After identifying a wide ureter, further imaging tests are performed to determine whether obstruction and reflux are present. A VCUG or nuclear cystogram will diagnose vesicoureteral reflux of the affected or contralateral kidney. A DTPA or MAG3 radionuclide study will indicate differential renal function and may diagnose ureteral obstruction. However, these studies may not be sufficient to identify obstruction, particu-larly if the megaureter is particularly massive or associated with severe hydronephrosis. In these cases, a urodynamic study of the upper urinary tract

(Whitaker test) is done to diagnose and quantify the severity of obstruction.

Nursing Management. Because the obstructed primary megaureter threatens the growth and development of the kidney it serves, surgery is required to relieve obstruction.[91,103] Early surgery is usually advocated to minimize the damage caused by the obstruction and maximize subsequent renal growth. In contrast, when obstruction is mild or absent and vesicoureteral reflux is diagnosed, conservative therapy is initiated. Prophylactic antibiotics are begun to prevent urinary tract infection and ongoing monitoring of upper urinary tract function is instituted. The parents are taught to monitor their infant for signs and symptoms of urinary tract infection. In addition to education about the causes and treatment options for megaureter, the urologic nurse teaches the family about the dosage and administration of suppressive antibiotics and the significance of ongoing monitoring of renal function via ultrasonography or radionuclide scanning. Parents also benefit from reassurance that in the absence of obstruction, a megaureter does not compromise renal function or the growth and development of the kidney.

In some cases, a nonrefluxing unobstructed megaureter may be diagnosed in an older child or adult. In this case, no medical intervention is warranted, but the nurse should teach the family to monitor their child for signs and symptoms of urinary tract infection. The urologic nurse should counsel the parents of an infant or younger child or infant who is diagnosed with an unobstructed nonrefluxing megaureter that repeat monitoring of the urinary system using ultrasonography or radionuclide scanning will be necessary. They can also be reassured that dilation of the ureter often diminishes with time and maturation of the urinary system.

Vesicoureteral Reflux

Vesicoureteral reflux occurs when a defect of the ureterovesical junction causes retrograde movement of urine from the lower to upper urinary tracts. Retrograde urine flow caused by a congenital defect in the ureterovesical junction development is called primary reflux and cases attributable to obstruction or voiding dysfunction are described as secondary. See Chapter 14 for a detailed discussion of vesicoureteral reflux and its relationship to urinary tract infection and renal growth and development.

ANOMALIES OF THE BLADDER AND URETHRA

Prior to week 5 of normal embryogenesis, the urinary, reproductive, and gastrointestinal structures empty into a common cloacal chamber. Separation of these chambers is complex and relies in part on regression of the cloacal membrane through apoptosis during a critical time frame. Migration of mesoderm between the ectoderm, which will evolve into the anterior abdominal wall, and the endoderm, which will evolve into abdominal or pelvic organs, will cause premature rupture of the cloaca.[105] Some researchers have hypothesized that early rupture of the cloacal membrane results in cloacal exstrophy, now called OEIS (omphalocele, imperforate anus, exstrophy, and spinal defects), although later rupture leads to a milder form, resulting in classic bladder exstrophy in the absence of these other defects.[106] In contrast, others believe that OEIS is a distinctive defect.

Cloacal exstrophy (OEIS) is a very rare and particularly severe anomaly that includes omphalocele (failure of abdominal wall closure with externalization of the bowel), bladder exstrophy (externalized bladder that does not close into its normal spherical configuration), imperforate anus (defect of the rectum, anus, and pelvic floor support structures), pelvic bone defects (diastasis or widening of the pubic bones), and spinal defects (myelomeningocele).[107] Defects are also common in the prenatal development of the cardiovascular and pulmonary systems, as well as the craniofacial structures. Cloacal exstrophy is rare, occurring once in every 200,000 to 400,000 births,[108] and discussions of nursing management in this chapter will be limited to the comparatively more common defects, bladder exstrophy and epispadias.

Bladder Exstrophy and Epispadias

Bladder exstrophy, sometimes called classic exstrophy, is a more common defect of pelvic chamber separation and lower urinary tract development seen in 1 in 10,000 to 50,000 births.[106,109] It is characterized by externalization of the posterior bladder wall, with failure of organ closure (Figure 12-13). Boys are more commonly affected than girls (4:1 male to female). The bladder neck is open and the urethra is splayed (spread open) to the level of the bladder outlet (epispadias). In the boy, the penis is

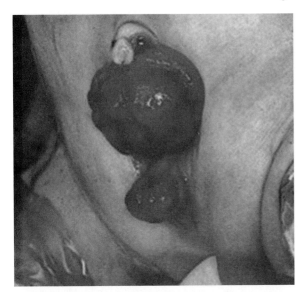

Fig. 12-13 Bladder exstrophy in a male demonstrating externalization of the posterior bladder wall, splaying of the urethra, and a bifid scrotum. (From Wein AJ, Kavoussi LR, Novick AC, Partin AW, Peters CA [eds]: Campbell-Walsh Urology, 9th edition. Philadelphia: Saunders-Elsevier, 2007, p 3401.)

broad and shortened, the cavernous bodies are also splayed, and the dorsum of the penis usually contains a chordee (fibrous band). The distance between the penis and scrotum is abnormally long and the scrotum is widened. The ejaculatory ducts and seminal vesicles are unaffected in most cases, but abnormalities of the bladder and proximal urethra predispose males to retrograde ejaculation and impaired fertility.

Girls with exstrophy also have externalization of the urinary bladder and a splayed urethra, leading to continuous urinary incontinence in addition to a bifid clitoris, depressed mons pubis, and widely separated labia majora and minora.[110] The labia minora are often poorly formed but the vagina and female reproductive organs remain intact.

Both genders have a widened symphysis pubis (pelvic diastasis). When severe, it affects normal gait and pelvic floor support structures, including the levator ani muscle and endopelvic fascia. Absence of the umbilicus also occurs. While its absence may appear trivial to parents, physicians, or nurses, it is often considered disfiguring by patients with bladder exstrophy.

Epispadias is a more limited but significant defect that is clearly related to classic exstrophy and possibly to OEIS.[106,109] It is characterized by failure of urethral closure to the level of the bladder neck. In this case, the entire urethra is splayed and the overlying skin is open, rendering the urethral sphincter mechanism nonfunctional. The bladder body is preserved, but continuous urinary incontinence is an inevitable result and bladder capacity is compromised because of chronic urine loss. Defects of the external genitalia are similar to those seen in classic exstrophy. The incidence of isolated epispadias is 2.4 in 100,000 births[111]; most cases are associated with exstrophy. Female exstrophy is more rare, occurring in approximately 1 in 480,000 live births,[112] a figure that has not changed.

Assessment. Prenatal ultrasound performed between weeks 16 and 20 can detect the presence of bladder exstrophy.[113] This is seen as absence of the urinary bladder, low-set umbilical cord, semisolid mass protruding from the abdominal wall, widened iliac crests, and/or anteriorly displaced scrotum and small penis in males. At birth, physical examination will reveal externalization of the bladder, pelvic diastasis, and characteristic malformations of the external genitalia.

Nursing Management. Caring for the patient with exstrophy requires multiple staged surgical reconstruction procedures and ongoing care of the many sequelae associated with this complex and challenging anomaly. Ideally, parental counseling and planning for care begin during the prenatal period or immediately following birth. It continues throughout the life of the patient and focuses around several goals, including protection of the exposed bladder mucosa, protection of the perineal skin, establishing urinary continence, prevention and management of urinary tract infections, repair of pelvic bone defects to ensure optimal gait and pelvic girdle function, repair of genital defects, and psychosocial support of the child and family.

The urologic nurse often interacts with the parents of a child with exstrophy prior to birth. Counseling with a pediatric urologist who will manage the child's exstrophy following birth is strongly recommended. This session is likely to include discussion of anticipated outcomes of exstrophy, including continuous urinary incontinence during early life and the likelihood that continence may remain a challenge throughout childhood. The significance of pelvic diastasis and a rationale for early treatment with traction or osteotomies is explained, and the impact of the

TABLE 12-3 Staged Surgical Management of the Child with Bladder Exstrophy[109,110,113,114]

APPROXIMATE AGE	PROCEDURE	DESCRIPTION
First days of life	Bladder reconstruction (Jeffs procedure, Mitchell repair; single-stage closure and epispadias repair)	Bladder internalized and closed (reconstructed to its typical spherical shape); epispadias repair also may be completed at this stage
First days of life (older than 72 hr)	Osteotomy	Open surgical correction of pelvic diastasis; nonsurgical approaches advocated in some cases
12-18 mo	Corporal lengthening and urethroplasty in boys (modified Cantwell-Ransley repair, Mitchell penile disassembly technique)	Corpora cavernosa lengthened, urethra tubularized (epispadias repair), but no attempt made to construct functional sphincter mechanism
12-18 mo	Urethroplasty, vulvoplasty, and clitoroplasty in girls	Urethra tubularized to repair epispadias; repair of vulva and clitoris may be completed by plastic surgeon with expertise in genital reconstruction
4-8 yr	Young-Dees-Leadbetter procedure	Bladder neck constructed from bladder base; urethral angle with respect to bladder may be altered to maximize continence
4 yr or older	Additional surgical procedures when primary closure and bladder neck reconstruction are not adequate to preserve renal function and ensure continence	• Repeat repair of dehiscence of primary bladder closure in cases of dehiscence • Repeat bladder neck reconstruction to enhance urethral closure and continence further • Suburethral collagen injection to promote urethral closure and continence • Artificial urinary sphincter to enhance urethral closure and continence • Bladder neck closure with appendicovesicostomy to enhance continence if above procedures fail to achieve adequate continence • Augmentation enterocystoplasty to enhance bladder capacity, alleviate low bladder wall compliance, and preserve renal function • Continent urinary diversion if above procedures fail to provide adequate bladder wall compliance and sufficient continence

disorder on sexual function and fertility in boys is presented. When educating parents of a girl, parents are counseled that internal reproductive organs are not usually affected but that structures of pelvic support are compromised, rendering the patient at higher risk for uterine prolapse. The pediatric urologist will outline a typical strategy for staged surgical intervention (Table 12-3), emphasizing that the approach to each child must be individualized.[109,110,113,114]

Learning that an expected child has a significant anomaly is emotionally distressing and this anxiety, when combined with the complexity of the care required to manage this defect, can overwhelm the parents. In our experience, parents frequently contact the urologic nurse by telephone, requesting clarification of information presented during initial counseling and to ask additional questions. The urologic nurse can optimize parents' ability to comprehend and retain information by providing written materials and websites that summarize the information provided and by reinforcing information given during any subsequent telephone conversations. Nevertheless, although it is important to reinforce information and reassure the parents that exstrophy is not associated with a poor or guarded prognosis, it is also important to avoid predicting outcomes related to continence, fertility, or severity of the defects because these are highly individualized.

The surgical management of bladder exstrophy is complex and requires a staged procedure approach.[115] Table 12-3 outlines a typical schedule of surgeries for the child with exstrophy. Physical care of the child with exstrophy begins at birth. The bladder mucosa should be covered with a protective barrier to prevent drying and scarring prior to initial surgical closure. Plastic wrap has been advocated, but a thin-film hydrated gel dressing protects the bladder mucosa and prevents dehydration.[109] The dressing is changed on a daily basis. Antibiotic therapy is usually administered prior to initial closure and osteotomy during the first week of life. Following initial closure, the child may have ureteral stents placed to allow the bladder to heal prior to filling with urine and an indwelling catheter. The stents and catheter should be securely fixed after surgery to avoid traction against suture lines.

Prolonged immobilization of the pelvis is recommended; the child may have a spica cast and soft or fixed traction may be applied for approximately 3 weeks. The urologic nurse should regularly monitor the newborn for abdominal distention and promptly contact the physician if distention occurs, because this places traction on and threatens the anatomic integrity of the bladder closure.

A successful outcome to initial closure surgery is also enhanced by adequate pain control and nutritional intake. The urologic nurse should closely monitor the neonate for postoperative pain and administer analgesics on a routine schedule in consultation with physician during the initial postoperative period. Consultation with a nutritionist may be indicated if the newborn does not feed well, because inadequate nutrition slows healing and threatens the integrity of the newly created anastomotic sites in the bladder and urethra.

Following initial closure, the urologic nurse should advise parents that their child will leak urine on a relatively continuous basis, given the absence of a functional sphincter mechanism. Judicious use of moisture barriers, combined with routine diaper changes and skin cleansing, will minimize the risk of perineal dermatitis from excessive urine exposure. Parents also should be taught that the relative risk of occasional perineal dermatitis is high because of the presence of continuous urine dribbling and does not indicate poor care of the child.

Parents are taught to recognize signs and symptoms of a urinary tract infection and the need for ongoing monitoring of urinary tract function by a pediatric urologist. As the child reaches age 12 to 18 months, education about genital repair and urethral reconstruction is provided. Parents are again reminded that this procedure is not intended to achieve continence, but will improve the appearance of the external genitalia and tubularize the urethra.

When the child is 4 to 8 years of age, the family is prepared for bladder neck reconstruction. The parents and child are advised that the surgery is designed to improve continence, although complete bladder control often is not achieved by a single procedure. They are further counseled that an indwelling catheter will be left in place for approximately 2 to 4 weeks after surgery to promote healing of the reconstructed bladder neck and proximal urethra.

Beginning early in life, and continuing throughout childhood, adolescence, and adulthood, patients with exstrophy and their families often rely on the urologic nurse to address psychosocial concerns related to exstrophy. Concerns about self-care and body image deficits often present in younger children and may persist into adolescence. Given these issues, and the need for multiple reparative surgeries, it is not surprising that children with exstrophy often experience significant anxiety disorders that affect family interactions, school performance, and social relationships.[116] The urologic nurse should encourage parents to express feelings about guilt or anxiety related to caring for a child with exstrophy, combined with reassurances that these feelings are common and have no negative ramifications. Parents may be encouraged to teach the child to participate in self-care and family tasks within the child's abilities to maximize the patient's self-esteem. Issues related to body image and sexual function often become apparent during adolescence.[117] Encouraging the patient to express feelings related to self-image, combined with professional counseling in selected cases, enables the adolescent to grapple with the special challenges presented by a birth defect that affects the external genitalia. From a urologic perspective, the nurse can also act as an advocate for the patient, encouraging aggressive management of continence and preservation of renal function by ensuring that adequate consideration is given to plastic reconstruction of the genitalia when planning care (including construction of an umbilicus) and by acting as an empathetic listener when patients, parents, and siblings express feelings and fears related to this challenging disorder.

Longitudinal data concerning the outcomes of patients with exstrophy or epispadias are generally encouraging.[113,117] Continence rates in adolescents and adults vary from 67% to 95% when patients with urinary diversions are included. Although studies measuring quality of life and psychological adjustment have demonstrated challenges and problems in many children and adolescents, adults with exstrophy tend to report good psychosocial adjustment, high employment rates, and integration into family life. Most adult men with exstrophy report engaging in sexual activity (53% to 100%), although documented fertility rates are lower (4% to 20%). Women with exstrophy are capable of becoming pregnant and bearing children; they should be advised of their increased risk for pelvic organ prolapse and of the possibility of requiring cesarean section when delivering a child.

Urethral Obstruction: Urethral Valves and Polyps

A urethral valve is a thin membrane of tissue that occludes the urethral lumen and obstructs urinary outflow in males.[118] Three types of valves have been described.[119] A type I valve is a thin membrane of tissue that arises from the posterior edge of the verumontanum and terminates near the proximal border of the membranous urethra. A type III valve is a ringlike membrane of tissue located just distal to the verumontanum. Type II valves have been described as obstructing urethral folds, but they are no longer considered to be a clinically relevant entity.[118] The embryonic origin of the type I valve is unclear but the type III valve is known to represent incomplete regression of the urogenital membrane. The incidence of urethral valves is estimated as between 1 in 8000 to 25,000 live births.[120] Most of these (95%) are type I and 5% are type III valves. Urethral valves almost always lead to significant

adverse effects, including ureterohydronephrosis. In some patients, compromised prenatal renal function causes oligohydramnios and pulmonary hypoplasia.

Other congenital causes of urethral obstruction include anterior urethral valves[121] and prostatic urethral polyps. Anterior valves are structurally similar to those located in the posterior urethra, except that they occur in the anterior urethra, which is embryologically distinct from its posterior portion. They are extremely rare and associated with a urethral diverticulum. Our knowledge of this condition arises primarily from case reports. The largest single experience reported 17 subjects.[122]

Congenital polyps are also a rare cause of urethral obstruction. Researchers from the Mayo Clinic reviewed all records of children diagnosed with urethral polyps between 1957 and 1992 and identified only 12 cases.[123] They were found most commonly in boys and were located in the posterior urethra or at the verumontanum, composed of fibroepithelial tissue. Polyps are even rarer in girls; as of 2008, less than 10 cases had been published in the medical literature.[124] Two of the polyps were transitional cell epithelium, fibroepithelial tissue, and an inflamed periurethral gland.

The clinical relevance of these anomalies is directly related to the severity of the obstruction that they produce. Lesions that provide severe obstruction, such as posterior urethral valves, compromise both upper and lower urinary tract function, and there is growing evidence that the adverse effects persist over time, despite successful relief of the obstructive lesion during early life.[125] The term *valve bladder syndrome* has been used to describe the deleterious effects of congenital urethral obstruction.[118,125] This syndrome is characterized by renal tubular dysfunction caused by damage during embryogenesis. As a result, patients with valve bladder syndrome have urine-concentrating defects, causing them to produce as much as 3 L of urine/day. This polyuria leads to frequent daytime voiding frequency, nocturia or enuresis, and diurnal urgency or urge urinary incontinence. In addition, chronically high intravesical volumes tend to overdistend the bladder and promote decompensation of the detrusor muscle. Ureteral peristalsis is also impaired because of a combination of dilation and ureteral wall scarring secondary to infection or iatrogenic causes. Finally, the bladder itself tends to be of low compliance, with diminished sensations of bladder filling and compromised contractility. This predisposes the patient to incomplete bladder emptying, which further compromises the upper urinary tract because intravesical pressures remain elevated, despite micturition.

Assessment. Because of the progressively deleterious effects of urethral obstruction during embryogenesis, the diagnosis is ideally established during the prenatal period. Posterior urethral valves are suspected when prenatal ultrasound in a male fetus reveals pelvicaliectasis, dilation of the entire ureteral length, and a large bladder.[126] These findings, however, do not necessarily indicate valves as the underlying cause of the obstruction.[127] Ultrasonic identification of a dilated posterior urethra (keyhole sign) and analysis of the fetal urine increase the accuracy of prenatal diagnosis.

After birth, the neonate with posterior urethral valves usually has a palpable abdominal mass caused by enlargement of the bladder (megacystis) and hydroureteronephrosis of the upper urinary tracts. Micturition, which usually occurs during the first hours of life and should occur in all infants within the first 12 to 24 hours, is often delayed. The urinary stream will be weak and the neonate may strain or grunt when voiding. Assessment of the neonate also includes an evaluation of pulmonary function, which may be compromised if obstruction has been severe and is associated with oligohydramnios.

The diagnosis is confirmed by the VCUG, with careful imaging of the posterior urethra. Posterior urethral valves are visualized as thin wisps of tissue as they fold down and obstruct the urethra during micturition (Figure 12-14); ideal views are obtained just after the start of voiding and after removal of the filling catheter. Dilation of the proximal urethra, just proximal to the valves, is also common. The VCUG is also used to grade vesicoureteral reflux, identify the severity of trabeculation, assess postvoid urinary residual, and detect diverticula that may serve as an energy dissipation chamber and protect the upper urinary tracts. Additional imaging studies include ultrasonography to assess the severity of hydronephrosis and parenchymal volume. A MAG3 radionuclide study is performed to evaluate differential renal function and drainage.[126]

Diagnosis of posterior urethral valves is sometimes not made until later in life. These children may be diagnosed with signs and symptoms of renal

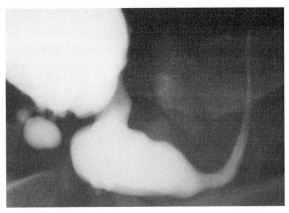

Fig. 12-14 Voiding cystourethrogram demonstrating posterior urethral valves in a male infant. Note the dilation of the posterior urethra and bladder diverticulum. (From Wein AJ, Kavoussi LR, Novick AC, Partin AW, Peters CA [eds]: Campbell-Walsh Urology, 9th edition. Philadelphia: Saunders, 2007; p 3586.)

insufficiency, although most present with lower urinary tract symptoms, including urinary incontinence, poor force of stream, and incomplete bladder emptying.[128] When compared with a group of children diagnosed at birth, they were found to be less likely to experience detrusor overactivity, but their renal function was no less compromised than those diagnosed during infancy.

Anterior urethral valves associated with severe bladder outlet obstruction produce similar clinical manifestations as those seen with posterior valves.[121] Their cause is unknown but it has been hypothesized that the distal lip of a ruptured syringocele may function as a flap valve, leading to anterior urethral obstruction.[129] In contrast to posterior urethral valves, anterior valves tend to produce milder obstruction and often escape detection during the neonatal period. Instead, they are typically diagnosed when evaluating the older child who presents with recurring urinary tract infections, urinary incontinence, or a poor urinary stream.[121]

Urethral polyps also may cause severe obstruction and clinical manifestations similar to those of posterior valves. Because of their rarity, they are often initially diagnosed as urethral valves. However, in addition to obstructive lower urinary tract symptoms, they frequently produce hematuria and are rarely seen in girls.[123] A VCUG will differentiate a urethral polyp from a valve, and a definitive diagnosis is confirmed by cystoscopy.

Clinical manifestations of the valve bladder syndrome include daytime voiding frequency and enuresis, particularly in younger boys, or nocturia, more common in older boys. Bothersome urgency and urge urinary incontinence are common. Results of a bladder log (voiding diary) usually reveal frequent micturition, large voided volumes, and high-volume fluid intake. Urodynamic testing is critical to the ongoing assessment of valve bladder syndrome, accompanied by ongoing monitoring of renal function using ultrasonography, radionuclide studies, and serum creatinine level measurement.[118,125] Urodynamic testing is used to determine bladder capacity and bladder wall compliance, identify any residual obstruction, and determine the cause of incomplete bladder emptying and urinary incontinence. Imaging studies and serum creatinine level determination are used to monitor renal function, which is often compromised from birth because of prenatal obstruction.

Nursing Management. Valve bladder syndrome has been reported to exist in varying degrees of severity in most patients diagnosed with posterior urethral valves and in some persons with anterior valves or urethral polyps. Left untreated, this syndrome can lead to renal failure, despite successful diversion and eventual ablation of obstruction during childhood.[130] Therefore, urologic management focuses both on immediate removal of the obstructive lesion and ongoing assessment and intervention designed to preserve renal function and prevent the deleterious effects associated with valve bladder syndrome.

Immediate management of congenital urethral obstruction focuses on removing the obstruction. Endoscopic ablation of urethral valves or a polyp is the treatment of choice.[126] A 7-French cystoscope with a 2- or 3-French working port is preferred for the procedure because it allows adequate visualization and access to the posterior urethra of most neonates, even when premature. Antibiotic prophylaxis is typically begun prior to the procedure and is extended for a brief period after treatment to prevent urinary infection. A transient indwelling catheter will be placed during the procedure; it usually remains in place for 24 to 48 hours. When the catheter is in place, the urologic nurse should monitor urine output and patency. Parents are advised that urine may be pink or blood-tinged, but that passage of bright red blood or clots is not expected and should be reported to the physician promptly. It is important to monitor the patient's urinary elimination after catheter removal, preferably by direct observation of the urinary stream.

Vesicostomy is the creation of a small vesicocutaneous fistula that bypasses the bladder outlet and allows urine to drain directly into a diaper placed relatively high on the infant's lower abdomen. It provides good urine drainage and bypasses the obstructing valves. However, it has been associated with higher creatinine levels and shorter stature patients when compared with those treated with primary valve ablation.[131] Therefore, it is now performed only in infants who are unable to tolerate primary valve ablation. In selected cases, the pediatric urologist may elect to perform a high diversion, such as a cutaneous ureterostomy or pyelostomy.[132] However, the indications for this procedure remain controversial, particularly in regard to its ability to minimize renal damage.[126]

Nursing management of the patient with a vesicostomy or higher urinary diversion focuses on assessment of patency of the cutaneous diversion, adapting diapering techniques to contain urine output from the diversion, and protection of the adjacent skin. Creation of a vesicostomy is associated with very minimal blood loss, and the urine is anticipated to be pink-tinged only. Passage of clots is unexpected and parents are advised to promptly contact the physician if this occurs. For the infant with a vesicostomy, a slightly large diaper with a high front is typically adequate to contain urine output. Cutaneous ureterostomies or pyelostomies terminate higher on the abdomen or on the flank and often require the use of two diapers. One is placed over the perineal area as usual, and a second is cut, attached to the primary diaper, and used to cover the cutaneous diversion. Parents are counseled that incontinence-associated diaper dermatitis can occur over any area that is covered by a containment device and exposed to urine. They are also advised that exposure of adjacent skin to continuous urine leakage from the diversion increases the risk of dermatitis. Regular diaper changes, combined with gentle cleansing with a perineal cleanser containing a moisturizer—as compared with scrubbing with soap and water—and application of a skin protectant, will prevent or reduce the severity of moisture-related skin damage commonly associated with a cutaneous diversion.

Following initial management or bypass of the obstructive lesion, the focus of care shifts to the prevention of complications and preservation of optimal renal function. The urologic nurse should emphasize that ongoing monitoring of renal function, using a combination of imaging studies and blood tests, is critical to the child's long-term health, even after the initial obstruction has been successfully eliminated. Parents are taught the signs and symptoms of urinary tract infection and expectations concerning mastery of urinary continence. In addition, some researchers now advocate aggressive bladder emptying via scheduled daytime voiding and nocturnal emptying, either arising from sleep to urinate or intermittent catheterization once during the early morning hours, to minimize the deleterious effects of polyuria.[133] Children with valve bladder syndrome and incomplete bladder emptying should be taught a double-voiding technique (micturition, followed by a 2- to 3-minute rest period and repeated urination) or intermittent catheterization if double-voiding is not effective. Overnight catheter drainage may improve daytime urinary incontinence, diminish urinary tract infection frequency, and slow or arrest renal deterioration.[134]

Megalourethra and Ureteral Duplication

Megalourethra is an abnormal dilation of the distal urethra in males; its cause is unknown.[126] It may arise from abnormal tubularization of the distal urethral folds. It may be associated with obstruction in certain cases; surgical repair is indicated when a megalourethra produces voiding dysfunction or obstruction.

Urethral duplications are very rare; approximately 175 cases have been reported in the medical literature.[135] Several types occur; the most common is an incomplete duplication with a blind channel in addition to a urethra traveling from the bladder to the penis.[136] Less common types include complete urethral duplication, leading to a single or two distinct meatus, and complete caudal duplication, involving duplication of the penis. Careful exploration of each urethra is necessary prior to surgical reconstruction of this rare anomaly.

Hypospadias

Hypospadias is an abnormal opening of the male urethra distal to the sphincter mechanism.[137] The position of this opening varies significantly. Distal hypospadias affects the glans penis just proximal to the location of the normal meatus, and distal hypospadias defects are found at the penoscrotal junction or perineum just beneath the scrotum. Hypospadias may be associated with a chordee, a fibrous band causing ventral curvature of the penis. The risk of an associated chordee is highest when the opening is proximal to the normal location of the meatus. The incidence of hypospadias is approximately 1 in 250 to 300 births. However, the incidence of hypospadias is rising, possibly because of the use of chemicals that exert antiandrogenic activity over the developing fetus,[138] an increase in premature births,[139] use of an intracytoplasmic sperm injection (ICSI) to achieve pregnancy,[140] advanced maternal age at the time of delivery,[141] or maternal gestational diabetes.[142] In addition to these risk factors, hypospadias shows both familial and racial predispositions, and genetic factors are hypothesized to play an important causative role.

The severity of hypospadias is determined by the location of the urethral meatus and the magnitude of penile angulation noted when erect.[143] First-degree hypospadias is characterized by a urethral meatus that lies within the glans penis; it is typically located on its dorsal aspect in the nonerect penis. Second-degree hypospadias is characterized by a urethral meatus on the penile shaft and a third-degree defect is located between the penoscrotal junction and perineum (Figure 12-15). Approximately 80% are first-degree, 15% are second-degree, and 5% are third-degree hypospadias. Specific intersex states are associated with hypospadias, including adrenogenital syndrome, mixed gonadal dysgenesis, true hermaphroditism, and male pseudohermaphroditism. Boys with hypospadias are also at increased risk for cryptorchidism and the presence of a prostatic utricle.

Assessment. With increasing sophistication in prenatal ultrasound, a growing number of cases of hypospadias are now diagnosed prior to birth.[144] Nevertheless, because hypospadias is a subtle defect and not associated with obstruction, it is often initially detected on newborn examination. Abnormality of the foreskin is often seen on initial inspection, followed by careful examination of the glans penis, penile shaft, penoscrotal junction, and perineum for a urethral meatus. A careful examination is demanded because the meatus is often the size of a pinhole, although it does not obstruct urine outflow. Direct observation of the

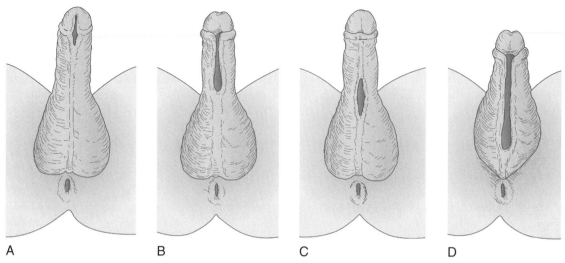

Fig. 12-15 Classification of hypospadias. **A,** Glandular (first degree). **B,** Coronal (second degree). **C, D,** Penoscrotal or perineal (third degree). (From Carlson B: Human Embryology and Developmental Biology, 3rd edition. St Louis: Mosby, 2005; p 424.)

urinary stream may be helpful for diagnosis, but imaging studies of the upper urinary tracts are not indicated unless the child has additional signs or symptoms suggesting urinary obstruction or hydronephrosis. After locating the meatus, the examiner evaluates the infant for cryptorchidism or signs of an intersex state.

Nursing Management. Left unrepaired, a hypospadias interferes with urination, causing a downward stream rather than the normal stream from the tip of the glans penis, and it impedes fertility potential. Therefore, surgical repair is considered necessary.[144] Surgical reconstruction of hypospadias incorporates three principal components—correction of chordee, urethral reconstruction and location of the meatus in its normal position, and cosmetic reconstruction of the penis itself.[143,145,146] Over 300 different procedures have been described, but one-stage procedures are generally preferred for most cases of first- and second-degree hypospadias, although third-degree defects are typically managed with more complicated procedures by a pediatric urologist with extensive experience in this type of procedure. Complications associated with hypospadias repair include persistence of the chordee, meatal stenosis, hair growth within the urethra (when hair-bearing skin is used for urethral reconstruction), fistulae, and urethroceles. Fistulae are particularly problematic, with 20% of patients experiencing

a fistula after initial repair and 25% experiencing persistence or recurrence after two repairs.[146]

During the immediate postoperative period, the child will have a relatively bulky perineal dressing and a suprapubic catheter. The penis itself may be wrapped by gauze and surrounded by a self-adhering elastic tape, and the bed sheet may be placed on a semicircular frame to prevent the contact of bed clothing with the surgical area. The urologic nurse monitors the catheter for patency and the urine for signs of excessive bleeding. The dressing is regularly assessed for environmental contamination, but dressing changes are done only in consultation with the physician. Younger children may require restraints to prevent inadvertent contact with the dressings or suprapubic tube. In rare cases, the suprapubic tube may become dislodged. If this occurs, the urologic nurse must contact the physician but no efforts to replace the tube or insert a urethral catheter should be made without consulting with the urologist.

In addition to providing physical care for the child undergoing surgical repair of hypospadias, nursing management of these children focuses on addressing psychosocial concerns of the patient and family. At the time of initial diagnosis, the urologic nurse can reassure the parents that surgical repair is expected to correct voiding problems, restore a normal appearance to the penis, and restore normal fertility potential.

The timing of surgical repair is individualized, but it is typically scheduled between 6 and 18 months.[147] This is based on a number of considerations, including anesthetic risks, technical surgical considerations, and psychological implications for the child and family. Families can be further reassured that hypospadias repair has not been found to be associated with deleterious effects on psychosexual development during later childhood[148] or adulthood.[149,150]

Although the vast majority of children with hypospadias are successfully managed during infancy or early childhood, a small but clinically relevant minority will undergo multiple unsuccessful surgical repairs into late adolescence or adulthood.[151] Sometimes mislabeled as *hypospadias cripples*, these individuals may experience persistent hypospadias defects, fistulae, urethral strictures, penile curvature, or stones. Surgical repair after many previous surgeries is technically challenging and the risk of additional complications is high. Therefore, patients seeking additional management should be referred to a urologist with significant clinical expertise and experience in this challenging practice area.

Intersex and Genital Anomalies

The term *intersex* refers to any infant born with ambiguous genitalia.[152] Intersex anomalies may represent an abnormality of chromosomal gender or phenotypic sex. They are classified according to genotypic and phenotypic characteristics. A hermaphrodite is an infant with both ovarian and testicular tissue. In contrast, a pseudohermaphrodite has ambiguous genitalia, with exclusively ovarian tissue. Similarly, a pseudohermaphrodite has indistinct genitalia but exclusive testicular tissue. Mixed gonadal dysgenesis refers to an infant with testicular tissue and streaks of ovarian tissue, and gonadal dysgenesis indicates streaks of both testicular and ovarian tissue. Female pseudohermaphroditism occurs in approximately 1 in 5000 to 15,000 live births, and male pseudohermaphroditism is diagnosed in 1 in 20,000 to 64,000 live births. True hermaphroditism and mixed gonadal dysgenesis are comparatively rare; their incidence is unknown.

Female pseudohermaphroditism is the most common form of intersex anomaly; more than 95% of cases are caused by congenital adrenal hyperplasia investing the clitoris and labia majora, with features that resemble a penis and scrotal folds, respectively

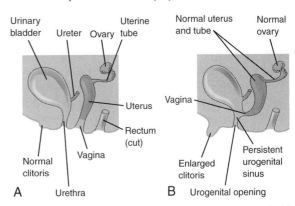

Fig. 12-16 Female pseudohermaphroditism in a 6-year-old girl caused by congenital adrenal hyperplasia. (From Moore K, Persaud TVN: The Developing Human, 7th edition. Philadelphia: Saunders, 2003; p 317.)

(Figure 12-16). Despite these external features, these infants are chromosomal females, with a 46XX genotype. Additional causes of female pseudohermaphroditism include excessive maternal androgens, virilizing tumors in the mother, or idiopathic cases.

A male pseudohermaphrodite has a 46XY genotype and exclusively testicular tissue, but the external genitalia show incomplete development.[153] Causes of male pseudohermaphroditism include gonadotrophic failure resulting from enzymatic defects blocking the conversion of androsterone to testosterone, Leydig cell agenesis, and 5α-reductase deficiencies. Additional causes include complete or partial androgen insensitivity caused by receptor or postreceptor defects, dysgenetic testes, and persistent müllerian duct syndrome. The underlying cause profoundly affects the prognosis for gender assignment, fertility potential, and the characteristics of reproductive organs in the male pseudohermaphrodite. For example, males with complete androgen insensitivity are likely to have external genitalia that are so completely feminized that their chromosomal gender is rarely recognized at birth. Instead, male pseudohermaphroditism is discovered incidentally when a testis is found within an inguinal hernia. In contrast, the clinical manifestations of incomplete androgen insensitivity vary from totally feminized external genitalia to male-appearing genitalia. In the latter case, the diagnosis is made when these males experience infertility and gynecomastia as they reach early adulthood.

Anomalies other than those related to intersex disorders may affect the embryonic development of the male reproductive system.[152] For example, the scrotum may be hypoplastic or may develop in an ectopic position, such as the inner thigh, perineum, or pubic region lateral to the penis. These defects usually present as an added feature to a more common and clinically relevant anomaly, such as bilateral undescended testes associated with scrotal hypoplasia or cloacal exstrophy associated with scrotal ectopia. Similarly, a bifid scrotum is a rare isolated defect; instead, it is usually present in intersex states.

Unilateral absence or atresia of the vas deferens occurs in approximately 1% of births. Bilateral absence is more rare; it is seen in about 10% of men undergoing evaluation for infertility with azoospermia. It is also associated with absence of the epididymis. In addition to an association with defects of the vas deferens, congenital anomalies of the epididymis also may occur in males with undescended testes, particularly when the testes are located in an intraabdominal position.

Assessment. Certain intersex states may be detected on prenatal ultrasonography,[154] but most cases are detected during newborn examination. The diagnosis of an intersex state begins with a physical examination of the newborn's genitalia.[152] The size and the shape of the penis are carefully observed, because a well-developed penis suggests adequate (or high) circulating levels of androgens and the presence of 5α-reductase receptors in the genitalia. The position of the urethral meatus is observed, particularly because of the relationship between hypospadias and intersex states. Scrotal presence and symmetry are also inspected, because asymmetry generally indicates the presence of at least one functioning testis. The neonate's skin is examined for abnormal pigmentation, particularly of the areola of the nipples or genitalia, possibly indicating hyperpigmentation caused by adrenal hyperplasia. The abdomen is palpated for masses, possibly indicating imperforate anus or cloacal defects. Although this evaluation may strongly suggest a diagnosis, the urologic nurse is strongly cautioned against referring to the child with an intersex state by any term that implies a male or female identity, or speculating on the probable diagnosis before a definitive diagnosis and plan of care have been promulgated. A careful family history also provides valuable clues to a possible diagnosis. Parents are queried about genital defects in the father or infertility in either parent, a sibling, or other close relatives.

After the history and physical examination, a buccal smear is obtained to elucidate genotypic gender. The sample is examined to identify the presence of a Barr body, indicating an inactive second X chromosome. Alternatively, fluorescein staining may be used to detect the presence of a Y chromosome. Although these tests are useful for screening, complete karyotype studies are indicated when evaluating a neonate with an intersex state.

Laboratory studies for the newborn with ambiguous genitalia include metabolic studies to evaluate for hypoglycemia, hyponatremia, hyperkalemia, or metabolic acidosis. The presence of these disorders increases the likelihood of congenital adrenal hyperplasia leading to female pseudohermaphroditism, particularly when the buccal smear shows no evidence of an active Y chromosome. The physician also may order endocrine studies, including a human chorionic gonadotropin stimulation test in newborns with nonpalpable gonads and abnormal testosterone levels.

An abdominopelvic ultrasonogram is obtained to determine the presence and location of gonadal tissue and to identify müllerian structures lying behind the bladder. Radiographic imaging of the vagina may be combined with a VCUG to determine the presence of a vagina, its size and configuration, and its relationship to any urogenital sinus.

Endoscopic examination of the vagina and bladder also may be carried out, particularly prior to any surgical reconstruction. Gonadal biopsy, laparoscopy, or laparotomy may be done in selected cases.

Nursing Management. Management of the child with ambiguous genitalia begins at the time of initial diagnosis and is multidisciplinary.[155] Gender is perhaps the most basic category applied by humans to identify others and it is natural for parents to "assign" a gender to their child. However, it is important for the urologic nurse to avoid any gender assignment until the evaluation is completed and a plan of care is formulated. Although gender-specific labels such as he or she are avoided, any dehumanizing reference, such as "it," is always avoided.

Female pseudohermaphroditism may be managed medically with hydrocortisone.[156] Administration of hydrocortisone replaces corticosteroid deficiencies and prevents overstimulation of the adrenals by adrenocorticotropin-stimulating hormone (ACTH). For hyponatremic infants, sometimes called salt wasters, or those with abnormally elevated renin levels, mineralocorticoid therapy with 9α-fluorohydrocortisone is indicated. Medical treatment is combined with feminizing surgery at an early age.[152] If the mother of a child with female pseudohermaphroditism becomes pregnant again, treatment with dexamethasone, initiated during the fifth week of pregnancy, will reduce the risk of abnormal virilization of subsequent girls.

The indications for surgical repair in children with intersex states continue to evolve; a consensus from an international conference has stated that surgery should be reserved for cases of severe virilization and be performed in conjunction with repair of the common urogenital sinus, when appropriate.[157] A detailed discussion of the various surgical techniques and related nursing care is beyond this scope of this chapter. It should be noted that the decision to assign a gender and pursue surgical or other treatment is especially complex and distressful to parents and care providers. Therefore, it must be based on meaningful input from an interdisciplinary team, including those in nursing, urology, pediatrics, endocrinology, genetics, and child psychology. At the center of this consultation are the infant and parents, who are anxious to resolve this most basic and profound issue of identity. A number of issues will influence their feelings about gender assignment and their child, including personal preference and opinions of family and close friends. Culture also exerts a profound influence on gender and the significance of bearing a child with an intersex anomaly.[158] The urologic nurse can serve a unique role as an advocate for the parents, ensuring that parental views and values are known and considered whenever issues of gender assignment are confronted. In addition, the nurse is in a unique position to advocate the infant's perspective to parents and family members, particularly in light of evidence suggestive that gender reassignment based on primarily surgical considerations may fail, leading to assignment of female gender to children with male genotypes.[159]

Cryptorchidism

Cryptorchidism is a hidden testis; it occurs when the developing testis fails to migrate from prenatal intraabdominal origins to an intrascrotal position. The risk for cryptorchidism is profoundly influenced by age. It incidence in premature boys is approximately 9% to 30% and its incidence in male infants delivered at term is 3% to 6%.[160,161] Following delivery, some cryptorchid testes will descend spontaneously, usually within the first 3 months of life. By 1 year of age, its incidence has diminished to approximately 1% to 2%. In addition to age, endocrine disorders such as intersex states associated with defects in gonadotropin production, androgen synthesis, or its action increase the risk of cryptorchidism, as do defects affecting the genitofemoral nerve. They are also characteristic of the prune-belly syndrome (see Chapter 13).

Undescended testes are classified according to their location with respect to the scrotum (Figure 12-17). Abdominal testes are not palpable; they are found at or above the internal inguinal ring. Canalicular testes are located within the inguinal canal; they often lie at the top of the scrotum. Ectopic testes are found outside the normal pathway of descent (see Chapter 1 for a detailed discussion of normal testicular descent). They may be located in the perineum, femoral canal, superficial inguinal pouch, suprapubic area, or contralateral hemiscrotum. The most common location is the superficial inguinal pouch, found just lateral to the external inguinal ring.

Retractile testes are fully descended, but move freely between the scrotum and groin. Retraction of the testis is provoked by contraction of the cremaster muscle in response to a decline in ambient temperature when the scrotum is exposed. Differentiation of retractile from cryptorchid testes is critical because the former requires no intervention, whereas the latter must be surgically placed in the scrotum to

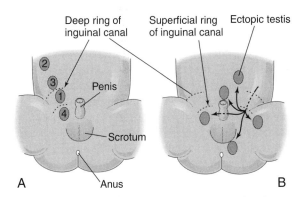

Fig. 12-17 Cryptorchid testes. **A,** Intraabdominal and canalicular testes. **B,** Ectopic cryptorchid testes. (From Moore K, Persaud TVN: The Developing Human, 7th edition. Philadelphia: Saunders, 2003; p 324.)

maximize fertility potential and reduce the risk of testicular malignancy.

Assessment. Palpation of the testes is an acquired physical examination skill that is aided by a reasonably warm room, warm hands, and persistence. The child may be placed in a supine position to enhance descent of the testes into the scrotum; alternatively, he may be held in the mother's lap to reduce anxiety or seated in a cross-legged position. Gentle pressure using the thumb and forefinger may assist the clinician to move the testis into the hemiscrotum, or gentle pressure may be applied to the femoral artery of the groin.[162] Although absence of either testicle raises the possibility of cryptorchidism, it does not diagnose the condition. Instead, repeated efforts must be made, particularly over the first year of life, to palpate and document the presence of a testis in each hemiscrotum. Palpation of each testis in the scrotum at least once indicates the presence of retractile rather than undescended testes; this phenomenon persists to puberty in some boys and is particularly common during the fifth and sixth years of life. The ability to milk the testis into the scrotum, followed by retraction to a nonpalpable position, also diagnoses a retractile testis. It is sometimes thought of as a normal variant, but it is important to remember that retractile testes carry a 32% risk for becoming cryptorchid, especially if the spermatic cord feels tight or inelastic on palpation.[163] In contrast, a testicle that can be palpated on examination but manipulated no further than the upper scrotum is called a gliding testis and indicates a cryptorchid state. Similarly, a testis that remains nonpalpable, despite multiple physical examinations, is assumed to be cryptorchid.

When a testis is not palpable in the scrotum, it is assumed to be cryptorchid or retractile—and not absent—until proven otherwise. Imaging studies may be useful in locating hidden testes only in selected cases.[161,162] Ultrasonography provides a rapid and inexpensive method of diagnosing a cryptorchid testis, but its sensitivity is limited. CT and MRI tend to be more accurate, but they are expensive and of questionable value when compared with laparoscopic localization or use of the human chorionic gonadotropin (HCG) provocation test. HCG is a hormone that has proved useful in stimulating testicular descent and in provoking an endocrinologic response in boys with testicular tissue.[164] The test dosage varies

by physician preference and body weight, but a typical dose might be a total dosage of 2000 units of HCG administered as divided intramuscular injections. The drug is given three times weekly for 3 weeks. Palpation for testicular descent is completed at least 1 week after completing the full treatment course. Descent of the testis is considered therapeutic, although those with partially descended or undescended testes will be schedule to undergo laparoscopy to identify the testis and determine management.

Laparoscopy, with or without HCG stimulation, can be used to identify and locate nonpalpable testes.[162] It is useful for selected cases of cryptorchidism and can help identify and treat the cryptorchid testis during the same procedure. However, it is not useful for routine localization in the nonpalpable testis because scrotal exploration is usually sufficient to locate and treat undescended testes.[165]

Nursing Management. Medical treatment relies on surgical repair, orchiopexy or orchidopexy, or hormonal stimulation to ensure that the testes are located in the scrotum. The timing of treatment is balanced by the likelihood of spontaneous testicular descent over time versus damage to the testis when it remains above the scrotum. In the full-term child, definitive treatment is instituted after 6 months. In premature infants, the age at treatment is adjusted based on a full-term pregnancy. Hormonal therapy with intramuscular HCG will lead to permanent descent in 20% to 65% of cases.[162] Alternatively, nonpalpable (intraabdominal) or ectopic testes require surgical intervention. Orchiopexy involves surgical exploration through an inguinal, suprainguinal (muscle splitting), or lower abdominal incision, identification of the undescended testis, and transfer to the appropriate hemiscrotum. See Chapter 18 for a detailed discussion of the nursing management of the child undergoing orchiopexy.

Nursing management of these children begins with reassurance to the parents that the undescended testis is usually located and successfully moved into its normal position with appropriate medical or surgical intervention. However, they are also counseled that the cryptorchid testis is at an increased risk for malignancy and infertility. The risk of infertility is affected by the length of time the testis remains above the scrotum and its location with respect to the hemiscrotum. In general, intraabdominal testes are more severely affected than canalicular testes, and those that remain outside the scrotum longer than 6 to 12 months prior to treatment are more severely affected than those that are managed sooner. Bilateral is worse than unilateral cryptorchidism because both testes are adversely affected. The magnitude of this risk is unclear, however; some researchers have reported no increased risk in boys with one undescended testis, irrespective of its size at the time of repair,[165] but others have detected a higher and clinically relevant risk in boys with a unilateral intraabdominal testis.[166] Therefore, the urologic nurse should advise parents of the potential risk while reassuring them that many males with one or even bilateral cryptorchid testes as children are capable of bearing children as adults. The nurse can also counsel the parents that problems with fertility as an adult are managed by urologists who specialize in this condition.

Males with cryptorchid testes are also at increased risk for germ cell testicular tumors; this risk involves the affected and contralateral testis.[167,168] Although the magnitude of this risk is unknown, it clearly affects only a very small proportion of males with a history of cryptorchidism. Urologic nursing management begins by informing parents of this slightly increased risk in consultation with the physician. As the child ages, he is taught the warning signs and symptoms of testicular cancer, including a persistent dull ache or sensation of pressure in the scrotum. Males with cryptorchidism are also taught to perform testicular self-examination on a monthly basis (see Chapter 8).

SUMMARY

Congenital anomalies affect adult and pediatric urologic patients. Many common defects produce few or no bothersome symptoms or sequelae, although others profoundly influence physical health and psychosocial well-being. Nursing management has two major goals: (1) to enable the patient to manage adverse physical effects associated with a genitourinary birth defect; and (2) to assist the patient and family in adjusting to any associated psychological or social distress caused by a defect that could compromise homeostatic function of the body's internal environment, sexual function, or even personal identity as a male or female.

REFERENCES

1. Rabinowitz R: General considerations of congenital anomalies. In Gillenwater JY, Grayhack JT, Howards SS, Duckett JW (eds): Adult and Pediatric Urology, 3rd edition. St Louis: Mosby, 1996; pp 2061-74.
2. Bakarat AJ, Drougas JG: Occurrence of congenital abnormalities of kidney and urinary tract in 13,775 autopsies. Urology, 1991; 38:347-50.
3. Dorland's Illustrated Medical Dictionary. 31st edition. Philadelphia: Saunders, 2007: p 39.
4. Koff SA, Mutabagani KH: Anomalies of the kidneys. In Gillenwater JY, Grayhack JT, Howards SS, Mitchell ME (eds): Adult and Pediatric Urology, 4th edition. Philadelphia: Lippincott Williams & Wilkins, 2002; pp 2129-54.
5. Kitagwa H, Pringle KC, Zucollo J, Koike J, Nakada K, Moriya H, Seki Y: Early fetal obstructive uropathy produces Potter's syndrome in the lamb. Journal of Pediatric Surgery, 2000; 35:1549-53.
6. Rodriguez-Garcia R: Bilateral renal agenesis (Potter's syndrome) in a girl born to a hyperthyroid mother who received methimazole in early pregnancy. Ginecologica y Obstetricia de Mexico, 1999; 67:587-9.
7. Carles D, Dally D, Serville F, Maugey-Laulom B, Alberti EM, Tissot H, Weichold W, Wursten-Guitton F: Cystic adenomatoid malformation of the lung, bilateral renal agenesis and left heart hypoplasia. An unusual association in Potter's syndrome. Annales de Pathologie, 1992; 12:367-70.
8. Hjort C, Larsen CO, Nathan E: Potter's sequence. Phenotype, pathogenesis, etiology and hereditary aspects. Ugeskrift for Laeger, 1992; 154:488-91.
9. Chittmittrapap S, Spitz L, Kiley EM, Brereton RJ: Esophageal atresia and associated anomalies. Archives of Disease in Childhood, 1989; 64:364-8.
10. Forrester MB, Merz RD: Risk of selected birth defects with prenatal illicit drug use, Hawaii, 1986-2002. Journal of Toxicology and Environmental Health Part A, 2007; 70:7-18.
11. Gloor JM, Ogburn PL Jr., Breckle RJ, Morgenstern BZ, Milliner DS: Urinary tract anomalies detected by prenatal ultrasound examination at Mayo Clinic, Rochester. Mayo Clinic Proceedings, 1995; 70:526-31.
12. Dhundiraj KM, Madhukar DN, Ambadasrao PG, Wamanrao KS, Prem ZM: Potter's syndrome: a report of 5 cases. Indian Journal of Pathology & Microbiology, 2006; 49:254-7.
13. Hill LM, Nowak A, Hartle R, Tush B: Fetal compensatory renal hypertrophy with a unilateral functioning kidney. Ultrasound in Obstetrics and Gynecology, 2000; 15:191-3.
14. Seeman T, Patzer L, John U, Dusek J, Vondrák K, Janda J, Misselwitz J: Blood pressure, renal function, and proteinuria in children with unilateral renal agenesis. Kidney & Blood Pressure Research, 2006; 29:210-5.
15. Cascio S, Paran S, Prem P: Associated urological anomalies in children with unilateral renal agenesis. Journal of Urology, 1999; 162:1081-3.
16. Krzemien G, Roszkowska-Blaim M, Kostro I, Wojnar J, Karpinska M, Sekowska R: Urological anomalies in children with renal agenesis or multicystic dysplastic kidney. Journal of Applied Genetics, 2006; 47(2):171-6.
17. Sy WM, Seo IS, Sze PC, Kimmel MA, Homs CJ, McBride JG, Smith KF: A patient with three kidneys: a correlative imaging case report. Clinical Nuclear Medicine, 1999; 24:264-6.
18. N'Guessan G, Stephens FD: Supernumerary kidney. Journal of Urology, 1983; 130:649-53.
19. Koureas AP, Panourgias EC, Gouliamos AD, Trakadas AJ, Vlahos LJ: Imaging of a supernumerary kidney. European Radiology, 2000; 10:1722-3.
20. Unal M, Erem C, Serce K, Tunder C, Bostan M, Gikce M: The presence of both horseshoe kidney and a supernumerary kidney associated with coarctation of the aorta. Acta Cardiologica, 1995; 50:155-60.
21. Flyer MA, Haller JO, Feld M, Kantor A: Ectopic supernumerary kidney: another cause of a pelvic mass. Abdominal Imaging, 1994; 19:374-5.

22. Bernik TR, Ravnik DJ, Wallack MK: Ectopic supernumerary kidney, a cause of para-aortic mass: case report and review. American Surgeon, 2001; 67:657-9.

23. Winyard P, Chitty L: Dysplastic and polycystic kidneys: diagnosis, associations and management. Prenatal Diagnosis, 2001; 21:924-35.

24. Granthan JJ, Nair V, Winklhofer F: Cystic diseases of the kidney. In Brenner BM (ed): The Kidney, 6th edition. Philadelphia: Saunders, 2000; pp 1699-1730.

25. Lippert MC: Renal cystic disease. In Gillenwater JY, Grayhack JT, Howards SS, Mitchell ME (eds): Adult and Pediatric Urology, 4th edition. Philadelphia: Lippincott Williams & Wilkins, 2002; pp 868-77.

26. Quan A: Fetopathy associated with exposure to angiotensin-converting enzyme inhibitors and angiotensin receptor antagonists. Early Human Development, 2006; 82(1):23-8.

27. Torres VE, Harris PC: Mechanisms of disease: autosomal dominant and recessive polycystic kidney diseases. Nature Clinical Practice Nephrology, 2006; 2(1):40-55.

28. Vora N, Perrone R, Bianchi DW: Reproductive issues for adults with autosomal dominant polycystic kidney disease. American Journal of Kidney Disease, 2008; 51:307-18.

29. Granthan JJ: Polycystic kidney disease: from the bedside to the gene and back. Current Opinion in Nephrology and Hypertension, 2001; 10:533-42.

30. Harris RA, Gray DW, Britton BJ, Toogood GJ, Morris PJ: Hepatic cystic disease in an adult polycystic kidney disease transplant population. Australian and New Zealand Journal of Surgery, 1996; 66:166-8.

31. Rohan J, Gonwa TA, Testa G, Abbasoglu O, Goldstein R, Husberg BS, Levy MF, Klintmalm GB: Liver and kidney transplant for polycystic kidney disease. Transplantation, 1998; 66:529-32.

32. Zerres K, Mucher G, Becker J, Steinkamm C, Rudnik-Schoneborn S, Heikkila P, Raopla J, et al: Prenatal diagnosis of autosomal recessive polycystic kidney disease (ARPKD): molecular genetics, clinical experience and fetal morphology. American Journal of Medical Genetics, 1998; 76:137-44.

33. Zerres K, Rudnik-Schoneborn S, Steinkamm C, Becker J, Mucher G: Autosomal recessive polycystic kidney disease. Journal of Molecular Medicine, 1998; 76:303-9.

34. Yang J, Zhang S, Zhou Q, Guo H, Zhang K, Zheng R, Xiao C: PKHD1 gene silencing may cause cell abnormal proliferation through modulation of intracellular calcium in autosomal recessive polycystic kidney disease. Journal of Biochemistry and Molecular Biology, 2007; 40:467-74.

35. Gunay-Aygun M, Avner ED, Bacallao RL, Choyke PL, Flynn JT, Germino GG, Guay-Woodford L, Harris P. Heller T, et al: Autosomal recessive polycystic kidney disease and congenital hepatic fibrosis: summary statement of a first National Institutes of Health/Office of Rare Diseases conference. Journal of Pediatrics, 2006; 149(2):159-64.

36. Lonergan GJ, Rice RR, Suarez ES: Autosomal recessive polycystic kidney disease: radiologic-pathologic correlation. Radiographics, 2000; 20:837-55.

37. Davis ID, MacRae Dell K, Sweeney WE, Avner ED: Can progression of autosomal dominant or autosomal recessive polycystic kidney disease be prevented?. Seminars in Nephrology, 2001; 21:430-40.

38. Bardaji A, Martinez-Vea A, Valero A, Guiterriz C, Garcia C, Ridao C, Oliver JA, Richart C: Cardiac involvement in autosomal dominant polycystic kidney disease: a hypertensive heart disease. Clinical Nephrology, 2001; 56:211-20.

39. Salehipour M, Jalaeian H, Salahi H, Bahador A, Davari HR, Nikeghbalian S, et al: Are large nonfunctional kidneys risk factors for posttransplantation urinary tract infection in patients with end-stage renal disease due to autosomal dominant polycystic kidney disease? Transplantation Proceedings, 2007; 39:887-8.

40. Gray M: Are cranberry juice or cranberry juice products effective in the prevention or management of urinary tract infection? Journal of Wound, Ostomy and Continence Nursing, 2002; 29:122-6.

41. Ng, CS, Yost A, Streem SB: Nephrolithiasis associated with autosomal dominant polycystic kidney disease: contemporary urological management. Journal of Urology, 2000; 163:726-9.

42. Winyard P, Chitty L: Dysplastic and polycystic kidneys: diagnosis, associations and management. Prenatal Diagnosis, 2001; 21:924-35.

43. Belk RA, Thomas DFM, Mueller RF, Godbole P, Markham AF, Weston MJ: A family study of the natural history of prenatally detected multicystic dysplastic kidney. Journal of Urology, 2002; 167:666-9.

44. Attar R, Quinn F, Winyard PJ, Mouriquand PD, Foxall P, Hanson MA, Woolf AS: Short-term urinary flow impairment deregulates PAX2 and PCNA expression and cell survival in fetal sheep kidneys. American Journal of Pathology, 1998; 152:1225-35.

45. Aslam M, Watson AR. Trent & Anglia MCDK Study Group. Unilateral multicystic dysplastic kidney: long term outcomes. Archives of Disease in Childhood, 2006; 91:820-3.

46. Mesrobian HG, Rushton HG, Bulas D: Unilateral renal agenesis may result from in utero regression of multicystic renal dysplasia. Journal of Urology, 1993; 150:793-4.

47. Wacksman J, Phipps L: Report of the Multicystic Kidney Registry: preliminary findings. Journal of Urology, 1993; 150:1870-2.

48. Konda R, Sato H, Ito S, Sakai K, Kimura N, Nagura H: Renin-containing cells present predominantly in scarred areas but not dysplastic regions in multicystic dysplastic kidney. Journal of Urology, 2001; 166:1910-4.

49. Strife JL, Souza AS, Kirks DR, Strife CF, Gelfand MJ, Wacksman J: Multicystic dysplastic kidney in children: U.S. follow-up. Radiology, 1993; 186:785-8.

50. Roach PJ, Paltiel HJ, Perez-Atayde A, Tello RJ, Davis RT, Treves ST: Renal dysplasia in infants: appearance on 99mTc DMSA scintigraphy. Pediatric Radiology, 1995; 25:472-5.

51. Cuckow PM, Nyirady P, Winyard PJ: Normal and abnormal development of the urogenital tract. Prenatal Diagnosis, 2001; 21:908-16.

52. Seeman T, John U, Blahova K, Vondrichova H, Misselwitz JJ: Ambulatory blood pressure monitoring in children with unilateral multicystic dysplastic kidney. European Journal of Pediatrics, 2001; 160:78-83.

53. Steven LC, Li AG, Driver CP, Mahomed AA: Laparoscopic nephrectomy for unilateral multicystic dysplastic kidney in children. Surgical Endoscopy, 2005; 19(8):1135-8.

54. Collura G, De Dominicis M, Patricolo M, Caione P: Hydronephrosis caused by malrotation in a pelvic ectopic kidney with vascular anomalies. Urologia Internationalis, 2004; 72(4):349-51.

55. Guarino N, Tadini B, Camardi P, Silvestro L, Lace R, Bianchi M: The incidence of associated urological abnormalities in children with renal ectopia. Journal of Urology, 2004; 172(4 Pt 2):1757-9.

56. Jefferson JP, Persad RA: Thoracic kidney:a rare form of renal ectopia. Journal of Urology, 2001; 165:504.

57. Stein JP, Kurzock EA, Freeman JA, Esrig D, Ginsberg DA, Grossfield GD, Hardy BE: Rigid intrathoracic renal ectopia: a case report and review of the literature. Techniques in Urology, 1999; 5:166-8.

58. Al Attia HM: Cephalad renal ectopia, duplication of pelvicalyceal system and patent ductus arteriosus in an adult female. Scandinavian Journal of Nephrology and Nephrology, 1999; 33:257-9.

59. Navarro A, Jimenez J, Rios T, Mestanza F, Aguirre I, Urquizo R: Unusual cause of lung and renal disease in a baby with trisomy 21. Pediatric Pulmonology, 2005; 40(2):173-4.

60. Sriprasad S, Poulsen J, Muir G, Kane P, Coptcoat MJ: Laparoscopic removal of multicystic dysplastic pelvic kidney. Journal of Endourology, 2001; 15:805-7.

61. Kocak M, Sudakoff GS, Erickson S, Begun F, Datta M: Using MR angiography for surgical planning in pelvic kidney renal cell carcinoma. AJR American Journal of Roentgenology, 2001; 177:659-60.

62. Kupeli B, Isen K, Biri H, Sinik Z, Alkibay T, Karaoglan U, Bozkirli I: Extracorporeal shockwave lithotripsy in anomalous kidneys. Journal of Endourology, 1999; 13:349-52.

63. Watterson JD, Cook A, Sahajpal R, Bennett J, Denstedt JD: Percutaneous nephrolithotomy of a pelvic kidney: a posterior approach through the greater sciatic foramen. Journal of Urology, 2001; 166:209-10.

64. Matlaga BR, Kim SC, Watkins SL, Kuo RL, Munch LC, Lingeman JE: Percutaneous nephrolithotomy for ectopic kidneys: over, around, or through. Urology, 2006; 67(3):513-7.

65. Strauss S, Dushnitsky T, Peer A, Manor H, Libson E, Lebsenart PD: Sonographic features of horseshoe kidney: review of 34 patients. Journal of Ultrasound Medicine, 2000; 19:27-31.

66. Talpallikar MC, Sawant V, Hirugade S, Borwankar SS, Sanghani H: Wilms' tumor arising in a horseshoe kidney. Pediatric Surgery International, 2001; 17:465-6.

67. Talpallikar MC, Sawant V, Hirugade S, Borwankar SS, Sanghani H: Wilms' tumor arising in a horseshoe kidney. Pediatric Surgery International, 2001; 17:465-6.

68. Isobe H, Takashima H, Higashi N, Murakami Y, Fujita K, Hanazawa K, Fujime M, Matsumoto T: Primary carcinoid tumor in a horseshoe kidney. International Journal of Urology, 2000; 7:184-8.

69. Begin LR, Guy L, Jacobson SA, Aprikian AG: Renal carcinoid and horseshoe kidney: a frequent association of two rare entities—a case report and review of the literature. Journal of Surgical Oncology, 1998; 68:113-9.

70. Kapur VK, Sakalkale RP, Samuel KV, Meisheir IV, Bhagwat AS, Pamprasad A, et al: Association of extrarenal tumor with a horseshoe kidney. Journal of Pediatric Surgery, 1998; 33:935-7.

71. Cho JY, Lee YH, Toi A, Macdonald B: Prenatal diagnosis of horseshoe kidney by measurement of the renal pelvic angle. Ultrasound in Obstetrics and Gynecology, 2005; 25(6):554-8.

72. Yohannes P, Smith AD: The endourological management of complications associated with horseshoe kidney. Journal of Urology, 2002; 168:5-8.

73. Uzzo RG, Hsu THS, Goldfarb DA, Taylor RJ, Novick AC, Gill IS: Strategies for the transplantation of cadaveric kidneys with congenital fusion anomalies. Journal of Urology, 2001; 165:761-5.

74. Stroosma OB, Kootstra G, Schurnik GW: Management of aortic aneurysm in the presence of a horseshoe kidney. British Journal of Surgery, 2001; 88:500-9.

75. Buyukdereli G, Burhas H, Ozogul S, Recep T: Tc-99m DMSA and Tc-99m DTPA imaging in the diagnosis of crossed renal ectopia. Clinical Nuclear Medicine, 2001; 26:257-8.

76. McDonald JH, McClellan DS: Crossed renal ectopia. American Journal of Surgery, 1957; 93:995-1002.

77. Matlaga BR, Miller NL, Terry C, Kim SC, Kuo RL, Coe FL, et al: The pathogenesis of calyceal diverticular calculi. Urological Research, 2007; 35:35-40.

78. Kasap B, Kavukcu S, Soylu A, Turkmen M, Secil M: Megacalycosis: report of two cases. Pediatric Nephrology, 2005; 20(6):828-30.

79. Gomex TE, Pais E, Mendez R, Montero M, Vela D, Carames J, Candal J: Use of Tc-99m DTPA in the follow-up of two pediatric patients diagnosed with megacalycosis or Pugivert's disease. Archivos Espanoles de Urologica, 1997; 50:762-6.

80. Pereira AJG, Gurtaby AI, Escobal TV, Ibarluzea GJG, Catalina J: Megacalycosis and lithiasis. Archivos Espanoles de Urologica, 1995; 48:310-4.

81. Schneider K, Martin W, Helmig FJ, Fendel H: Infundibulopelvic stenosis—evaluation and diagnostic imaging. European Journal of Radiology, 1988; 8:172-4.

82. Hussmann DA, Kramer SA, Malek RS, Allen TD: Infundibulopelvic stenosis: a long-term follow up. Journal of Urology, 1994; 152:837-40.

83. Williams B, Tareen B, Resnick MI: Pathophysiology and treatment of ureteropelvic junction obstruction. Current Urology Reports, 2007; 8:111-7.

84. Zhang PL, Peters CA, Rosen S: Ureteropelvic junction obstruction: morphological and clinical studies. Pediatric Nephrology, 2000; 14:820-6.

85. Rooks VJ, Lebowitz RL: Extrinsic ureteropelvic obstruction from a crossing renal vessel: demography and imaging. Pediatric Radiology, 2001; 31:120-4.

86. Kajbafzadeh AM, Payabvash S, Salmasi AH, Monajemzadeh M, Tavangar SM: Smooth muscle cell apoptosis and defective neural development in congenital ureteropelvic junction obstruction. Journal of Urology, 2006; 176(2):718-23.

87. Hosgor M, Karaca I, Ulukus C, Ozer E, Ozkara E, Sam B, Ucan B, Kurtulus S, Karkiner A, Temir G: Structural changes of smooth muscle in congenital ureteropelvic junction obstruction. Journal of Pediatric Surgery, 2005; 40(10):1632-6.

88. Zeltser IS, Liu JB, Bagley DH: The incidence of crossing vessels in patients with normal ureteropelvic junction examined with endoluminal ultrasound. Journal of Urology, 2004; 172(6 Pt 1):2304-7.

89. Capello SA, Kogan BA, Giorgi LJ Jr, Kaufman RP Jr: Prenatal ultrasound has led to earlier detection and repair of ureteropelvic junction obstruction. Journal of Urology, 2005; 174(4 Pt 1):1425-8.

90. Reddy PP, Mandell J: Prenatal diagnosis: therapeutic implications. Urologic Clinics of North America, 1998; 25:171-80.

91. Cooper CS, Snyder HM III, Noe WH: The ureter. Ureteral anomalies. The wide ureter. In Gillenwater JY, Grayhack JT, Howards SS, Mitchell ME (eds): Adult and Pediatric Urology, 4th edition. Philadelphia: Lippincott Williams & Wilkins, 2002; pp 2155-2208.

92. Fallon E, Ercole B, Lee C, Best S, Skenazy J, Monga M: Contemporary management of ureteropelvic junction obstruction: practice patterns in Minnesota. Journal of Endourology, 2005; 19(1):41-4.

93. Nordmark B: Double formations of the pelves of the kidneys and the ureters: embryology, occurrence and clinical significance. Acta Radiologica, 1948; 30:267-367.

94. Glassberg KI, Braren V, Duckett JW, Jacobs EC, King LR, Lebowitz RL, Perlmutter AD, Stephens FD: Suggested terminology for duplex systems, ectopic ureters and ureteroceles. Journal of Urology, 1984; 132:1153-4.

95. Geavlete P, Nita G, Georgescu D, Mirciulescu V: European classification and endourologic therapy in proximal incomplete ureteral duplication. European Urology, 2001; 39:304-7.

96. Limura A, Yi SQ, Terayama H, Naito M, Buhe S, Oguchi T, et al: Complete ureteral duplication associated with megaureter and ureteropelvic junction dilatation: report on an adult cadaver case with a brief review of the literature. Annals of Anatomy, 2006; 188:371-5.

97. Slaughenhoupt BL, Mitcheson HD, Lee DL: Ureteral duplication with lower pole ectopia to the vas: a case report of an exception to the Weigert-Meyer rule. Urology, 1997; 42:269-71.

98. Hsu THS, Goldfarb DA: Blind-ending ureteral triplication. Journal of Urology, 1998; 159:1295-6.

99. Bouhafs A, Dubois R, Chaffagne P, Laboure S, Valla JS, Dodat H: Two rare case reports of ureteral triplication. Annales d'Urologie, 2002; 36:42-4.

100. Shankar KR, Vishwanath N, Rickwood AML: Outcome of patients with prenatally detected duplex system ureterocele; natural history of those managed expectantly. Journal of Urology, 2001; 165:1226-8.

101. Upadhyay J, Bolduc S, Braga L, Farhat W, Bagli DJ, McLorie GA, Khoury AE, El-Ghoneimi A: Impact of prenatal diagnosis on the morbidity associated with ureterocele management. Journal of Urology, 2002; 167:2560-5.

102. Jankowski JT, Palmer JS: Holmium:yttrium-aluminum-garnet laser puncture of ureteroceles in neonatal period. Urology, 2006; 68(1):179-81.

103. Shokier AA, Nijman RJM: Primary megaureter: current trends in diagnosis and treatment. BJU International, 2000; 86:861-8.

104. Report of working party to establish an international nomenclature for the large ureter. Birth Defects: Original Article Series, 1977; 13:3-8.

105. Qi BQ, Beasley SW, Williams AK, Fizelle F: Apoptosis during regression of the tailgut and septation of the cloaca. Journal of Pediatric Surgery, 2000; 35:1556-61.

106. Metcalfe PD, Schwarz RD: Bladder exstrophy: neonatal care and surgical approaches. Journal of Wound Ostomy and Continence Nursing, 2004; 31:284-92.

107. Vasudevan PC, Cohen MC, Whitby EH, Anumba DO, Quarrell OW: The OEIS complex: two case reports that illustrate the spectrum of abnormalities and a review of the literature. Prenatal Diagnosis, 2006; 26(3):267-72.

108. Keppler-Noreuil K, Gorton S, Foo F, Yankowitz J, Keegan C: Prenatal ascertainment of OEIS complex/cloacal exstrophy - 15 new cases and literature review. American Journal of Medical Genetics. Part A, 2007; 143:2122-8.

109. Grady RW, Mitchell ME: Exstrophy and epispadias anomalies. In Gillenwater JY, Grayhack JT, Howards SS, Mitchell ME (eds): Adult and Pediatric Urology, 4th edition. Philadelphia: Lippincott Williams & Wilkins, 2002; pp 2270-2310.

110. Caione P, Zavaglia D, Capozza N: Pelvic floor reconstruction in female exstrophic complex patients: different results from males? European Urology, 2007; 52:1777-82.

111. Epidemiology of bladder exstrophy and epispadias: a communication from the International Clearinghouse for Birth Defects Monitoring Systems. Teratology, 1987; 36:221-7.

112. Dees JE: Congenital epispadias with incontinence. Journal of Urology, 1949; 62:513-22.

113. Cacciari A, Pilu GL, Mordenti M, Ceccarelli PL, Ruggeri G: Prenatal diagnosis of bladder exstrophy: what counseling?. Journal of Urology, 1999; 161:259-61.

114. Grady RW, Mitchell ME: Newborn exstrophy closure and epispadias repair. World Journal of Urology, 2000; 16:200-4.

115. Gray M: Nursing interventions for alterations in urinary function. In Broadwell DB, Parrish RS, Saunders RC (eds): Child Health Nursing. Philadelphia: Lippincott, 1993; pp 1243-1320.

116. Reiner WG, Gearhart JP: Anxiety disorders in children with epispadias—exstrophy. Urology, 2006; 68(1):172-4.

117. Mukherjee B, McCauley E, Hanford RB, Aalsma M, Anderson AM: Psychopathology, psychosocial, gender and cognitive outcomes in patients with cloacal exstrophy. Journal of Urology, 2007; 178:630-5.

118. Close CE: The valve bladder. In Gillenwater JY, Grayhack JT, Howards SS, Mitchell ME (eds): Adult and Pediatric Urology, 4th edition. Philadelphia: Lippincott Williams & Wilkins, 2002; pp 2311-8.

119. Casale AJ: Posterior urethral valves and other urethral anomalies. In Wein AJ, Kavoussi LR, Novick AC, Partin AW, Peters CA (eds): Campbell-Walsh Urology, 9th edition. Philadelphia: Saunders, 2007; pp 3583-3603.

120. Kimura T, Miyazato M, Kawai S, Hokama S, Sugaya K, Ogawa Y: Urethral polyp in a young girl: a case report. Hinyokika kiyo. Acta Urologica Japonica, 2007; 53:657-9.

121. van Savage JG, Khoury AE, McLorie GA, Bagli DJ: An algorithm for management of anterior urethral valves. Journal of Urology, 1997; 158:1030-2.

122. Williams DI, Retik AB: Congenital valves and diverticula of the anterior urethra. British Journal of Urology, 1969; 41:228-34.

123. Gleason PE, Kramer SA: Genitourinary polyps in children. Urology, 1994; 44:106-9.

124. Lamaghewage AK, Kelsey A, Gough DCS: Urethral polyp in a girl. British Journal of Urology, 1998; 82:456-7.

125. Glassberg KI: The valve bladder syndrome: 20 years later. Journal of Urology, 2001; 166:1406-14.

126. Brock JW, Adams MC: The male urethra. In Gillenwater JY, Grayhack JT, Howards SS, Mitchell ME (eds): Adult and Pediatric Urology, 4th edition. Philadelphia: Lippincott Williams & Wilkins, 2002; pp 2380-2404.

127. Abbott JF, Levine D, Wapner R: Posterior urethral valves: inaccuracy of prenatal diagnosis. Fetal Diagnosis and Therapy, 1998; 13:179-82.

128. Ziylan O, Oktar T, Ander H, Korgali E, Rodoplu H, Kocak T: The impact of late presentation of posterior urethral valves on bladder and renal function. Journal of Urology, 2006; 175(5):1894-7.

129. McLellan DL, Gaston MV, Diamond DA, Lebowitz RL, Mandell J, Atala A, Bauer SB: Anterior urethral valves and diverticula in children: a result of ruptured Cowper's duct cyst? BJU International, 2004; 94(3):375-8.

130. Ghanem MA, Wolffenbuttel KP, De Vylder A, Nijman RJ: Long-term bladder dysfunction and renal function in boys with posterior urethral valves based on urodynamic findings. Journal of Urology, 2004; 171(6 Pt 1):2409-12.

131. Krueger RP, Hardy BE, Churchill BM: Growth in boys with posterior urethral valves. Primary resection versus temporary diversion. Urologic Clinics of North America, 1980; 7:265-72.

132. Churchill BM, McLorie GA, Khoury AE, Merguerian PA, Houle AM: Emergency treatment and long-term follow-up of posterior urethral valves. Urologic Clinics of North America, 1990; 17:343-60.

133. Koff SA, Mutabagani KH, Jayanthi VR: The valve bladder syndrome: pathophysiology and treatment with nocturnal bladder emptying. Journal of Urology, 2000; 167:291-7.

134. Nguyen MT, Pavlock CL, Zderic SA, Carr MC, Canning DA: Overnight catheter drainage in children with poorly compliant bladders improves post-obstructive diuresis and urinary incontinence. Journal of Urology, 2005; 174(4 Pt 2):1633-6.

135. Sanchez MM, Vellibre RM, Castelo JL, Arias MP, Sarmiento RC, Costa AR: A new case of male Y-type urethral duplication and review of literature. Journal of Pediatric Surgery, 2006; 41(1): e69-e71.

136. Effmann EL, Lebowitz RL, Collodny AH: Duplication of the urethra. Radiology, 1976; 119:179-85.

137. Baskin LS: Hypospadias and urethral development. Journal of Urology, 2000; 163:951-6.

138. Baskin LA, Himes K, Colborn T: Hypospadias and endocrine disruption: is there a connection? Environmental Health Perspectives, 2001; 109:1175-83.

139. Gatti JM, Kirsch AJ, Troyer WA, Perez-Brayfield MR, Smith EA, Sherz HC: Increased incidence of hypospadias in small for gestational age infants in a neonatal intensive care unit. BJU International, 2001; 87:548-50.

140. Buckett WM, Chian RC, Holzer H, Dean N, Usher R, Tan SL: Obstetric outcomes and congenital abnormalities after in vitro maturation, in vitro fertilization, and intracytoplasmic sperm injection. Obstetrics and Gynecology, 2007; 110:885-91.

141. Fisch H, Golden RJ, Libersen GL, Hyun GS, Madsen P, New MI, Hensle TW: Maternal age as a risk factor for hypospadias. Journal of Urology, 2001; 165:934-6.

142. Aberg A, Westbom L, Kallen B: Congenital malformations among infants whose mothers had gestational diabetes or preexisting diabetes. Early Human Development, 2001; 61:85-95.

143. Snodgrass W, Baskin LS, Mitchell ME: Hypospadias. In Gillenwater JY, Grayhack JT, Howards SS, Mitchell ME (eds): Adult and Pediatric Urology, 4th edition. Philadelphia: Lippincott Williams & Wilkins, 2002; pp 2510-32.

144. Devesa R, Munoz A, Torrents M, Comas C, Carrera JM: Prenatal diagnosis of isolated hypospadias. Prenatal Diagnosis, 1998; 18:779-88.

145. Fisch M: Urethral reconstruction in children. Current Opinion in Urology, 2001; 11:253-5.

146. Wilcox DT, Ransley PG: Medicolegal aspects of hypospadias. BJU International, 2000; 86:327-31.

147. American Academy of Pediatrics: Timing of elective surgery on the genitalia of male children with particular reference to the risks, benefits, and psychological effects of surgery and anesthetics. Pediatrics, 1996; 97:590-4.

148. Sandberg DE, Meyer-Bahlburg HF, Hensle TW, Levitt SB, Kogan SJ, Reda EF: Psychosocial adaptation of middle childhood boys with hypospadias after genital surgery. Journal of Pediatric Psychology, 2001; 26:465-75.

149. Aho MO, Tammela OK, Somppi EM, Tammela TL: Sexual and social life of men operated in childhood for hypospadias and phimosis. A comparative study. European Urology, 2000; 37:95-101.

150. Mondaini N, Ponchietti R, Bonafe M, Biscioni S, Di Loro F, Agostini P, Salvestrini F, Rizzo M: Hypospadias: incidence and effects on psychosexual development as evaluated with the Minnesota Multiphasic Personality Inventory test in a

sample of 11,649 young Italian men. Urologia Internationalis, 2002; 68:81-5.

151. Barbagli G, De Angelis M, Palminteri E, Lazzeri M. Failed hypospadias repair presenting in adults. European Urology, 2006; 49(5):887-95.

152. Diamond DA: Sexual differentiation: Normal and abnormal. In Wein AJ, Kavoussi LR, Novick AC, Partin AW, Peters CA (eds): Campbell-Walsh Urology, 9th edition. Philadelphia: Saunders, 2007; pp 3799-3829.

153. Neri G, Opitz J: Syndromal (and nonsyndromal) forms of male pseudohermaphroditism. American Journal of Medical Genetics, 1999; 89:201-9.

154. Cheikhelard A, Luton D, Philippe-Chomette P, Leger J, Vuillard E, Garel C, Polak M, Nessman C, Aigrain Y, El-Ghoneimi A: How accurate is the prenatal diagnosis of abnormal genitalia? Journal of Urology, 2000; 164:984-7.

155. Parisi MA, Ramsdell LA, Burns MW, Carr MC, Grady RE, Gunther DF, et al: A Gender Assessment Team: experience with 250 patients over a period of 25 years. Genetics in Medicine: Official Journal of the American College of Medical Genetics, 2007; 9:348-57.

156. Anhalt H, Neely EK, Hintz RL: Ambiguous genitalia. Pediatrics in Review, 1996; 17:203-20.

157. Lee PA, Houk CP, Ahmed SF, Hughes IA: International Consensus Conference on Intersex organized by the Lawson Wilkins Pediatric Endocrine Society and the European Society for Pediatric Endocrinology. Consensus statement on management of intersex disorders. International Consensus Conference on Intersex. Pediatrics, 2006; 118(2):e488-e500.

158. Kuhnle U, Krahl W: The impact of culture on sex assignment and gender development in intersex patients. Perspectives in Biology and Medicine, 2002; 45:85-103.

159. Glassberg KI: Gender assignment and the pediatric urologist [editorial]. Journal of Urology, 1999; 161:1308-10.

160. Leissner J, Filipas D, Wolf HK, Fisch M: The undescended testis: considerations and impact on fertility. BJU International, 1999: 885-6.

161. Schneck FX, Bellinger MF: Abnormalities of the testes and scrotum and their surgical management. In Wein AJ, Kavoussi LR, Novick AC, Partin AW, Peters CA (eds): Campbell-Walsh Urology, 9th edition. Philadelphia: Saunders, 2007; pp 3761-98.

162. Kogan SJ, Hadziselmovic F, Howards SS, Huff D, Snyder HM: Pediatric andrology. In Gillenwater JY, Grayhack JT, Howards SS, Mitchell ME (eds): Adult and Pediatric Urology, 4th edition. Philadelphia: Lippincott Williams & Wilkins, 2002; pp 2565-2621.

163. Agarwal PK, Diaz M, Elder JS: Retractile testis—is it really a normal variant? Journal of Urology, 2006; 175(4):1496-9.

164. Bukowski TP, Sedberry S, Richardson B: Is human chorionic gonadotropin useful for identifying and treating nonpalpable testis? Journal of Urology, 2001; 165:221-3.

165. Williams EV, Appanna T, Foster ME: Management of the impalpable testis: a six year review together with a national experience. Postgraduate Medical Journal, 2001; 77:320-2.

166. Lee PA, Coughlin MT, Bellinger MF: No relationship of testicular size at orchiopexy with fertility in men who previously had unilateral cryptorchidism. Journal of Urology, 2001; 166:236-9.

167. Hadziselimovic F, Hocht B, Herzog B, Buser MW: Infertility in cryptorchidism is linked to the stage of germ cell development at orchidopexy. Hormone Research, 2007; 68:46-52.

168. Ritchie ML, Shamberger RC: Pediatric urologic oncology. In Wein AJ, Kavoussi LR, Novick AC, Partin AW, Peters CA (eds): Campbell-Walsh Urology, 9th edition. Philadelphia: Saunders, 2007; pp 3870-3906.

Multisystem Anomalies: Spinal Dysraphisms, Prune-Belly Syndrome, Sacral Agenesis, and Imperforate Anus

A number of anomalies lead to urologic dysfunction via direct effects on urinary embryogenesis and indirect effects on the pelvic floor muscles or the nerves that modulate nervous system function. The management of these challenging anomalies requires a multidisciplinary approach, ongoing assessment of needs and coping skills, and close communication among care providers in the acute care setting, rehabilitation facility, and community. Urologic nurses have the skills to assess both the child's and family's needs in the acute care, rehabilitation, and community settings; to work with a multidisciplinary health care team; and to enable the family to coordinate information from various specialists into a rational program of care in terms of renal function, urinary and fecal continence, and additional challenges.

SPINAL DYSRAPHISMS

Dysraphism is defined as a defective closure. In the context of congenital anomalies of the nervous system, it can be defined as a defective closure of the neural folds.[1] The word dysraphism arises from a Greek term *raphe*, meaning structure. Spinal dysraphism is a defect or malformation of the structures of the developing nervous system, caused by failure of neural fold fusion. Because the brain and spinal cord develop by fusion (closure) of primitive nervous tissue, malformations also may be described as neural tube defects.[2,3] Actually, a neural tube defect is any anomaly that affects primary neurulation—embryogenesis of the neural tube that will form the brain and spinal cord—but the term is sometimes used to include any defect associated with differentiation or incomplete closure of the dorsal midline structures, including the spinal tissues, meninges, vertebrae, muscles, and/or skin. Neural tube defects can be categorized into two major types, open and closed spinal dysraphisms (Figure 13-1). Open spinal dysraphisms are characterized by exposure of the nervous tissues through a congenital bony defect,

whereas closed defects are covered by skin.[4] Sometimes mislabeled as occult dysraphisms, as many as 86% will have cutaneous manifestations, such as hemangiomas, hairy nevi, dimples, fat pads, or discolored skin patches (Figure 13-2).[4] Although cutaneous lesions and related stigmata do not reliably predict the presence of a spinal dysraphism, their presence should lead to spinal ultrasound being done to determine the presence of underlying neural tube anomalies,[5] especially when two or more lesions are found.[6] Table 13-1 reviews common dysraphisms that may profoundly affect urinary system function. This section will focus on the most common of these defects, myelomeningocele.

Epidemiology

The incidence of neural tube defects is approximately 0.6 per 1000 live births in the United States,[7] 0.9 per 1000 live births in Ontario, Canada,[8] and 1.17 per 1000 live births in Nova Scotia.[9]

The cause of spinal dysraphism is probably multifactorial and a number of risk factors have been identified. Epidemiologic studies have demonstrated that the incidence of neural tube defects is higher in families from northern (cooler) climates, but no seasonal variability in the incidence of spinal dysraphism has been found.[10] Familial predisposition has been hypothesized, based on varying relative risks among racial or ethnic groups and familial tendencies, with the risk of having a second child with a neural tube rising to approximately 2% to 5% when one sibling is affected.[11] Others have linked neural tube defects to Meckel's syndrome (an autosomal recessive disorder), trisomies 13 and 18, and cloacal exstrophy. Folic acid deficiency is an important and modifiable risk factor that has been implicated in the development of anencephaly, spina bifida, and encephalocele.[3,7,12] Controlled and observational studies have shown that if all pregnant women were to take a multivitamin with the B vitamin folic acid,

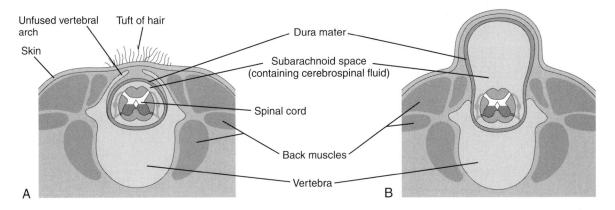

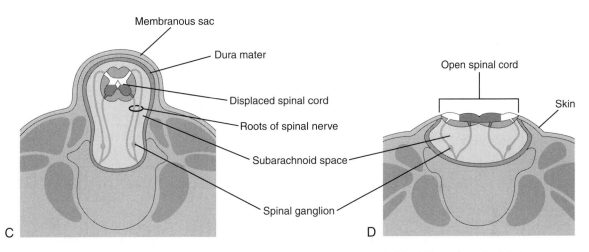

Fig. 13-1 Spinal dysraphisms. **A,** Closed spinal dysraphism is characterized by failure of vertebral fusion; this defect is also called spinal bifida occulta. **B,** Open spinal dysraphism containing meninges and cerebrospinal fluid; this defect is commonly referred to as a meningocele. **C,** Open dysraphism contains meninges, cerebrospinal fluid, and elements of the spinal cord; this defect is also called a myelomeningocele. **D,** Open defect with incomplete closure of spinal cord; this defect is also called myeloschisis. Note that myelomeningocele and myeloschisis are collectively referred to as spinal bifida cystica because of the cystlike sac over the incompletely closed neural tube that is present at birth. (From Moore K, Persaud TVN: The Developing Human, 7th edition. Philadelphia: Saunders, 2003; p. 437.)

the risk of neural tube defects could be reduced by 50% to 75%.[7,9,13-15] It is recommended that all women who plan to become pregnant take a folic acid supplement and continue this at least into the third trimester, when most neural tube formation is completed. It is not well understood why the preconceptual period is so important.

Additional risk factors include established diabetes mellitus in the mother and use of the anticonvulsants valproic acid or carbamazepine.[16] Associated factors include maternal obesity, maternal hyperthermia, and frequent or severe diarrhea during pregnancy.

Pathophysiology

Myelodysplasia—meningocele, lipomeningocele, myelomeningocele—can occur at any level along the spinal column although almost 90% of the involvement is lumbar, lumbosacral, or sacral. Myelomeningocele accounts for 90% of all open spinal dysraphisms[12] and 85% have an associated Arnold-Chiari malformation affecting the aqueductal system, which circulates cerebrospinal fluid from the brain to the spinal cord (Table 13-2). The magnitude of neurologic deficits is influenced by which neural elements are present in the meningocele sac, asymmetry of the defect, and

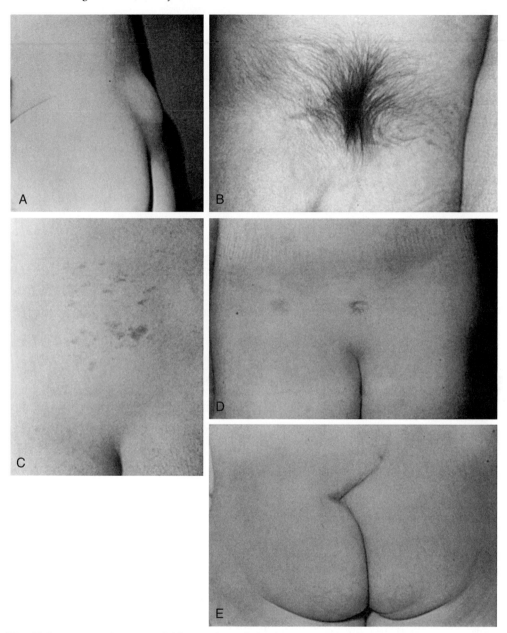

Fig. 13-2 Cutaneous lesions in children with myelodysplasia. **A,** Fatty mass associated with lipomeningocele. **B,** Hairy patch of lower back. **C,** Dermal vascular formation. **D,** Dimple affecting lower back associated with slight curvature of gluteal line. **E,** Abnormal gluteal cleft. (From Walsh PC, Retik AB, Vaughan ED, Wein AJ [eds]: Campbell's Urology, 8th edition. Philadelphia: Saunders, 2002; p. 2246.)

involvement of spinal segments above or below the primary deformity. Knowledge of the bony vertebral defect provides little insight into the type or severity of neurologic deficits. These deficits are also affected by the Arnold-Chiari defect, growth and development of the bony spine, intercurrent urinary tract infections, and interventions such as repair of the original defect, spinal cord tethering, or revision of a ventriculoperitoneal shunt. Therefore, it is necessary to treat each child's defect as unique and to avoid predicting function or relying on vertebral defects when making decisions about care.

TABLE 13-1 Congenital Spinal Dysraphisms[2,3]

DEFECT	CLINICAL CHARACTERISTICS
Anencephaly	Profound neural tube defect resulting in congenital absence of the brain; many are stillborn, the remaining victims die in neonatal period
Open Spinal Dysraphisms	
Myelomeningocele (spina bifida cystica)	Protrusion of spinal cord and meninges segment caused by failure of neurulation through bony vertebral defect; neural elements contained within thin sac that protrudes from sac; most common dysraphism (90% of dysraphisms and 99% of all open defects)
Myeloschisis (myelocele)	Similar to myelomeningocele but neural elements do not expand and form protruding sac
Chiari II malformation	Anomaly of hindbrain characterized by narrowed posterior cranial fossa and caudal displacement of fourth ventricle and brainstem; occurs with all open spinal dysraphisms; may or may not require placement of ventriculoperitoneal shunt
Closed Spinal Dysraphisms	
Lipomyelomeningocele, lipomyeloschisis	Fatty tissue protrudes through posterior spina bifida into spinal canal, tethering spinal cord; lipomyelomeningocele presents with protruding sac but lipomyeloschisis has no protrusion; collectively, account for about 75% of all closed dysraphisms; lipomyeloschisis occurs twice as frequently as lipomyelomeningocele
Meningocele	Posterior protrusion of meninges and cerebrospinal fluid through posterior spina bifida defect; accounts for less than 3% of closed dysraphisms; Chiari II malformation occasionally occurs with posterior meningocele. Anterior meningoceles (rare) herniate through anterior defect; not associated with identifiable cutaneous lesions but associated with caudal regression syndrome
Intrasacral meningocele	Rare defect; protrusion of arachnoid membrane through dural defect located at bottom of thecal sac
Spinal Cord Malformations	
Diastematomyelia with septum (type I spinal cord malformation)	Cleft in thoracic or lumbar cord, dividing it into two hemicords, each housed in its own meningeal sac; is associated with cutaneous signs of spinal dysraphism (e.g., hairy tuft, dyschromic skin patches), vertebral anomalies; comprise about 25% of all these types of defects
Diastematomyelia without septum (type II spinal cord malformation)	Similar to type I defects, but both hemicords housed in single meningeal sac; bony and cutaneous manifestations similar to those of type I defects; accounts for approximately 75% of malformations
Caudal regression syndrome	Describes various defects associated with hypogenesis or agenesis of the lower spinal column; defects leading to caudal regression syndrome include OEIS (**o**mphalocele, cloacal **e**xstrophy, **i**mperforate anus, **s**pinal deformity), anorectal malformation and presacral mass, teratoma, and/or meningocele

TABLE 13-2 Arnold-Chiari Malformations

TYPE	FEATURES
1	Seen in 20% of children with myelomeningocele; elongation and protrusion of medullary and cerebellar tissue through foramen magnum into cervical spinal cord
2	Seen in 80% of patients with myelomeningocele; hydrocephalus may be stable or progressive; signs and symptoms of progressive hydrocephalus include bulging anterior fontanelle, dilated scalp veins, "setting sun" eyes, irritability, nausea, vomiting, increasing head circumference; may be associated with hindbrain dysfunction characterized by feeding difficulties, choking, stridor, apnea, vocal cord paralysis, pooling of secretions, upper limb spasticity

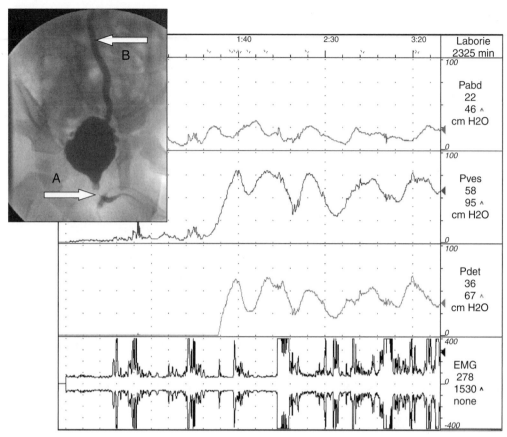

Fig. 13-3 Videourodynamics in a 1-month-old male infant with myelomeningocele reveals preservation of detrusor contractions, but the infant also has (**A**) detrusor sphincter dyssynergia and (**B**) vesicoureteral reflux.

Because of the profound spinal and brain defects associated with myelodysplasia (and myelomeningocele in particular) the risk of neuropathic bladder dysfunction and subsequent upper urinary tract distress is extremely high (Figure 13-3).[12] Newborn evaluation will reveal urinary tract abnormalities in 10% to 15%, including hydronephrosis in 3%, obstructive uropathy in 10%, and vesicoureteral reflux in 3% to 5%. When urodynamic studies are used to characterize lower urinary tract function, 43% will have absence of detrusor contractions and 18% will have low bladder wall compliance. Pelvic floor muscle electromyography (EMG) reveals vesicosphincter dyssynergia in 45% and evidence of muscle denervation in 36% (Figure 13-4).

As the child grows and his or her nervous system develops, neuropathic bladder dysfunction will continue to evolve.[12] By age 3 years, almost three out of four children with vesicosphincter dyssynergia and/or low bladder wall compliance will demonstrate upper urinary tract distress and deterioration in renal function. The likelihood of clinically relevant neuropathic bladder dysfunction by age 5 is significant. In addition to infants born with dyssynergia or abnormal detrusor function, approximately 32% of those with normal bladder function at birth will develop dyssynergia, low bladder wall compliance, or the ability to evacuate the bladder via a detrusor contraction.

When the child with myelodysplasia approaches school age, issues of continence arise. Surprisingly little is known about the risk of urinary incontinence (UI) in these children. Among children with open defects and profound motor deficits, it is presumed that the incidence of UI approaches 100%.[12] Even in children with more limited neurologic defects who retain the ability to ambulate independently or with the aid of ankle braces, the continence rate remains low, 7% in one study of 45 school-age children.[17] Even fewer studies are available that examine UI

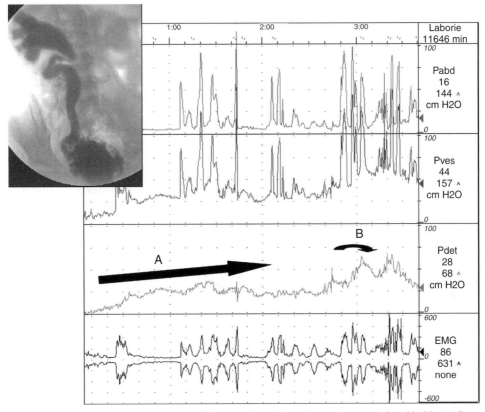

Fig. 13-4 Videourodynamics in a 4-year-old boy with myelomeningocele reveals low bladder wall compliance (**A**) and neurogenic detrusor overactivity with detrusor sphincter dyssynergia. Note the severe trabeculation of the bladder, with multiple diverticula and right vesicoureteral reflux, indicating upper urinary tract distress.

rates in young adults with myelomeningocele. One study of young adult patients has revealed a continence rate of 8%.[18]

Assessment Overview

Diagnosis of a neural tube defect may occur at birth or during the prenatal period. Measurement of the maternal serum alpha-fetoprotein level may raise a suspicion of a neural tube defect, but it does not diagnose the condition. Instead, measurement of alpha-fetoprotein levels via amniocentesis is combined with ultrasound to diagnose a neural tube defect.[19] Neural tube defects may be identified on prenatal ultrasound as early as week 12 of gestation,[20] which may be particularly important for the family facing the anxiety associated with unfavorable maternal serum alpha-fetoprotein levels.[21] Testing is especially valuable for the high-risk family, such as those with previous pregnancies or children with neural tube defects. Neonates with known myelomeningocele may be delivered by cesarean section in an attempt to minimize trauma to the neurologic system, although the evidence supporting this practice is mixed.[22,23]

Open spinal dysraphism is characterized by a protruding sac lying over the spinal column that contains meninges and elements of the spinal cord. Whether delivered by cesarean section, based on knowledge of open spinal dysraphism, or vaginally, without knowledge of a defect, each neonate should undergo a detailed neurologic examination. Of particular interest for the urologic nurse is the abdominal wall tone, lower extremity function, anal sphincter tone, and function of the sacral reflex arc, reflected by the presence or absence of the bulbocavernosus reflex.[12,24] This evaluation also encompasses diagnosis of associated Arnold-Chiari malformations, hydrocephalus, or other defects of the brain. The presence of an

Arnold-Chiari defect is particularly important because it displaces the cerebellum, brainstem, and fourth ventricle, causing hydrocephalus (see Table 13-2).[8] Unless hydrocephalus is promptly relieved by placement of a ventriculoperitoneal shunt, function of the posterior fossa of the brain is impaired and vital functions, including respiration, are compromised.

Assessment of the Neonate. Urologic assessment often occurs after initial repair of the myelomeningocele and placement of a ventriculoperitoneal shunt. It focuses on evaluation of renal function and initial characterization of lower urinary tract function. Physical assessment of the abdomen is completed to detect apparent enlargement of the kidneys (bilateral abdominal mass) and bladder distention (midline mass of the lower abdomen), and to determine whether a gentle Crede's maneuver produces urine loss. Observation of spontaneous micturition is an important assessment that is often completed by the nurse; this observation should include the force of the stream, presence of intermittency, and whether micturition occurs when the infant is quiet or only with crying or other actions that raise abdominal pressure.

Renal function is further evaluated by ultrasound and serum creatinine level measurement. The ultrasonogram is scrutinized for parenchymal size and the presence of hydronephrosis and bladder wall thickness. A urinalysis is performed and urine culture completed, when indicated. A voiding cystourethrogram is obtained to assess lower urinary tract anatomy, including trabeculation of the bladder wall, urethral anatomy, and vesicoureteral reflux.

Urodynamic testing may be combined with voiding cystourethrography (videourodynamics; see Figure 13-3) or it may be completed separately. The goal of testing is to identify hostile neurogenic bladder dysfunction, which increases the risk of upper urinary tract distress. Urinary tract distress is characterized by trabeculation of the bladder, vesicoureteral reflux, hydronephrosis, ureteral dilation, and compromised renal function (renal deterioration). These conditions predispose the infant to urinary stasis and pyelonephritis. Infection of the upper urinary tracts, in turn, leads to scarring, loss of parenchyma, and deterioration of renal function. Urodynamics is completed with the child in a supine position. Although uroflowmetry is not technically feasible, cystometrography, combining measurement of intravesical, abdominal, and detrusor pressures, is combined with sphincter EMG to evaluate lower urinary tract function.

Filling cystometry determines bladder capacity, compliance of the bladder wall, detrusor response to bladder filling, urethral resistance, and urinary residual volume. Bladder capacity in the neonate is approximately 15 ml, and residuals greater than 5 ml are excessive.[12] Because of the small vesical capacity, bladder wall compliance cannot be measured as ml/cm H_2O, but it can be qualitatively assessed by observing the slope of the detrusor line during cystometric filling. Detrusor response is assessed by observing whether cystometric filling provokes a detrusor contraction. The construct "detrusor overactivity" does not apply to urodynamic testing in the neonate, because spontaneous contractions are physiologic at this age. Nevertheless, absence of a detrusor contraction (detrusor areflexia) indicates a clinically relevant defect of the sacral micturition center. Sphincter EMG reveals one of four patterns: (1) coordinated relaxation of the sphincter mechanism during detrusor contraction; (2) paradoxic contraction of the sphincter during detrusor contraction (vesicosphincter dyssynergia); (3) increasing electromyographic activity during bladder filling in the presence of detrusor areflexia (nonrelaxing sphincter response); or (4) quiet pattern electromyogram throughout bladder filling (denervated sphincter). In the neonate, the risk of upper urinary tract distress increases when vesicosphincter dyssynergia exists, or when low bladder wall compliance coexists with significant urethral resistance to urinary outflow, such as that seen with detrusor areflexia and a nonrelaxing or denervated sphincter producing a detrusor leak point pressure of 40 cm H_2O or higher (see Figure 13-4). A low risk of upper urinary tract distress is associated with preservation of detrusor contractions and coordinated sphincter response to micturition or a denervated sphincter response to bladder filling, combined with a low detrusor leak point pressure (Table 13-3). Diagnosis of hostile neurogenic bladder dysfunction indicates the need for a more aggressive bladder management program than diaper containment alone to relieve upper urinary tract distress *before* renal deterioration occurs.

Assessment During Infancy and Early Childhood. Because growth and development of the child, as well as initial urologic and neurologic

TABLE 13-3 Urodynamic Findings in the Neonate with Myelomeningocele

FINDINGS	DESCRIPTION
Detrusor response	Detrusor contractions present in 57%; especially those with thoracic or upper lumbar lesions
	Absence of detrusor contractions (detrusor areflexia) in 43%; 18% will have low bladder wall compliance
Electromyographic response	Preservation of detrusor-striated sphincter coordination in 19%
	Detrusor-sphincter dyssynergia or failure of sphincter relaxation with bladder filling in 45%
	Denervation pattern—quiet pattern electromyogram during bladder filling, absence of bulbocavernosus reflex in 36%
Urodynamic findings	Preservation of detrusor contractions and coordination between detrusor and striated sphincter (risk of upper urinary tract distress or deterioration, 15%)
	Preservation of detrusor contractions but detrusor sphincter dyssynergia (risk of upper urinary tract distress or deterioration, 60%)
	Detrusor areflexia with low bladder wall compliance (risk of upper urinary tract distress or deterioration, 25%)
	Detrusor areflexia with quiet electromyographic response to bladder filling (risk of upper urinary tract distress or deterioration, 30%)

management, profoundly influence urinary and nervous system function, assessment is an ongoing process. Routine surveillance includes urinalysis, measurement of a postvoid urinary residual, imaging of the upper urinary tracts (renal ultrasound), serum creatinine level determination, assessment of bowel function, and/or urodynamic testing.[12,24] The frequency of specific evaluations is influenced by the results of baseline testing. Infants with preservation of detrusor contractions and coordination between detrusor and sphincter response to micturition may undergo urinalysis, postvoid residual measurement, and a serum creatinine level determination every 3 to 4 months for the first year, and every 6 to 12 months up to the third year of life. Upper urinary tract imaging and a voiding cystourethrogram or radionuclide cystogram are usually obtained every 3 to 4 months during the first year of life, and every 6 to 12 months thereafter. Urodynamic testing may be completed annually or whenever routine monitoring indicates upper urinary tract distress. Specific signs of upper urinary tract distress include a febrile urinary tract infection (pyelonephritis), ureterohydronephrosis, vesicoureteral reflux, and trabeculation of the bladder wall (see Figure 13-4).

Assessment of the School-Age Child. In addition to ongoing evaluation to prevent upper urinary tract distress, issues of continence are significant for the school-age child with myelomeningocele.[12] Urodynamic testing should be completed between the fifth and sixth years of life to characterize the detrusor response to bladder filling and urethral resistance. Denervation of the pelvic floor muscles often produces intrinsic sphincter deficiency and stress UI. The results of urodynamic testing are used to determine a bladder management program that both preserves optimal upper urinary tract function and maximizes continence. A conservative program is tried initially, but further urodynamic testing may be indicated if this program fails to achieve continence and surgery is contemplated.

Assessment of the Adolescent and Young Adult. The tremendous physical and psychosocial problems faced by persons with spina bifida as they approach adulthood remained largely unrecognized until the dawn of this century. Close neurologic and urologic monitoring, often including urodynamic testing, is indicated during adolescence because rapid growth and development may change neurologic or urologic function. Although ongoing evaluation of urinary and fecal continence using the principles described above continues into adolescence and young adulthood, assessment of the adolescent and young adult also incorporates issues of sexual function and the need for independence. Raising these issues usually provokes anxiety for the person affected by myelodysplasia and her or his family, but the need for the teenager and young adult to establish an identity as a sexual being and interdependent young adult, as compared with a relatively dependent child, is the same as that experienced by anyone in this age group. Research into sexual function has revealed that 72% of young adult males with myelodysplasia are capable of a penile erection and 67% are capable of ejaculation.[25] Furthermore, a survey of young adults using the International Index of Erectile Function has revealed that 40% of young men with myelomeningocele had engaged in intercourse within the previous month.[26] Nevertheless, approximately 75% experience erectile dysfunction, usually manifested as an inability to maintain an erection. Even less is known about sexual function in young adult women with spinal dysraphisms and fertility. Between 70% and 80% of women with myelodysplasia are capable of bearing children, and as many as 39% of males claim that they have fathered children.[27-29] Sexual problems are reported by 52%; these are more prevalent among young adults with ventriculoperitoneal shunts.[30] In addition to these findings, almost all persons with myelodysplasia state a desire to marry and bear children.[12]

Management

The primary goals of urologic management of children and adults with myelomeningocele or other neural tube defects are (1) preservation of optimal renal function by prevention of upper urinary tract distress, (2) prevention of urinary tract infection, and (3) maintenance of social continence. Additional goals of particular importance to urologic nursing management include prevention of chronic constipation, impaction, and fecal incontinence and assisting the adolescent and young adult with myelodysplasia in addressing issues related to sexual function and independence.

Bladder Management. Initial decisions about bladder management are made during the first days of life, but they will be modified as the child grows, as urinary and nervous system function evolve, and as the goals of urologic management change. In addition, because of the variable nature of the anomaly and the unique influences of growth and development on urinary system function, management for each child remains highly

individualized.[31] Urine elimination in the newborn includes diaper containment, although intermittent catheterization may be begun prior to completing a furologic evaluation if the neonate does not void spontaneously. Intermittent catheterization, usually combined with anticholinergic therapy, is also begun in neonates at risk for upper urinary tract distress. Prompt institution of an intermittent catheterization program is justified because it reduces the incidence of upper tract deterioration in children with dyssynergia from 50% to 10%.[32] Intermittent catheterization also reduces the risk of vesicoureteral reflux in infants with dyssynergia or low bladder wall compliance and increases the likelihood that low-grade reflux will resolve.[12]

Initially, parents or care providers are taught to perform catheterization using a clean technique. The infant is catheterized every 4 hours around the clock, but this schedule is gradually reduced to every 4 hours while awake or a four times daily schedule as the child grows. When the child is sufficiently mature enough to assume responsibility, usually around 6 to 7 years or age, he or she is taught to perform self-catheterization. Catheters may be cleaned with soap and water and reused, instead of reliance on a single-use sterile catheter.[33] Bacteriuria is common in children managed by intermittent catheterization, but the incidence of clinically relevant symptomatic urinary tract infection is approximately 30%.[34] Complication rates associated with intermittent catheterization are low; complications include transient urethral bleeding, meatitis, epididymitis, and creation of a false passage in the bulbar urethra.[12,35]

Intermittent catheterization is frequently combined with anticholinergic therapy to increase bladder capacity and reduce the magnitude of low bladder wall compliance and the frequency of high pressure detrusor contractions. Infants are begun on liquid oxybutynin, 0.2 mg/kg/dose, two to four times daily.[36] Bauer recommends 1.0 mg/year of age, every 12 hours in children older than 12 months; older children may be managed with alternative agents such as long-acting oxybutynin, tolterodine, propantheline, or hyoscyamine.[12] Intravesical instillation of oxybutynin may reduce side effects but must be weighed against the demands of obtaining specially formulated oxybutynin or having to crush tablets, dissolve them in sterile water, and instill this preparation several times daily.[37,38]

Parents or care providers are taught to monitor children for side effects of anticholinergics, including dry mouth, constipation, and heat intolerance. Young children may not complain of dry mouth, but saliva is necessary for healthy teeth and gums; children who are on anticholinergics are at risk for dental caries and impaired swallowing. Heat intolerance leads to flushing and parents should be counseled to monitor their child for signs of heat intolerance, particularly on warm humid days. Constipation is common among children with myelodysplasia because of a neurogenic bowel, and a regular bowel management program is especially important when anticholinergics are administered.

Intermittent catheterization also forms the cornerstone of continence management in the child with myelodysplasia. In some children, the combination of intermittent catheterization and anticholinergic provide adequate continence, but most school-age children also experience stress UI because of denervation and incompetence of the urethral sphincter mechanism. An α-adrenergic agonist such as pseudoephedrine may be administered to increase urethral resistance and prevent UI.[12] However, more aggressive interventions are often necessary when this regimen fails to achieve social continence.

If intermittent catheterization and pharmacotherapy fail to prevent upper urinary tract distress or achieve social continence, surgical intervention is warranted.[12] A vesicostomy may be created in the infant who experiences progressive upper urinary tract distress or deterioration.[39,40] The vesicostomy can be managed by application of a high-riding diaper during infancy, allowing the child to grow and develop prior to performance of more extensive surgical reconstruction. In the older child, a urinary bladder that creates upper urinary tract distress may be managed by augmentation enterocystoplasty using a detubularized segment of small bowel (see Chapter 18). Gastrocystoplasty, enlargement of the bladder using a segment of the stomach, has been advocated as an alternative to gastrocystoplasty but is no longer widely used because of significant long-term complications, including hyponatremic, hypochloremic metabolic acidosis,[41] and hematuria-dysuria syndrome.[42]

Several techniques are used to manage stress UI.[12] Suburethral collagen may be injected transurethrally, thus avoiding the need for a surgical incision.[43]

However, repeated injections are required to maintain continence. The bladder neck may be reconstructed surgically using a technique advocated by Kropp and Angwafo.[44] The technique requires urethral lengthening by formation of a tube using the bladder, which is reimplanted back into the bladder through a submucosal tunnel. A subsequent modification attempts to render self-catheterization easier by using an anterior bladder wall flap sutured to the posterior wall, creating a flap valve that promotes continence.[45] An artificial sphincter may be implanted that significantly increases urethral resistance.[46] However, it also tends to lower bladder wall compliance, which must be promptly managed to avoid deterioration of renal function.[12]

Urinary diversion with bladder neck closure may be completed using the Mitrofanoff procedure (Figure 13-5).[47] The bladder neck is closed and the appendix is brought to the umbilicus or abdominal wall, creating a small catheterizable stoma that is easily covered with a small dressing to prevent mucus from staining overlying clothing. Low bladder wall compliance or severe neurogenic detrusor overactivity may be relieved by augmentation

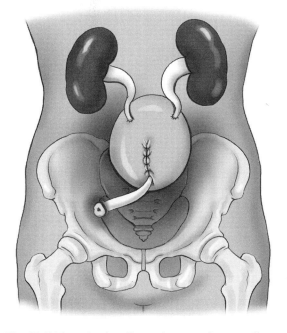

Fig. 13-5 The Mitrofanoff procedure uses the appendix, or a ureteral segment in selected cases, to create a catheterizable continent stoma that is brought to the umbilicus or suprapubic area.

enterocystoplasty. Alternatively, a ureteral segment or segment of small bowel (Mainz transverse retubularized sigmoidvesicostomy) may be substituted for the appendix in selected cases.[48] Postoperatively, an indwelling catheter is left in the stoma for approximately 2 to 3 weeks to allow anastomotic healing. Intermittent catheterization begins as soon as the indwelling catheter is removed. Complications include stomal stenosis and bladder perforation at the anastomotic segment, between the bowel and bladder cuff.[49] Intravesical calculi may form when an augmented bladder is not irrigated daily. The reservoir rarely ruptures spontaneously, particularly if a regular intermittent catheterization regimen is followed.[50]

Vesicoureteral Reflux. Vesicoureteral reflux is managed using principles similar to those applied to children with normal neurologic function. Low-grade reflux (grades 1 to 3) is managed by clean intermittent catheterization and anticholinergic pharmacotherapy; promoting bladder emptying by Crede's maneuver is contraindicated because this increases urethral resistance and exacerbates rather than alleviates retrograde urine movement.[12] In addition, prophylactic antibiotics are given to prevent pyelonephritis (see Chapter 14). Reimplantation of the ureters is indicated in children with high-grade reflux, recurring UTI, or upper urinary tract deterioration. However, hostile neurogenic bladder dysfunction must be relieved prior to antireflux surgery by intermittent catheterization and anticholinergic therapy, or at the time of reimplantation by augmentation enterocystoplasty. The impact of surgical interventions that increase urethral resistance, such as a Kropp procedure or implantation of an artificial urinary sphincter, must be considered carefully, because these techniques tend to lower compliance and may exacerbate existing reflux.

Bowel Management. The normal propulsive tone of the bowel is impaired in children with spina bifida, and only 14% of younger children with spina bifida have bowel control.[51] This results in bowel management challenges that can be frustrating for children, parents, and healthcare professionals. Bowel management is further complicated by the Arnold-Chiari syndrome, which affects swallowing and feeding. Individualized routines, along with intervention at birth and maintaining a timed regimen of fiber, oral stool softeners, suppositories,

and occasional enemas, are the key to effective management. If a bowel routine is not established, chronic constipation or fecal impaction may occur, leading to megacolon, recurring urinary tract infections, lethargy, poor appetite, and fecal incontinence.

Bowel management typically begins with gentle disimpaction using one or multiple enemas. Adequate fluid intake and fiber from dietary sources (Table 13-4) are encouraged to minimize formation of hardened stool, but a scheduled defecation program must be established that routinely evacuates stool from the bowel and prevents involuntary defecation episodes.[52] These programs must be individualized and establishing a predictable bowel routine usually requires a period of days to weeks. The program usually incorporates abdominal or perineal massage to provoke a peristaltic wave; anorectal digital stimulation is used when these methods are not adequate. A glycerin or bisacodyl suppository may be administered to provoke anal evacuation, or a low-volume enema (100 to 150 ml), with or without a glycerin or contact laxative, may be used if necessary. Oral laxatives may be used in some patients. Alternatives include isosmotic laxatives, hyperosmotic solutions, and a senna preparation (Table 13-5).[53]

Attempts to trigger defecation are made approximately 20 minutes after a meal. Successful defecation can be achieved but not without commitment on the part of the parents and child. The urologic nurse should support the family, particularly as they seek to identify and establish a successful bowel management program. Parents and patients are advised that even the most successful bowel regimen may be interrupted by incontinent episodes that can provoke feelings of embarrassment and failure. Children with

TABLE 13-4 Common Dietary Fiber Sources

TYPE OF FOOD	SOURCE
Whole grains	Wheat, rye, oat, millet, buckwheat, all-bran cereal, shredded wheat cereal, popcorn, brown rice
Fruits	Apples, blackberries, raspberries, strawberries, peaches, pears, bananas, apricots
Vegetables	Beans, lentils, asparagus, carrots, garlic, broccoli, Brussels sprouts, acorn squash, zucchini

myelodysplasia may experience multiple surgical procedures; hospitalization can be a source of frustration for parents who have their child on a satisfactory bowel routine at home, only to have it completely altered by the hospital routine. Hospital-based nurses can prevent or ease this frustration by inquiring about the child's bowel routine and incorporating it during the child's care during hospitalization as closely as possible.

Antegrade colonic enemas may be used in children who cannot be adequately managed by more conservative means.[54] To perform antegrade irrigation, a surgical channel to the large bowel is formed (both left and right colons may be selected), usually using the appendix. The parents are then taught to perform antegrade colonic irrigations to improve bowel evacuation and prevent fecal soiling.

Latex Precautions. Children with myelomeningocele have a high incidence of severe latex allergy (15%) and an even higher incidence of latex hypersensitivity (48%).[55] The cause of this problem is not understood, but repeated exposure to latex products (especially the powder from latex gloves) during the first few months of life appears to play a role. Hypersensitivity reactions to latex among children with myelomeningocele often include rhinitis, conjunctivitis, bronchospasm, anaphylaxis, and cardiac arrest. Because of the prevalence of these reactions and the risk of anaphylaxis, all children with spina bifida are managed in a latex-free environment and parents or care providers are taught to avoid using products containing latex in the immediate environment.[56] Box 13-1 lists common latex-containing medical equipment and supplies.

TABLE 13-5 Dosage Guidelines for Stool Softeners and Stimulants

TYPE OF AGENT	GUIDELINES AND DOSAGE
Stool Softeners	
Mineral oil (plain)*	Age 4-7 yr or <28 kg: 10 ml at bedtime
	Age >7 yr or >28 kg: 20 ml at bedtime
Mineral oil with phenolphthalein (Agoral), flavored*	Age 4 to 7 yr or <28 kg: 5 ml at bedtime
	Age >7 yr or >28 kg: 10 ml at bedtime
Lactulose	0.5-1.0 ml/kg bid
	Adolescents: 15 ml bid (maximum dose, 90 ml/day)
Laxatives	
Barley malt soup extract (Maltsupex), liquid or powder	Age 4-7 yr or <28 kg: 5-10 ml at bedtime
	Age >7 yr or >28 kg: 5-10 ml bid
Phillips' Milk of Magnesia (MOM) or Haley's M-O (75% MOM and 25% mineral oil)	1 ml/kg bid
	Adolescents: 60 ml bid (1 tablet MOM = 2.5 ml liquid)
Sennosides (Senokot)	Age 4-7 yr or <28 kg: 2.5-5 ml of syrup bid
	Age >7 yr or >28 kg: 5-10 ml of syrup bid *or* 2.5-5 ml of granules bid *or* 1-2 tablets bid
Senna concentrate (Fletcher's Castoria)	Age <5 yr: 5-10 ml at bedtime
	Age >5 yr: 10-15 ml at bedtime
Dulcolax	Age >5 yr: 1 5-mg tablet at bedtime
	Age >12 yr: 2 5-mg tablets at bedtime
Rectal Suppositories	
Glycerin suppository	Use prn to stimulate defecation
Dulcolax suppository	10 mg—use with children >2 yr to stimulate defecation
Enemas	
Mineral oil enema	30-60 ml/9 kg prn to soften stool
	Adolescents: 120 ml prn to soften stool
Sodium phosphate (Fleet) enema	30-60 ml/9 kg prn to stimulate defecation
	Adolescents: 120 ml (maximum dose, 240 ml) prn to stimulate defecation

*If mineral oil is used, multivitamin supplementation is recommended because of potential for reduced absorption of fat-soluble vitamins.

Sexuality. Sexual dysfunction may affect both males and females with myelodysplasia.[12] Males with lesions affecting spinal level S1 or lower are more likely to have preservation of erectile function, whereas 50% of those with higher lesions will experience erections adequate for sexual activity.[12] Women with myelodysplasia are typically able to conceive children, although little is known about the influence of myelodysplasia on their sexual function. Although the likelihood of sexual activity is inversely proportional to the severity of neurologic impairment,[57] it must be remembered that counseling about sexual function must made available for all adolescents and young adults with myelodysplasia.

BOX 13-1 Common Latex-Containing Medical Equipment and Supplies

. . . .

Electrocardiogram pads
Tape
Foley catheters
Dilating catheters
Surgical drains
Nasogastric tubes
Surgical or examination gloves
Reservoir bags
Blood pressure cuffs
Tourniquets
Face masks
Ventilators, hoses, and bellows
Injection ports of IV tubing and IV bags
Stoppers in medication vials and syringes
Floating disk valves on some IV burette chambers

Urologic management of children with myelomeningocele occurs in the context of an overall rehabilitation program. Nevertheless, communication among specialists managing the child with a neural tube defect may be inadequate, leading to replication of services or conflicting approaches to general management. When managing any patient with a neural tube defect, the urologic nurse should remain aware of the goals and interventions provided by others caring for each patient, and assist the individual to understand and incorporate urologic services into their overall rehabilitation program. In addition, the urologic nurse should direct the family to resources for those coping with spina bifida; these can provide invaluable assistance when coping with the demands created by this multisystem anomaly (Box 13-2).

PRUNE-BELLY SYNDROME

Prune-belly syndrome (PBS), sometimes called triad or Eagle-Barrett syndrome, is characterized by deficiency of the abdominal muscles, dilation of the urinary tract (large bladder; hydronephrosis; and tortuous, wide ureters), and bilateral cryptorchidism (Figure 13-6).[58] Along with these trademark characteristics, PBS is also associated with respiratory, gastric, musculoskeletal, and cardiovascular anomalies. The full triad of symptoms only occurs in males; however, some female infants (approximately 3% of all cases) will have the abdominal wall defects and urinary tract dilation characteristic of full-blown PBS (Table 13-6). A classification system for PBS advocated by Woodard is presented in Table 13-7.[58]

BOX 13-2 Resources for Parents and Children

. . . .

Organizations

Spina Bifida and Hydrocephalus Association of Canada: English—www.sbhac.ca. Accessed March 4, 2008.

Spina Bifida Association of America—http://www.spinabifidaassociation.org/site/c.liKWL7PLLrF/b.2642297/k.5F7C/ Spina_Bifida_Association.htm. Accessed March 4, 2008.

Association of Spina Bifida and Hydrocephalus UK – www.asbah.org/. Accessed March 4, 2008.

Books and Publications

Woodbine House: The Special-Needs Collection—books on disabilities and related topics; www.woodbinehouse.com. Accessed March 4, 2008.

SBAA Publications—many booklets and pamphlets; http://www.spinabifidaassociation.org/site/apps/ka/ec/category.asp? c=liKWL7PLLrF&b=2705387&en=grKHIYOHI8LGKVNAI7LGIZPKIpI1J3NxFaKSK9NLIiJMLYOMLvF. Accessed March 4, 2008.

The incidence of PBS is 1 in 35,000 to 50,000 live births.[58] One in every 23 boys born with PBS is a twin; other high-risk groups include blacks and children born to younger mothers. However, clinical experience has suggested that the incidence of PBS may be declining, possibly as a result of prenatal ultrasonography.

PBS is usually diagnosed during neonatal examination because of the absence of abdominal musculature, resulting in the characteristic flabby, wrinkled, "prune belly"[58] (Figure 13-7) Nevertheless, some infants will have more subtle deficiencies of abdominal musculature, more closely resembling a pot-bellied rather than prune-belly appearance seen with the full-blown syndrome. They also tend to have less severe urinary system anomalies. Palpation of the scrotum is completed, which will reveal bilateral absence of the testes. Because the testes are typically intraabdominal, the likelihood that they will spontaneously descend is extremely low.

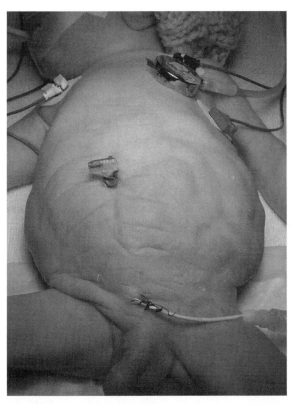

Fig. 13-6 Prune-belly syndrome in a newborn. (From Wein AJ, Kavoussi LR, Novick AC, Partin AW, Peters CA [eds]: Campbell-Walsh Urology, 9th edition. Philadelphia: Saunders-Elsevier, 2007; p 3486.)

In addition to a careful physical examination, the initial evaluation focuses on cardiopulmonary function.[58] After cardiopulmonary function is stabilized, urologic assessment proceeds with a serum creatinine and electrolyte level determination, as well as ultrasonography to characterize the extent of urinary tract dilation. A radionuclide imaging study, either a ^{99m}Tc-mercaptoacetyltriglycine (MAG3) or dimercaptosuccinic acid (DMSA) study, is completed at about age 4 to 6 weeks. A diethylenetriaminepentaacetic acid (DTPA) scan or Whitaker test may be completed to evaluate

TABLE 13-6 Genitourinary Tract Anomalies of the Prune-Belly Syndrome

ORGAN OR STRUCTURE AFFECTED	DESCRIPTION
Urethra	Dilated appearance of proximal urethra caused by prostatic hypoplasia; congenital megalourethra may occur, causing dilation of *anterior* urethra, with normal-caliber distal urethra; urethral atresia seen occasionally, associated with poor prognosis
Accessory sex organs	Prostate hypoplastic; may see absence of atresia of seminal vesicles, vas deferens
Bladder and urachus	Bladder is large, may have hourglass configuration on voiding cystourethrogram; compliance of bladder wall usually high but detrusor contraction strength usually compromised; lateral displacement of ureteric orifices in 70%; apex of bladder may be attached to umbilicus, with patent urachus
Ureters	Dilated, tortuous, elongated ureter; dilation may be segmental, interspersed with sections of normal caliber; distal ureter most severely affected; vesicoureteral reflux seen in 85%
Kidneys	Hydronephrosis, renal dysplasia occur in more than 50%
Testicles	Bilateral cryptorchidism; testes typically intraabdominal; infertility, azoospermia common

TABLE 13-7 Woodard Classification System for Prune-Belly Syndrome

TYPE	DESCRIPTION
I	Oligohydramnios, pulmonary hypoplasia, or pneumothorax; may have urethral obstruction of patent urachus and clubfoot
II	Typical external features and uropathy of full-blown syndrome but no immediate problem with survival; may have mild or unilateral renal dysplasia; may or may not develop urosepsis or gradual azotemia
III	External features may be mild or incomplete; uropathy less severe, renal function stable

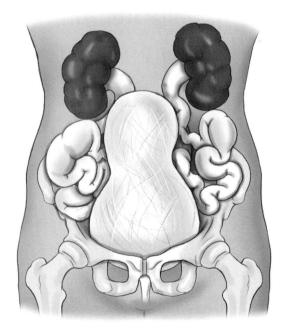

Fig. 13-7 Schematic drawing of PBS showing absence of abdominal musculature, bladder distention, gross ureteric dilatation, and hydronephosis (Source Jeanne Robinson November 1, 2007, doc A1912-13-08.)

upper urinary tract drainage, particularly if urinary tract infection or massive hydronephrosis is compromising renal function. Ongoing evaluation includes repeated measurement of the serum creatinine level.[59]

Initial evaluation is followed by ongoing assessment of renal and urinary system function with a combination of urinalysis, serum creatinine or other blood studies, and imaging studies such as ultrasonography or radionuclide scan throughout infancy and childhood. Follow-up evaluation is critical because of the risk for urinary stasis, infection, and potentially reversible renal deterioration.

Care is given in a medical center with expertise in managing this unusual syndrome and a multidisciplinary team capable of addressing the healthcare needs of the child with PBS. The urologic goals of treatment are preservation of renal function, prevention of urinary tract infection, correction of cryptorchidism when present, and reconstruction of the abdominal wall. Although surgical intervention is not typically indicated for the infant with PBS, obstruction may occur that demands prompt and aggressive intervention to avoid further renal deterioration. Orchidopexy is typically performed during early infancy. Early timing is preferential for the boy with PBS because the testes are more easily mobilized into the scrotum, and because later surgery is associated with a much higher risk of significant subfertility.[60]

External support devices may be obtained that provide support for the abdominal wall, but most patients prefer surgery to provide a more cosmetically pleasing appearance to the abdominal wall. Abdominoplasty is also advocated because it improves micturition and defecation efficiency. Surgical repair involves a transverse lower abdominal incision to remove lax tissue. The most abnormal segments of redundant abdominal wall are excised with care to preserve the motor nerves to the retained lateral and upper abdominal walls and musculature.

SACRAL AGENESIS

Sacral agenesis, also called caudal regression syndrome, is characterized by complete or total absence of the sacrum, hemisacrum, coccyx, and at least two vertebrae of the sacral spinal column.[61] In the pediatric neurologic literature, sacral agenesis comprises one aspect of a larger set of defects described as crural-vesical gluteal dystrophy syndrome.[62] Vertebral defects are characteristically found in the lower (sacral) vertebrae, but the lumbar cord also may be affected (lumbosacral agenesis) and the thoracic cord is rarely involved. It is divided into four types—partial agenesis is seen in types 1 and 2, type 3 is characterized by total absence of the sacral vertebrae, and type 4 is characterized by lumbosacral agenesis.[63]

It is a rare disorder, with a reported incidence of 0.09% to 0.43%.[64] Maternal diabetes is a major risk factor, yielding a 1% risk of sacral agenesis with each pregnancy.[12] In addition, the incidence of delivering a child with sacral agenesis when the mother is affected is 12% to 16%. One variant of the disorder is called Currarino syndrome, or autosomal dominant sacral agenesis.[65] Children with Currarino syndrome have absence of sacral vertebrae S2-S5 only, as well as anorectal malformations, a presacral mass, and neuropathic bladder dysfunction.

Assessment

Diagnosis typically occurs in one of two settings. More than 75% are diagnosed during early infancy based on physical findings, including flattened buttocks causing a shortened gluteal cleft, orthopedic abnormalities (especially clubfoot), and neurologic deficits. However, others will have a normal newborn neurologic examination and they are usually diagnosed between ages 4 and 5 years because of unsuccessful toilet training.[12] Motor deficits correspond closely to the level of the associated vertebral anomaly, but sensations are usually preserved.[61] A kidney, ureter, and bladder (KUB) study may reveal abnormal gas patterns and raise a suspicion of sacral agenesis, but lateral x-rays of the lower spine or spinal magnetic resonance imaging (MRI) should be used to confirm the diagnosis.

Neuropathic Bladder Dysfunction. Because sacral agenesis affects the spinal cord, neuropathic bladder dysfunction is found in almost all children with sacral agenesis.[66] Assessment of the urinary system begins with a history and physical examination, focusing on lower urinary tract symptoms. Older children with sacral agenesis will have voiding frequency, urgency, and dribbling UI.[12] Constipation, fecal soiling, or spotting and recurring urinary tract infection are also common. Videourodynamic testing, or multichannel urodynamics and voiding cystourethrography, is necessary to characterize lower urinary tract function. In one series of 22 children seen over a period of 20 years, urodynamic evaluation revealed neurogenic detrusor overactivity in 91%, vesicosphincter dyssynergia in 64%, and

clinically relevant postvoid residual urine in 68%.[69] The bladder neck was open in 68% but the prevalence of stress UI was not reported. Evidence of upper urinary tract distress was found in almost 50%, including vesicoureteral reflux in 45%, renal scarring in 32%, and elevated creatinine level or decreased glomerular filtration rate in 14%.

Treatment

Management principles in the child with sacral agenesis are similar to those outlined for spinal dysraphism. Early diagnosis is important because of the risk of upper urinary tract distress and renal function deterioration when management is delayed. In addition to preventing or arresting upper urinary tract distress and urinary tract infection, maintenance of social continence is achieved by a combination of scheduled toileting, pharmacotherapy, and/or intermittent catheterization.[12,67] Surgical intervention is necessary in select children and may include augmentation enterocystoplasty or ureteral reimplantation for reflux. Bowel management also must be carefully assessed and a bowel program instituted, when indicated, to prevent constipation and fecal incontinence and reduce the risk of urinary tract infection.

In addition to urinary system disorders, the urologic nurse should remember that sacral agenesis is a multisystem anomaly and its optimal management requires a multidisciplinary team. Key players usually include gastroenterologists and pediatric surgeons to manage anorectal disorders and neurosurgeons to assess for operable disorders, such as a tethered spinal cord or lipomeningocele to arrest progressive neurologic damage.[68]

Management

Management is directed to the specific lesion identified by urodynamic testing. Intermittent catheterization and anticholinergics should be prescribed as indicated. Children with sacral agenesis have bowel dysfunction similar to that in children with spina bifida. Early bowel management is critical to optimize the remaining function and maintain fecal continence.

IMPERFORATE ANUS (RECTAL ATRESIA)

Imperforate anus—rectal atresia—describes one aspect of a constellation of anorectal malformations associated with fecal and urinary incontinence and sexual dysfunction in children.[12,69] In addition, 30% to 45% of children will have spinal defects. Various classification systems have been advocated; the Wingspread classification system is useful for the urologic nurse (Table 13-8).[70] This divides anorectal anomalies into low lesions, primarily affecting structures inferior to the levator ani; intermediate lesions, primarily affecting structures at or below the levator ani; and high lesions, affecting structures well above the pelvic floor. Imperforate anus may occur alone or as part of a constellation of abnormalities called VATER or VACTERL syndrome (**v**ertebral, **a**nal, **c**ardiac, **t**racheo**e**sophageal fistula, **r**enal, **l**imb). Imperforate anus also occurs with cloacal anomalies in girls or the Townes-Brock syndrome[71]—external ear anomalies, hearing loss, preaxial polydactyly, triphalangeal thumbs, renal malformations, and rectal atresia. The cause of imperforate anus is not yet completely understood, but genetic mutations are strongly suspected[71, 72] and a porcine model has been constructed that indicates that abnormal development of the cloacal membrane may play a role.[73]

Urologic involvement depends on the level of the lesion. About 20% of infants with low lesions will have urologic anomalies as compared with 60% with high (supralevator) lesions. Common urologic disorders associated with imperforate anus include vesicoureteral reflux, neuropathic bladder with incontinence and/or urinary retention, renal agenesis, renal dysplasia, perineal or prostatic fistulae, and cryptorchidism. Spinal defects often include a tethered cord, increasing the risk for secondary neuropathic bladder dysfunction.[12]

Assessment

Newborn assessment begins with inspection of the perineum, paying careful attention to the anus and any fistulae from the bowels, and neurologic examination, looking for spinal defects. Urologic evaluation is begun after bowel elimination is established and the neonate is medically stable. Similar to the child with a spinal dysraphism, it incorporates serum creatinine and electrolyte level determination, urinalysis, and imaging of the upper urinary tracts. Infants with a spinal anomaly also undergo videourodynamic testing or voiding cystourethrography and multichannel urodynamics.

Management

A double-barrel colostomy is usually performed to ensure a patent gastrointestinal tract. Approximately 1 month after the initial diverting colostomy, definitive repair of the anorectal malformations is completed and the colostomy closed and large bowel reanastomosed in a third surgery.[69] More recently, primary repair has been advocated because it avoids the initial colostomy and final closure procedures, but a comparison of long-term functional results using this versus the staged approach has not been completed.[74]

Urologic nursing management focuses on the same three goals described for spinal dysraphisms: (1) preservation of optimal renal function; (2) prevention or prompt management of urinary tract infections; and (3) social continence. Many children will have neurogenic detrusor overactivity with detrusor-sphincter dyssynergia (reflex urinary incontinence). This condition may be managed by

TABLE 13-8 Wingspread Classification of Anorectal Malformation

DEFECT	HIGH (SUPRALEVATOR) (36%)*	INTERMEDIATE (INFRALEVATOR) (14%)	LOW (SUBLEVATOR) (47%)
Male	Anorectal agenesis; rectourethral fistula*; rectal atresia	Rectovestibular urethral fistula; anal agenesis, no fistula	Anocutaneous fistula; anal stenosis
Female	Anorectal agenesis; rectovaginal fistula†; rectal atresia	Rectovestibular atresia; rectovaginal fistula; anal agenesis without fistula	Anovestibular fistula; anocutaneous fistula; anal stenosis

*Remaining 1% are cloacal anomalies.

†Defect may or may not occur.

Modified from Bauer SB: Voiding dysfunction in children: neurogenic and non-neurogenic. In Walsh PC, Retik AB, Vaughan ED, Wein AJ (eds): Campbell's Urology, 8th edition. Philadelphia: Saunders, 2002; p 2251.

intermittent catheterization, usually in combination with antimuscarinic pharmacotherapy. Others will have poor detrusor contraction strength with sphincter incompetence, which is also frequently managed by intermittent catheterization supplemented by α-adrenergic agonist drug therapy to increase urethral resistance. Regardless of the urologic defects, it should be remembered that a bladder management program must be combined with ongoing bowel management to maximize fecal and urinary incontinence care.

SUMMARY

Nurses coordinate care for children and families who experience a wide range of needs throughout different stages of growth and development, and the numerous hospitalizations they encounter. The urologic nurse uses her or his skills to assist the family in maximizing independence and self-care while maintaining an optimal level of health, through client education, knowledge of best practices and resources, and continuous assessment of individuals and families.

REFERENCES

1. Dorlands Illustrated Medical Dictionary, 31st edition. Philadelphia: Saunders, 2007; p 589.
2. Tortoir-Donati P, Rossi A, Biancheri R, Cama A: Magnetic resonance imaging of spinal dysraphism. Topics in Magnetic Resonance Imaging, 2001; 12:375-409.
3. Hasenau SM, Covington C: Neural tube defect defects: prevention and folic acid. MCN American Journal of Maternal Child Nursing, 2002; 27:87-91.
4. Schropp C, Sorensen N, Collmann H, Krauss J: Cutaneous lesions in occult spinal dysraphism—correlation with intraspinal findings. Childs Nervous System, 2006; 22(2):125-31.
5. Henriques JG, Pianetti G, Henriques KS, Costa P, Gusmao S: Minor skin lesions as markers of occult spinal dysraphisms—prospective study. Surgical Neurology, 2005; 63(Suppl 1):S8-S12.
6. Guggisberg D, Hadj-Rabia S, Viney C, Bodemer C, Brunelle F, Zerah M, Pierre-Kahn A, de Prost Y, Hamel-Teillac D, et al: Skin markers of occult spinal dysraphism in children: a review of 54 cases. Archives of Dermatology, 2004; 140(9):1109-15.
7. Rosenberg IH: Folic acid and neural tube defects—time for action? New England Journal of Medicine, 1992; 327:1875-7.
8. Gucciardi E, Pietrusiak MA, Reynolds DL, Rouleau J: Incidence of neural tube defects in Ontario, 1986-1999. Canadian Medical Association Journal, 2002; 167:237-40.
9. Persad VL, Van den Hof MC, Dube JM, Zimmer P: Incidence of open neural tube defects in Nova Scotia after folic acid fortification. Canadian Medical Association Journal, 2002; 167:241-5.
10. Siffel C, Alverson CJ, Correa A: Analysis of seasonal variation of birth defects in Atlanta. Birth Defects Research, 2005; 73(10):655-62.
11. Byrne J, Cama A, Reilly M, Vigliaoro M, Levato L, Boni L, et al: Multigenerational maternal transmission in Italian families with neural tube defects. American Journal of Medical Genetics, 1996; 18:303-10.
12. Yeung CK, Sihoe JDY, Bauer SB: Voiding Dysfunction in Children: Non-Neurogenic and Neurogenic. In Wein AJ, Kavoussi LR, Novick AC, Partin AW, Peters CA (eds): Campbell-Walsh Urology, 9th edition. Philadelphia: Saunders, 2007; pp 3604-55.
13. Centers for Disease Control and Prevention (CDC): Spina bifida and anencephaly before and after folic acid mandate—United States, 1995-1996 and 1999-2000. MMWR Morbidity and Mortality Weekly Report, 2004; 53(17):362-5.
14. Werler MM, Shapiro S, Mitchell AA: Preconceptual folic acid exposure and risk of occurrent neural tube defects. Journal of the American Medical Association, 1993; 269:1257-61.
15. Williams LJ, Rasmussen SA, Flores A, Kirby RS, Edmonds LD: Decline in the prevalence of spina bifida and anencephaly by race/ethnicity: 1995-2002. Pediatrics, 2005; 116(3):580-6.
16. Mitchell LE, Adzick NS, Melchionne J, Pasquariello PS, Sutton LN, Whitehead AS: Spina bifida. Lancet, 2004; 364(9448):1885-95.
17. Mevorach RA, Bogaert GA, Baskin LS, Lazzaretti CC, Edwards MS, Kogan BA: Lower urinary tract function in ambulatory children with spina bifida. British Journal of Urology, 1996; 77:593-6.
18. Peeker R, Damber JE, Hjalmas K, Sjodin JG, Zweigbergk M: The urological fate of young adults with myelomeningocele: a three-decade follow-up study. European Urology, 1997; 32:213-7.
19. Bell WO, Nelson LH, Block SM, Rhoney JC: Prenatal diagnosis and pediatric neurosurgery. Pediatric Neurosurgery, 1996; 24:134-7.
20. Blumenfeld Z, Siegler E, Bronshtein M: The early diagnosis of neural tube defects. Prenatal Diagnosis, 1993; 13:863-71.
21. Ennever FK, Lave LB: Parent preferences and prenatal testing for neural tube defects. Epidemiology, 1995; 6:8-16.
22. Benson JT, Dillard RG, Burton BK: Open spina bifida: does cesarean delivery improve prognosis? Obstetrics and Gynecology, 1988; 71:532-4.
23. Hogge WA, Dungan JS, Brooks MP, Dilks SA, Abbitt PL, Thiagarajah S, Ferguson JE: Diagnosis and management of prenatally detected myelomeningocele: a preliminary report. American Journal of Obstetrics and Gynecology, 1990; 163:1061-5.
24. Sutherland RW, Gonzales ET: Current management of the infant with myelomeningocele. Current Opinion in Urology, 1999; 9:527-31.
25. Decter RM, Furness PD 3rd, Nguyen TA, McGowan M, Laudermilch C, Telenko A: Reproductive understanding, sexual functioning and testosterone levels in men with spina bifida. Journal of Urology, 1997; 157:1466-8.
26. Game X, Moscovici J, Game L, Sarramon JP, Rischmann P, Malavaud B: Evaluation of sexual function in young men with spina bifida and myelomeningocele using the International Index of Erectile Function. Urology, 2006; 67(3):566-70.
27. Cass AS: Urinary tract complications in myelomeningocele patients. Journal of Urology, 1976; 115:102-4.
28. Bomalaski MD, Teague JL, Brooks B: The long-term impact of urological management on the quality of life of children with spina bifida. Journal of Urology, 1995; 154:778-81.
29. Laurence KM, Beresford A: Continence, friends, marriage and children in 51 adults with spina bifida. Developmental Medicine and Child Neurology, 1975; Suppl(35):123-8.
30. Verhoef M, Barf HA, Vroege JA, Post MW, Van Asbeck FW, Gooskens RH, Prevo AJ: Sex education, relationships, and sexuality in young adults with spina bifida. Archives of Physical Medicine and Rehabilitation, 2005; 86(5):979-87.
31. Lemelle JL, Guillemin F, Aubert D, Guys JM, Lottmann H, Lortat-Jacob S, Moscovici J, Mouriquand P, Ruffion A, Schmitt M: A multicenter evaluation of urinary incontinence management and outcome in spina bifida. Journal of Urology, 2006; 175(1):208-12.
32. Geraniotis E, Koff SA, Enrile B: The prophylactic use of clean intermittent catheterization in the treatment of infants and young children with myelomeningocele and neurogenic bladder dysfunction. Journal of Urology, 1988; 139:85-6.
33. Getliffe K, Fader M, Allen C, Pinar K, Moore KN: Current evidence on intermittent catheterization: Sterile single-use catheters or clean reused catheters and the incidence of UTI. Journal of Wound, Ostomy and Continence Nursing, 2007; 34:289-296.

34. Cohen RA, Rushton HG, Belman AB, Kass EJ, Majd M, Shaer C: Renal scarring and vesicoureteral reflux in children with myelodysplasia. Journal of Urology, 1990; 144:541-5.

35. Campbell JB, Moore KN, Voaklander DC, Mix LW: Complications associated with clean intermittent catheterization in children with spina bifida. Journal of Urology, 2004; 171(6 Pt 1):2420-2.

36. Turkoski BB, Lance BR, Bonfiglio MF: Drug Information Handbook for Advanced Practice Nursing, 8th edition. Hudson, Ohio: Lexi-Comp, 2007.

37. Buyse G, Waldeck K, Verpoorten C, Bjork H, Casaer P, Andersson KE: Intravesical oxybutynin for neurogenic bladder dysfunction: less systemic side effects due to reduced first pass metabolism. Journal of Urology, 1998; 160(3 Pt 1):892-6.

38. Palmer LS, Zebold K, Firlit CF, Kaplan WE: Complications of intravesical oxybutynin chloride therapy in the pediatric myelomeningocele population. Journal of Urology, 1997; 157:638-40.

39. Morrisroe SN, O'Connor RC, Nanigian DK, Kurzrock EA, Stone AR: Vesicostomy revisited: the best treatment for the hostile bladder in myelodysplastic children? BJU International, 2005; 96(3): 397-400.

40. Lee MW, Greenfield SP: Intractable high-pressure bladder in female infants with spina bifida: clinical characteristics and use of vesicostomy. Urology, 2005; 65(3):568-71.

41. Gosalbez R Jr, Woodard JR, Broecker BH, Warshaw B: Metabolic complications of the use of stomach for urinary reconstruction. Journal of Urology, 1993; 150:710-2.

42. Nguyen DH, Mitchell ME, Horowitz M, Bagli DJ, Carr MC: Demucosalized augmentation gastrocystoplasty with bladder auto-augmentation in pediatric patients. Journal of Urology, 1996; 156:206-9.

43. Kassouf W: Collagen injection for treatment of urinary incontinence in children. Journal of Urology, 2001; 165:1666-8.

44. Kropp KA, Angwafo FF: Urethral lengthening and reimplantation for neurogenic incontinence in children. Journal of Urology, 1986; 135:533-6.

45. Salle JL, de Fraga JC, Amarante A, Silveira ML, Lambertz M, Schmidt M, Rosito NC: Urethral lengthening with anterior bladder wall flap for urinary incontinence: a new approach. Journal of Urology, 1994; 152:803-6.

46. Spiess PE: Is an artificial sphincter the best choice for incontinent boys with spina bifida? Review of our long term experience with the AS-800 artificial sphincter. Canadian Journal of Urology, 2002; 9:1486-91.

47. Mitrofanoff P: Trans-appendicular continent cystostomy in the management of the neurogenic bladder. Chirurgie Pediatrique, 1980; 21:297-305.

48. Duckett JW, Snyder HM 3rd: Continent urinary diversion: variations on the Mitrofanoff principle. Journal of Urology, 1986; 136:58-62.

49. Stein R, Fisch M, Ermert A, Schwarz M, Black P, Filipas D, Hohenfellner R: Urinary diversion and orthotopic bladder substitution in children and young adults with neurogenic bladder: a safe option for treatment? Journal of Urology, 2000; 163:568-79.

50. Mitchell ME: Reconstruction of the urinary tract: general principles. In Gillenwater JY, Grayhack JT, Howards SS, Duckett JW (eds): Adult and Pediatric Urology, 4th edition. St Louis: Mosby, 2002; pp 2405-14.

51. Lie HR, Lagergren J, Rasmussen F, Lagerkrist B, Hagelsteen J, Borjeson M-C, et al: Bowel and bladder control of children with myelomeningocele: a Nordic study. Developmental Medicine and Child Neurology, 1991; 33:1053-61.

52. Corazziari E, Badiali D, Inghilleri M: Neurologic disorders affecting the anorectum. Gastroenterology Clinics of North America, 2001; 30:253-68.

53. Jinbo A, Stark M: Bowel and bladder management in children. In Doughty DB (ed): Urinary and Fecal Incontinence: Nursing Management, 3rd edition. St Louis: Mosby, 2006; pp 491-545.

54. Lemelle JL, Guillemin F, Aubert D, Guys JM, Lottmann H, Lortat-Jacob S, Moscovici J, Mouriquand P, Ruffion A, Schmitt M: A multicentre study of the management of disorders of defecation in patients with spina bifida. Neurogastroenterology and Motility, 2006; 18(2):123-8.

55. Rendeli C, Nucera E, Ausili E, Tabacco F, Roncallo C, Pollastrini E, Scorzoni M: Latex sensitization and allergy in children with myelomeningocele. Childs Nervous System, 2006; 22(1):28-32.

56. Nieta A, Mazon A, Pamies R, Lanuza A, Munoz A, Estornell F, Garcia-Ibarra F: Efficacy of latex avoidance for primary prevention of latex sensitization in children with spina bifida. Journal of Pediatrics, 2002; 140:370-72.

57. Joyner BD, McLorie GA, Khoury AE: Sexuality and reproductive issues in children with myelomeningocele. European Journal of Pediatric Surgery, 1998; 8:29-34.

58. Caldemone AA, Woodard JR: Prune-belly syndrome. In Wein AJ, Kavoussi LR, Novick AC, Partin AW, Peters CA, editors: Campbell-Walsh Urology, 9th edition. Philadelphia: Saunders, 2007; pp 3482-96.

59. Noh PH, Cooper CS, Winkler AC, Zderic SA, Snyder HM 3rd, Canning DA: Prognostic factors for long-term renal function in boys with the prune-belly syndrome. Journal of Urology, 1999; 162:1399-401.

60. Woodard JR, Parrott TS: Orchiopexy in the prune belly syndrome. British Journal of Urology, 1978; 50:348-51.

61. Ashwal S: Congenital structural defects. In Swaiman KE, Ashwal S (eds): Pediatric Neurology: Principles and Practice, 4th edition. St Louis: Mosby, 2006; pp 234-300.

62. Gregoire A, Zerdani S: Lumbo-sacral agenesis. Pediatria Medica e Chirurgica, 2001; 23:89-98.

63. Renshaw TS: Sacral agenesis. Journal of Bone and Joint Surgery, 1978; 60:373-83.

64. Guzman L, Bauer SB, Hallett M, Khoshbin S, Colodny AH, Retik AB: Evaluation and management of children with sacral agenesis. Urology, 1983; 22:506-10.

65. Lynch SA, Wang Y, Strachan T, Burn J, Lindsay S: Autosomal sacral agenesis: Currarino syndrome. Journal of Medical Genetics, 2000; 37:561-6.

66. Boemers TM, Beek FJ, van Gool JD, de Jong TP, Bax KM: Urologic problems in anorectal malformations. Part 1: urodynamic findings and significance of sacral anomalies. Journal of Pediatric Surgery, 1996; 31:407-10.

67. Wilmshurst JM, Kelly R, Borzyskowski M: Presentation and outcome of sacral agenesis: 20 years' experience. Developmental Medicine and Child Neurology, 1999; 41:806-12.

68. Muthukumar N: Surgical treatment of nonprogressive neurologic deficits in children with sacral agenesis. Neurosurgery, 1996; 38:1133-8.

69. Pena A, Hong A: Advances in the management of anorectal malformations. American Journal of Surgery, 2000; 180:370-6.

70. Shaul DB, Harrison EA: Classification of anorectal malformation: initial approach, diagnostic test and colostomy. Seminars in Pediatric Surgery, 1997; 6:187-95.

71. Lam FW, Chan WK, Lam ST, Chu WP, Kwong NS: Proximal 10q trisomy: a new case with anal atresia. Journal of Medical Genetics, 2000; 37:E24.

72. Keegan CE, Mulliken JB, Wu BL, Korf BR: Townes-Brocks syndrome versus expanded spectrum hemifacial microsomia: review of eight patients and further evidence of a "hot spot" for mutation in the SALL1 gene. Genetics in Medicine, 2001; 3:310-3.

73. Finnigan DF, Fisher KR, Vrablic O, Halina WG, Partlow GD: A proposed mechanism for intermediate atresia ani (AA), based on a porcine case of AA and hypospadias. Birth Defects Research, 2005; 73(6):434-9.

74. Levitt MA, Pena A: Outcomes from the correction of anorectal malformations. Current Opinion in Pediatrics, 2005; 17(3):394-401.

CHAPTER 14

Urinary Tract Infections and Vesicoureteral Reflux

As noted in Chapter 5, urinary tract infection (UTI) is prevalent in adults. However, most cases in adults occur in community-dwelling women, are associated with characteristic symptoms including dysuria and suprapubic pain, are characterized as simple (not associated with fever, voiding dysfunction, or an imminent risk to upper urinary tract function), and respond to 3 to 7 days of empirical therapy. In contrast, UTI in the pediatric population is associated with vague and nonspecific symptoms, is more likely to be associated with a fever or vesicoureteral reflux (VUR), and may require a more extensive evaluation to identify and present secondary complications such as recurring pyelonephritis, renal scarring, hypertension, or renal insufficiency.[1] This chapter will review the epidemiology, pathophysiology, assessment, and management of UTI and VUR in the pediatric population.

URINARY TRACT INFECTION

The basic terminology used to describe UTI in children is similar to that used for adult patients[2] (see Chapter 5). Bacteriuria is the presence of bacteria in the urine. Asymptomatic bacteriuria is defined as the presence of bacteria in the urine without added signs or symptoms of UTI. Similar to adults, its mere presence does not create justification for further evaluation or treatment. A UTI is defined as an inflammatory response of the urinary epithelium (urothelium) to invasion by a pathogen; it is also referred to as a symptomatic UTI, but the clinical manifestations of a UTI in a child differs from that seen in adults. Pyelonephritis describes a cluster of signs and symptoms used to describe a UTI that involves the upper urinary tracts and renal parenchyma in particular.

In contrast to the adult population, pediatric UTI may be categorized as initial or recurrent. This comparatively simplistic classification schema is more useful than the more complex classification system used for adults because of the unique clinical features of UTI in children and their propensity to be associated with fever, VUR, or pyelonephritis. An initial UTI is defined as the first symptomatic episode and a recurrent UTI is defined as one that occurs after an initial or previous episode. Similar to adults, the classic definition of recurrent UTI remains current today and is further classified as a reinfection, an episode that occurs after an initial or previous UTI has been successfully eradicated; an unresolved UTI; unrelenting bacteriuria because of ineffective therapy; or a persistent UTI, bacterial persistence caused by an anatomic defect or foreign object such as a stone that provides safe harbor for pathogens, despite appropriate antimicrobial therapy.[3] An afebrile UTI occurs in the absence of a fever, whereas as compared to febrile UTI, which is associated with a fever of 100.5° (38.0° C) or higher. Although research and clinical experience have suggested that a febrile UTI implies the presence of a true pyelonephritis (infection involving the upper urinary tracts) in adults, children may experience UTI in the absence of upper urinary tract infection.[1]

Epidemiology

Even though UTI is the most common reason for referral to a pediatric urology practice, surprisingly little is known about its prevalence and incidence in infants and children younger than 18 years. During the first year of life, almost 3% of boys and slightly less than 1% of girls will experience bacteriuria.[4] During the first 60 days of life, uncircumcised male infants are especially at risk for febrile UTI[5-7] but breast-feeding has been found to exert a protective effect in girls and boys.[8] A meta-analysis of more than 402,000 boys demonstrates that circumcision exerts a protective effect against UTI.[9] However, given a 1% incidence, 111 circumcisions must be performed to prevent one UTI. In addition, male infants undergoing circumcision by a Mohel (person of the Jewish faith who is ordained to perform circumcision in accordance with religious guidelines) have been found to have a higher rate of UTI as compared with infants circumcised by a physician, possibly because of difference in techniques used to wrap the penile shaft and achieve hemostasis.[10]

Following the first 60 days of life, the incidence and prevalence of UTI in girls exceed those of boys, and this trend persists into adulthood. Estimates of the incidence of UTI in girls vary from 1% to 10%, whereas the approximate incidence in boys falls to about 1%-1.6%.[1,11-13] In addition, the risk for a first-time and recurring UTI rises even more in girls as they enter into adolescence but decreases in boys.

Natural History

Potential long-term consequences of pediatric UTI include renal scarring, hypertension, proteinuria, and an increased risk for pyelonephritis as an adult.[14] Approximately 17% of children who experience UTI (especially febrile infections) will develop one or more renal scars.[1] Factors associated with an increased risk for renal scar formation include age; genetic factors such as a P1 blood group phenotype, which provides resistance to P fimbriae produced by some bacterial strains; angiotensin-converting enzyme genetic polymorphisms; and VUR. High levels of the inflammatory cytokine IL8 are often seen in children with UTI, VUR, renal scarring, and renal insufficiency, but the associated gene has not been found to be elevated in these patients or their siblings.[14a] The greatest risk for scar formation occurs during the first 4 years of life, and the subsequent risk for significant renal injury increases with each febrile UTI.[1,15] However, even among older children, the presence of VUR increases the risk for subsequent scarring. Women with renal scarring have been found to be at greater risk for pyelonephritis as adults.[16,17] This risk is particularly high during pregnancy and can lead to deleterious effects for the mother and a greater risk for mental retardation in the fetus unless promptly managed.[18] In addition, the number of pyelonephritis episodes has been found to increase proportionally with the severity of underlying scarring.[16,17]

Scarring has been associated with long-term changes in renal anatomy, as evidenced by a small renal mass that persists into adulthood, prompting fears of compromised renal function or hypertension.[19] However, several follow-up studies spanning 16 to 26 years following the onset of an initial childhood UTI have shown no increased risk for renal insufficiency and no substantial reduction in glomerular filtration rates, even in cases of moderately severe or severe renal scarring.[12,17,20] Furthermore, two of these studies have found no increased risk for hypertension,[12,20] and one found a low rate (5.5%) of hypertension in a group of 97 women followed by a nephrologist for 13 to 18 years.[16] Nevertheless, these studies follow subjects only into young adulthood, and the lifetime risk is unknown.

Etiology and Pathophysiology

The pathogenesis of pediatric UTI is complex and is not well understood. As in the adult patient, the development of a UTI represents a complex relationship between host resistance and bacterial virulence. Among community-dwelling children, *Escherichia coli* is the most common pathogen associated with UTI.[21] The number of pediatric UTIs attributable to *E. coli* varies from 57% to 89%, followed by a gram-positive pathogen (*Enterococcus*), 4% to 19%.[22-25] Other gram-negative species, such as *Proteus*, *Klebsiella*, *Enterobacter*, and *Pseudomonas* species, comprise less than 10% of total isolates. Even when community-dwelling children with a history of urinary system anomalies or existing disease of the urinary system, including end-stage renal disease, were compared with children without a known history of renal disease, *E. coli* emerged as the predominant species (40%) followed by *Enterococcus* species, which accounted for 20% of isolates.[23] In contrast, the characteristics of pathogens associated with nosocomial UTI differed from those affecting community-dwelling children. Among a group of 1045 children cared for in pediatric critical care units in the United States between 1992 and 1997, *E. coli* accounted for only 19% of all isolates, whereas *Enterococcus* species accounted for 10%. *Pseudomonas aeruginosa* was found in 13%, *Enterobacter* was found in 10%, and *Candida albicans* (a fungal species) accounted for 14%.[26] These findings reinforce the necessity of culture and sensitivity testing when managing a nosocomial UTI in a child, as well as some important differences when isolates in community-dwelling children are compared with isolates found in community-dwelling adult women.

Two virulence factors are strongly associated with an increased risk for producing a symptomatic UTI in children—fimbriae production and the ability to cause mannose-resistant hemagglutination.[11] When these two attributes coexist in a single strain of bacteria, the resulting infection is more likely to produce a fever in the child, irrespective of bacterial invasion of the upper urinary tracts. Nevertheless, the presence of these virulence factors also increases the risk for acute pyelonephritis and subsequent renal scarring.

Associated Factors

Multiple host susceptibility factors influence a child's risk for UTI (Table 14-1). Although most of these factors are constitutional, several are modifiable and of particular interest to urologic nurses.

Voiding Dysfunction. Voiding dysfunction is a nonspecific term used to describe various lower urinary tract symptoms often seen in neurologically normal children, including diurnal frequency or infrequent daytime voiding, urgency, urinary incontinence, dribbling or interrupted urinary stream, postvoid dribbling, and pain with urination. Lower urinary tract symptoms are frequently associated with fecal elimination abnormalities, such as encopresis or constipation.[27-30] Urodynamic characteristics of voiding dysfunction include sensory urgency, detrusor overactivity, and dyssynergia between detrusor muscle contraction and striated sphincter muscles.

TABLE 14-1 Host Susceptibility Factors Affecting the Risk for Urinary Tract Infection (UTI) in Infants and Children[21,31,77]

FACTOR	INFLUENCE ON UTI RISK
Gender and age	Males: First 3 months of life, overall risk diminishes with increasing age
	Females: Less than males during neonatal period; overall risk increases with age up to adolescence
Periurethral colonization	Males: Associated with uncircumcised phallus, particularly during infancy when foreskin cannot be retracted
	Females: Common in girls and adolescents with recurring UTI; risk possibly exacerbated with sexual activity
Genetic and familial factors	Humoral, cellular immunity factors modify risk*
	Familial patterns often seen in girls with recurring UTI but voiding or fecal elimination dysfunction (constipation, infrequency) more common than anatomic anomalies
	Familial patterns seen in boys and girls with vesicoureteral reflux; screening for vesicoureteral reflux recommended with strong family history
Fecal colonization	Increased risk in children with fecal incontinence, especially when managed by containment device (e.g., diaper), and those with encopresis, chronic constipation
Genitourinary anomalies	Increased risk for urinary stasis and obstruction, with resulting UTI; presence of UTI often leads to diagnosis of underlying anomaly
Neurogenic bladder dysfunction	Urinary incontinence, retention, obstruction associated with neurogenic bladder, increased risk of UTI
Voiding dysfunction	Infrequent voiding, overactive bladder dysfunction, non-neurogenic vesicosphincter dyssynergia lead to incomplete bladder emptying, turbulence of urinary outflow, increased risk for UTI
Approaching puberty in females	Risk for pyelonephritis, renal scarring, febrile UTI during pregnancy may be increased in young women who have persistent vesicoureteral reflux as they enter puberty

*See Chapter 5 for a more detailed discussion.

Voiding dysfunction characteristics usually associated with recurring UTI, febrile UTI, and VUR are infrequent voiding, low fluid intake, and stool retention.[31] Urodynamic characteristics most commonly seen in these children are detrusor overactivity associated with vesicosphincter dyssynergia. See Chapter 15 for a detailed discussion of voiding dysfunction in children and its management.

Dysfunctional Fecal Elimination. A number of researchers have observed an association among voiding dysfunction, abnormal bowel elimination (encopresis or constipation), VUR, and UTI.[28-30] Also, several studies have demonstrated that treatment of constipation or encopresis resolves abnormal lower urinary tract symptoms in as many as 63% of patients.[28,29] Although clinical reports have clearly demonstrated a correlation among these conditions, they do not establish a cause and effect relationship or elucidate the nature of underlying relationships. The complexity of these factors was illustrated in a noncontrolled study that compared two comparatively large groups of children, one with history of a febrile UTI before 2 years ($N = 123$) and another seen in a hospital emergency department with high fever but negative urine culture ($N = 125$). No differences were found in the prevalence of voiding dysfunction based on results of a dysfunctional elimination instrument.[32] Nevertheless, despite a lack of knowledge concerning the precise nature of these relationships, best practice recommendations strongly support assessing all children with recurrent UTI for dysfunctional urine and bowel elimination patterns.

A dysfunctional voiding score has been developed and validated. It deserves special mention as a potentially valuable adjunct to the urologic nursing assessment of children with voiding or bowel elimination disorders and UTI (Figure 14-1).[33] The score has been tested prospectively by patient interview; application and testing in studies using urodynamics as the gold standard are now required.

Vesicoureteral Reflux. VUR is defined as the retrograde movement of urine from the lower to upper urinary tracts. Reflux is closely related to UTI in the pediatric population because its presence gives ready access to bacterial colonization and infection of the upper urinary tracts; it is strongly associated with febrile UTI and an increased risk for urosepsis unless promptly and effectively treated. See later,

"Vesicoureteral Reflux," to gain a greater understanding of its relationship to UTI in the pediatric population.

Route of Infection

In the adult population, the ascending urethral route is by far the most common origin for UTI. However, it has been suggested that most UTIs occurring during the first 2 months of life may be associated with a hematogenous route in the presence of a systemic infection.[1] Similar to adults, UTIs occurring after this age are more likely to represent ascending bacterial infection, generally representing pathogens commonly found in the gastrointestinal tract and perianal region.

Diagnosis

Clinical Manifestations. The signs and symptoms of UTI in children vary widely according to age. Infants and toddlers younger than 2 years have nonspecific symptoms, such as fever, irritability, poor feeding, vomiting, and diarrhea, and are initially evaluated in the context of an unknown febrile illness in a primary care clinic rather than a pediatric urologic service. Approximately 10% of these children will have a UTI, and the rest will have various nonurologic disorders, such as gastroenteritis, or a systemic viral disorder.[14,34] Hematuria is uncommon, but parents will occasionally report bloodstains in the diaper. Scrotal swelling accompanied by epididymitis is sometimes seen in male infants. Some of these cases are caused by intrinsic obstruction distal to the ejaculatory ducts or extrinsic blockage caused by ureteral duplication, resulting in an upper pole ureter draining ectopically into the ejaculatory duct.[21]

At some point between 2 and 4 years, children develop the ability to localize pain to the suprapubic area and to report bothersome lower urinary tract symptoms, such as dysuria or burning. Additional lower urinary tract symptoms include an acute onset of daytime voiding frequency, nocturia, dysuria (reported by less than 50% of children younger than 4 years), suprapubic pain, and hesitancy. A new onset of enuresis may indicate UTI, but it is also associated with pinworm infestation, urethritis, or severe emotional distress (see Chapter 16). Upper tract symptoms include fever, flank pain, vomiting, malaise, diarrhea, and upper or central abdominal pain. However, these symptoms are extremely nonspecific

---

Dysfunctional Voiding Symptom Score

Diganosis

This test will help us understand the problems you have going to the bathroom. Think about your bathroom habits during the past month. Then circle your answer to each of the following questions.

1. I have had wet clothes or wet underwear during the day.
   Almost never   Less than 1/2 the month   About 1/2 the month   Almost every day   Don't know

2. My underwear is soaked when I wet myself.
   Almost never   Less than 1/2 the month   About 1/2 the month   Almost every day   Don't know

3. I do not go poo (have a bowel movement) every day.
   Almost never   Less than 1/2 the month   About 1/2 the month   Almost every day   Don't know

4. I have to push for my bowel movements to come out.
   Almost never   Less than 1/2 the month   About 1/2 the month   Almost every day   Don't know

5. I have to push to pee.
   Almost never   Less than 1/2 the month   About 1/2 the month   Almost every day   Don't know

6. I only pee 1 or 2 times each day.
   Almost never   Less than 1/2 the month   About 1/2 the month   Almost every day   Don't know

7. I can hold onto my pee by crossing my legs, squatting, or doing the "pee dance."
   Almost never   Less than 1/2 the month   About 1/2 the month   Almost every day   Don't know

8. I cannot wait when I have to pee.
   Almost never   Less than 1/2 the month   About 1/2 the month   Almost every day   Don't know

9. It hurts when I pee.
   Almost never   Less than 1/2 the month   About 1/2 the month   Almost every day   Don't know

10. For parents to answer:
Has your child had something stressful happen to him or her during the past month? (Circle yes or no.)
   Yes   No

Examples of stressful things are:
New baby brother or sister
Moved to a new home
Moved to a new school
Problems with school, such as tests or friends
Abuse (sexual, physical, or emotional)
Problems at home, such as divorce, separation, or death
Special events, such as accident or injury to your child or a close family member

---

For staff to complete:

0 points for every "almost never" answer   _____

1 point for every "less than 1/2 month" answer _____

2 points for every "about 1/2 month" answer   _____

3 points for every "almost every day" answer   _____

3 points if answer to #10 is "yes"   _____

Total points: _____

Fig. 14-1 Dysfunctional voiding scale. (Modified from Upadhyay J, Bolduc S, Bägli D, McLorie GA, Khoury AE, Farhat W: Use of the Dysfunctional Voiding Symptom Score to predict resolution of vesicoureteral reflux in children with voiding dysfunction. Journal of Urology, 2003; 169:1842-6.)

TABLE 14-2 Nursing Assessment of the Child With Suspected Urinary Tract Infection (UTI)

PARAMETER	DESCRIPTION
Social history	Age of the child, siblings, and birth order, occupation of parent(s), living accommodation, caregiver(s) other than parent
Urinalysis and urine culture	Critical to accurate diagnosis of UTI in infant or child; culture must be obtained before treatment begins; urine observed for color, odor, specific gravity, volume
Chief complaint and history of present illness	Why is the patient here today? What has triggered his or her visit? UTI symptoms in infants are nonspecific, classic signs rarely discernible; fever is most common; irritability, poor feeding, vomiting, diarrhea are reported in less than 50% of infants with UTI
Past medical history	Congenital urinary tract abnormalities are risk factors for UTI. Was prenatal ultrasound done? What were the results? Was there previous catheterization? Is there a history of constipation?
Family history	Risk factors for UTI—siblings or mother who have or have had renal anomalies, VUR, history of UTI
Physical examination	Assess for height, weight, and growth parameters. Observe for jaundice in infants. Check blood pressure for hypertension or hypotension. Check for signs of sepsis—tachycardia, tachypnea, hypotension, fever. Assess for hydration—skin turgor, eye sockets; obtain serum creatinine and electrolyte levels when indicated. Abdominal examination may reveal renal mass or tenderness, enlarged bladder, costovertebral (flank) pain, or constipated stool. Check genitalia for vestibulitis, vaginitis, perineal skin condition, phimosis, vaginal adhesions, and signs of sexual abuse. Assess the lower back and spine for signs suggesting spinal anomalies, including sacral dimples, pitting, hairy tuft, or fat pad.

and common to other conditions, including gastroenteritis and bacterial or viral infections.[35]

Physical Examination. The physical examination is often nonspecific. Even with proven pyelonephritis, only 27% of younger children will report localized flank pain.[14] A renal mass is sometimes palpable in an infant or very young child with significant hydronephrosis complicated by pyelonephritis. Ureterocele, ectopic ureter, urethral discharge, labial adhesions, or vaginal abnormalities are rarely seen on perineal examination in girls, and an acutely swollen and tender scrotum is seen in boys when UTI coexists with epididymitis. Even with a negative physical examination, all children with suspected UTI should undergo additional investigation. Table 14-2 summarizes the nursing assessment of the child with a suspected UTI.

Diagnostic Testing. Urinalysis and urine culture are the primary tools for diagnosing a UTI in an infant or child. Obtaining a usable urine specimen is critical to this diagnosis; Table 14-3 describes

options for obtaining usable specimens in infants and children. A UTI is diagnosed in a pediatric patient when the urinalysis reveals bacteriuria and pyuria, and the culture grows 10^5 CFU/ml or more in a bag specimen or less in a catheterized specimen[11] (Table 14-4). Additional evaluation is indicated for children with an initial febrile UTI and those with recurring afebrile infections.

Best practice standards among pediatric urologists and the official recommendation of the American Academy of Pediatrics state that a renal ultrasound and voiding cystourethrogram (VCUG) should be obtained after an initial febrile UTI.[36] The optimal timing of obtaining VCUG is not yet known. Some pediatric urologists suggest that the VCUG should be obtained within 7 days of diagnosis because it is postulated to be more likely to reveal reflux, but at least one retrospective chart review of children younger than 5 years admitted with a first episode of UTI has failed to find any differences in overall detection

TABLE 14-3 Collecting a Urine Specimen in a Child

TECHNIQUE	PROCEDURE AND ACCURACY OF TECHNIQUE
Collection bag	Collection bag is positioned over the cleansed and dried perineum and left in place until the child voids and an adequate quantity is collected in the bag.
	Urine specimens from bag collection have been found to be unusable in infants younger than 2 months.[78]
	A negative urinalysis and urine culture may be more helpful than a positive result.[79]
	A study comparing a urine specimen collected in plastic specimen bags versus catheterization found evidence of contamination of 55%-69% of 7584 specimens collected in an emergency department or outpatient pediatric diagnostic center of an acute care facility.[80]
Urine collection pad	Urine is obtained from a clean pad applied to the child after perineal cleansing.
	Mixed evidence exists concerning this practice. A small prospective trial has found acceptable reproducibility when a urine collection pad was compared with a clean catch technique in infants,[81] but others have found contamination in more than 60%.[79,82]
Clean catch specimen	The child is asked to void into a specimen cup. Younger children may be assisted by a parent after adequate explanation of the procedure. Older children can be instructed to provide a midstream urine specimen (see Chapter 5).
	Several authors have described clean catch techniques. The diaper is removed and the infant is stimulated to urinate into a foil-lined bowl; considerable patience may be required while awaiting micturition.[81,83]
	Research comparing contamination of clean catch urine specimens consistently has shown superiority to collection bag procedures in young children (prior to toilet training), as noted above.
	Research comparing contamination rates is primarily limited to adults but supports this method as comparable to catheterization when performed with meticulous technique.[83]
Urethral catheterization	A urethral catheter is inserted into the bladder using sterile technique; the procedure must be performed by skilled professionals only
	The sensitivity of urethral catheterization in children is 95% and its specificity is 99% when compared with suprapubic aspiration.[36]
Suprapubic aspiration	The suprapubic skin is cleansed and a 21- or 22-gauge needle is inserted into the abdomen 1-2 cm until urine is obtained. The specimen is collected into a syringe.
	Suprapubic aspiration is the gold standard for collecting urine specimens in infants and children.[1,83]

rates when early and late imaging studies were completed.[37]

Some researchers question the necessity of routinely conducting ultrasonography after an initial febrile UTI in children aged 1 to 24 months. Hoberman and colleagues[38] evaluated 309 children with a first febrile UTI using ultrasonography and voiding cystourethrography. All were found to have VUR and pyelonephritis but a paucity of underlying anomalies was identified on ultrasonography that indicated the need for treatment other than sensitivity-guided antimicrobial therapy. Therefore, Hoberman's group questioned the necessity of ultrasonography, because findings did not change or modify their initial treatment. Instead, they suggested that advances in prenatal ultrasound and identification of anomalies in utero may be adequate to identify infants with severe VUR and associated anomalies who do require aggressive therapy.

In response to this study,[39] Stapleton has cautioned adoption of the protocol without careful consideration of the history and previous evaluation. In children older than 24 months with a UTI, the recommendations are currently not standard of care.

TABLE 14-4 Urine Culture Criteria for Diagnosis of Urinary Tract Infection (UTI)[1]

METHOD OF COLLECTION	COLONY COUNT	PROBABILITY OF INFECTION (%)
Suprapubic aspiration	Gram-negative bacilli—any number; gram-positive bacilli—few thousand or more	>99%
	Staphylococcus aureus uncommon but genuine pathogen, should be treated; organisms such as *S. aureus* most likely contaminants	
Catheterization	$>10^5$	95%;
	10^4 to 10^5	Highly likely
	10^3 to 10^4	Suspicious repeat
	$<10^3$	Unlikely
Clean void male	$>10^4$	Accuracy unknown, suspected to be similar to female
Clean void female	10^5	80% (in one specimen), 90% (in two specimens), 95% (in three specimens)
	$\geq 10^4$	Suspicious, repeat if symptomatic; if asymptomatic, UTI unlikely
	$<10^4$ or presence of more than one organism	UTI unlikely

Stapleton has noted that the authors did not report whether the mothers underwent prenatal ultrasonography, typically performed at 18 weeks' gestation. Prenatal ultrasound may identify clinically significant lesions in the infant and be treated much earlier than at onset of the first UTI. Thus, part of history taking should include questions on prenatal imaging of the developing kidneys. Stapleton has recommended that urinary tract ultrasonography be completed for children with UTI who do not respond to antimicrobial therapy, have an associated palpable abdominal mass, and/or have hydronephrosis on renal ultrasound. Finally, it was also cautioned in this study that findings should not be applied to children older than 24 months until further studies have been completed that weigh the contribution of ultrasonography to the evaluation of an initial febrile UTI.

Treatment

Treatment of a UTI in a child centers on eradication of bacteria using antimicrobial drugs. If the child is ill and pyelonephritis is suspected, empirical antibiotic treatment is initiated as soon as a urine specimen is obtained, followed by adjustment of the antibiotic under the guidance of culture and sensitivity testing.

The choice of antibiotic depends on the age of the child and the ability and willingness to take oral medications, any history of medication hypersensitivity, severity of the UTI, and ability to tolerate any oral fluids or medications.

Traditionally, parenteral antibiotics have been the preferred method, particularly by pediatric nephrologists who have been guided by the concern of renal damage associated with acute pyelonephritis.[40] However, a randomized clinical trial comparing an oral third-generation cephalosporin with parenteral antibiotics revealed no difference in initial treatment efficacy or in the number or severity of renal scars noted on follow-up dimercaptosuccinic acid (DMSA) scan.[41] Nevertheless, initial treatment with parenteral antimicrobials is indicated for infants when an oral medication cannot be readily administered or tolerated. A systematic review of the literature reveals that, while limited, existing data strongly suggest that daily treatment with a parenteral aminoglycoside such as gentamicin is effective for the management of febrile UTI in infants.[41a]

Among older children, a systematic review of the literature[42] has revealed that treatment with oral cefixime or a 2- to 4-day course of intravenous therapy followed by oral therapy is equally effective in eradicating febrile UTI. No differences in renal damage or duration of fever were found when these treatment options were compared. Administration of a short course of parenteral antibiotics also may be indicated for infants or children who exhibit signs of an unresolved UTI caused by bacterial resistance or poor absorption resulting from nausea and vomiting when taking an oral agent.

Treatment with an oral antimicrobial agent has traditionally been prescribed for 7 to 14 days in febrile UTI.[43] However, newer evidence has emerged that supports the efficacy of a short course of antibiotic therapy (2 to 4 days) for children with afebrile UTI. A systematic review has evaluated 10 trials of children with afebrile UTI, and no significant difference in efficacy was noted when a short course of oral antibiotic therapy (2 to 4 days) was compared with a longer course (7 to 14 days).[44] There was also no significant difference between short and standard duration when recurring UTI was treated. Therefore, long-term treatment is usually reserved for children with febrile or complicated UTI, and it remains a strong consideration when treating afebrile UTI in infants up to 24 months of age, given their higher risk for subsequent renal scarring.

Selection of an oral antibiotic prior to obtaining results from a urine culture, or for empirical therapy, is influenced by the age of the child, presence of complicating factors such as a fever, and knowledge of patterns of urine isolates within a specific community or region. Fluoroquinolones have been avoided in younger children because of the potential risk of musculoskeletal problems, such as slipped epiphysis and ruptured Achilles tendon.[45] However, clinical experience with children with cystic fibrosis has demonstrated a potential role for fluoroquinolones in certain cases and further study is needed to determine whether this drug class can be safely administered to children. Because of its known safety profile, a penicillamine such as ampicillin or amoxicillin may be considered. However, there is growing evidence of bacterial resistance by *E. coli* species, affecting as many as 49% to 53% of isolates.[46-48] Increasing bacterial resistance to trimethoprim-sulfamethoxazole has also been reported, but the rates are significantly lower than those associated with ampicillin (15%).[46] Because of these trends, some have recommended nitrofurantoin or a cephalosporin for empirical or initial therapy when treating an uncomplicated UTI

in a community-dwelling child.[46,47] Table 14-5 outlines the choices, doses, and contraindications for antibiotic treatment of UTI in children.

Urologic nursing management focuses on enabling the parents to ensure that the child receives regular and adequate antibiotic medications and on helping the family respond to the need for hospitalization or outpatient administration of parenteral antibiotics. For the very ill child, management will require immediate hospital admission, rehydration with intravenous fluids, and administration of intravenous antibiotics. Although essential to the care of the infant or child, the demands of hospital admission are significant. These may include disruption of work schedules for one or both parents, arrangements for care for siblings, and arrangements for transportation to and from an acute care facility. These challenges also may apply if the child is scheduled to receive parenteral antibiotics on an outpatient basis. Anticipatory guidance in making arrangements may help many families meet these challenges, but it may be necessary to contact a social worker for assistance, particularly in the case of a single working parent with other children and few support mechanisms.

Counseling about the importance of regular and complete administration of antibiotic medications should be accompanied by strategies to enable children to consume the drug safely and completely to ensure maximal benefit (see Clinical Highlights for Expert and Advanced Practice: Enabling Families to Administer Oral Medications to an Infant or Child).

Similar to adults, recurring UTIs are common in children[1]. Although the cause of recurring infections in children is unclear, several interventions have been found effective in certain cases. These include aggressive management of voiding dysfunction and administration of suppressive or prophylactic antimicrobials for the prevention of pyelonephritis and renal scarring in children with grade II and higher VUR. Aggressive treatment of encopresis or constipation is also advocated. Treatment begins with administration of oral laxatives combined with scheduled defecation. However, children who do not respond to oral laxatives may be treated by more aggressive means such as colonic washout enemas using 20 ml/kg of water daily for the first 2 weeks, followed by washout enemas administered 3 times weekly for 6 to 12 months.[49] Chapter 15 discusses the

TABLE 14-5 Oral and Parenteral Antibacterial Agents for Pediatric Urinary Tract Infection (UTI)

DRUG	ACTION	INDICATION	DOSAGE	SIDE EFFECTS	CONTRAINDICATIONS
Sulfonamide	Blocks conversion of para-aminobenzoic acid to dihydrofolic acid	Used to treat multiple gram-negative organisms, including *Escherichia coli*	120-150 mg/kg in four to six divided doses	Few; jaundice in neonate; long-term use affects gut flora	Sulfa allergy; hypersensitivity with Stevens-Johns syndrome
Trimethoprim-sulfamethoxazole (TMP-SMX)	Interferes with dihydrofolic acid reductase; induces phase variation of fimbriated *E. coli* to nonfimbriated	Used to treat many gram-negative and gram-positive organisms; used especially for prophylaxis	TMP, 6-12 mg/kg; SMX, 30-60 mg/kg in two divided doses; uroprophylaxis, TMP, 2 mg/kg	Neutropenia, thrombocytopenia (clinical significance unknown)	
Nitrofurantoin	Probably interferes with bacterial Krebs cycle	Effective against multiple gram-negative organisms; prophylaxis against *E. coli*, enterococci; not effective for *Klebsiella, Proteus, Pseudomonas*	Child >3 mo: 5-7 mg/kg/day in three or four divided doses	Nausea and vomiting with nitrofurantoin alone, but not with macrocrystals	Can cause hemolytic anemia in children with decreased renal function, neonates
Nalidixic acid	Interferes with DNA synthesis	Used to treat UTI associated with *Proteus* species	55 mg/kg/day in four divided doses		
Methenamine, mandelic acid, hippuric acid	Methenamine in acidic urine converted to bactericidal formaldehyde; mandelic and hippuric acid are urinary acidifiers	Used for prophylaxis	100 mg/kg in four doses × 1 day, then 50 mg/kg; action enhanced by addition of ascorbic acid to maintain urine, pH <5.5	Dysuria in high doses; hemorrhagic cystitis (very rare)	Renal failure

Drug	Action	Clinical use	Dosage	Adverse effects	Contraindications
Penicillins—penicillin G, ampicillin, amoxicillin, carbenicillin, ticarcillin	Block mucopeptide synthesis in cell wall so that bacterium is unprotected from high osmotic pressures	Limited activity owing to increasing antibiotic-resistant species, used to treat some gram-negative and gram-positive UTI; ampicillan is most widely used	Ampicillin 50-100 mg/kg/day every 6 hr; uroprophylaxis—20 mg/kg daily, especially for children 2 mo of age or younger	Diarrhea because of poor absorption from GI tract; amoxicillin causes less diarrhea	Penicillin allergy
Cephalosporins (oral)—first generation: cephalexin, cephradine; second generation: cefaclor; cefadroxil; third generation: cefixime		Used to treat multiple gram-negative and gram-positive organisms	25-50 mg/kg/day every 6 hr; uroprophylaxis—cephalexin, 20 mg/kg/day, especially for children 2 mo of age or younger		
Cephalosporins (parenteral)—many first-, second-, and third-generation choices		Used to treat febrile UTI caused by E. coli, Klebsiella, Proteus; not effective for Pseudomonas			
Aminoglycosides—gentamycin, tobramycin, amikacin	Interfere with protein synthesis by binding proteins of bacterial ribosomes; gentamycin most widely used pediatric amino-glycoside	Complicated gram-negative UTI; gentamycin and tobramycin effective against Pseudomonas; amikacin effective against new emerging strains of Pseudomonas	5-7.5 mg/kg/day every 8-12 hr, depending on renal function	Ototoxicity, nephrotoxicity (especially if given with cephalosporins); monitor serum creatinine level	

Clinical Highlights for Expert and Advanced Practice: Enabling Families to Administer Oral Medications to an Infant or Child[84,85]

Background

Safe and effective administration of an oral medication requires knowledge, preparation, and skill, and may be particularly challenging for inexperienced parents. This process is enhanced by clear and concise instruction to parents and care providers concerning dosing and scheduling, techniques for administering and ensuring that an adequate dosage has been consumed, and monitoring for therapeutic responses and adverse side effects.

Administering an Oral Drug

- Liquid suspensions should be prescribed for younger children whenever possible. A medication should be selected that requires fewer daily doses when possible.
- Verbal and written instructions concerning dosage, administration, and scheduling of a medication should be backed up by demonstration of a first dosage (particularly for inexperienced or anxious parents).
- Parents are advised to administer antibiotic medications for the entire duration, as prescribed by the pediatric urologist.
- Advise parents to draw medicine up in an oral syringe, dropper, or similar device and teach them to hold the infant or child upright to avoid gagging. Parents can be counseled to place the child in an infant seat, stroller, or high chair when administering medications. The oral syringe or dropper should be placed in the side of the child's mouth, about halfway back. The liquid should be given slowly and the device rinsed thoroughly between administrations.
- When a suspension cannot be administered, parents should be counseled about alternative strategies for giving a capsule or powdered formulation, such as mixing in 5 to 10 ml of pudding, chilled or frozen grape juice, or similar juice to disguise any disagreeable taste. Parents are further advised to avoid mixing with a larger amount because the child may not be able to consume the entire portion, thus receiving only a partial dosage.
- The specific dosage should be specified in a manner that allows parents to identify the volume of suspension to be administered readily and clearly.
- Switching from a liquid to a pill is enhanced by demonstrating the procedure. Advise the parent to teach the child to take pills by illustrating how she or he self-administers a vitamin or other pill. Children may begin practicing with a pill-shaped candy such as a small mint or a sprinkle-type candy for cake or ice cream.

Safety

- Teach parents to store all medications in a safe place, such as a locked or childproof cabinet.
- Parents should be advised to keep all medications in their original container to ensure accurate recognition of each type of medication consumed by any family member.
- Parents are counseled to inform all healthcare providers and the school nurse about the child's medication.
- Discard any unused medication after the prescribed course has been completed.

management of voiding dysfunction and related bowel elimination problems; the remainder of this chapter will review the management of VUR.

VESICOURETERAL REFLUX

VUR is defined as retrograde flow of urine from the lower urinary tract—from the bladder vesicle across the ureterovesical junction and into the ureter and renal pelvis (Figure 14-2).[50] Although our understanding of the causes and pathophysiology of VUR continues to evolve, it is typically subdivided into two broad categories, primary and secondary. Primary VUR is defined as a congenital defect that renders the ureterovesical junction incompetent; secondary VUR is an acquired condition associated with voiding dysfunction or a neurogenic bladder that compromises ureterovesical junction competence.

Grading System

VUR varies significantly in its magnitude, and these differences profoundly affect its natural history and optimal management. Several classification schemas for VUR have been proposed. The most widely accepted is the International Classification System promulgated by an International Reflux Study Committee in 1981, and it will be used throughout this text.[51] Table 14-6 illustrates and describes the five grades of VUR outlined by the committee.

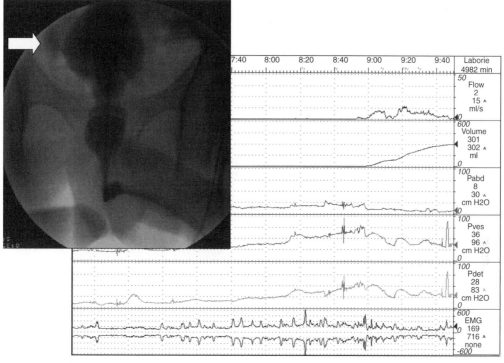

Fig. 14-2 Videourodynamic testing in a child with vesicoureteral reflux (*arrow*), detrusor overactivity, and detrusor sphincter dyssynergia.

Epidemiology

The overall incidence of VUR in the general population is slightly higher than 10%,[50] but it is seen in as many as 70% of children presenting with UTI. The incidence of primary VUR is about 1% to 2% in the general population, and it occurs in 36% to 40% of siblings of affected children.[52] VUR presenting in the context of a symptomatic UTI in girls aged 2 to 7 years outnumbers boys by a ratio of 5:1. In contrast, VUR is more common in very young boys (0 to 2 years) and it tends to be of moderate to high grade (III to V).

Etiology and Pathophysiology

Primary VUR is caused by a congenital deficiency of the longitudinal muscle of the intravesical ureter that results in an incompetent one-way valvular mechanism.[50] As noted, the incidence of VUR in siblings is high, indicating a possible genetic basis for the disorder. Existing evidence strongly suggests that the genetic factors that predispose children to VUR are heterogenous, and involve multiple genes within the human genome.[50,50a,50b] Fortunately, as these children age, the length of the submucosal tunnel usually increases, which often leads to spontaneous resolution of VUR, particularly when it is low grade.

Secondary reflux is closely associated with voiding dysfunction and neurogenic bladder. In classic studies, several urodynamic factors have been identified that, when combined, profoundly raise the risk for secondary VUR.[53-55] They are low bladder wall compliance and an elevated detrusor leak point pressure. The risk is greatest when the bladder wall compliance is lower than 10 ml/cm H_2O and the detrusor leak point pressure is 40 cm H_2O or higher, resulting in sustained detrusor pressures of 40 cm H_2O or higher during bladder filling and storage. Children with myelomeningocele and neurogenic bladder dysfunction are at very high risk for secondary VUR. In addition, voiding dysfunction, characterized by a combination of detrusor overactivity and vesicosphincter dyssynergia, also raises the risk for VUR. A particularly severe form of voiding dysfunction in children, called the Hinman or Hinman-Allen syndrome, is characterized by high-grade VUR, recurring

TABLE 14-6 International Classification System for Grading Vesicoureteral Reflux

CLASSIFICATION	DEPICTION	DESCRIPTION	CHANCE OF SPONTANEOUS RESOLUTION (%)
Grade I		Contrast is visible in distal ureter. Ureter is not dilated. Contrast does not reach renal pelvis.	80-85
Grade II		Contrast is visible in entire ureter and renal pelvis. Ureter or pelvis are not dilated. Calices remained cupped.	80-85
Grade III		Contrast is visible in entire ureter and renal pelvis. Ureter or pelvis show mild-to-moderate dilation. Calices are mildly blunted.	50
Grade IV		Contrast is visible in entire ureter and renal pelvis, which is significantly dilated. Mild tortuosity of ureteral course and moderate blunting of renal calices is easily observed.	9-30
Grade V		Contrast visible in entire ureter and renal pelvis. Ureter and renal pelvis are massively dilated and ureter is tortuous. There is a loss of papillary impression and intrarenal reflux.	12

Modified from Atalla A, Keating MA: Vesicoureteral reflux and megaureter. In Walsh P, Retik AB, Vaughan ED, Wein AJ (eds): Campbell's Urology, 8th edition. Philadelphia: Saunders, 2002; p 2060.

pyelonephritis, renal scarring, and end-stage renal disease in the absence of neurologic disease.[56]

Reflux Nephropathy

Reflux nephropathy is defined as thinning of the renal parenchyma, distortion of the pelvicalyceal system (described on imaging studies as clubbing), hydronephrosis, and impaired renal growth associated with localized renal scars or generalized atrophy. The risk for reflux nephropathy is proportionally related to the grade of VUR, affecting less than 10% of patients with grade I or II VUR, 17% of those with grade III, 25% of children with grade IV, and 50% of those with grade V.[50] As noted, scarring has been associated with increased long-term risks for

hypertension, proteinuria, renal insufficiency, and predisposition to pyelonephritis during pregnancy, although the incidence and magnitude of these risks have been found to be lower than previously believed. Although sterile VUR has been implicated in the development of antenatal scars, additional scarring or atrophy occurs only in the presence of a UTI in the infant or older child. Therefore, to avoid progressive renal scarring and its attendant long-term risks, it is necessary to prevent UTI in children with known VUR, particularly in those with high-grade reflux.

Infection-related scars develop after a pyelonephritis episode and have been historically described as adhering to a "big bang phenomenon."[50] This has been characterized as parenchymal damage during an episode of pyelonephritis, followed by the development of one or more scars and loss of nephrons. The mechanisms whereby renal scars develop is unknown, but it is known that the risk for scarring is greatest in children younger than 1 year of age and when the first febrile UTI occurs before age 4 years. Aging appears to act as a protective factor. In addition, several factors, including elevated serum levels of procalcitonin and matrix metalloproteinase inhibitor 1 (MMP-1), have been associated with an increased likelihood of renal scarring.[57]

Children with VUR are also at increased risk for ureteropelvic junction obstruction. Specifically, high-grade VUR is associated with a fivefold increase in likelihood for developing ureteropelvic junction obstruction when compared with children with low-grade VUR.[58] The precise nature of this relationship is unknown; obstruction may occur as a secondary phenomenon because of kinking or angulation of the ureteropelvic junction when VUR causes significant dilation and tortuosity of the ureters, or it may develop simultaneously because of an as yet unidentified but shared congenital defect.

Diagnosis

Diagnosis of VUR is based on imaging. VUR is diagnosed when a cystogram, VCUG, or radionuclide cystogram reveals retrograde movement of contrast materials or radionuclide tracers from the lower to upper urinary tracts (Figure 14-3). The cystogram and VCUG require catheterization and injection of radiographic contrast material into the bladder, and radionuclide cystography relies on computer analysis of radionuclide materials following catheterization. Either study can be used to identify and grade VUR and to detect associated ureteropelvic junction obstruction. A VCUG is generally preferred over a plain cystogram because many cases of VUR will not be revealed prior to detrusor contraction and micturition. The VCUG also allows imaging of the posterior urethra during micturition, which may provide information about associated voiding dysfunction, urethral valves, or other conditions affecting the lower urinary tract. Videourodynamic testing also may reveal VUR while simultaneous diagnosing voiding dysfunction. However, it must be remembered that the fluoroscopic imaging routinely performed during videourodynamic testing focuses on the lower urinary tract and bladder outlet, rather than

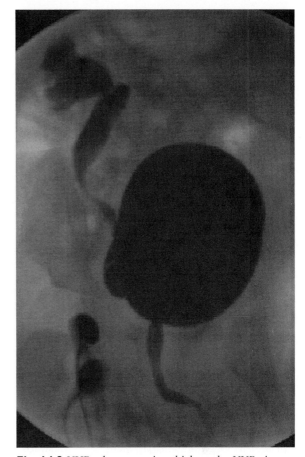

Fig. 14-3 VUR demonstrating high-grade VUR in an infant.

on the upper tracts. In addition, videourodynamic testing is ideally completed in an upright (sitting or standing) position to reproduce lower urinary tract symptoms and evaluate micturition better, whereas an imaging study specifically aimed at diagnosing VUR is optimally performed with the child in a supine position.

Because radionuclide imaging does not provide the detailed anatomy obtained with radiographic studies, VCUG is preferred for the initial evaluation of VUR. It avoids the need for infusion of iodine-bound contrast media and is the procedure of choice for children hypersensitive to them.[64] In addition, radionuclide cystourethrography is also used to follow the progress of VUR over time (Table 14-7).

In addition to routine preparation for obtaining a radionuclide cystogram or VCUG, the urologic nurse

TABLE 14-7 International Classification System for Grading Vesicoureteral Reflux Based on Results of Radionuclide Cystography

CLASSIFICATION	DEPICTION	DESCRIPTION	CORRESPONDING GRADE USING INTERNATIONAL CLASSIFICATION SYSTEM
Grade I		Radionuclide tracer is visible in ureter. Renal pelvis is not visualized.	Grade I
Grade II		Radionuclide tracer substances visible in ureter and renal pelvis. There is no grossly apparent evidence of dilation of renal pelvis.	Grades II-III
Grade III		Radionuclide tracer substances visible in ureter and renal pelvis. Evidence of dilation and/or tortuosity of ureter and renal pelvis grossly apparent.	Grades IV-V

Modified from Atalla A, Keating MA: Vesicoureteral reflux and megaureter. In Walsh P, Retik AB, Vaughan ED, Wein AJ (eds): Campbell's Urology, 8th edition. Philadelphia: Saunders, 2002; p 2061.

should ensure that the child is not overhydrated, because a brisk diuresis may blunt retrograde urine flow and mask low-grade reflux.[50] The study should not be scheduled immediately following a diagnostic test that requires intravenous injection of contrast materials or radionuclide tracers, because this will confound the examiner's ability to diagnose VUR accurately. Even though imaging studies obtained during an active UTI may reveal VUR not seen on subsequent studies, this practice is avoided because of the increased risk for adverse events associated with catheterization and retrograde filling of a refluxing urinary system.

Clinical Manifestations. Sterile VUR does not produce bothersome symptoms, and it is most commonly diagnosed during the evaluation of febrile and afebrile UTI evaluation during childhood. Chronic renal failure and hypertension are rare presenting symptoms in North America, although they sometimes occur in areas in which access to health care is limited, such as rural areas of developing countries. VUR may also be found on assessment for recurring UTI or voiding dysfunction.

Screening. VUR also may be detected within the context of a screening examination. The most common scenarios are prenatal ultrasonography and screening siblings of children with known reflux.

Prenatal ultrasonography. Prenatal ultrasound is designed to screen for a number of potential anomalies, including those affecting the urinary system. With increases in the number of women who undergo prenatal screening, and advances in the quality of this imaging, high-grade VUR associated with ureterohydronephrosis can be accurately identified and early intervention instituted when indicated. In males, primary VUR accounts for 15% to 20% of all prenatally detected cases of uropathy.

Screening of siblings with vesicoureteral reflux. Because of the familial nature of primary VUR, siblings of children with VUR are known to be at higher risk for the disorder than siblings of children without VUR.[59] In a systematic literature review[60] that included 1768 siblings of children with VUR, 32% were found to have VUR. Two thirds had low-grade reflux (I or II) and 2% had high-grade reflux (IV or V), and individual studies have found that 30% or more of siblings of children with VUR will be found to have the condition.[60-62] Because of this increased risk, many U.S. pediatric urologists advocate screening siblings of children with VUR, whereas others (including most pediatric urologists in

Europe) do not advocate routine screening.[63] To resolve this controversy, research is needed to determine whether treatment of asymptomatic siblings of children with VUR will reduce their risk of renal scarring or long-term complications associated with VUR. Until this information is obtained, the decision to screen siblings should be determined individually, based on the clinical judgment of the physician, acting in close consultation with the family.

Evaluation of Renal Function. The assessment of VUR also includes an evaluation of renal function. A serum creatinine level is obtained to rule out renal insufficiency or renal failure. A renal ultrasound is useful for the detection of hydronephrosis, renal parenchymal mass, massive ureteral enlargement, and thickening of the bladder wall. Ultrasonography offers several advantages as an initial test for uropathy: (1) it does not require intravenous injection of radiographic materials or radionuclide tracing substances; (2) it does not expose the child to any radiation; and (3) it can be completed in the pediatric urologist's office. However, it is also associated with significant limitations, including the inability to measure differential renal function and a lack of anatomic detail, particularly with respect to the ureters. To overcome these limitations, the child with VUR and evidence of reflux nephropathy may undergo radionuclide study such as a MAG3, dynamic renal scans, diethylenediaminetetraacetic acid (DTPA), or DMSA scanning. DTPA or MAG3 scans are particularly useful when ureteropelvic junction obstruction is suspected. These scans also provide an estimate of differential function, which is useful when extensive scarring or renal atrophy creates severe damage to one or both kidneys. A DMSA scan is particularly useful for measuring differential renal function and imaging focal renal scarring, but it lacks the ability to diagnose ureteropelvic junction obstruction.

Treatment

Management decisions in children with VUR are complex and based on a number of factors, including reflux grade; age at diagnosis; renal function; complicating or associated conditions such as voiding dysfunction, ureteropelvic junction obstruction, ureteral duplication, or other urinary tract anomalies; documented history and assessment of susceptibility to UTI; and likelihood of spontaneous resolution. Treatment usually involves surgical correction or medical management. Nevertheless, it is important

to remember that neither of these broad categories is mutually exclusive and pursuit of one course does not preclude the other, depending on the course of VUR in an individual child.

Medical Management. Medical management is based on knowledge that sterile VUR has not been found to produce scarring or compromise renal function after the prenatal period and spontaneous remission, particularly in younger children and those with lower grades of VUR. Therefore, prophylactic or suppressive antibiotics are administered to prevent symptomatic UTI and the associated risk for scarring. The duration of a prophylactic antibiotic treatment varies, but such decisions are based more on expert opinion and clinical experience rather than on evidence from randomized controlled trials. Prophylactic antibiotics may be administered from 10 weeks to 12 months or longer. A systematic literature review has noted that antibiotics clearly reduce the risk of recurrent UTI when compared with placebo.[65] Nitrofurantoin was found to be more effective than trimethoprim in preventing recurrent UTI over a 6-month period, but patients receiving nitrofurantoin were also more likely to discontinue the drug because of side effects—mainly gastrointestinal—than patients receiving trimethoprim. The review concluded that most published studies to date have been poorly designed, with biases known to overestimate the true treatment effect. Large, properly randomized, double-blinded trials are needed to determine the efficacy of long-term antibiotics for the prevention of UTI in susceptible children. Usual practice recommendations for prophylactic antibiotics are trimethoprim-sulfamethoxazole (TMP-SMX), nitrofurantoin, or sulfisoxazole given once daily.

The urologic nurse should advise parents to administer a suppressive antibiotic near bedtime to ensure highest levels of drug during the longest period of urinary stasis. Prophylaxis is usually begun when VUR is diagnosed or strongly suspected and continues until age 5 years in girls, age 4 years in boys, or until 12 months have elapsed since the last symptomatic UTI. Prophylaxis also may be discontinued when a VCUG is obtained indicating spontaneous resolution of VUR, reduction in severity to grade I, and/or correction of reflux following surgical correction or endoscopic injection with a submucosal bulking agent. Treatment is typically combined with routine urine surveillance, and parents are counseled to ensure that an adequate urine specimen is obtained and tested for infection whenever a febrile illness or symptoms of a UTI develop.

Both medical and surgical management of VUR have been associated with a spurt in renal growth, particularly when a cycle of recurring febrile UTI is interrupted.[66] Clinicians have long observed a similar spurt in overall growth (increases in height and weight), although a randomized clinical trial has failed to detect significant gains in height or weight.[67]

Urotherapy is the term often used by pediatricians and pediatric urologists to describe a comprehensive program for bladder and bowel elimination problems. A urotherapy program typically includes fluid and dietary alterations, counseling about toileting behaviors, aggressive treatment of bowel elimination disorders, and pelvic floor muscle rehabilitation. Bowel elimination problems such as encopresis or constipation are initially managed by evacuation of the bowel using laxatives or enemas, followed by a scheduled, prompted defecation schedule and ongoing use of stool softeners or laxatives until defecation frequency and stool consistency are normalized. This program is complemented by ensuring that the child consumes adequate fluids and dietary fiber. Effective defecation is also encouraged by teaching the child optimal positioning on toilet and allowing adequate time for complete rectal evacuation.

Scheduled voiding is combined with efforts to ensure that the child spends adequate time emptying the bladder. Girls are counseled to sit with their legs spread apart and to place their feet firmly on the floor or a solid surface. Antimuscarinic drugs may be prescribed to relieve symptoms of detrusor overactivity. Children who fail to respond to initial treatment may undergo urodynamic testing to characterize voiding dysfunction better.

Despite appropriate antibiotic therapy, approximately 21% will experience recurring infections, and children and families must be taught to self-monitor for signs and symptoms of UTI, and febrile UTI in particular.[50] The need for routinely obtaining a VCUG to document resolution of VUR in older children continues to evolve. Radio-nuclide cystography may be used to evaluate VUR routinely in children 2 years or younger, and in those with higher grades of reflux in particular. Although the risk for hypertension has been found to be lower than once believed, routine blood pressure monitoring is strongly recommended. Routine evaluation of renal function is indicated for children with VUR and extensive renal scarring or other evidence of reflux nephropathy.

Surgery. Reimplantation of the ureters, sometimes called ureteroneocystostomy, requires surgical manipulation of the distal ureter to create a nonrefluxing ureterovesical junction. Surgery resolves VUR in more than 90% of cases and reduces the risk of subsequent febrile UTI to approximately 10%, less than half the risk associated with medical therapy. Nevertheless, surgery carries significant risks, including those associated with anesthesia, urinary tract obstruction, breakthrough UTI, and recurring VUR. Thus, the decision to pursue surgical correction must be individualized. Generally accepted indications for treatment include the following: (1) breakthrough UTI despite prophylactic antibiotic therapy; (2) nonadherence to prophylactic antibiotic therapy; (3) VUR complicated by ureteropelvic junction obstruction, ureterocele, ureteral duplication, or similar defects; (4) progressive reflux nephropathy evidenced by failure of renal growth and progressive renal scarring, with deterioration of renal function affecting one or both kidneys; and (5) VUR that persists in girls as they reach full linear growth near puberty.[50]

Open surgery. The choice of surgical procedure is based on the severity of the VUR, presence of anatomic defects, and surgeon's training and preference. In cases in which the ureter is not significantly dilated and the bladder mucosa allows a tunnel at least four or five times the diameter of the implanted ureter, the surgeon may use any one of a number of intravesical procedures, such as the Cohen cross-trigonal, Politano-Leadbetter, Gil-Vernet, or Glenn-Anderson technique.[68] Alternatively, extravesical techniques may be used for ureteroneocystostomy, such as the Lich-Gregoir procedure. Extravesical techniques are widely used in Europe and sometimes used in the United States. Extravesical ureteroneocystostomy often involves detrusorrhaphy, or the incision and reconstruction of a small segment of detrusor to ensure creation of an ample submucosal tunnel. However, this technique is usually avoided when a bilateral reimplantation is required because of a small but significant risk (approximately 16%) of transient urinary retention. Laparoscopic techniques have also been used for ureteral reimplantation, but have not proved superior to open procedures and are not widely used. See Chapter 18 for a more detailed discussion of the nursing management of children undergoing surgical correction of VUR.

Endoscopic procedures. Because the ureterovesical junction is readily accessible to endoscopic management, pediatric urologists have investigated the potential role of a number of materials that could be implanted into the subtrigonal mucosa to correct VUR. The first report of a subtrigonal injection was by O'Donnell and Puri,[69] who injected polytetrafluoroethylene (Teflon paste) in what is now referred to as the STING procedure. In a long-term follow-up of children with grades IV or V reflux treated with subtrigonal Teflon injection, VUR was eradicated or converted to grade I or II in 50% of patients.[70] It was noted that no migration of the Teflon product occurred, but this finding differs from those who have found migration of particles after submucosal injection of polytetrafluoride paste (Teflon).[71] A number of alternative substances have been used, including glutaraldehyde, cross-linked bovine collagen (GAX collagen),[72] polydimethylsiloxane (Macroplastique),[73] and autologous chondrocytes.[74] One material, dextranomer–hyaluronic acid (Deflux), has gained considerable popularity in North America.[75] In a report of 180 children, 72% were successfully treated with a single injection, and resolution of VUR varied from 90% in grade I VUR to 65% in grade IV. Advantages of these procedures include avoidance of a surgical incision and the need for hospitalization. These advantages must be carefully weighted against their most important limitation, durability, when deciding on a management plan for VUR.[76]

SUMMARY

Urinary infection and VUR are closely related in children, and these conditions have been found to be associated with voiding dysfunction and bowel elimination disorders in many patients. Urologic nursing management includes supporting patients and families as they undergo treatment for each of these conditions, and providing education about the magnitude and nature of short-and long-term complications associated with these clinically relevant but readily treatable conditions.

REFERENCES

1. Shortliffe LMD: Infection and inflammation of the pediatric genitourinary tract. In Wein AJ, Kavoussi LR, Novick AC, Partin AW, Peters CA (eds): Campbell-Walsh Urology, 9th edition. Philadelphia: Saunders, 2007; pp 3232-68.

2. Schaeffer AJ, Schaeffer EM: Infections of the urinary tract. In Wein AJ, Kavoussi LR, Novick AC, Partin AW, Peters CA (eds): Campbell-Walsh Urology, 9th edition. Philadelphia: Saunders, 2007; pp 223-303.

3. Stamey TA: Clinical classification of urinary tract infections based upon origin. Southern Medical Journal, 1975; 68:934-9.

4. Wettergren B, Jodal U, Jonasson G: Epidemiology of bacteriuria during the first year of life. Acta Paediatrica, 1985; 74:925-33.

5. Zorc JJ, Levine DA, Platt SL, Dayan PS, CG, Krief W, Schor J, et al: Clinical and demographic factors associated with lower urinary tract infection in young febrile infants. Pediatrics, 2005; 116(3):644-8.

6. Bachur R: Pediatric urinary infection. Clinical Pediatric Emergency Medicine, 2004; 5(1):28-36.

7. Singh-Grewal D, Macdessi J, Craig J: Circumcision for the prevention of urinary tract infection in boys: a systematic review of randomized trials and observational studies. Archives of Diseases in Childhood, 2005; 90:853-8.

8. Marild S, Hannsson S, Jodal U, Oden A, Svedberg K: Protective effect of breastfeeding against urinary tract infection. Acta Paediatrica, 2004; 93(2):164-8.

9. Harel L, Straussburgr R, Jackson S, Amer J, Tiqwa P: Influence of circumcision technique on the frequency of urinary tract infections in neonates. Pediatric Infectious Disease Journal, 2002; 21:879-80.

10. Singh-Grewal D, Macdessi J, Craig J: Circumcision for the prevention of urinary tract infection in boys: a systematic review of randomized trials and observational studies. Archives of Disease in Childhood, 2005; 90:853-8.

11. Schroeder AR, Newman TB, Wasserman RC, Finch SA, Pantell RH: Choice of urine collection methods for the diagnosis of urinary tract infection in young, febrile infants. Archives of Pediatrics and Adolescent Medicine, 2005; 159(10):915-22.

12. Craig JC: Urinary tract infection: new perspectives on a common disease. Current Opinion in Infectious Disease, 2001; 14:309-13.

13. Smith G: Management of urinary tract infection. Current Pediatrics, 2004; 14(7):556-62.

14. Jahnukainen T, Chen M, Celsi G: Mechanisms of renal damage because of infection. Pediatric Nephrology, 2005; 20(8):1043-53.

14a. Kuroda S, Puri P: Lack of association of IL8 gene polymorphisms with familial vesico-ureteral reflux. Pediatric Surgery International, 2007; 23(5):441-5.

15. Winberg J: Commentary: progressive renal damage from infection with or without reflux. Journal of Urology, 1992; 148(5 Pt 2): 1733-4.

16. Martinell J, Claesson I, Lidin-Janson G, Jodal U: Urinary infection, reflux and renal scarring in females continuously followed for 13-38 years. Pediatric Nephrology, 1995; 9(2):131-6.

17. Beetz R, Mannhardt W, Fisch M, Stein R, Thuroff JW: Long-term follow-up of 158 young adults surgically treated for vesicoureteral reflux in childhood: the ongoing risk of urinary tract infections. Journal of Urology, 2002; 168(2):704-7.

18. McDermott S, Callaghan W, Szwejbka L, Mann H, Daguise V: Urinary tract infections during pregnancy and mental retardation and developmental delay. Obstetrics and Gynecology, 2000; 96(1):113-9.

19. Jacobson SH, Eklof O, Lins LE, Wikstad I, Winberg J: Long-term prognosis of post-infectious renal scarring in relation to radiological findings in childhood—a 27-year follow-up. Pediatric Nephrology, 1992; 6(1):19-24.

20. Wennerstrom M, Hansson S, Hedner T, Himmelmann A, Jodal U: Ambulatory blood pressure 16-26 years after the first urinary tract infection in childhood. Journal of Hypertension, 2000; 18: 485-91.

21. Rickwood AMK: Urinary infection. In Thomas DFM, Rickwood AMK, Duffy PG (eds): Essentials of Paediatric Urology. London: Martin Dunitz, 2002; pp 35-43.

22. Haller M, Brandis M, Berner R: Antibiotic resistance of urinary tract pathogens and rationale for empirical intravenous therapy. Pediatric Nephrology, 2004; 19(9):982-6.

23. Ladhani S., Gransden W: Increasing antibiotic resistance among urinary tract isolates. Archives of Disease in Childhood, 2003; 88(5):444-5.

24. McLoughlin TG Jr, Joseph MM: Antibiotic resistance patterns of uropathogens in pediatric emergency department patients. Academic Emergency Medicine, 2003; 10(4):347-51.

25. Prais D, Straussberg R, Avitzur Y, Nussinovitch M, Harel L, Amir J: Bacterial susceptibility to oral antibiotics in community-acquired urinary tract infection. Archives of Disease in Childhood, 2003; 88(3):215-8.

26. Richards MJ, Edwards JR, Culver DH, Gaynes RP: Nosocomial infections in pediatric intensive care units in the United States. National Nosocomial Infections Surveillance System. Pediatrics, 1999; 103(4):e39.

27. Farhat W, Bägli D, Capolicchio G, O'Reilly S, Merguerian PA, Khoury A, et al: The Dysfunctional Voiding Scoring System: quantitative standardization of dysfunctional voiding symptoms in children. Journal of Urology, 2000; 164:1011-5.

28. Loening-Baucke V: Urinary incontinence and urinary tract infection and their resolution with treatment of chronic constipation of childhood. Pediatrics, 1997; 100(2 Pt 1):228-32.

29. Grafstein NH, Combs AJ, Glassberg KI: Primary bladder neck dysfunction: an overlooked entity in children. Current Urology Reports, 2005; 6(2):133-9.

30. McKenna LS, McKenna PH: Modern management of nonneurologic pediatric incontinence. Journal of Wound, Ostomy and Continence Nursing, 2004; 31(6):351-6.

31. Mingin GC, Hinds A, Nguyen HT, Baskin LS: Children with a febrile urinary tract infection and a negative radiologic workup: factors predictive of recurrence. Urology, 2004; 63(3):562-5.

32. Shaikh N, Hoberman A, Wise B, Kurs-Lasky M, Kearney D, Naylor S, et al: Dysfunctional elemination syndrome: is it related to urinary tract infection or vesicoureteral reflux diagnosed early in life? Pediatrics, 2003; 112:1134-7.

33. Upadhyay J, Bolduc S, Bägli D, McLorie GA, Khoury AE, Farhat W: Use of the Dysfunctional Voiding Symptom Score to predict resolution of vesicoureteral reflux in children with voiding dysfunction. Journal of Urology, 2003; 169:1842-6.

34. Cohen AL, Rivara FP, Davis R, Christakis DA: Compliance with guidelines for the medical care of first urinary tract infections in infants: a population-based study. Pediatrics, 2005; 116(4):1051-2.

35. Rushton HG, Pohl HG: Urinary tract infections in children. In Belman AB, King LR, Kramer SA (eds): Clinical Pediatric Urology. London: Martin Dunitz, 2002; pp 261-329.

36. Giorgi LJ, Jr, Bratslavsky G, Kogan BA: Febrile urinary tract infections in infants: renal ultrasound remains necessary. Journal of Urology, 2005; 173(2):568-70.

37. Mahant S, To T, Friedman J: Timing of voiding cystourethrogram in the investigation of urinary tract infections in children. Journal of Pediatrics, 2001; 139:568-71.

38. Hoberman A, Charron M, Hickey RW, Baskin M, Kearney DG, Wald ER: Imaging studies after a first febrile urinary tract infection in young children. New England Journal of Medicine, 2003; 348:195-202.

39. Stapleton FB: Imaging studies for childhood urinary tract infections. New England Journal of Medicine, 2003; 348:251-2.

40. Cornu C, Cochat P, Collet J-P, Delair S, Haugh MC, Rolland C: Survey of the attitudes to management of acute pyelonephritis in children. Pediatric Nephrology, 1994; 8:275-7.

41. Hoberman A, Wald ER, Hickey RW, Baskin M, Charron M, Majd M, et al: Oral versus initial intravenous therapy for urinary tract infections in young febrile children. Pediatrics, 1999; 104(1 Pt 1):79-86.

41a. Shahid M, Cooke R: Is a once daily dose of gentamicin safe and effective in the treatment of UTI in infants and children? Archives of Disease in Childhood, 2007; 92(9):823-4.

42. Bloomfield P, Hodson EM, Craig JC: Antibiotics for acute pyelonephritis in children. Cochrane Database of Systematic Reviews, 2003; (4):CD003772.

43. Keren R, Chan E: A meta-analysis of randomized, controlled trials comparing short and long course antibiotic therapy for urinary tract infections in children. Pediatrics, 2002; 109:E70-E80.

44. Michael M, Hodson EM, Craig JC, Martin S, Moyer VA: Short versus standard duration oral antibiotic therapy for acute urinary tract infection in children. Cochrane Database of Systematic Reviews, 2003; (1):CD003966.

45. Chalumeau M: Fluoroquinolone safety in pediatric patients: a prospective, multicenter, comparative cohort study in France. Pediatrics, 2003; 111(6 Pt 1):E714-9.

46. Bonsu BK, Shuler L, Sawicki L, Dorst P, Cohen DM: Susceptibility of recent bacterial isolates to cefdinir and selected antibiotics among children with urinary tract infections. Academic Emergency Medicine, 2006; 13(1):76-81.

47. Abelson Storby K, Osterlund A, Kahlmeter G: Antimicrobial resistance in *Escherichia coli* in urine samples from children and adults:a 12 year analysis. Acta Paediatrica, 2004; 93(4):487-91.

48. Byington CL, Rittichier KK, Bassett KE, Castillo H, Glasgow TS, Daly J, Pavia AT: Serious bacterial infections in febrile infants younger than 90 days of age: the importance of ampicillin-resistant pathogens. Pediatrics, 2003; 111(5 Pt 1):964-8.

49. Chrzan R, Klijn AJ, Vijverberg MAW, Sikkel F, de Jong TPVM: Colonic washout enemas for persistent constipation in children with recurrent urinary tract infections based on dysfunctional voiding. Journal of Urology, 2008; 179(3):947-51.

50. Khoury A, Bagli DJ: Reflux and megaureter. In Wein AJ, Kavoussi LR, Novick AC, Partin AW, Peters CA (eds): Campbell-Walsh Urology, 9th edition. Philadelphia: Saunders, 2007; pp 3243-81.

50a. Kelly H, Molony CM, Darlow JM, Pirker ME, Yoneda A, Green AJ, Puri P, Barton DE: A genome-wide scan for genes involved in primary vesicoureteric reflux. Journal of Medical Genetics, 2007; 44(11):710-7.

50b. van Eerde AM, Koeleman BP, van de Kamp JM, de Jong TP, Wijmenga C, Giltay JC: Linkage study of 14 candidate genes and loci in four large Dutch families with vesico-ureteral reflux. Pediatric Nephrology, 2007; 22(8):1129-33.

51. Medical versus surgical treatment of primary vesicoureteral reflux: report of the International Reflux Study Committee. Pediatrics, 1981; 67(3):392-400.

52. Tombesi M, Ferrari CM, Bertolotti JJ: Renal damage in refluxing and non-refluxing siblings of index children with vesicoureteral reflux. Pediatric Nephrology, 2005; 20(8):1201-2.

53. McGuire EJ, Woodside JR, Borden TA, Weiss RM: Prognostic value of urodynamic testing in myelodysplastic patients. Journal of Urology, 2002; 167(2 Pt 2):1049-54.

54. Ghoneim GM, Roach MB, Lewis VH, Harmon EP: The value of leak pressure and bladder compliance in the urodynamic evaluation of meningomyelocele patients. Journal of Urology, 1990; 144(6):1440-2.

55. Ghoneim GM, Bloom DA, McGuire EJ, Stewart KL: Bladder compliance in meningomyelocele children. Journal of Urology, 1989; 141(6):1404-6.

56. Bogaert G, Beckers G, Lombaerts R: The use and rationale of selective alpha blockade in children with non-neurogenic neurogenic bladder dysfunction. International Brazilian Journal of Urology, 2004; 30(2):128-34.

57. Prat C, Dominguez J, Rodrigo C, Gimenez M, Azuara M, Jimenez O, Gali N, Ausina V: Elevated serum procalcitonin values correlate with renal scarring in children with urinary tract infection. Pediatric Infectious Disease Journal, 2003; 22(5):438-42.

58. Bomaslaski MD, Hirschl RB, Bloom DA: Vesicoureteral reflux and ureterolepvic junction obstruction: association, treatment options and outcome. Journal of Urology, 1997; 157(3):969-74.

59. Chertin B, Puri P: Familial vesicoureteral reflux. Journal of Urology, 2003; 169:1804-8.

60. Hollowell JG, Greenfield SP: Screening siblings for vesicoureteral reflux. Journal of Urology, 2002; 168(5):2138-41.

61. Ataei N, Madani A, Esfahani ST, Kejbafzadeh A, Ghaderi O, Jalili S, Sharafi B: Screening for vesicoureteral reflux and renal scars in

siblings of children with known reflux. Pediatric Nephrology, 2004; 19(1):1127-31.

62. Noe HN: The long-term result of perspective sibling reflux screening. Journal of Urology, 1992; 148(5 Pt 2):1739-42.

63. Giel DW, Noe HN, Williams MA, Lottmann H, Rushton HG, Nguyen D: Ultrasound screening of asymptomatic siblings of children with vesicoureteral reflux: a long-term follow-up study. Journal of Urology, 2005; 174(4 Pt II):1602-5.

64. Westwood ME, Whiting PF, Cooper J, Watt IS, Kleijnen J: Further investigation of confirmed urinary tract infection (UTI) in children under five years: a systematic review. BioMed Central Pediatrics, 2005; 5(2):4.

65. Williams GJ, Lee A, Craig JC: Long-term antibiotics for preventing recurrent urinary tract infection in children. Cochrane Database of Systematic Reviews, 2006; (4):CD001534pub2.

66. Olbing H, Hirche H, Koskimies O, Lax H, Seppanen U, Smellie JM, Tamminen-Mobius T, Wikstad I: Renal growth in children with severe vesicoureteral reflux: 10-year prospective study of medical and surgical treatment: the International Reflux Study in Children (European branch). Radiology, 2000; 216(3):731-7.

67. Wingen A-M, Koskimies O, Olbing H, Seppanen J, Tamminen-Mobius T: Growth and weight gain in children with vesicoureteral reflux receiving medical versus surgical treatment: 10-year results of a prospective, randomized study. Acta Paediatrica, 1999; 88(1):56-61.

68. Ellsworth PI, Crendon M, McCollough MF: Surgical management of vesicoureteral reflux. AORN Journal Online, 2000; 71(3):496-513.

69. O'Donnell B, Puri P: Treatment of vesicoureteric reflux by endoscopic injection of Teflon. British Medical Journal, 1984; 289(6436):7-9.

70. Chertin B, De Caluwé D, Puri P: Endoscopic treatment of primary Grades IV and V vesicoureteral reflux in children with subureteral injection of polytetrafluoroethylene. Journal of Urology, 2003; 169:1847-9.

71. Aaronson IA, Rames RA, Greene WB, Walsh IG, Hasal UA, Garen PD: Endoscopic treatment of reflux: migration of Teflon to the lungs and brain. European Journal of Urology, 1993; 23:394-9.

72. Frey P, Berger D, Jenny P, Herzog B: Subureteral collagen injection for the endoscopic treatment of vesicoureteral reflux in children. Follow-up study of 97 treated ureters and histological

analysis of collagen implants. Journal of Urology, 1992; 148(2 Pt 2):718-23.

73. Dodat H, Valmalle AF, Weidmann JD, Collet F, Pelizzo G, Dubois R: Endoscopic treatment of vesicorenal reflux in children. Five-year assessment of the use of Macroplastique. Progres en Urologie, 1998; 8(6):1001-6.

74. Diamond DA, Caldamone AA: Endoscopic correction of vesicoureteral reflux in children using autologous chondrocytes: preliminary results. Journal of Urology, 1999; 162(3 Pt 2):1185-8.

75. Lendvay TS, Sorensen M, Cowan CA, Joyner BD, Mitchell MM, Grady RW: The evolution of vesicoureteral reflux management in the era of dextranomer/hyaluronic acid copolymer: a pediatric health information system database study. Journal of Urology, 2006; 176(4 Pt 2):1864-7.

76. Chertin B, Puri P: Endoscopic management of vesicoureteral reflux: does it stand the test of time? European Urology, 2002; 42(6):598-606.

77. Shortliffe LMD: Pediatric urinary tract infections. In Gearhart JP, Rink RC, Mouriquand PDE (eds): Pediatric Urology. Philadelphia: Saunders, 2001; pp 237-58.

78. Falcao MC, Leone CR, D'Andrea RA, Berardi R, Ono NA, Vaz FA: Urinary tract infection in full-term newborn infants: value of urine culture by bag specimen collection. Revista do Hospital das Clinicas; Faculdade de Medicina Da Universidade de Sao Paulo, 1999; 54(3):91-6.

79. Ahmad T, Vickers D, Campbell S, Coulthard MG: Urine collection from disposable nappies. Lancet, 1991; 338:674-6.

80. Al-Orifi F, McGillivray D, Tange S, Kramer MS: Urine culture from bag specimens in young children: are the risks too high? Journal of Pediatrics, 2000; 137:221-6.

81. Lewis J: Clean-catch versus urine collection pads: a prospective trial. Pediatric Nursing, 1998; 10(1):15-6.

82. Macfarlane PI, Houghton C, Hughes C: Pad urine collection for early childhood urinary-tract infection. Lancet, 1999; 354(9178):571.

83. Liao JC, Churchill BM: Pediatric urine testing. Pediatric Clinics of North America, 2001; 48:1425-40.

84. Li SF, Lacher B, Crain EF: Acetaminophen and ibuprofen dosing by parents. Pediatric Emergency Care, 2000; 16(6):394-7.

85. McMahon SR, Rimsza ME, Bay RC: Parents can dose liquid medication accurately. Pediatrics, 1997; 100(3 Pt 1):330-3.

Dysfunctional Voiding

The phrase often quoted by pediatric nurses and other clinicians, "children are not merely little adults" can be applied to many disorders, and it is particularly true for dysfunctional voiding. For example, as noted in Chapter 6, most adults suffering from urinary incontinence (UI) experience stress, urge, or mixed incontinence. Approximately 50% experience stress UI; pure urge UI is the least common among these three types that collectively account for 90% of all cases in adults.[1,2] In contrast, pure urge UI is more common in children than stress or mixed UI, nighttime urinary incontinence (enuresis) is the most prevalent form of urine loss in neurologically normal children, and detrusor sphincter dyssynergia, an unusual finding in adults without neurologic impairment, is fairly common in younger children in particular. This chapter will define the evolving concept of dysfunctional elimination syndromes in children and provide a detailed review of the causes, pathophysiology, assessment, and management of daytime incontinence in the neurologically normal child using the standardized terminology from the International Children's Continence Society.[3] In this section, Chapter 16 focuses on the diagnosis and management of monosymptomatic enuresis in children, and Chapter 13 focuses on the management of dysfunctional voiding in children with neural tube defects and imperforate anus.

OVERVIEW OF DYSFUNCTIONAL VOIDING IN CHILDREN

Dysfunctional voiding is a broad term used to describe various lower urinary tract symptoms in children, including enuresis, overactive bladder (OAB) syndrome, detrusor sphincter dyssynergia, non-neurogenic neurogenic bladder (Hinman's syndrome), infrequent voiding or decreased voiding frequency, postmicturition dribble, and giggle incontinence (Table 15-1).[4] However, based on an increased sensitivity to associations among dysfunctional voiding, functional bowel elimination symptoms, urinary tract infection (UTI), and vesicoureteral reflux, the term *dysfunctional voiding* ultimately may be replaced by a taxonomy of dysfunctional elimination syndromes that recognizes these associations and overlapping principles of diagnosis and treatment.[3-6]

Epidemiology

Unlike adults, voiding symptoms in children are frequently divided into nocturnal versus daytime; nocturnal symptoms typically refer to monosymptomatic enuresis, and the presence of daytime symptoms implies bothersome urgency, UI, or a less common lower urinary tract symptom experienced during waking hours. Daytime lower urinary tract symptoms affect 7% to 21% of school-age girls and 3% to 7% of school-age boys.[7,8] When children undergoing evaluation and treatment of dysfunctional voiding are analyzed, OAB syndrome, characterized by bothersome urgency, with or without urge UI and usually accompanied by frequent urination, is the most prevalent form. In one study, OAB affected 76% of a group of 226 children undergoing evaluation and treatment in a pediatric urologic service.[9] Of these, 79% experienced urge UI, as compared with 37% of adults in another study.[10] When these symptoms are combined with closely related disorders labeled by the authors as extraordinary daytime frequency, giggle incontinence, or transient dysfunctional voiding, the prevalence of OAB rises to 88.6%.

Fortunately, the prevalence of dysfunctional voiding declines with age. In one study of 1176 children, the prevalence of daytime UI dropped from 12.5% in children aged 11 to 12 years to 3% when they reached 15 to 16 years,[11] similar to an epidemiologic survey of 6917 Japanese schoolchildren aged 7 to 11years.[12] Whereas the overall prevalence of daytime UI in the Japanese children was 6.3%, when stratified by age, the prevalence of 9% among 7-year-olds as compared with 2% of the 12-year-olds was noted.

TABLE 15-1 Voiding Dysfunction Disorders in Children

COMMON NAME	SIGNS AND SYMPTOMS	URODYNAMIC CHARACTERISTICS
Overactive bladder (OAB)	Bothersome urgency, usually associated with frequent urination, enuresis, or nocturia, with or without daytime urinary incontinence	Small bladder capacity with sensory urgency, detrusor overactivity
Non-neurogenic neurogenic bladder (Hinman or Hinman-Allen syndrome)	Urinary incontinence and retention, recurring urinary tract infection (UTI), vesicoureteral reflux, ureterohydronephrosis on renal imaging studies, signs of renal insufficiency in advanced cases	Detrusor overactivity, dyssynergia, low bladder wall compliance, poor contraction strength may occur in advanced cases
Giggle incontinence	Urine loss during episodes of laughter, often associated with symptoms of overactive bladder	Normal or small bladder capacity with sensory urgency; urodynamically demonstrated detrusor overactivity not present in giggle incontinence
Postmicturition dribble	Urine loss immediately following micturition	Normal
Infrequent voiding (decreased daytime voiding frequency)	Postpones micturition for prolonged periods of time (8-12 hr), recurring UTI common	Large capacity bladder with delayed or diminished sensations of bladder filling, large postvoid residuals, poor detrusor contraction strength in advanced cases

Follow-up interviews with 98 parents and 51 patients followed at least 6.5 years in a pediatric urology practice in the northeastern United States have revealed that 91% achieve continence within 3 years of their initial evaluation and 86% deny bothersome urinary urgency.[13]

Stress incontinence, perhaps the most prevalent type of UI in adults, is less common in children. This discrepancy is partly attributable to the absence of well-known risk factors such as pregnancy, vaginal delivery, and menopausal status, or other as yet unknown risk or protective factors that almost certainly exert an influence. Although data on the relationship between age and incontinence are sparse, a pattern apparently related to age has emerged. For example, although less than 5% of elementary school-age children (12 years or younger) reported UI,[9,12] 15% of a group of 332 Canadian teenage girls reported stress UI symptoms and 17% reported urge incontinence.[14]

Stress UI has been noted in female adolescents with cystic fibrosis (CF)[15] and in teenage girls and young adult women involved in certain athletic activities.[16,17] An association between stress UI and chronic obstructive pulmonary disease has been observed in adult women, hypothesized to arise from chronic coughing, a condition shared by teenage girls with CF. In a survey of 55 female teenagers with CF, 84% reported urine loss provoked by coughing, whereas only 18% reported bothersome urgency and 9% reported episodes of urge UI.[15] Eliasson and coworkers[16] have surveyed 35 females aged 12 to 22 years who regularly competed in trampoline events. Of these, 80% reported urine loss while using the trampoline, despite evidence of good pelvic floor muscle strength. Bø and Borgen[17] queried 660 adolescent and young adult athletes who regularly participated in organized sport and compared findings to 765 nonathlete controls. Although 41% of female athletes reported urine loss when engaging in activities requiring considerable physical exertion, such as running or gymnastics, 39% of nonathletes also admitted to stress UI, a nonsignificant difference. Of note was a statistically significant difference between the prevalence of UI in female athletes with eating disorders compared with those who reported normal eating habits. The mechanism behind this difference is unknown.

Associated Factors. As noted in Chapter 14, fecal elimination disorders, UTIs, and vesicoureteral reflux often coexist with dysfunctional voiding, although evidence of cause and effect has not been established.[9,18-21] However, a number of researchers have demonstrated that treatment of fecal elimination disorders such as encopresis or chronic constipation often alleviates and may relieve dysfunctional voiding, UTI risk, and vesicoureteral reflux, raising persistent questions about whether these conditions act as risk factors or are merely sequelae of a common underlying disorder, such as pelvic floor muscle dysfunction.[19,20] Nevertheless, these observations do demonstrate that an important clinical link exists among these disorders, affecting evaluation and treatment.

Attention-deficit/hyperactivity disorder (ADHD) is a relatively common learning disorder, affecting approximately 3% to 5% of children in the United States.[22] The diagnosis is based on clinical manifestations, including inattention, impulsivity, and excessive motor activity present before age 7 years, and occurring in at least two separate environmental settings (e.g., school and home). In a study of 153 6-year-olds, children with ADHD were 4.5 times more likely to have daytime urinary incontinence than unaffected children and 2.7 times more likely to have enuresis.[23] Duel and colleagues[24] have compared a group of 28 children with ADHD with a cohort of 22 unaffected children and also reported significantly higher rates of daytime urinary incontinence, enuresis, OAB, and constipation in affected children. Both studies have recommended screening children with ADHD for dysfunctional voiding.

A number of other conditions have been associated with dysfunctional voiding in children. These are outlined in Table 15-2.[25-40]

Etiology and Pathophysiology

Although the basic sequence of events that leads to continence and the many factors associated with delayed or incomplete toilet training have been defined, surprisingly little is known about the causes of dysfunctional voiding in children.

Detrusor Overactivity and Overactive Bladder Dysfunction. Research and overwhelming clinical experience in children and adults have shown a clear relationship between disorders affecting the nervous system and lower urinary tract function,[41] but the underlying causes of persistent detrusor overactivity, voiding frequency, and/or urge UI in children who have no apparent disorders of the nervous system remain unclear. Several hypotheses have been put forward: (1) delayed maturation of the central nervous system; (2) genetic factors leading to lifelong overactive bladder dysfunction; (3) de novo detrusor overactivity caused by a transient insult to the lower urinary tract such as intrauterine obstruction; and (4) sequelae of a functional disorder of the pelvic floor muscles, possibly affecting bladder and bowel dysfunction.[4,6,42,43]

Even less is known about transient bothersome urgency associated with daytime voiding frequency, defined as eight or more voids daily.[3] It typically develops between the fourth and fifth years of life and usually occurs without an apparent precipitating event, persisting for weeks to months. Clinical evaluation reveals absence of UTI, UI, or urinary retention. Symptoms of urgency and frequency usually resolve spontaneously, again without any apparent precipitating event. Emotional distress has been identified as a possible cause but no persuasive evidence supporting this hypothesis has been reported. Seasonal variations may affect prevalence, and hypercalciuria is seen in approximately one third of cases, but neither of these observations has led to further knowledge about the causes of this puzzling but self-limited dysfunctional voiding.

Detrusor Sphincter Dyssynergia and the Non-Neurogenic Neurogenic Bladder. As noted in Chapter 2, the sphincter mechanism remains closed during bladder filling and storage, and opens during micturition to allow efficient evacuation of urine. However, approximately 33% of normal neonates demonstrate an interrupted voiding pattern, along with detrusor sphincter dyssynergia—contraction of the pelvic floor and striated sphincter muscles, leading to voiding interruption and incomplete bladder emptying—on urodynamic testing.[44] The problem gradually resolves within the first year. The developmental processes that account for this resolution are unknown, but maturation of the pontine micturition center remains a strong possibility. A minority of otherwise normal infants will experience significant ureterohydronephrosis and often high-grade vesicoureteral reflux (Figure 15-1).[45,46] Among male infants in particular, vesicoureteral reflux has been observed

TABLE 15-2 Childhood Disorders Associated with Dysfunctional Voiding

DISORDER	CHARACTERISTICS OF DYSFUNCTIONAL VOIDING
Congenital Anomalies	
Ureterocele[26]	Chronic urinary retention, obstruction or poor detrusor contraction strength in approximately 20%; unclear whether dysfunctional voiding represents sequela of disease or complication of surgical repair or unroofing
Posterior urethral valves[25]	Dysfunctional voiding in 34%; most common symptoms are overactive bladder dysfunction, enuresis, with increasing risk of urinary incontinence (UI) as child ages
Bladder exstrophy and epispadias[27]	Severe stress UI because of congenital absence of urethral closure and formation of sphincter mechanism; continuous UI in exstrophy because of failure of closure of bladder vesicle; risk for obstruction following surgical repair of bladder neck anomaly
Imperforate anus[28-30]	Dysfunctional voiding in approximately 24%; principal risk factor appears to be spinal and vertebral anomalies—mainly sacral agenesis, occult spina bifida, sacral lipoma, syringomyelia, tethered spinal cord
Nervous System Disorders	
Cerebral palsy[31,32]	Daytime UI in 24%; incomplete bladder emptying in smaller proportion who tend to attain continence later than unaffected children; factors associated with dysfunctional voiding include cognitive deficits, spastic paraplegia or quadriplegia; urodynamic evaluation reveals detrusor overactivity, detrusor sphincter dyssynergia
Central nervous system tumors[35]	UI typically associated with detrusor overactivity; detrusor sphincter dyssynergia may occur in lesions at or below the brainstem
Neoplasms of pelvis with neuromuscular tissue elements[34]	Sacrococcygeal teratoma, ganglioneuroma, yolk sac tumor, neuroblastoma, myofibroblastic bladder sarcoma associated with dysfunctional voiding, including detrusor overactivity and detrusor sphincter dyssynergia
Spina bifida occulta[33]	Dysfunctional voiding in 43% of symptomatic children; proportion in general population with dysfunctional voiding unknown; features include urinary retention, UI, detrusor overactivity, deficient detrusor contraction strength
Mental retardation, including Down syndrome, William's syndrome[36,37,39]	Significant mental retardation (IQ less than 70) associated with delayed attainment of continence and elevated risk of UI; approximately 37% of one cohort of 132 children had daytime UI at age 7 years and 17% at age 20 years; Down syndrome has not been linked to increased risk for UI unless associated with severe cognitive deficits or spinal cord problems, such as atlantoaxial dislocation; dysfunctional voiding noted in 32% of small group of children with Williams syndrome
Neuromuscular Disorder	
Duchenne muscular dystrophy[40]	Dysfunctional voiding in approximately 50%; enuresis, daytime UI with detrusor overactivity and detrusor sphincter dyssynergia, stress UI with urethral sphincter incompetence

to occur during high-pressure detrusor contractions, whereas reflux tended to occur without any elevation in female infants.[45] Nevertheless, given the presence of interrupted voiding patterns in up to one third of neonates with normal upper urinary tracts, it is not possible to conclude a cause-and-effect relationship between these observations.

Although detrusor sphincter dyssynergia is an uncommon finding in neurologically normal adults, it occurs in approximately 20% of children with detrusor overactivity[47] and may be associated with other dysfunctional elimination syndromes, such as constipation.[48] Neurologic abnormalities are not common in these children, and most respond well

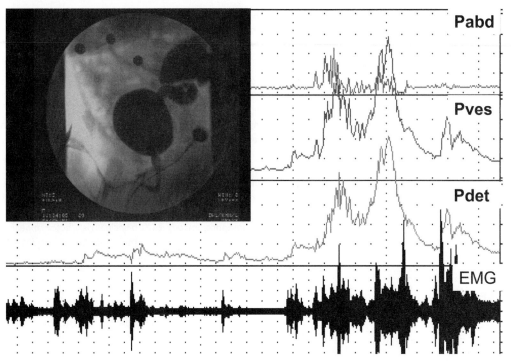

Fig. 15-1 Videourodynamic tracing demonstrates detrusor sphincter dyssynergia associated with high-grade detrusorureteral reflux and ureterohydronephrosis in a neonate. *EMG*, Electromyogram; *Pabd*, rectal pressure/abdominal pressure; *Pves*, intravesical pressure; *Pdet*, detrusor pressure.

to pelvic floor muscle rehabilitation (PFMR).[49] Dyssynergia is thought to reflect a functional disorder rather than a neurologic lesion.

In contrast, a small group of children experience a condition known as the non-neurogenic neurogenic bladder, or the Hinman-Allen or Hinman's syndrome.[50] Clinical manifestations of the syndrome include daytime UI, enuresis, interrupted voiding, and recurring UTI. Urologic evaluation reveals a thickened and trabeculated bladder wall, vesicoureteral reflux, and ureterohydronephrosis, often combined with renal insufficiency or renal failure. Constipation, fecal soiling, or encopresis are also common, and may reflect underlying pelvic floor muscle hypertonicity. It has been postulated that psychological factors and familial distress may separate these children from others who experience OAB, often with dyssynergia, but fail to develop the severe urologic complications characteristic of the non-neurogenic neurogenic bladder. These include a high prevalence of sexual abuse and personality abnormalities,[51] as well as familial alcoholism, verbal physical abuse, and intolerance for failure.[50]

The most severe of these may merit neurosurgical evaluation and intervention. Cutaneous findings in the lumbar spine region, such as hairy patch, sacral dimple, or a cutaneous malformation, may herald underlying bony or spinal cord abnormalities. In these cases, spinal cord surgery and release of the tethered cord may result in improvement in up to 50% of patients.[52] This concept has been applied to patients with severe non-neurogenic neurogenic bladders without apparent abnormalities on magnetic resonance imaging (MRI), currently referred to as occult tethered cord syndrome.[53-56] However, it must be emphasized that neurosurgical intervention should only be considered for the most severe cases, only after failure of maximal medical management and with urodynamic evidence of neuropathic dysfunction.[54]

Giggle Incontinence. The term *giggle incontinence* has been attributed to MacKeith,[57] who described it as involuntary urination during a fit of laughter. Estimates of prevalence have varied, from 8%[58] to as high as 25%.[59] Urologic and urodynamic testing results should be normal. If urodynamic evaluation reveals OAB, then the term *giggle incontinence* should not be applied, according to the International Children's Continence Society (ICCS).[3] Some have hypothesized that giggle incontinence may be mediated by the central nervous system,[60] but other researchers argue that existing evidence suggests that bladder function is completely normal and that giggle incontinence must be differentiated from the more common OAB or other symptoms.

Postmicturition Dribble. Postmicturition dribble is uncontrolled urine loss immediately after urination. The volume is typically small, but many children (and adults) find the problem distressing. Among girls, it usually occurs when urine refluxes into the vaginal vault during micturition and subsequently drains as the girl rises from the toilet. In boys, it usually occurs when a small volume of urine is trapped in the bulbous urethra that drains as the boy moves away from the toilet.

Voiding Postponement. Voiding postponement or infrequent voiding is more common in girls and is characterized by postponed urination for prolonged periods, often 8 to 12 hours.[4] It may be caused by denervation of the lower urinary tract, possibly caused by congenital factors such as spina bifida occulta or megacystis from transient bladder outlet obstruction in utero. Alternatively, it may represent the outcome of habitual voiding postponement, often caused by unwillingness or fear of urinating while at school or in a public restroom. Urodynamic testing usually reveals a large-capacity bladder with delayed and/or diminished sensations of bladder filling. Voiding pressure flow studies usually reveal adequate detrusor contraction strength and no dyssynergia, except for advanced cases, in which detrusor contractility is compromised and residual volumes are large.

Assessment

Evaluation of pediatric dysfunctional voiding begins with a focused history involving the child and parents, guardians, or regular care providers. Lower urinary tract symptoms should be queried, including daytime voiding frequency, UI while awake, enuresis, bothersome urgency, pain, and hematuria. Toddlers void about 11 times daily and schoolchildren average five or six voids while awake.[61] Among adults, urinary frequency is said to exist when a person voids more often than every 2 hours while awake,[62] or more than eight times daily,[63] but these figures have not been normalized for children. Most children

achieve daytime urinary continence by age 4 years, but 15% will experience enuresis through the fifth year of life (see Chapter 16).[4]

Bothersome urgency can be defined as a sudden strong desire to urinate that interrupts normal activities and subsides only after voluntary (or involuntary) urination occurs. It applies to children who have attained bladder control or have reached the age of 5 years, whichever comes first. Parents often interpret urgency as "waiting until the last moment" or "forgetting to go to the toilet," especially if the child reports no desire to urinate when prompted and then has a sudden and strong desire soon afterward. Urgency is usually accompanied by voiding frequency while awake. Adults typically report nocturia, but children are more likely to experience enuresis, as well as daytime wetting episodes. Children who experience urgency also may exhibit characteristic holding maneuvers in an attempt to prevent UI, such as squatting and placing a heel against the perineum (Vincent's curtsy), or grasping the penis and pants and twisting in an attempt to occlude the urethra.[64] Holding postures or maneuvers are typically more apparent in younger children and become more subtle as the child ages and is more self-aware of the potential social embarrassment associated with these gestures.

Queries about UI episodes should identify whether the child experiences leakage while awake, or whether daytime incontinence occurs only when napping. Enuresis, or urinating without awakening, should be differentiated from awakening from sleep because of the desire to urinate. Questions about which factors provoke UI are helpful, although younger children in particular may be unable to identify these or specific maneuvers that provoke UI. Because most UI in children is associated with OAB, most will report urinary leakage with a sudden urge to urinate; some state that urination occurs without obvious urgency or is induced by giggling or laughter. Damp underclothing while awake is more likely to indicate OAB than stress UI. Dribbling after voiding should be specifically queried and differentiated from urine loss prior to a voluntary void.

Pain is not commonly associated with OAB dysfunction or UI in children, unless it is complicated by a UTI or similar process. Whereas older children are usually able to localize urinary tract pain to the suprapubic area or urethra, toddlers and very young children may only be able to describe global discomfort or a "tummy ache."

Grossly visible hematuria is uncommon in children but microscopic hematuria is not, and it may indicate any one of a number of nonmalignant conditions, including a UTI. Although hematuria does not entail the same risk for genitourinary malignancy as in adults, a reasonable evaluation of its cause is mandatory.

The child and parents are also asked about fecal elimination habits, including the frequency of defecation, soiling of underclothing (staining), and frank fecal incontinence. Signs and symptoms of constipation or encopresis also may include abdominal or stomach pain relieved by defecation, passage of large stools that clog the toilet, difficulty evacuating stool, and passage of blood in the stool. Because as many as 42% of parents may be unaware of their child's bowel elimination habits,[64a] the results of the oral history should be augmented with repeated questioning after a 7-14 day bowel elimination diary or other strategies to diagnose constipation.

Farhat and colleagues[18] have designed a 10-item instrument designed to quantify dysfunctional voiding in children (see Figure 14-1). The instrument includes nine items to be completed by the child and one to be completed by parents or guardians. Construct validity is reported, although further psychometric testing is recommended to confirm the validity and reliability of this instrument.

A review of systems incorporates congenital defects affecting the urinary or neurologic system and history of neuromuscular or urologic disorders likely to affect voiding. Parents should be asked about febrile illnesses of unknown origins, because they may indicate a potentially unrecognized UTI or reflux (see Chapter 14).

Physical Examination. The physical examination focuses on identification of contributing factors, including evidence of previously undetected nervous anomalies. The lower back and buttocks are inspected for cutaneous lesions, which are found in 90% of children with occult dysraphic states.[41] These include a small fatty mass in the lower back, hairy patch, dermal vascular lesions, dimple, or asymmetry of the anal cleft (see Figure 13-2). The abdominal examination focuses on evidence of urinary retention or retention of stool in the rectal vault or large colon, which may be easily palpable in the younger child.

The child's height and weight are measured and body mass index calculated since obesity has been linked to lower response rates to treatment and greater risk of poor adherence to behavioral elements of the diagnostic and treatment regimen.[41a]

Diagnostic Testing. Urinalysis and urine culture are the only laboratory tests routinely indicated for all types of dysfunctional voiding.[4] Urodynamic testing is not indicated for the routine evaluation of OAB in children, regardless of the presence of UI.[65] Although it provides an accurate and reproducible assessment of voiding function, it does not alter initial treatment, which is primarily based on symptoms. However, urodynamic testing is valuable for children who fail to respond to an adequate trial of conservative treatment, those with evidence of urinary retention or decompensation of the bladder, when an anatomic defect of the lower urinary tract such as a large diverticulum or undetected urethral valves is suspected, or when surgical repair is anticipated.

Imaging of the upper urinary tract is indicated when upper urinary tract distress or a congenital anomaly is suspected. Ultrasonography of the urinary system and/or voiding cystourethrography may be performed when the child has a history of recurring UTI or febrile UTI in particular. Imaging is particularly important in the child with a non-neurogenic neurogenic bladder because this syndrome is associated with a significant risk of upper tract distress and renal insufficiency.

Imaging studies of the spine are indicated for select children with dysfunctional voiding. Indications are not universally agreed on, but imaging is usually recommended when dysfunctional voiding is associated with urinary retention and impaired sensations of bladder filling, or when the child exhibits cutaneous evidence of an occult spinal dysraphism.[66]

Treatment

Treatment is directed toward the bothersome lower urinary tract symptoms, but also is profoundly influenced by the underlying pathophysiology, presence of complicating factors such as UTI, vesicoureteral reflux, associated factors such as encopresis or constipation, and/or the presence of a congenital defect, such as urethral valves or an occult spinal dysraphism.

Overactive Bladder Dysfunction. Behavioral and/or pharmacologic interventions are pursued initially, particularly because they sometimes alleviate or relieve dysfunctional voiding. Collectively, these interventions are referred to as urotherapy by pediatric clinicians. The principal components of urotherapy are behavioral and pharmacologic management of constipation, fluid and dietary alterations, scheduled toileting, pelvic muscle rehabilitation, and pharmacotherapy. A randomized clinical trial in 72 children reveals that combined therapy (behavioral interventions and antimuscarinic therapy) provides superior results when compared to behavioral interventions alone or drug therapy alone.[66a] A formal education for urotherapy is offered in Sweden, but no comparable program yet exists in North America.[7]

The child and family are counseled concerning relationships among constipation, frequently coexisting with encopresis, UI, and the risk for UTI or vesicoureteral reflux. If no constipation is present, behavioral management begins with changes in fluid consumption, scheduled toileting, with particular focus on voiding habits while at school, and toileting behaviors designed to ensure routine and complete bladder emptying.

Education about fluid intake focuses on total volume consumed on a daily basis, scheduling, and beverage selection. Because of the highly variable demands for fluids placed on the human body based on physical activity and environment, it is not possible to provide a strict recommendation for daily fluid intake. Nevertheless, an average intake of 30 ml/kg/day (about ½ ounce/pound/day), originally recommended in 1980, is still the guideline for the moderately active person living in a moderate climate.[67] This type of weight-based guideline is particularly helpful when counseling children and families because it provides the flexibility to adjust goals based on the child's weight and activity. Fluid intake should be spread evenly throughout the day as much as possible; children and families should be specifically counseled not to withhold fluids while at school, because the child might then consume large volumes over a brief period after school. This pattern of fluid intake is discouraged because it often leads to brisk diuresis and provokes UI. Limiting fluid intake for 1 to 2 hours prior to sleep may reduce the risk for enuresis when daytime and nighttime UI coexist.

Families and children are also advised to reduce beverages or foods containing bladder irritants, especially caffeine, because of its association with frequent urination, urgency, and urge UI.[62] The urologic nurse should provide information about common and sometimes unsuspected products containing caffeine, such as certain carbonated beverages, powdered drinks, and many over-the-counter medications.

If present, constipation should be aggressively managed because its successful resolution benefits both bowel and bladder function. The North American Society of Pediatric Gastroenterology supports disimpaction as the initial step when managing chronic constipation, defined as "a delay or difficulty in defecation present for two or more weeks and sufficient to cause distress to the patient."[68] Disimpaction may be achieved by one or two 150-ml phosphate enemas, a mineral oil enema followed by a phosphate enema, or a hyperosmolar milk of molasses enema (ratio of 1:1 milk to molasses), using 200 to 600 ml or until the child perceives pressure or discomfort in the rectum. Alternatively, an oral agent can be administered that avoids the need for enemas. Polyethylene glycol 3350, with or without electrolytes (MiraLax, PEG 3350), is a powdered substance that is reconstituted with water to make a tasteless solution; this is usually well tolerated when mixed with 8 ounces of juice or a flavored drink mix. A randomized clinical trial of 40 children has demonstrated that a dosage regimen using 1.0 to 1.5 g/kg day of polyethylene glycol 3350 resulted in effective bowel cleansing in 95% within a 3-day period.[69] Adverse side effects included nausea and vomiting in 5%, diarrhea in 13%, and sensations of bloating in 18%. No significant alterations in fluid and electrolyte balance occurred during this trial.

Disimpaction is followed by a maintenance regimen consisting of a scheduled toileting program.[70] Maintenance requires working with the child and parents to identify a suitable time for defecation, ideally based on the child's habits prior to the onset of encopresis and constipation or following meals to maximize the tendency to evacuate the bowels in response to the gastroenteric reflex. The child should be comfortably seated with his or her feet supported on the floor or a foot stool. She or he should sit for approximately 5 minutes to promote stool evacuation; the parents and child should keep a diary of bowel elimination patterns and episodes of encopresis or fecal incontinence (soiling). Children with short attention spans may be allowed to read while on the toilet, provided that they primarily focus on the goal at hand, bowel evacuation. A reward system is recommended to assist the child in achieving regular and complete bowel elimination. Behavioral interventions are complemented by the regular use of a defecation stimulant. Alternatives include milk of magnesia, mineral oil, lactulose, sennosides (Senokot), sorbitol, and polyethylene glycol 3350. Each of these agents enables the child to produce a soft formed stool and the choice of product should be based on side effect profile, family or clinician preference and familiarity, and tolerability when taken over a prolonged period. For example, mineral oil has been shown to be effective in preventing constipation and preserve fat-soluble vitamin stores. However, children vary in their tolerance of mineral oil and it is contraindicated for children with gastroesophageal reflux or those with neurodevelopmental disorders because of the risk of aspiration and pneumonia. PEG 3350, without electrolytes, can be safely used as a maintenance agent for children with chronic constipation for as long as 12 months.[71] However, when daily doses of PEG 3350, milk of magnesia, or lactulose were compared in a group of 49 children, those receiving PEG 3350 were more likely to experience stool soiling, but were also more likely to tolerate PEG 3350 than milk of magnesia.[70]

Scheduled toileting is recommended for all patients with OAB and is particularly important for children, because they are often unwilling to toilet prior to perceiving a strong urge or unable to toilet at will in many situations. Care must go beyond merely determining a reasonable toileting schedule. Instead, the urologic nurse is often called on to engage in more aggressive advocacy, including providing letters to teachers and others to ensure that the child has adequate access to toileting facilities at school or in other environments in which institutional rules and policies typically limit access.[72] A routine toileting schedule every 2 to 3 hours while awake is strongly recommended to help the child avoid the precipitous urgency and accompanying detrusor overactivity that provokes UI.

Pharmacotherapy should be viewed as complementary to behavioral interventions. Several antimuscarinic or anticholinergic medications are now available for children with OAB. See Table 6-9 for detailed information about dosage, administration, and potential side effects. Although the variety of medications used to treat OAB in adults has grown considerably over the past decade, not all are specifically labeled for children. For example, oxybutynin is available in an immediate-release formulation (as a tablet or liquid), extended-release formulation (specially designed pill-like delivery system only), or transdermal formulation (adhesive matrix patch). However, only the immediate-release formulation's U.S. Food and Drug Administration (FDA) label includes data about its use in children. Tolterodine is also available in extended- and immediate-release formulations, but its FDA label does not contain specific data about its safety and efficacy in children. Nevertheless, several studies have evaluated the use of tolterodine[73,74] and extended-release oxybutynin[75,76] in children and reported positive results. Therefore, the decision to prescribe any of these agents to a child is based on individualized assessment, counseling with the child and family, and clinician judgment.

Urologic nursing management related to pharmacotherapy includes dosage, schedule of administration, evaluating effectiveness, and monitoring side effects. The most common side effect of these agents tends to be dry mouth. Other side effects occur much less frequently, but are significant for certain patients. They include constipation, which may exacerbate existing bowel elimination disorders, flushing and heat intolerance, especially in children who live in warm and humid climates and play or work outdoors for prolonged periods, and central nervous system effects, often described as nightmares or changes in behavior at home or in school.[73,75,77,78] Therapy may persist for several months to years, but children and parents can be advised of the natural history of pediatric dysfunctional voiding and the likelihood that symptoms tend to diminish or disappear as the child ages.

Overactive Bladder Dysfunction with Detrusor Sphincter Dyssynergia. Because of its intimate relationship with the respective sphincter mechanisms, pelvic floor muscle dysfunction complicates bladder and bowel elimination. In addition to the behavioral and pharmacologic interventions described for OAB, a program of PFMR can be instituted to establish coordinated sphincter function and optimize bladder function. Simple interventions include teaching children to allow adequate time when urinating and to focus on establishing and maintaining a continuous urinary stream.[79] Girls can be taught to squat over the toilet rather than sit on it to enable them to observe and establish a continuous flow pattern more easily. In other cases, a more sophisticated PFMR program can enable the child to gain mastery over the pelvic floor muscles[79] (see, Clinical Highlights for Advanced and Expert Practice: Pelvic Floor Muscle Rehabilitation for Dysfunctional Voiding in Children).

Non-Neurogenic Neurogenic Bladder. Formal PFMR is necessary for the successful management of the non-neurogenic neurogenic bladder, and it should be complemented by psychological support and counseling involving the child and optimally the entire family.[62] Similar to the management of OAB with detrusor sphincter dyssynergia, the goal of treatment is to teach the child to identify and relax the pelvic floor and striated sphincter muscles consistently and effectively, and long enough to achieve complete bladder emptying. Aggressive management of constipation is also critical, as is treatment of any UTI. Antimuscarinic therapy may be used following PFMR, but it may exacerbate urinary retention if dyssynergia is not adequately addressed before beginning treatment. In some cases α-adrenergic blocking agents such as tamsulosin or alfuzosin have also been used to promote bladder emptying.[80]

Children with prolonged or advanced dysfunction may have a severely trabeculated bladder, poor detrusor contraction strength, and low bladder wall compliance.[81] In addition to a detailed evaluation of upper urinary tract function, these children may require intermittent catheterization to ensure effective bladder emptying. However, the secondary psychological effects of the non-neurogenic neurogenic bladder often make teaching self-intermittent catheterization a formidable challenge. Close consultation with a psychologist, psychiatrist, or mental health professional is strongly recommended. High-grade vesicoureteral reflux, ureterohydronephrosis, and renal insufficiency or renal failure may accompany advanced cases and require multidisciplinary involvement, including pediatric nephrology.[82]

Transient Daytime Urgency and Frequency Without Urinary Incontinence. Education and reassurance are combined with behavioral interventions when managing transient daytime symptoms of OAB. After excluding underlying pathology, the child and parents are reassured that symptoms are transient and self-limiting. The child and family are also instructed to maintain adequate fluid intake, avoid bladder irritants, and go to the toilet on a fixed schedule if possible. They also should be counseled that pharmacotherapy is not effective in the treatment of this puzzling symptom syndrome.

Giggle Incontinence. Giggle incontinence usually responds to behavioral interventions or pharmacotherapy. It may be managed by tricyclic antidepressants, aimed at resolving the underlying central nervous system dysfunction. Alternatively, when symptoms of OAB are present, behavioral and pharmacologic interventions are implemented, similar to those described above. In one series of children with suspected giggle incontinence, OAB was present in 95% and treatment resulted in cessation of incontinence in 89%.[58]

Postmicturition Dribble. Parents and children are reassured that the condition does not indicate a serious underlying pathology. Girls who experience postmicturition dribble because of vaginal reflux may be taught to urinate by facing the back of the toilet, allowing them to separate the labia more effectively. Alternatively, a girl may be taught to void in the usual position, sitting forward on the toilet to completion, and then to lean forward and touch her hands to her toes to evacuate the vaginal vault.[4] Boys with postmicturition dribble can be taught to allow adequate time for urination and to milk urine from the urethra gently to evacuate the bulbous urethra.

Decreased Voiding Frequency. Scheduled toileting is critical when managing infrequent voiding. However, children are taught to void *more* rather than less frequently, in direct contrast to typical practice when managing OAB. In addition, aggressive management of constipation and/or encopresis is completed to promote effective bladder emptying and prevent UTI.

SUMMARY

Although the characteristics of pediatric dysfunctional voiding are significantly different than those seen in adults, principles of therapy are similar. They include a combination of behavioral and selective pharmacotherapy and aggressive management of coexisting bowel elimination disorders. Collectively, these interventions have been labeled as urotherapy by many in the pediatric urology community. This label seems appropriate because it emphasizes the value of combination therapy and the contributions of the urologic nurse.

Clinical Highlights for Advanced and Expert Practice: Pelvic Floor Muscle Rehabilitation for Dysfunctional Voiding in Children

Introduction

Pelvic floor muscle rehabilitation (PFMR) is a mainstay of urotherapy in children with dysfunctional voiding. It is usually undertaken in children with overactive bladder dysfunction complicated by non-neurologic detrusor sphincter dyssynergia or a non-neurogenic neurogenic bladder. Any child who does not have a neurologic disorder is theoretically a candidate for PFMR, but age remains an important consideration. We have found that children who are 6 years of age or older usually respond well to PFMR, although we have successfully used these methods on highly selected children as young as 4 years. Pelvic muscle rehabilitation can be divided into three distinctive but inseparable components—biofeedback, muscle training, and neuromuscular re-education.

Biofeedback

Biofeedback is the use of visual, auditory, or tactile signals to alert the child to previously unnoticed muscle function. The goal is to teach the child to identify, isolate, contract, and relax the pelvic floor muscles. Identification is defined as the ability to contract (squeeze) the pelvic muscles and isolation is the ability to squeeze these muscles without simultaneous contraction of the abdominal, thigh, or hip muscles. When working with children in particular, computer-assisted biofeedback is invaluable, because it provides an effective and reliable method for rapidly teaching muscle identification and isolation. McKenna and associates[79,83] have designed an interactive computer game that is an entertaining and effective tool that provides biofeedback and promotes muscle training. Alternatives to computer-assisted biofeedback include asking girls to sit backward on the toilet while actively observing the urinary stream.

Muscle Training

Improving muscle strength and endurance is often a primary goal of PFMR in adults—thus, the terms *Kegel exercises* and *pelvic floor muscle exercises*. However, many children with dysfunctional voiding have adequate muscle strength. In these cases, the principal goal of muscle training shifts from strength to skill training to ensure that the child is able to relax the pelvic floor muscles effectively during micturition or contract the muscles during urge suppression. When teaching children to relax the pelvic floor muscles to interrupt a pattern of functional dyssynergia, a graded program composed of 5 to 10 contractions/day is used. The child is taught to contract the pelvic floor muscles for a period of 5 or 6 seconds, followed by increasing longer periods of relaxation, beginning at 10 seconds and progressively building to 30 to 60 seconds.

Neuromuscular Re-education and Skill Training

Neuromuscular re-education is the process of teaching a child to contract and/or relax the pelvic floor muscles in ways that optimize lower urinary tract or bowel elimination. Two maneuvers are most often taught—pelvic floor muscle relaxation during micturition and urge suppression. Relaxation during urination can be taught by asking the child to squeeze the pelvic floor muscles immediately prior to the onset of voiding and then slowly counting to 30 during micturition. Children should try to complete the entire count, even if the urinary stream cuts off before the count is finished, and to complete urination if they reach 30 before the urine stream stops (this situation rarely occurs). We encourage children to complete this maneuver no more than once or twice daily, but many parents report that they have observed their children quietly counting during multiple voids, even when not actively encouraged to do so. This maneuver helps the child relax the pelvic floor and striated sphincter muscle throughout urination, and to allow adequate time to evacuate the bladder completely.

   The second technique is urge suppression. Urge suppression requires children to respond to a precipitous desire to urinate in a structured fashion. They are taught to stop and complete three to five quick flick contractions (a strong 1- to 4-second contraction, followed by a brief but equally long pause) while breathing slowly and deeply until the urge subsides. Children are then taught to walk to the bathroom at a normal pace and urinate. Children are discouraged from postponing urination because the next occurrence of a precipitous urge episode is more likely to result in urinary leakage. This technique is more difficult to teach than muscle relaxation with voiding, but we have had good success when working with older motivated children (about 7 or 8 years or older).

Measuring Outcomes

Success with muscle relaxation can be measured by uroflow studies or combined uroflow-sphincter electromyography. As seen, in Figure 15-2A, baseline evaluation reveals an interrupted flow pattern, and Figure 15-2B demonstrates a continuous flow pattern following four sessions of computer-enhanced PFMR. The efficacy of bladder evacuation can be monitored by a bladder ultrasound, which provides a noninvasive and accurate assessment of postvoid residual volumes.

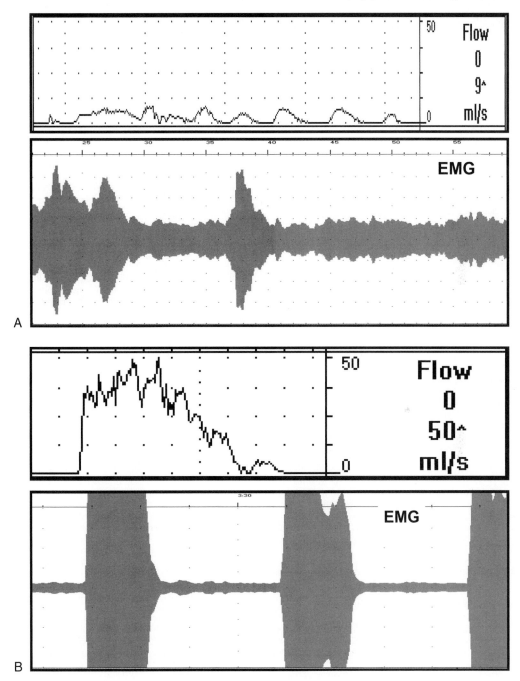

Fig. 15-2 Uroflow studies of 7-year-old girl diagnosed with non-neurogenic neurogenic bladder undergoing pelvic floor muscle rehabilitation. **A,** Baseline evaluation reveals interrupted flow pattern *(top tracing)* and inability to identify, contract, and relax the pelvic floor muscles demonstrated by surface electromyography (EMG; *lower tracing*). Postvoid residual volume is approximately 150 ml. **B,** After 4 weeks of therapy, her flow pattern is now continuous and her EMG shows the ability to identify, contract, and relax the pelvic muscles with precision. Her residual volume is now less than 10 ml.

REFERENCES

1. Palmer MH: Stress urinary incontinence: prevalence, etiology and risk factors in women at three life stages. American Journal for Nurse Practitioners, 2004; (Supplement):5-14.
2. Minassian VA, Drutz HP, Al-Badr A: Urinary incontinence as a worldwide problem. International Journal of Gynecology and Obstetrics, 2003; 82(3):327-38.
3. Nevéus T, von Goutard A, Hoebeke P et al: The standardization of terminology of lower urinary tract function in children and adolescents: report from the Standardization Children's Continence Society. Journal of Urology, 2006; 176:314-24.
4. Feldman AS, Bauer SB: Diagnosis and management of dysfunctional voiding. Current Opinion in Pediatrics, 2002; 18(2):2261-83.
5. Chen JJ, Mao W, Homayoon K, Steinhardt GF: A multivariate analysis of dysfunctional elimination syndrome, and its relationships with gender, urinary tract infection and vesicoureteral reflux in children. Journal of Urology, 2004; 171(5):1907-10.
6. Greenfield SP, Wan J: The relationship between dysfunctional voiding and congenital vesicoureteral reflux. Current Opinion in Urology, 2000; 10(6):607-10.
7. Hellstrom AL, Hanson E, Hansson S, Hjalmas K, Jodal U: Micturition habits and incontinence in 7-year-old Swedish school entrants. European Journal of Pediatrics, 1990; 149(6):434-7.
8. Chandra M: Voiding and its disorders in children. In Trachtman H, Gauthier B (eds): Monographs in Clinical Pediatrics. Amsterdam: Harwood Academic, 1998; pp 217-29.
9. Hellerstein H, Linebarger S: Voiding dysfunction in pediatric patients. Clinical Pediatrics, 2003; 42(1):43-9.
10. Stewart WF, Van Rooyen JB, Cundiff GW, Abrams P, Herzog AR, Corey R, Hunt TL, Wein AJ: Prevalence and burden of overactive bladder in the United States. World Journal of Urology, 2003; 20(6):327-36.
11. Swithinbank LV, Brookes ST, Shepherd AM, Abrams P: The natural history of urinary symptoms during adolescence. British Journal of Urology, 1998; 81(Suppl 3):90-3.
12. Kajiwara M, Inoue K, Usui A, Kurihara M, Usui T: The micturition habits and prevalence of daytime urinary incontinence in Japanese primary school children. Journal of Urology, 2004; 171(1):403-7.
13. Saedi NA, Schulman SL: Natural history of voiding dysfunction. Pediatric Nephrology, 2003; 18:894-7.
14. Alnaif B, Drutz HP: The prevalence of urinary and fecal incontinence in Canadian secondary school teenage girls: questionnaire study and review of the literature. International Urogynecology Journal, 2001; 12(2):134-8.
15. Nixon GM, Glazner JA, Martin JM, Sawyer SM: Urinary incontinence in female adolescents with cystic fibrosis. Pediatrics, 2002; 110(2 Part 1):e22.
16. Eliasson K, Larsson T, Mattsson E: Prevalence of stress incontinence in nulliparous elite trampolinists. Scandinavian Journal of Medicine and Science in Sports, 2002; 12(2):106-10.
17. Bø K, Borgen JS: Prevalence of stress and urge urinary incontinence in elite athletes and controls. Medicine and Science in Sports and Exercise, 2001; 33(11):1797-1802.
18. Farhat W, Bägli D, Capolicchio G, O'Reilly S, Merguerian PA, Khoury A: The Dysfunctional Voiding Scoring System: quantitative standardization of dysfunctional voiding symptoms in children. Journal of Urology, 2000; 164:1011-5.
19. Loening-Baucke V: Prevalence, symptoms and outcomes of constipation in infants and toddlers. Journal of Pediatrics, 2005; 146(3):359-63.
20. Koff SA, Wagner TT, Jayanthi VR: The relationship among dysfunctional elimination syndromes, primary vesicoureteral reflux and urinary tract infections in children. Journal of Urology, 1998; 160(3 Pt 2):1019-22.
21. Mazzola BL, von Vigier RO, Marchand S, Tonz M, Bianchetti MG: Behavioral and functional abnormalities linked with recurrent urinary tract infections in girls. Journal of Nephrology, 2003; 16(1):133-8.
22. American Academy of Pediatrics: Clinical practice guideline: diagnosis and evaluation of the child with attention-deficit/hyperactivity disorder. Pediatrics, 2000; 105(5):1158-70.
23. Robson WL, Jackson HP, Blackhurst D, Leung AK: Enuresis in children with attention-hyperactivity disorder. Southern Medical Journal, 1997; 90(5):503-5.
24. Duel BP, Steinberg-Epstein R, Hill M, Lerner M: A survey of voiding dysfunction in children with attention deficit-hyperactivity disorder. Journal of Urology, 2003; 170(4 Pt 2):1521-4.
25. Lal R, Bhatnagar V, Mitra DK: Urinary continence following posterior urethral valves treatment. Indian Journal of Pediatrics, 1999; 66(1):49-54.
26. Sherman ND, Stock JA, Hanna MK: Bladder dysfunction after bilateral ectopic ureterocele repair. Journal of Urology, 2003; 170(5):1975-7.
27. Mouriquand PD, Buban JT, Feyaerts A, Jandric M, Timsit M, Mollard P, Mure PY, Basset T: Long-term results of bladder neck reconstruction for incontinence in children with classical bladder exstrophy or incontinent epispadias. BJU International, 2003; 92(9):997-1002.
28. Kakizaki H, Nonomura K, Asano Y, Shinno Y, Ameda K, Koyanagi T: Preexisting neurogenic voiding dysfunction in children with imperforate anus: problems in management. Journal of Urology, 1994; 151(4):1041-4.
29. Boemers TM, Beek FJ, van Gool JD, de Jong TP, Bax KM: Urologic problems in anorectal malformations. Part 1: urodynamic findings and significance of sacral anomalies. Journal of Pediatric Surgery, 1996; 31(3):407-10.
30. Boemers TM, de Jong TP, van Gool JD, Bax KM: Urologic problems in anorectal malformations. Part 2: functional urologic sequelae. Journal of Pediatric Surgery, 1996; 31(5):634-7.
31. Karaman M, KY C, Caskurlu T, Guney S, Ergenekon E: Urodynamic findings in children with cerebral palsy. International Journal of Urology, 2005; 12(8):717-20.
32. Roijen LE, Postema K, Limbeek VJ, Kuppevelt VH: Development of bladder control in children and adolescents with cerebral palsy. Developmental Medicine and Child Neurology, 2001; 43(2):103-7.
33. Silveri M, Capitanucci ML, Capozza N, Mosiello G, Silvano A, Gennaro MD: Occult spinal dysraphism: neurogenic voiding dysfunction and long-term urologic follow-up. Pediatric Surgery International, 1997; 12(2-3):148-50.
34. Mosiello G, Gatti C, De Gennaro M, Capitanucci ML, Silveri M, Inserra A, Milano GM, De Laurentis C, Boglino C: Neurovesical dysfunction in children after treating pelvic neoplasms. BJU International, 2003; 92(3):289-92.
35. Soler D, Borzyskowski M: Lower urinary tract dysfunction in children with central nervous system tumors. Archives of Diseases in Childhood, 1998; 79(4):344-7.
36. Chaudhry V, Sturgeon C, Gates AJ, Myers G: Symptomatic atlantoaxial dislocation in Down's syndrome. Annals of Neurology, 1987; 21(6):606-9.
37. von Wendt L, Simila S, Niskanen P, Jarvelin MR: Development of bowel and bladder control in the mentally retarded. Developmental Medicine and Child Neurology, 1990; 32(6):515-8.
38. Eyman RK, Grossman HJ, Chaney RH, Call TL: The life expectancy of profoundly handicapped people with mental retardation. New England Journal of Medicine, 1990; 323(9):584-9.
39. Schulman SL, Zderic S, Kaplan P: Increased prevalence of urinary symptoms and voiding dysfunction in Williams syndrome. Journal of Pediatrics, 1996; 129(3):466-9.
40. MacLeod M, Kelly R, Robb SA, Borzyskowski M: Bladder dysfunction in Duchenne muscular dystrophy. Archives of Disease in Childhood, 2003; 88(4):347-9.
41. Bauer SB: Neuropathic dysfunction of the lower urinary tract. In Wein AJ, Kavoussi LR, Novick AC, Partin AW, Peters CA (eds): Campbell-Walsh Urology, 9th edition. Philadelphia: Saunders, 2007; pp 3625-55.
41a. Guven A, Giramonti K, Kogan BA. The effect of obesity on treatment efficacy in children with nocturnal enuresis and voiding dysfunction. Journal of Urology, 2007; 178(4 Part 1):1458-62.

42. McKenna PH, Herndon CD: Voiding dysfunction associated with incontinence, vesicoureteral reflux and recurrent urinary tract infections. Current Opinion in Urology, 2000; 10(6):599-606.

43. Nijman RJ: Pediatric voiding dysfunction and enuresis. Current Opinion in Urology, 2000; 10(5):365-70.

44. Sillen U: Bladder function in healthy neonates and its development during infancy. Journal of Urology, 2001; 166(6):2376-81.

45. Sillen U, Bachelard M, Hansson S, Hermansson G, Jacobson B, Hjalmas K: Video cystometric recording of dilating reflux in infancy. Journal of Urology, 1996; 155(5):1711-5.

46. Podesta ML, Castera R, Ruarte AC: Videourodynamic findings in young infants with severe primary reflux. Journal of Urology, 2004; 171(2 Pt 1):829-33.

47. Berry A: Helping children with dysfunctional voiding. Urologic Nursing, 2005; 25(3):193-201.

48. Erdem E, Lin A, Kogan BA, Feustel PJ: Association of elimination dysfunction and body mass index. Journal of Pediatric Urology, 2007; 2(4):364-7.

49. Porena M, Costantini E, Rociola W, Mearini E: Biofeedback successfully cures detrusor-sphincter dyssynergia in pediatric patients. Journal of Urology, 2000; 163(6):1927-31.

50. Allen TD: Forty years experience with voiding dysfunction. BJU International, 2003; 92(Supplement 1):15-22.

51. Gray M: Sphincter re-education for pediatric voiding dysfunction complicated by dyssynergia. In Association for Continence Advice International Conference, Bournemouth, United Kingdom, April 1993.

52. Khoury AE, Hendrick EB, McLorie GA, Kulkarni A, Churchill BM: Occult spinal dysraphism: clinical and urodynamic outcome after division of the filum terminale. Journal of Urology, 1990; 144(2 Part II):426-8.

53. Selcuki M, Vatansever S, Inan S, Erdemli E, Bagdatoglu C, Polat A: Is a filum terminale with a normal appearance really normal? Childs Nervous System, 2003; 19(1):3-10.

54. Metcalfe PD, Luerssen TG, King SJ: Treatment of the occult tethered spinal cord for neuropathic bladder: results of sectioning the filum terminale. Journal of Urology, 2006; 176(5):1826.

55. Guerra LA, Pike J, Milks J, Barrowman N, Leonard M: Outcome in patients who underwent tethered cord release for occult spinal dysraphism. Journal of Urology, 2006; 176(5):1729-32.

56. Wehby MC, O'Hollaren PS, Abtin K, Hume JL, Richards BJ: Occult tight filum terminale syndrome: results of surgical untethering. Pediatric Neurosurgery, 2004; 40(2):51-7.

57. MacKeith RC: Micturition induced by giggling. Guys Hospital Reports, 1964; 113:250-60.

58. Chandra M, Saharia R, Shi Q, Hill V: Giggle incontinence in children: a manifestation of detrusor instability. Journal of Urology, 2002; 168(5):2184-7.

59. Christmas TJ, Noble JG, Watson GM, Turner-Warwick RT: Use of biofeedback in treatment of psychogenic voiding dysfunction. Urology, 1991; 37:43-5.

60. Sher PK, Reinberg Y: Successful treatment of giggle incontinence with methylphenidate. Journal of Urology, 1996; 156(2 Pt 2):656-8.

61. Goellner MH, Ziegler EE, Fomon SJ: Urination during the first three years of life. Nephron, 1981; 28(4):174-8.

62. Gray M, Marx RM, Peruggio M, Patrie J, Steers WD: A model for predicting motor urge urinary incontinence. Nursing Research, 2001; 50:116-22.

63. Sampselle CM: Teaching women to use a voiding diary. American Journal of Nursing, 2003; 103:311-9.

64. Kondo A, Kato K, Takita T, Otani T: Holding postures characteristic of unstable bladder. Journal of Urology, 1985; 134(4):702-4.

64a. Akyol I, Adayener C, Senuki T, Baykal K, Iseri C: An important issue in the management of elimination dysfunction in children: parental awareness of constipation. Clinical Pediatrics, 2007; 46(7):601-3.

65. Soygur T, Arikan N, Tokatli Z, Karaboga R: The role of video-urodynamic studies in managing non-neurogenic voiding dysfunction in children. BJU International, 2004; 93(6):841-3.

66. Wraige E, Borzyskowski M: Investigation of daytime wetting: when is spinal cord imaging indicated? Archives of Disease in Childhood, 2002; 87(2):151-5.

66a. Ayan A, Topsakal K, Gokce G, Gulteken EY: Efficacy of a combined treatment and behavioral modification as a first line treatment for nonneurogenic and nonanatomical voiding dysfunction in children: a randomized clinical trial. Journal of Urology, 2007; 177:2325-9.

67. National Academy of Sciences, Food and Nutrition Board. Recommended Daily Allowances. 9th edition. Washington DC: National Academy of Sciences, 1980.

68. Loening-Baucke V: Encopresis. Current Opinion in Pediatrics, 2002; 14:570-5.

69. Youssef NN, Peters JM, Henderson W, Shultz-Peters S, Lockhart DK, Di Lorenzo C: Dose response of PEG 3350 for the treatment of childhood fecal impaction. Journal of Pediatrics, 2002; 141(3):410-4.

70. Loening-Baucke V, Pashankar DS: A randomized, prospective, comparison study of polyethylene glycol 3350 without electrolytes and milk of magnesia for children with constipation and fecal incontinence. Pediatrics, 2006; 118(2):528-35.

71. Erickson BA, Austin JC, Cooper CS, Boyt MA: Polyethylene glycol 3350 for constipation in children with dysfunctional elimination. Journal of Urology, 2003; 170(4 Part 2):1518-20.

72. Cooper CS, Abousally CT, Austin JC, Boyt MA, Hawtery CE: Do public schools teach voiding dysfunction? Results of an elementary school teacher survey. Journal of Urology, 2003; 170(3):956-8.

73. Raes A, Hoebeke P, Segaert I, Van Laecke E, Dehoorne J, Vande Walle J: Retrospective analysis of efficacy and tolerability of tolterodine in children with overactive bladder. European Urology, 2004; 45(2):240-4.

74. Nijman RJ: Role of antimuscarinics in the treatment of nonneurogenic daytime urinary incontinence in children. Urology, 2004; 63(3 Suppl 1):45-50.

75. Youdim K, Kogan BA: Preliminary study of the safety and efficacy of extended-release oxybutynin in children. Urology, 2002; 59(3):428-32.

76. Reinberg Y, Crocker J, Wolpert J, Vandersteen D: Therapeutic efficacy of extended release oxybutynin chloride, and immediate release and long-acting tolterodine tartrate in children with daytime urinary incontinence. Journal of Urology, 2003; 169(1):317-9.

77. Valsecia ME, Malgor LA, Espindola JH, Carauni DH: New adverse effect of oxybutynin: "night terror." Annals of Pharmacotherapy, 1998; 32(4):506.

78. t'Veld BA, Kwee-Zuiderwijk WJ, van Puijenbroek EP, Stricker BH: Neuropsychiatric adverse effects attributed to use of oxybutynin. Nederlands Tijdschrift voor Geneeskunde, 1998; 142(11):590-2.

79. McKenna LS, McKenna PH: Continence care. Modern management of nonneurologic pediatric incontinence. Journal of Wound, Ostomy and Continence Nursing, 2004; 31(6):351-6.

80. Austin PF, Homsy YL, Masel JL, Cain MP, Casale AJ, Rink RC: Alpha-adrenergic blockade in children with neuropathic and non-neuropathic voiding dysfunction. Journal of Urology, 1999; 162(3 Pt 2):1064-7.

81. Ewalt DH, Bauer SB: Pediatric neurourology. Urologic Clinics of North America, 1996; 23(3):501-9.

82. Ozcan O, Tekgul S, Duzova A, Aki F, Yuksel S, Bakkaloglu A, Erkan I, Bakkaloglu M: How does the presence of urologic problems change the outcome of kidney transplantation in the pediatric age group. Transplantation Proceedings, 2006; 38(2):552-3.

83. Herndon CD, Decambre M, McKenna PH: Interactive computer games for treatment of pelvic floor dysfunction. Journal of Urology, 2001; 166(5):1893-8.

The term *enuresis* is broadly defined as any involuntary loss of urine.[1] However, the International Children's Continence Society (ICCS) recommends that the term should be applied only to intermittent episodes of incontinence while sleeping.[2] Previously called nocturnal enuresis, they further recommend that the descriptor "nocturnal" be dropped and the term shortened to simply "enuresis." Enuresis is further categorized by its onset. Primary enuresis is defined as persistence of isolated bedwetting beyond the age that a child masters daytime urinary continence, and secondary enuresis is the occurrence of isolated bedwetting in a child who had previously achieved daytime and nighttime urinary control. This chapter will review primary and secondary enuresis in children. Bedwetting is also common in children who experience diurnal urinary incontinence, but that issue is discussed in Chapter 15.

DEVELOPMENT OF URINARY CONTINENCE AND THE EPIDEMIOLOGY OF ENURESIS

Although the age at which urinary continence is achieved varies among children, it nevertheless follows a predictable sequence. Three developmental milestones are critical for urinary continence: (1) increased bladder capacity; (2) control of the pelvic floor muscles and striated urinary sphincter; and (3) control over detrusor contractions.[3] During infancy, bladder function is characterized by frequent urination (approximately once every hour), continuous or interrupted voiding (often with dyssynergic sphincter muscle contraction during micturition), and frequent residual urine after micturition.[4] As the child enters the second year of life, bladder capacity increases significantly and the frequency of micturition falls to approximately 11 episodes/day, reflecting both a decrease in urine production and

an increase in bladder capacity.[5] Pelvic floor muscle and striated sphincter control usually occur around age 3 years. This is observed as voluntarily interruption of the urinary stream, but urinary incontinence persists. Detrusor control, the final milestone for urinary continence, is characterized by the absence of detrusor contractions until the child wishes to urinate, even in the presence of a desire to void. It requires maturation of modulatory areas in the brainstem, midbrain, and cerebral hemispheres and is typically mastered by the fourth to fifth years of life.[3] When these milestones are reached, daytime urinary continence occurs initially, followed by nighttime dryness.

However, although most children achieve urinary continence by age 4 to 5 years, approximately 18% of boys and 15% of girls will continue to experience enuresis.[6] The prevalence of enuresis gradually diminishes as the child ages; by age 12 years, it has declined to 6% of boys and 4% of girls, and it will fall to 1% to 2% by late adolescence or early adulthood.[7] When teaching patients and families about enuresis many clinicians quote the "laws of 15"[3]: (1) 15% of 5-year-old children have enuresis; (2) 15% of enuretics also have encopresis; (3) 15% become dry each year; and (4) 15% have secondary enuresis. However, these so-called laws are actually comprised of clinical observations that approximate common epidemiologic characteristics of enuresis, rather than specific research-based findings.

Etiology and Pathophysiology

The cause remains unknown, but various contributing factors have been identified. Genetic and familial factors profoundly influence the risk of primary or secondary enuresis.[8] Approximately 39% of fathers and 23% of mothers of children with enuresis have reported bedwetting during their childhoods. Furthermore, the risk of a child having enuresis is about 44% when one parent experienced isolated bedwetting as a child, 77% when both parents were enuretic, and 83% if both parents and one or more cousins, uncles, or aunts were affected.

Further evidence of a genetic basis for enuresis is found when monozygotic (identical) and dizygotic (fraternal) twins are studied. Genetic concordance studies, the likelihood that a specific disorder occurs because of genetic rather than environmental factors, have indicated a strong genetic predisposition for enuresis.[8,9] For example, in one study involving 11,220 subjects, the phenotypic variance attributed to genetic influence in persons with enuresis was 67% in males and 70% in females.[10]

Genetic predisposition for enuresis is autosomal dominant, and its penetrance is approximately 90%.[8] The specific genes that predispose children to enuresis are unknown. Possible defects have been located on the long arm of chromosome 13, in a region labeled ENUR1, the q11 region of chromosome 22, and the q region of chromosome 12.[11-13] Investigation of chromosome 13 has also focused on the *VPNP II* (vasopressin-neurophysin II) gene, which is known to cause diabetes insipidus. However, no linkage to primary enuresis was found.

Although there is strong evidence that genetic factors play an important role in monosymptomatic enuresis, approximately 15% to 30% are classified as sporadic cases, occurring in children with no familial history or known genetic predisposition, and not all children with a genetic predisposition will have enuresis.[8,13] Nongenetic factors associated with enuresis include urodynamic abnormalities, high urine production during sleep, arousal disorders affecting sleep patterns, obstructive airway disorders, maturational lag, and psychological distress.

The most common urodynamic abnormality associated with enuresis is a small bladder capacity.[13-15] This reduction in functional bladder capacity is associated with sensory urgency, but urodynamic evidence has revealed only a slightly elevated prevalence of overactive detrusor contractions among children with enuresis versus normal children.[16]

High-volume urine output has also been implicated as a cause of enuresis.[17-20] This defect has been linked to abnormalities in antidiuretic hormone (vasopressin) production or hypercalciuria and desmopressin (a drug that supplements antidiuretic hormone production); low-calcium diets have been found to relieve or ablate enuresis in some children.

Antidiuretic hormone is manufactured in the hypothalamus and released from the posterior pituitary; it acts on the kidneys to regulate urine production. In addition to responding to the proportion of water in the body's internal environment, vasopressin follows a circadian rhythm—it peaks during the early morning hours, limiting urine production and the need to interrupt sleep for micturition. Some researchers have hypothesized that enuresis may be caused by rapid bladder filling in response to insufficient vasopressin release,[17,18] possibly because of absorptive hypercalciuria and secondary release of aquaporin-2, a paracrine substance that increases urine dilution.[19,20] However, other studies have compared enuretics to normal children and failed to find differences in urine osmolarity, serum vasopressin levels, or urinary calcium concentrations.[21]

Immaturity of the brainstem has also been hypothesized as a cause of enuresis. Evaluation of prepulse inhibition (a noninvasive test reflecting maturation of brainstem function) comparing a group of continent children with a group of enuretic children revealed evidence of a lack of brainstem maturation in those with enuresis.[21a] Studies in animals have indicated that the brainstem, among other functions, is responsible for arousal from sleep in response to bladder filling.[22] Lack of arousal, in turn, has been linked to impaired vasopressin release resulting in bladder distension when asleep, and these factors are hypothesized to predispose affected children to enuretic episodes.[13] Early clinical studies demonstrated that enuretic episodes are *not* limited to the deeper stages of sleep,[23] but more recent studies have shown differences in individual cases, suggesting that arousal disorders may affect a subgroup of children with enuresis.[24,25] When children with enuresis and evidence of brainstem immaturity were measured after a period of 2 years, evidence of brainstem maturation when compared with continence controls had disappeared, suggesting brainstem maturation despite persistence of bedwetting episodes.[21a]

Obstructive sleep apnea (OSA) in children is most commonly associated with adenoidal or tonsillar hypertrophy.[26,27] These children have been shown to have nighttime polyuria[28] caused by increased sodium production and increased levels of the atrial natriuretic peptide, a hormone that stimulates urine production, possibly leading to a growing number of studies linking OSA to primary and secondary enuresis.[26,28,29]

Enuresis has been clinically described as arising from a maturational lag,[30] but others have cautioned against use of this description as vague and confusing.[31] In one review,[32] the concept of maturational lag was described as incorporating abnormalities of sleep arousal, bladder capacity, and response to distension with urine. Nevertheless, given the negative connotations of the term *maturational lag*, it is probably best avoided when describing the causes of enuresis to colleagues, patients, or families.

Psychological distress has been associated with enuresis.[33] Common precipitating events include the birth of a sibling, parental separation or divorce, physical or sexual abuse, a death in the family, or school-related problems. However, when behavioral disorders or psychological distress are assessed in children with enuresis, they typically precede the onset of bedwetting and are associated with *secondary* rather than primary enuresis.

Less than 1% of children with monosymptomatic enuresis have underlying urologic abnormalities such as urethral obstruction or a urinary tract infection.[3] Instead, the vast majority of these children experience bothersome lower urinary tract symptoms that occur both day and night.

Assessment

The routine evaluation of enuresis without daytime symptoms includes a focused history, physical assessment and urinalysis.[3] Questions about the onset of enuresis are used to differentiate primary from secondary bedwetting. Inquiry includes the frequency of enuresis, its perceived severity, and how the family and child are currently managing the problem. A family history for enuresis and a recent history of psychological distress or behavioral problems provide further information allowing differentiation of primary versus secondary enuresis. Daytime lower urinary tract symptoms, including voiding frequency, bothersome urgency, urinary incontinence, encopresis, or urinary tract infections are sought, particularly because these help differentiate isolated enuresis from polysymptomatic enuresis (see Chapter 15). The physical examination includes careful inspection of the abdomen, searching for evidence for bladder or bowel distension because of retention and encopresis. The lower back and buttocks are inspected for signs of

spinal dysraphism (see Chapter 13) and the perineal skin for integrity.

A urinalysis is obtained to screen for urinary tract infection (positive nitrites and leukocytes), diabetes mellitus (glucosuria), diabetes insipidus (very low specific gravity), urinary system tumor (hematuria), and renal disease (proteinuria). A urine culture or further tests are indicated only when urinalysis is abnormal.

Some pediatric urologists advocate renal ultrasonography, but studies have revealed that the occurrence of positive findings is less than 3%, an incidence equivalent to that found in age-matched children without urologic complaints.[34] Invasive tests, such as voiding cystourethrography or multichannel urodynamics, are not indicated in the routine evaluation of isolated bedwetting.[3]

Management

A number of treatment modalities have proved effective for primary enuresis.[35] Selection of an optimal program is influenced by a number of factors, including the preferences of the child and family and the child's age. Simple behavioral interventions are usually tried first, and a urologist or urologic nurse will be consulted if these prove ineffective.

Timing of Intervention. Because nighttime urinary continence is a developmental milestone, the timing of interventions should be discussed with the child and family. For example, some families may seek care for a child with persistent enuresis as early as age 3 to 4 years. In this case, parents may be reassured that nighttime urinary continence is not achieved by 85% of all children before the end of the fifth year of life.[3] In contrast, the school-age child with enuresis usually justifies prompt intervention, particularly if enuresis is frequent and the child is bothered or embarrassed by the condition.

Containment Therapies. Various containment devices are available for the child with enuresis, including absorptive underclothing, water-resistant bed coverings, or sleeping bag liners. Although these devices do not prevent or treat enuresis, they do protect mattresses from deep soiling and afford privacy for the child who participates in a sleepover with friends or an overnight camping experience. Families are taught about specific products and they also may be advised to search the Internet or consult with a local medical supply retailer to learn more about available product choices.

First-Line Behavioral Interventions. A number of simple or first-line behavioral interventions can be initiated by the child and family following an initial counseling session.[35-37] Restricting fluid intake 2 hours before bedtime may alleviate nocturnal urine production. Beverages containing caffeine, in particular, are avoided because of their potential to act as a bladder irritant.[38] The parents may be counseled to awaken the child one or more times during the night to urinate to empty the bladder before an enuretic episode occurs. Some clinicians have advocated a more aggressive approach for awakening the child for urination such as turning on lights, placing a cool moist washcloth on the child's face, or speaking in a loud but nonpunitive voice to awaken the child fully.[39] Others advocate a less aggressive approach, even if the child does not appear fully awake when helped to urinate.

The older child may be encouraged to become involved in managing enuresis by helping parents change bed linens and helping with cleaning and replacing soiled linens and pajamas. However, involvement with this task should be viewed as a self-management strategy and counseling should emphasize that enuresis is not a form of misbehavior indicating the need for punishment or sanctions.

A simple reward system can also be used to encourage nighttime continence. A calendar is constructed and goals for consecutive dry nights negotiated with the child and family. Dry nights are recorded on the calendar, usually with a star or other sticker indicating a worthy accomplishment, and parents are counseled to praise dry nights but avoid placing blame or criticizing nights marked by an enuretic episode.

Retention control training is a behavioral strategy designed to increase functional bladder capacity.[40,41] The child remains NPO for a period of 2 hours and urinates to empty the bladder completely. The patient is then asked to drink a specific volume of water; the volume is calculated by multiplying the child's weight in kilograms times 30 (for those less than 25 kg) or multiplying weight times 20 for children weighing more than 25 kg (the volume should never exceed 1000 ml). The child is asked to refrain from voiding as long as possible, and the voided volume is measured in a graduated container. This strategy can be repeated and the child is encouraged to retain fluids for progressively longer periods to increase functional bladder capacity. Although many children will require additional therapy, simple behavioral interventions resolve enuresis in some children,[36,37,39] and they provide safe adjunctive therapies for any child with primary or secondary bedwetting.

Moisture Alarms. Moisture alarms are incorporated into the clothing or bed covers and initiate an alarm when exposed to urine.[35,42] Various devices are commercially available and can be obtained from the Internet or a medical supply retailer. The family and child are advised of the purpose of the alarm, its installation, and care. Selecting the ideal moisture alarm is individualized, but devices that are economic, incorporated into the child's clothing, and easy to assemble and use are generally preferred over unnecessarily expensive devices or underpads that may not be activated until the enuretic episode is well underway. Parents are taught about the proper use of the device and the child is encouraged to activate the alarm while awake by placing moist fingers against the sensor. Most moisture alarms use an audible alarm, but some are designed to activate room lights and are preferred for the child who is hearing-impaired. The alarm is set before it is used overnight and the child is taught to turn the alarm off, arise, and urinate when it sounds. Therapy usually requires 4 to 6 weeks and can be combined with the calendar award system described earlier. The mechanism of action for moisture alarm therapy is not entirely understood. One study of 28 enuretic children older than 7 years has demonstrated a statistically significant and clinically relevant increase in bladder capacity after 12 weeks of treatment.[43] Another study of 37 children aged 5 to 13 years has found that alarm therapy not only improved enuresis, but also improved daytime voiding frequency while diminishing the number of urge incontinence episodes.[44] This again suggests that alarm therapy may improve bladder capacity by mechanisms that are not yet understood.

Although it seems logical that the alarm would condition children to awaken at night and urinate before an enuretic episode occurs, clinical observation has revealed that ablation of enuresis is the more common outcome. Regardless of the mechanism of action, alarm therapy has proved equally effective as pharmacotherapy during active treatment and its durability is better than that achieved by desmopressin or imipramine.[42] Success varies from

30% to as high as 87%. Predictors of success include selection of an alarm device that promptly and reliably sounds at the onset of urine loss and treatment duration (up to 12 weeks).[45] In contrast to the higher success rates achieved when behavioral and pharmacologic interventions are combined for the management of overactive bladder, the success rate of alarm therapy is not improved by the addition of a drug.[46] Relapse rates are lower than other treatment options, varying from 4% to 55%.[45]

Pharmacotherapy. Drugs may reduce the frequency of enuretic episodes by decreasing nocturnal urine production, altering sleep arousal responses, increasing bladder capacity, or inhibiting overactive detrusor contractions.[35] Two drugs are primarily used to manage enuresis, desmopressin and imipramine; alternatives include α-sympathomimetics, antimuscarinics, and diuretics.

Desmopressin (DDAVP) is an analogue of the antidiuretic hormone vasopressin.[47] It is hypothesized to reduce enuresis episodes by decreasing nocturnal urine production[47] or by diminishing nocturnal excretion of potassium chloride into the urine.[48] Administration does not affect bladder capacity. Desmopressin is available in several formulations, including a nasal spray and tablets.[49] Multiple studies have shown that it is effective in reducing the frequency of enuretic episodes over a relatively short term (2 to 12 weeks), although episodes are not eliminated competely in 75% of those treated.[3,50,51] Unlike imipramine, it is effective when given over a single night; this dosing schedule is useful when a child participates in a sleepover or travels overnight. Long-term studies have shown that desmopressin is effective when used continuously over periods of 6 months or longer, and that the risk for side effects is similar to that seen with short-term use.[51] In addition, long-term use does not affect vasopressin production after the drug is stopped, but a stepwise reduction in dosage is recommended to maximize the possibility of a cure following prolonged treatment. Nevertheless, the cure rate following treatment with desmopressin is relatively low, 18% to 38% after 6 months of treatment.

Desmopressin was originally available as a nasal spray only. A single puff delivers 10 μg and the usual dosage is 20-40 μg, or one or two puffs per nostril.[49] No more than three puffs per nostril should be given in a single night. The nasal spray must be stored in a refrigerator. The child should blow his or her nose to clear excess mucus and the medication may be withheld if rhinitis occurs. The cap is removed and the bottle tilted so that the spray pump tubing is immersed in the fluid remaining in the bottle. The child is taught to tilt her or his head back to maximize delivery to the nasal mucosa and avoid medication running from the nose or down the throat. A single puff is delivered to each nostril approximately 30 minutes prior to bedtime, and the child is taught not to lie down immediately after the medication is given to maximize absorption and avoid nasal irritation.

Some families and children find the nasal spray more difficult to administer as compared with tablets. In addition, it may produce nasal irritation, leading to unreliable absorption of the drug. Therefore, tablets are typically preferred. Tablets are administered 30 to 60 minutes before sleep; the usual dose is 200 to 400 μg.[49]

Regardless of the route of administration, parents and children are counseled that the drug reaches its peak efficacy within 8 hours of administration. The child may need to be awakened to urinate if expected to sleep for 10 hours or more to prevent an enuretic episode as the drug's serum level declines.

In addition to teaching dosage and administration, the urologic nurse should counsel patients about potential side effects, including nasal congestion and headache, the most common persisting side effect when therapy is discontinued after 6 months or longer.[51] The most serious side effect is water intoxication and hyponatremia. Water intoxication is prevented by counseling parents to reduce fluid intake to 2 ounces 2 hours before bedtime if the child weighs 75 pounds (34 kg), 3 ounces if the child weighs 76 to 100 pounds (35 to 46 kg), and 4 ounces if the child weighs more than 100 pounds (46 kg), and never to exceed 8 ounces during the night of administration, even in large adults or adolescents. The medication is avoided when the child has vomiting, diarrhea, or a fever because of the risk for alterations in fluid and electrolyte balance. Although very uncommon, hyponatremia and water intoxication may occur. Signs and symptoms of water intoxication include infrequent urination, confusion, lethargy, and seizures if not resolved promptly. If symptoms occur, parents should seek emergent care and provide health care professionals with details about fluid intake and recent dosages of desmopressin. Desmopressin is contraindicated in children with inherited thrombotic thrombocytopenic purpura (Upshaw-Schulman syndrome).[52]

Imipramine is a tricyclic antidepressant that has been used to manage enuresis and daytime urinary incontinence in children and adults.[3,35,49,53] Pharmacologic actions in the child with enuresis include its anticholinergic effects,[54,55] reduction of nocturnal urine output,[56] and possible alterations of sleep patterns or arousal responses.[57] The usual dosage is 25 mg for children up to 8 years of age and 50 to 75 mg in older children. The timing of the dose may be altered depending on when enuretic episodes are likely to occur; imipramine is given in the early afternoon to children who tend to wet the bed at 1 AM or earlier and it is given in the early evening to children who tend to wet after 1 AM. A period of 10 to 14 days is required to achieve maximal response; single-night dosing of imipramine is not effective. The drug may be administered continuously over a period of 3 months. It should then be discontinued for a brief period to determine whether enuresis occurs. Tapering may be necessary if the dosage is particularly high to avoid nausea, vomiting, irritability, and lethargy.

Side effects associated with imipramine can be significant. Common side effects include interference with sleep, irritability, depressed appetite, nausea, and vomiting.[3,56] In addition to teaching children and families about dosing, administration, tapering doses (as directed), and potential side effects, education must include drug safety and prevention of inadvertent ingestion by siblings. If an accidental overdose is ingested by a younger sibling, tricyclic antidepressants can cause cardiac suppression and death.

Desmopressin and imipramine have been used in combination for monosymptomatic and polysymptomatic enuresis.[58] A randomized clinical trial involving 158 patients has compared results of monotherapy (imipramine or desmopressin) with dual-agent therapy (desmopressin *and* oxybutynin). Children randomized to combination therapy were found to obain more benefit than when single-agent therapy was used for monosymptomatic or polysymptomatic enuresis. Nevertheless, treatment with multiple agents must be carefully weighed against the increased risk for adverse side effects.

Alternative medications include α-sympathomimetics, antimuscarinics, and diuretics. Oxybutynin has been evaluated in enuresis and found to have little benefit.[59] Symptom improvement occurs in as little as 5% of patients, and its role is probably limited to children with polysymptomatic enuresis (bedwetting combined with daytime urge urinary incontinence). α-Sympathomimetic agents have been investigated, often given in combination with an anticholinergic, but they also have not proved effective. Furosemide was administered to 63 children with primary enuresis during the late afternoon in an attempt to reduce nocturnal urine production. Although the children treated with the diuretic experienced a reduction in enuretic episodes, only 12% achieved total dryness as compared with 24% who were dry when managed by desmopressin.[60]

Psychological counseling is sometimes indicated for managing secondary enuresis associated with psychological distress or dysfunction.[3,52] Alternative therapies, such as hypnotherapy, may be used in highly selected cases, particularly for children with severe persistent enuresis that does not respond to traditional treatment options.

Surgery. Urologic procedures, such as Y-V plasty of the bladder outlet, have been used historically but are no longer considered viable treatment options.[3] Adenotonsillectomy has been advocated for children with lower urinary tract symptoms, including enuresis. In a study of 86 children with OSA and enuresis, Firoozi and colleagues[27] found that adenotonsillectomy leads to complete symptom relief in 33%, improved symptoms in 31%, and no change in 36%.

SUMMARY

Perhaps more than any other common disorder that affects children, enuresis serves to remind the urologic nurse of the importance of a stepwise evaluation and management plan, beginning with noninvasive simple programs and progressing to more invasive treatments only after simple interventions have proved ineffective. Using this approach, along with careful education of the child and family, enuresis can often be managed by behavioral interventions alone or can be combined with pharmacotherapy to alleviate symptoms until the problem spontaneously resolves or the child is conditioned to awaken at night and empty the bladder prior to occurrence of an enuretic episode.

REFERENCES

1. Dirck JH (ed): Stedman's Concise Medical Dictionary for the Health Professions, 6th edition. Philadelphia: Lippincott, Williams and Williams, 2007.

2. Neveus T, von Gontard A, Hoebeke P, Hjalmas K, Bauer S, Bower W, Jorgensen TM, Rittig S, Walle JV, Yeung CK, Djurhuus JC: The standardization of terminology of lower urinary tract function in children and adolescents: report from the Standardization Committee of the International Children's Continence Society. Journal of Urology, 2006; 176(1):314-24.

3. Yeung CK, Sihoe JD: Non-neuropathic dysfunction of the lower urinary tract. In Wein AJ, Kavoussi LR, Novick AC, Partin AW, Peters CA (eds): Campbell-Walsh Urology, 9th edition. Philadelphia: Saunders, 2007; pp 3604-55.

4. Sillen U: Bladder function in healthy neonates and its development during infancy. Journal of Urology, 2001; 166:2376-81.

5. Goellner MH, Ziegler EE, Fomon SJ: Urination during the first three years of life. Nephron, 1981; 28:174-8.

6. Hunskaar S, Burgio K, Diokno AC, Herzog AR, Hjalmas K, Lapitan MC: Epidemiology and natural history of urinary incontinence (UI). In Abrams P, Cardozo L, Khoury S, Wein AJ (eds): Incontinence: Second International Consultation on Incontinence, 2nd edition. Plymbridge, UK: World Health Organization, 2002; pp 167-201.

7. Feehan M, McGee R, Stanton W, Silva PA: A 6-year follow-up of childhood enuresis: prevalence in adolescence and consequences for mental health. Journal of Pediatrics and Child Health, 1990; 26:75-9.

8. von Gontard A, Schaumburg H, Hollmann E, Eiberg H, Rittig S: The genetics of enuresis: a review. Journal of Urology, 2001; 166:2438-43.

9. Bakwin H: Enuresis in twins. American Journal of Diseases of Children, 1971; 121(3):222-5.

10. Hublin C, Kaprio J, Partinen M, Koskenvuo M: Nocturnal enuresis in a nationwide twin cohort. Sleep, 1998; 21:579-85.

11. Eiberg H: Nocturnal enuresis is linked to a specific gene. Scandinavian Journal of Urology and Nephrology, 1995; 173(Supplement):15-7.

12. Loeys B, Hoebeke P, Raes A, Messiaen L, De Paepe A, Vande Walle J: Does monosymptomatic enuresis exist? A molecular genetic exploration of 32 families with enuresis/incontinence. BJU International, 2002; 90:76-83.

13. Norgaard JP, Djurhuus JC, Watanabe H, Stenberg A, Lettgen B: Experience and current status of research into the pathophysiology of nocturnal enuresis. British Journal of Urology, 1997; 79:825-35.

14. Yeung CK, Sit FK, To LK, Chiu HN, Sihoe JD, Lee E, Wong C: Reduction in nocturnal functional bladder capacity is a common factor in the pathogenesis of refractory nocturnal enuresis. BJU International, 2002; 90:302-7.

15. Esperanca M, Gerrard JW: Nocturnal enuresis: studies in bladder function in normal children and enuretics. Canadian Medical Association Journal, 1969; 101:324-7.

16. Norgaard JP, Hansen JH, Wildschiodz G, Sorensen S, Rittig S, Djurhuus JC: Sleep cystometrics in children with nocturnal enuresis. Journal of Urology, 1989; 141:1156-9.

17. Rittig S, Frøkiaer J: Basis and therapeutical rationale of the urinary concentrating mechanism. International Journal of Clinical Practice Supplement, 2007; (155):2-7.

18. Chiozza ML, Plebani M, Scaccianoce C, Biraghi M, Zacchello G: Evaluation of antidiuretic hormone before and after long-term treatment with desmopressin in a group of enuretic children. British Journal of Urology, 1998; 81(Supplement 3):53-5.

19. Valenti G, Laera A, Gouraud S, Pace G, Aceto G, Penza R, Selvaggi FP, Svelto M: Low-calcium diet in hypercalciuric enuretic children restores AQP2 excretion and improves clinical symptoms. American Journal of Physiology, 2002; 283:F895-903.

20. Valenti G, Laera A, Pace G, Aceto G, Lospalluti ML, Penza R, Selvaggi FP, Chiozza ML, Svelto M: Urinary aquaporin 2 and calciuria correlate with the severity of enuresis in children. Journal of the American Society of Nephrology, 2000; 11:1873-81.

21. Neveus T, Hansell P, Stenberg A: Vasopressin and hypercalciuria in enuresis: a reappraisal. BJU International, 2002; 90:725-9.

21a. Baeyens D, Roeyers H, Naert S, Hoebeke P, Vande Walle J: The impact of maturation of brainstem inhibition on enuresis: a startle eye blink modification study with 2-year followup. Journal of Urology, 2007; 178(6):2621-5.

22. Page ME, Akaoka H, Aston-Jones G, Valentino RJ: Bladder distension activates noradrenergic locus caeruleus neurones by an excitatory amino acid mechanism. Neuroscience, 1992; 51:555-63.

23. Norgaard JP, Hansen HH, Nielsen JB, Rittig S, Djurhuus JC: Nocturnal studies in enuretics. A polygraphic study of sleep-EEG and bladder activity. Scandinavian Journal of Urology and Nephrology, 1989; (Supplement 125):73-8.

24. Wolfish NM, Pivik RT, Busby KA: Elevated sleep arousal thresholds in enuretic boys: clinical implications. Acta Paediatrica, 1997; 86:381-4.

25. Freitag CM, Rholing D, Seifen S, Pukrop R, vin Gontard A: Neurophysiology of nocturnal enuresis: evoked potentials and repulse inhibition of the startle reflex. Developmental Medicine and Child Neurology, 2006; 48(4):278-84.

26. Sakai J, Frederick H: Secondary enuresis associated with obstructive sleep apnea. Journal of the American Academy of Child and Adolescent Psychiatry, 2000; 39:140-1.

27. Firoozi F, Batniji R, Aslan AR, Longhurst PA, Kogan BA: Resolution of diurnal incontinence and nocturnal enuresis after adenotonsillectomy in children. Journal of Urology, 2006; 175(5):1885-8.

28. Alexopoulos EI, Kostadima E, Pagonari I, Zintzaras E, Gourgoulianis K, Kaditis AG: Association between primary nocturnal enuresis and habitual snoring in children. Urology, 2006; 68(2):406-9.

29. Cinar U, Vural C, Cakir B, Topuz E, Karaman MI, Turgut S: Nocturnal enuresis and upper airway obstruction. International Journal of Pediatric Otorhinolaryngology, 2001; 59:115-8.

30. Skoog SJ: Primary nocturnal enuresis—an analysis of factors related to its etiology. Journal of Urology, 1998; 159:1338-9.

31. Robson WLM, Leung AKC: Re: Editorial: primary nocturnal enuresis—an analysis of factors related to its etiology. Journal of Urology, 1998; 160:1808-9.

32. Wolfish NM: Sleep/arousal and enuresis subtypes. Journal of Urology, 2001; 166:2444-7.

33. Robson WLM, Leung AKC: Secondary nocturnal enuresis. Clinical Pediatrics, 2000; 39:375-89.

34. Cayan S, Doruk E, Bozlu M, Akbay E, Apaydin D, Ulusoy E, Canpolat B: Is routine urinary tract investigation necessary for children with monosymptomatic primary nocturnal enuresis? Urology, 2001; 58:598-602.

35. Robson WL: Enuresis. Advances in Pediatrics, 2001; 48:409-38.

36. Robson LM, Leung AK: Urotherapy recommendations for bedwetting. Journal of the National Medical Association, 2002; 94:577-80.

37. Glazener CMA, Evans JHC: Simple behavioural and physical interventions for nocturnal enuresis in children. Cochrane Database of Systematic Reviews, 2002; (2):CD003637.

38. Gray M: Caffeine and urinary incontinence. Journal of Wound Ostomy and Continence Nursing, 2001; 28:66-9.

39. Klein NJ: Management of primary nocturnal enuresis. Urologic Nursing, 2001; 21:71-6.

40. Harris LS, Purhoit AP: Bladder training and enuresis: a controlled trial. Behavior Research and Therapy, 1977; 15:485-90.

41. Ronen T, Abraham Y: Retention control training in the treatment of younger versus older enuretic children. Nursing Research, 1996; 45:78-82.

42. Glazener CM, Evans JH, Peto RE: Treating nocturnal enuresis in children: review of evidence. Journal of Wound, Ostomy, & Continence Nursing, 2004; 31(4):223-34.

43. Taneli C, Ertan P, Taneli F, Genc A, Gunsar C, Sencan A, Mir E, Onag A: Effect of alarm treatment on bladder storage capacities in monosymptomatic nocturnal enuresis. Scandinavian Journal of Urology and Nephrology, 2004; 38(3):207-10.

44. Van Leerdam FJ, Blankespoor MN, Van Der Heijden AJ, Hirasing RA: Alarm treatment is successful in children with day- and night-time wetting. Scandinavian Journal of Urology and Nephrology, 2004; 38(3):211-5.

45. Butler RJ, Gasson SL: Enuresis alarm treatment. Scandinavian Journal of Urology, 2005; 39:349-57.

46. Naitoh Y, Kawauchi A, Yamao Y, Seki H, Soh J, Yoneda K, Mizutani Y, Miki T: Combination therapy with alarm and drugs for monosymptomatic nocturnal enuresis not superior to alarm monotherapy. Urology, 2005; 66(3):632-5.

47. Norgaard JP, Hashim H, Malmberg L, Robinson D: Antidiuresis therapy: mechanism of action and clinical implications. Neurourology & Urodynamics, 2007; 26(7):1008-13.

48. Unuvar T, Sonmez F: The role of urine osmolality and ions in the pathogenesis of primary enuresis nocturna and in the prediction of responses to desmopressin and conditioning therapies. International Urology and Nephrology, 2005; 37(4):751-7.

49. Karch AM: 2003 Lippincott Nursing Drug Guide. Philadelphia: Lippincott, 2003.

50. Glazener CMA, Evans JHC: Desmopressin for nocturnal enuresis in children. Cochrane Database of Systematic Reviews, 2000; (2):CD002112.

51. von Kerrobroeck PEV: Experience with the long-term use of desmopressin for nocturnal enuresis in children and adolescents. BJU International, 2002; 89:420-5.

52. Veyradier A, Meyer D, Loirat C: Desmopressin, an unexpected link between nocturnal enuresis and inherited thrombotic thrombocytopenic purpura (Upshaw-Schulman syndrome). Journal of Thrombosis and Haemostasis, 2006; 4(3):700-1.

53. Fritz GK, Rockney RM, Yeung AS: Plasma levels and efficacy of imipramine treatment for enuresis. Journal of the American Academy of Child and Adolescent Psychiatry, 1994; 33:60-4.

54. Sohn UD, Kim CY: Suppression of the rat micturition reflex by imipramine. Journal of Autonomic Pharmacology, 1997; 17:35-41.

55. Smellie JM, McGrigor VS, Meadow SR, Rose SJ, Douglas MF: Nocturnal enuresis: a placebo-controlled trial of two antidepressant drugs. Archives of Disease in Childhood, 1996; 75:62-6.

56. Hunsballe JM, Rittig S, Pedersen EB, Olesen OV, Djurhuus JC: Single-dose imipramine reduces nocturnal urine output in patients with nocturnal enuresis and nocturnal polyuria. Journal of Urology, 1997; 158:830-6.

57. Perlmutter AD: Enuresis. In Kelalsi AP, King LR, Belman AB (eds): Clinical Pediatric Urology, 2nd edition. Philadelphia: Saunders, 1985; pp 311-25.

58. Lee T, Suh HJ, Lee HJ, Lee JE: Comparison of effects of treatment of primary nocturnal enuresis with oxybutynin plus desmopressin, desmopressin alone or imipramine alone: a randomized controlled clinical trial. Journal of Urology, 2005; 174(3):1084-7.

59. Glazener CMA, Evans JHC: Drugs for nocturnal enuresis in children (other than desmopressin and tricyclics). Cochrane Database of Systematic Reviews, 2000; (3):CD002238.

60. Neveus T, Johansson E, Nydahl-Persson K, Peterson H, Hansson S: Diuretic treatment of nocturnal enuresis. Scandinavian Journal of Urology and Nephrology, 2005; 39(6):474-8.

CHAPTER

17 *Pediatric Oncology*

·····································

A diagnosis of cancer provokes fear and anxiety in a patient at any age, but this is especially true when the patient is a child. Significant advances in surgery, anesthesia, radiotherapy, and chemotherapy have improved our ability to treat childhood urologic cancers successfully. An increased understanding of the genetics of malignancies, especially Wilms' tumor, has been particularly significant. This chapter provides an overview of three of the most common urologic cancers of childhood—neuroblastoma, rhabdomyosarcoma, and Wilms' tumor.

NEUROBLASTOMA
·····································

Neuroblastomas arise from neural crest tissue that differentiates into the sympathetic nervous system and adrenal medulla. Tumor cells resemble embryonic neural cells (neuroblasts) but they have sparse stroma (connective and supportive cells). Neuroblastomas occur frequently in the mediastinal and retroperitoneal regions, but can be found anywhere along the sympathetic chain, including the neck, thorax, pelvis, and adrenal gland; 75% of neuroblastomas arise in the retroperitoneum, 50% in the adrenals, and 25% in the paravertebral ganglia. Depending on several factors (see later), neuroblastomas may regress spontaneously, evolve into benign neoplasms, or behave as an aggressive malignancy, with local tumor extension and distant metastases.[1]

Epidemiology and Genetics

Neuroblastoma is the most common tumor of infancy, with at least 40% diagnosed in the first year of life. It is the fourth most common malignancy in children.[2] It accounts for 8% to 10% of all childhood cancers. In the United States, the annual incidence is 10.4 cases/1,000,000[3]; in the United Kingdom, 8.6 cases/1,000,000[4]; and in Canada, 8.6 cases/1,000,000.[5] Over 50% of all cases occur in children younger than 2 years of age and 75% are diagnosed by the fourth year of life.

Risk and Protective Factors

Occupational exposures to electromagnetic fields have been examined in relationship to neuroblastoma but no strong evidence exists to support this hypothesis.[6] Paternal exposure to hydrocarbons, lacquer thinner, turpentine, wood dust, and solders also has been associated with a slightly increased risk of having a child with neuroblastoma.[7]

Neuroblastoma may have a familial component because of an autosomal dominant genetic predisposition. The median age at diagnosis of familial neuroblastoma is 9 months as compared with nonfamilial cases, in which it is 21 months. At least 20% of patients with familial neuroblastoma have bilateral adrenal or multifocal primary tumors. The risk for development of neuroblastoma in a sibling or offspring of a patient with neuroblastoma is lower than 6%.[8] Numerous chromosomal markers, also called biologic markers, have been associated with specific tumors that influence a tumor's biologic behavior[9,10] (Box 17-1). Of historical note, neuroblastoma was the first tumor for which treatment was guided not only by stage and histology of the tumor but also by its biologic markers.[1]

A retrospective study from Canada has provided evidence that fortification of cereals with folic acid reduces neuroblastoma risk.[11] Case-control studies have shown that breast-feeding also may be protective.[12,13]

Etiology and Pathophysiology

As noted, neuroblastomas vary significantly with respect to their propensity for local invasion and distant metastasis. The International Staging System for Neuroblastoma is presented in Table 17-1.[14]

Survival is excellent for patients with stage 1 tumors who undergo complete resection of the primary tumor (up to 100%); most stage 2 patients also have a good prognosis, even if there is incomplete excision of the tumor. Stages 0, 1, and 2 tumors found on screening that are smaller than 5 cm and do not involve major organs or vessels may regress spontaneously.[15] Stage 4S ("S" for special) is a distinct category referring to infants with small primary tumors along with liver, skin, and bone marrow

TABLE 17-1 International Neuroblastoma Staging System

· ·

STAGE	DEFINITION
0	In situ tumor (usually incidental finding on ultrasonography)
1	Tumor confined to adrenal organ or structure of origin
2A	Local tumor extends beyond organ or structure of origin; no spread to local lymph nodes
2B	Local tumor extends beyond organ or structure of origin; ipsilateral lymph nodes are positive for tumor but nonadherent
3	Tumor extends beyond midline*; regional lymph nodes may or may not be involved
4	Distant metastasis involves lymph nodes, bone, bone marrow, liver, skin, and/or other organs
4S	Localized primary tumor (as defined for stage 1, 2A, or 2B), with dissemination limited to skin, liver, and/or bone marrow (less than 10% tumor) in infants younger than 1 yr

*The midline is defined as the vertebral column. Tumors originating on one side and crossing the midline must infiltrate to or beyond the opposite side of the vertebral column.

metastases, but without bony metastases. Stage 4S is associated with a survival rate between 72% and 90% and many of these tumors regress spontaneously.[1] In contrast, the prognosis for children with an advanced stage 3 or 4 tumor is poor. Only 20% to 30% remain disease-free after 2 years, despite aggressive treatment.[16,17]

In addition to stage and grade of disease at diagnosis, prognosis is affected by multiple factors, including age, site of origin, and presence of molecular markers. Children diagnosed at age 1 year or younger have an improved survival rate compared with older children. In addition, those with thoracic and nonadrenal tumors have a better survival rate than children with tumors arising from the genitourinary tract or other sites. Approximately 30% of neuroblastomas are characterized by amplification of the *N-myc* oncogene status.[18] Its presence is strongly correlated with a greater likelihood of an advanced tumor at the time of diagnosis and poorer overall prognosis, irrespective of age or stage. Another molecular marker, MRP glycoprotein, is frequently detectable in advanced-stage neuroblastomas, and its presence is associated with increased resistance to chemotherapy.

In contrast to the expression of *N-myc* oncogene and MRP glycoprotein, the presence of CD44 glycoprotein is associated with a lower risk of local invasion or metastasis and improved long-term survival. CD44 and *N-myc* oncogene are inversely correlated in specific tumors. Another molecular marker, Trk (tyrosine kinase), is also associated with a more favorable prognosis.[18]

Assessment

Clinical Presentation. Neuroblastoma may be detected as a hard palpable mass by a parent during routine child care, such as bathing. In other cases, it is found during physical examination or as an incidental finding of an imaging study. Periorbital ecchymosis (raccoon eyes) occurs in selected cases. Some children complain of abdominal pain; those with metastatic disease may report bone or joint pain and refuse to walk because of pain. Tumor compression of the bowel and bladder can produce urinary retention and constipation. Thoracic lesions may cause cough or dyspnea, whereas direct extension of the tumor into the spinal canal may cause back pain and impaired

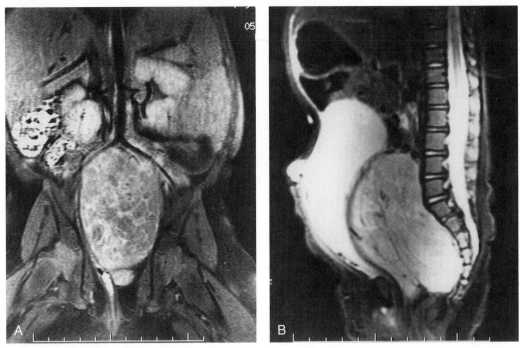

Fig. 17-1 Magnetic resonance imaging (MRI) of pelvic neuroblastoma showing (**A**) bifurcation of the aorta and the iliac vessels and relationship to the mass and (**B**) compression of the bowel and bladder. (From Wein AJ, Kavoussi LR, Novick AC, Partin AW, Peters CA [eds]: Campbell-Walsh Urology, 9th edition. Philadelphia: Saunders, 2007; pp 3872, 3873.)

voiding and bowel function. Spinal cord compression caused by tumor spread through the paravertebral ganglia occurs frequently, sometimes leading to paraplegia or quadriplegia (Figure 17-1).[19]

Metastases are often present at diagnosis and may present as a unique syndrome related to the hormonal and biochemical products produced by a neuroblastoma. For example, catecholamine release can cause symptoms that are similar to those of pheochromocytoma, including paroxysmal hypertension, palpitations, flushing, and headache. Tumors that secrete vasoactive intestinal peptide (VIP) may produce intractable watery diarrhea and hypokalemia.[20] Others can produce sudden jerky movements of the legs and feet (myoclonus), rapid multidirectional eye movements (opsoclonus), and ataxia caused by acute myoclonic encephalopathy. Myoclonic encephalopathy is postulated to occur because of the interaction between antibodies produced against the neuroblastoma and normal neural tissues.[1]

Screening. The urine may be screened for elevated levels of two catecholamines, homovanillic acid and vanillylmandelic acid.[10] Although screening has diagnosed low-stage tumors that spontaneously regress,[14] it has not significantly diminished the prevalence of advanced-stage disease.[21] A German study has concluded that screening at 1 year of age is not an effective preventive measure; earlier detection was not found to change the final outcome.[22]

Diagnosis

Laboratory Evaluation. Increased levels of metabolites secreted by the adrenals, including catecholamines vanillylmandelic acid and homovanillic acid, are found in 24-hour urine specimens in most children with neuroblastoma.[19] Twenty-four hour urine testing may be used to confirm a diagnosis of neuroblastoma or detect tumor relapse. A complete blood count may reveal anemia when the bone marrow is involved. Two bone marrow aspirates and two biopsies are typically obtained, although neuroblastoma-specific immunocytology of marrow aspirates will obviate the need for marrow biopsies in most patients.[1]

Ongoing research has identified several potential serum markers for neuroblastoma, including BIRC, a marker of cellular apoptosis; CDKN2D, indicating alterations in cell cycle physiology; and SMARCD3, which is released with DNA or RNA transcription.[13] Their role in the clinical evaluation and management of neuroblastoma continues to evolve.

Imaging Studies. Plain radiographs may demonstrate a calcified abdominal or posterior mediastinal mass. Skeletal survey or radionuclide bone scan will detect cortical bone metastases. Radionuclide scans of the bones using technetium 99m or radiolabeled iodine 131 *m*-iodobenzylguanidine (MIBG) are obtained when feasible. MIBG is specific in the diagnosis of neuroblastoma because the labeled material is taken up by the tumor cells.[20] Abdominal disease and liver metastasis are assessed by ultrasound, computed tomography (CT), or magnetic resonance imaging (MRI). MRI is particularly helpful in the diagnosis of intraspinal tumor extension.[1] In addition to its therapeutic value when the tumor is excised, surgery is used to confirm the diagnosis, stage, and grade of a neuroblastoma.[20]

Treatment

The treatment of neuroblastoma may include surgery, chemotherapy, radiation therapy, and bone marrow transplantation. Treatment choice depends on tumor stage, age, and biologic prognostic factors. The urologic nurse should inform the patient and the family of the purpose, therapeutic effects, and potential adverse side effects of each therapeutic option.

Stages 1, 2, 4S: Low-Risk Disease. The primary treatment of stages 1, 2A, and 2B tumors is complete surgical resection.[23] Surgery alone is used to treat infants and children with stage 1 neuroblastomas; chemotherapy is administered only if the tumor recurs or if further analysis reveals *N-myc* amplification and an unfavorable histology. Infants and children with stage 2A disease and infants with stage 2B disease are managed by surgical resection and postoperative chemotherapy.

In contrast, surgical resection has not shown significant benefit in children with stage 4S tumors.[18] Fortunately, these tumors tend to evolve into benign neoplasms or spontaneously regress without specific treatment.

Stages 3 and 4: High-Risk Disease. Chemotherapy is first-line treatment for high-risk disease.[1,18] Commonly used agents include cyclophosphamide, ifosfamide, vincristine, doxorubicin, cisplatin, carboplatin, etoposide, and melphalan. Preoperative chemotherapy is administered to shrink and consolidate the primary tumor and reduce lymph node metastases. Surgery is usually performed 13 to 18 weeks after chemotherapy is commenced; the delay is advocated because it allows the tumor time to shrink following chemotherapy, thus limiting the risk of operative complications. Nevertheless, even though preoperative chemotherapy has been found to reduce the overall risk for surgical complications, surgery is associated with significant adverse effects including tumor rupture, hemorrhage, injury to renal vessels, and neurologic deficits.[20] In addition, significant and persistent diarrhea often occurs after resection of tumors surrounding the celiac axis and superior mesenteric artery, possibly because of resection of the autonomic nerves.[1] Intraoperative radiation therapy has been attempted to spare normal adjacent tissues[24] but the results have been equivocal.[25]

Toxic side effects of chemotherapy agents used to treat neuroblastoma include radiation sensitivity (doxorubicin, thiotepa), nephrotoxicity (platinum compounds, ifosfamide), and cardiotoxicity (doxorubicin, cyclophosphamide).[25] The toxic effects and myelosuppression limit the amount of chemotherapy that can be given. An alternative for some children is autologous bone marrow transplantation. A remission rate as high as 50% has been reported in children with stage 4 disease who receive autologous bone marrow transplantation following chemotherapy or total-body irradiation.[1]

Hematologic side effects, sometimes severe, are increasingly being managed with transfusion of peripheral blood with stem and progenitor cells. Treatment has resulted in diminished infection risk, reduced need for transfusion of whole blood or platelets, and reduction in overall mortality. Because of these advances, the Neuroblastoma Committee of the U.S. Children's Oncology Group has released a position statement recommending collection of peripheral blood stem cells at the time of treatment initiation.[26]

Radiation therapy. Although neuroblastoma is a radiosensitive tumor, radiotherapy is generally avoided in stage 1 and 2 tumors because of limited benefit as well as a significant incidence of adverse side effects.[26] However, radiotherapy has been shown to diminish local tumor recurrence in higher grade tumors. It is useful when a stage 4S tumor produces hepatomegaly and respiratory distress. Radiation has also been used for palliation and pain control in terminal stages of illness, particularly when spinal cord compression occurs.[20]

As with all treatment options for childhood urologic malignancies, radiotherapy is associated with significant adverse side effects.[20] Younger children may require a short-duration general anesthetic to allow safe focused administration of radiation. Gastrointestinal irritation; organ damage, especially to the bladder, kidneys, and liver; and myelosuppression may occur, resulting in radiation proctitis, hemorrhagic cystitis, and mucositis. Growth arrest, vertebral damage, and scoliosis may occur, particularly when treating spinal cord involvement or compression.[20] Late side effects include neurodevelopmental delay, deterioration of vital organs, and secondary malignancies.[25] Newer techniques of delivering radiation therapy, including highly focused low-dose protocols[25] and proton beam therapy,[27] may reduce the risk for adverse side effects.

Neuroblastoma and Renal Cell Carcinoma. Survivors of abdominal neuroblastoma are at risk for long-term renal complications, particularly renal cell carcinoma.[28] Parents should be advised of this increased risk and of the importance of long-term surveillance.

GENITOURINARY RHABDOMYOSARCOMA

Rhabdomyosarcoma (Greek, *rhabdos*, rod; *myo*, muscle; *sarcoma*, connective tissue neoplasm) is a malignant neoplasm that arises from skeletal (striated) muscle.[29] The resulting tumors appear in diverse locations throughout the body and exhibit considerable histologic diversity. Rhabdomyosarcomas are typically divided into two major subtypes, embryonal and alveolar, although some tumors contain elements of both and tend to behave more like alveolar malignancies. Alveolar rhabdomyosarcomas are composed of loose aggregates of small round cells; they are clinically more aggressive than

embryonal tumors. Embryonal rhabdomyosarcomas are more well-differentiated (similar to mature muscle cells) than other major histologic variants; they resemble the developing muscle cells seen in a 6- to 8-week-old developing fetus. Less common histologic variants include botryoid tumors that arise as grapelike lesions in the mucosa of the vagina and urinary bladder and pleomorphic tumors that arise from muscle cells in the extremities of adults.

Rhabdomyosarcoma is the most common soft tissue sarcoma in infants and children; it accounts for 2% to 8% of all childhood and adolescent malignancies.[30,31] Of these, 15% to 20% of cases arise from the genitourinary system.[32] The most common genitourinary sites are prostate, bladder, and paratesticular structures (Figure 17-2). In contrast, tumors arising from the vagina and uterus are uncommon.[1] Advances in assessment and treatment have increased the overall 5-year survival rate from approximately 60% to almost 80%.[33,34]

Epidemiology

Of all rhabdomyosarcomas, 85% occur in children younger than 18 years. The annual incidence of rhabdomyosarcoma in the United States is 4.5/1,000,000 white children and 1.3/1,000,000 African American children.[29] Canada's annual incidence is 4.3/1,000,000;[5] the United Kingdom's is 5.3/1,000,000.[35] The incidence of rhabdomyosarcoma is somewhat lower in Asian children, affecting 4.0/1,000,000 children 0 to 14 years.[36] Boys are

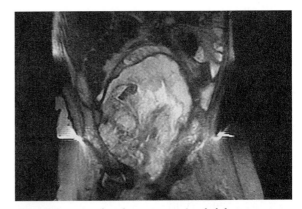

Fig. 17-2 MRI of a large prostatic rhabdomyosarcoma showing extension into the abdomen. (From Wein AJ, Kavoussi LR, Novick AC, Partin AW, Peters CA [eds]: Campbell-Walsh Urology, 9th edition. Philadelphia: Saunders, 2007; p. 3881.)

approximately 1.5 times more likely to develop rhabdomyosarcoma than girls. Its peak incidence is during the first 10 years of life and again at adolescence.[37,38]

Risk Factors

Most rhabdomyosarcoma occurs without any obvious risk factors. Known risk factors include children with neurofibromatosis, Beckwith-Wiedemann syndrome (BWS), or Li-Fraumeni syndrome, a genetic predisposition to the development of cancer.[39] A mutation of the *p53* tumor suppressor gene has been found in the tumors of all patients with Li-Fraumeni syndrome.[40] Tenuous evidence supports a possible association with types II and IIa spinal muscular atrophy.[41]

Etiology and Pathophysiology

Embryonal rhabdomyosarcomas arise from the genitourinary system and account for most paratesticular tumors.[30] They account for 60% to 70% of all rhabdomyosarcomas affecting children. Although the precise cause of embryonal rhabdomyosarcoma is unknown, a loss of genomic material on the short arm of chromosome 11p15 is common. Alveolar rhabdomyosarcoma is found in the trunk, extremity, perineal, or perianal region. Alveolar and embryonic rhabdomyosarcoma are associated with a translocation between chromosomes 1 or 2 and chromosome 13, forming a chimeric protein. Botryoid cell tumors represent a variant of embryonal rhabdomyosarcoma. They account for 10% of cases and typically arise from the genitourinary tract. Tumors of the bladder usually occur as a botryoid form, characterized by multiple protuberances similar to a bunch of grapes, and grow intraluminally at or near the trigone.[42,43]

Stage, Grade, and Clinical Grouping

The current stage and grade system from the International Rhabdomyosarcoma Study Group is summarized in Table 17-2. It is based on clinical findings, laboratory tests, and imaging studies.[1,44] Rhabdomyosarcomas arise from striated muscle cells, so their location varies widely. Therefore, they are also classified according to clinical groups, based on tumor location and origin. The four major clinical sites for rhabdomyosarcomas are (1) head and neck (especially periorbital), 35% to 40%, (2) genitourinary tract, 20%, (3) extremities, 15% to 20%, and (4) trunk, 10% to 15%.[45]

Assessment and Clinical Presentation

Proper assessment for determining the extent of disease includes chest x-ray, CT, and MRI of the primary site and regional lymph nodes, a bone scan, and bone marrow aspiration and/or biopsy.

Bladder or Prostate Tumors. Clinical manifestations of rhabdomyosarcoma arising from the bladder or prostate usually reflect ureteral or urethral obstruction. Specific signs and symptoms include urinary frequency, straining to void, acute urinary retention, and hematuria. On physical examination, an abdominal mass from the tumor or a distended bladder can be seen or palpated.[1]

Paratesticular Tumors. Paratesticular rhabdomyosarcoma is typically detected earlier than rhabdomyosarcoma at other genitourinary sites. They often present as a unilateral, painless, scrotal swelling or mass above the testis. On physical examination, a firm mass is palpated that is distinct from the testis. Ultrasound may be completed to confirm the solid nature of the lesion.

Vagina, Vulvar, and Uterine Tumors. Vaginal and vulvar rhabdomyosarcoma usually presents with

TABLE 17-2 Stage and Grade of Rhabdomyosarcoma[44]

STAGE OR GRADE	DESCRIPTION
Stage I	Favorable site, absence of nodal or distant metastases
Stage II	Unfavorable site, absence of nodal or distant metastases
Stage III	Unfavorable site, enlarged or positive nodes, absence of distant metastases
Stage IV	Any site, metastatic
Tumor	T_{site} 1—confined to site of origin
	T_{site} 2—fixation to surrounding tissues
	Size: ≤5 cm or ≥5 cm
Histology	G_1—favorable histology (embryonal, botryoid, spindle cell)
	G_2—unfavorable histology (alveolar, undifferentiated)
Regional lymph nodes	N_0—regional lymph nodes not clinically involved
	N_1—regional lymph nodes clinically involved
Metastases	M_0—no distant metastases
	M_1 site—metastases present

vaginal bleeding or discharge. A palpable mass may prolapse from the vagina. Uterine rhabdomyosarcoma may manifest in two ways, as a tumor originating from the cervix, with vaginal bleeding or mass, or as a tumor originating in the uterine body, with an abdominal mass.

Diagnosis

The diagnosis of rhabdomyosarcoma is based on the tumor site and histopathology. Standard histology plus electron microscopy, FDG-PET cytogenetics, immunohistochemistry, and DNA flow cytometry may all be necessary to confirm a diagnosis of rhabdomyosarcoma. In addition to initial biopsy, clinical staging; imaging studies with CT, MRI, FDG-PET, and ultrasound; and bone marrow examination are performed. [46] CT can delineate the extent of the tumor and evaluate pelvic and retroperitoneal nodes, especially in paratesticular tumors.

Bladder, Prostate, Vaginal, Vulvar, and Uterine Tumors. Imaging studies of the lower urinary tract may demonstrate a filling defect within the bladder or elevation of the bladder base. Cystoscopy may be completed to allow direct visualization of the tumor and assess bladder invasion, and transurethral biopsy specimens can be obtained. Vaginoscopy is performed when a vaginal tumor is suspected. Paratesticular tumors are usually evaluated by abdominopelvic CT to assess for retroperitoneal lymph node involvement. Diagnosis of a uterine tumor requires incisional or excisional biopsy, usually obtained during dilation and curettage and transvaginal biopsy.

Treatment

Treatment of the child with a genitourinary rhabdomyosarcoma focuses on eradicating the existing tumor, preventing local invasion or distant metastases, and preserving lower urinary tract function.[1] Therapy usually includes a combination of surgery, chemotherapy, and radiation. Chemotherapy often involves multiple agents, and children with higher grade tumors may be treated with a five-agent regimen that includes vincristine, doxorubicin, cyclophosphamide, ifosfamide, and etoposide.[47]

Bladder and Prostate Tumors. Partial resection of the bladder wall for primary tumors affecting the dome or sides of the bladder distant from the trigone is recommended as initial therapy or as a delayed procedure after chemotherapy. Residual disease and relapse are of concern after partial cystectomy, although the estimated 3-year survival rate of 79% is similar to that noted for all patients with primary bladder tumors. For patients with more extensive disease of the bladder or prostate, chemotherapy and radiotherapy are administered to shrink the tumor, followed by radical cystectomy or anterior pelvic exenteration, with preservation of the rectum.[6,38]

Paratesticular Tumors. Lesions involving the testis or spermatic cord are removed by radical inguinal orchiectomy, which includes resection of the entire spermatic cord.[48] Because of the high incidence of lymphatic spread, it is recommended that all patients have an abdominopelvic CT scan to evaluate lymph nodes. Even if no evidence of nodal involvement is detected on initial evaluation, the CT scan is repeated every 3 months. Unilateral retropubic lymph node dissection (RPLND) may be completed to stage the tumor, but a bilateral RPLND is associated with significant morbidity, such as intestinal obstruction, ejaculatory dysfunction, and edema of the lower extremities, and is not routinely done. Laparoscopic lymph node dissection may offer a less morbid alternative to RPLND.

Vaginal, Vulvar, and Uterine Tumors. Chemotherapy is the initial approach, with subsequent transvaginal biopsies to assess the response to treatment. Surgery with anterior pelvic exenteration is rarely necessary with effective chemotherapy and radiotherapy. If there is persistence of disease, delayed tumor resection is performed. This may consist of partial vaginectomy or vaginectomy with hysterectomy.[1]

WILMS' TUMOR

Wilms' tumor (nephroblastoma) is an embryonal neoplasm that arises from remnants of an immature kidney.[1] It is the most common renal tumor of childhood and represents 6% of all childhood cancers. The excellent outcome now expected for most children with this tumor is attributed to the combination of effective adjuvant chemotherapy, improved surgical and anesthetic techniques, and radiosensitivity of the tumor.[1]

Epidemiology

The annual incidence of Wilms' tumor in children younger than 15 years is about 7 to 10 cases/1,000,000 in the United States and 6.1 cases/1,000,000 in Canada.[5] More than 80% are identified before 5 years of age. The incidence appears lower in east Asian populations and higher in black populations.[49]

Risk Factors

Several studies have investigated potential occupation-, environment-, and lifestyle-related risk factors for Wilms' tumor, but few have been identified. A number of genitourinary anomalies, including hypospadias, cryptorchidism, renal fusion anomalies, male pseudohermaphroditism, and horseshoe kidney, are associated with an increased risk for Wilms' tumor.[50] In contrast to neuroblastoma, heredity plays only a minimal role, accounting for 1% to 2% of all cases.[51]

Etiology and Pathophysiology

Etiology. An autosomal dominant gene has been implicated in a few cases of Wilms' tumor. It has also been associated with some congenital anomalies and several chromosomal abnormalities (Box 17-2). These may increase the risk for a Wilms' tumor by interrupting tumor suppression mechanisms noted in unaffected individuals.[52] A comprehensive summary of the chromosomal abnormalities and present state of the science has been presented by Dome and colleagues.[52]

Pathology. Macroscopically, most Wilms' tumors are solitary lesions arising from the periphery of the renal cortex (Figure 17-3); some are multifocal, and approximately 7% will involve both kidneys.[52] The tumor may spread to the renal vein and can extend up the vena cava to the right atrium.[50] Microscopically, Wilms' tumor has a distinct cellular diversity compared with neuroblastoma; it has

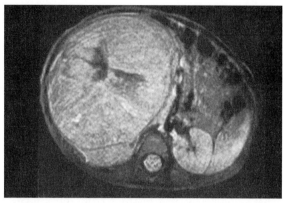

Fig. 17-3 MRI image of Wilms' tumor that was pretreated with chemotherapy. (From Wein AJ, Kavoussi LR, Novick AC, Partin AW, Peters CA [eds]: Campbell-Walsh Urology, 9th edition. Philadelphia: Saunders, 2007; p 3895.)

BOX 17-2 Genetic Factors Associated with Wilms' Tumor[1,4,49,54]

The following rare events are associated with Wilms' tumor (WT):
- Aniridia—incomplete formation of the iris of the eye
- WAGR syndrome (**W**ilms' tumor, **a**niridia, **g**enitourinary tract abnormalities, mental **r**etardation)
- Beckwith-Wiedemann syndrome (BWS)—congenital disorder characterized by larger than normal internal organs and hypoglycemia at birth
- Hemihypertrophy—one side of the body grows faster than the other
- Enys-Drash syndrome—characterized by abnormal renal function and pseudohermaphroditism
- Nephroblastomatosis—presence of small pockets of embryonal renal tissue under the capsule of the kidney; high risk of developing tumor

Chromosomal abnormalities associated with Wilms' tumor:
- Short arm chromosome 11 (band 11p13), which harbors the Wilms' tumor suppressor gene *WT1*
- Chromosome 11p15, which includes the suspected Wilms' tumor gene *WT2*
- Chromosome 16q
- Chromosome 1p
- Chromosome 7p
- P53 at chromosome 17p
- Nephrogenic rests—embryonic precursor cells with two subtypes, perilobar and intralobar; nephrogenic rests, dysplastic lesions of metanephric origin, now believed to represent precursor lesions

TABLE 17-3 Staging of Wilms' Tumor[4]

STAGE	PATIENTS AFFECTED (%)	DESCRIPTION
1	43	Tumor limited to kidney and completely removed; surface of renal capsule intact; no rupture before or during removal; no apparent residual tumor beyond margins
2	23	Tumor extends beyond kidney but completely removed; regional extension tumor (penetrates renal capsule); vessels outside kidney infiltrated or contain tumor thrombus; tumor may have been biopsied, or spillage of tumor confined to flank; no residual tumor beyond margins of excision
3	23	Residual nonhematogenous tumor confined to abdomen; occurrence of any the following—lymph node involvement in hilus, periaortic chains, or beyond; diffuse peritoneal spillage; implants onto peritoneal surface; extension beyond surgical margins grossly or microscopically; local infiltration into vital structures
4	10	Hematogenous metastases (lung, liver, bone, brain)
5	5	Bilateral renal tumors

been categorized by favorable and unfavorable histologic groups, which are used as guides for prognosis.[50,53] Favorable histology mimics normal kidney development and consists of three cell types—undifferentiated blastoid cells, differentiated epithelial tissue, and stroma (connective tissue). This is the "classic" Wilms' tumor. Unfavorable histology is characterized by anaplasia, a loss of cellular structure differentiation; tumors with unfavorable histology are typically more resistant to chemotherapy than those with favorable histology.

Stage and Grade

Staging of a Wilms' tumor is based on surgical findings, pathology, and the presence or absence of distant metastases. Staging allows treatment results to be evaluated and enables comparison of outcomes with other international and national groups. The staging system for Wilms' tumor, used by the National Wilms' Tumor Staging Group (Table 17-3),[1] is based primarily on surgical and histopathologic findings.

Assessment

Clinical Presentation. Most children will present with an asymptomatic abdominal or flank mass detected by a parent when dressing or bathing the child or by a healthcare professional during physical examination.[50] Other clinical manifestations may include hematuria, dysuria, hypertension caused by increased plasma renin levels, abdominal pain, fever,

anemia, and malaise.[54] Wilms' tumors may metastasize to the lungs, contralateral kidney, liver, bones, or brain. Lymphatic spread is a sign of advanced disease.[2,22] In rare cases, compression or invasion of the renal vein and inferior vena cava causes a varicocele, hepatomegaly (caused by hepatic vein obstruction), ascites, and congestive heart failure.[1]

Screening. Ultrasound is recommended for children known to be at increased risk for Wilms' tumor, including those with congenital anomalies associated with aniridia, hemihypertrophy, nephroblastomatosis, and BWS. Most researchers suggest that 3 to 4 months is the appropriate screening interval for children up to 10 years old. General screening is not recommended because of the low incidence of the disease.

Diagnosis

Laboratory Evaluation. Laboratory evaluation should include a complete peripheral blood count, platelet count, renal function tests, liver function tests, serum calcium level determination, and urinalysis. Bone marrow biopsy and aspiration complete the initial assessment. Table 17-4 summarizes the evaluation of the child for Wilms' tumor.[52]

Imaging Studies. Ultrasound of the abdominal mass and both kidneys is the first study performed and demonstrates the solid or cystic nature of the lesion, as well as its size and origin. Ultrasound will also allow examination of the inferior vena cava to exclude intracaval tumor extension. CT and MRI

TABLE 17-4 Assessment of Child for Wilms' Tumor

	ASSESSMENT PARAMETERS	TYPICAL ABNORMAL FINDINGS

History	A. Personal, family, and social history
	  1. Age of child
	  2. Employment of parent
	  3. Perinatal history
		A. Personal and social risk factors
		  1. Younger than 5 years
		  2. Often in a metal industry
		  3. Medications taken by mother during pregnancy, patient's birth weight abnormal, patient has recent weight loss

	B. Evaluation of genitourinary status	B. Recent trauma or infection, abdominal pain
Physical examination	A. Abdominal inspection and gentle examination by palpation	A. Large, movable abdominal mass; hepatomegaly
	B. Examination of child for associated physical features	B. Presence of aniridia, hemihypertrophy, or characteristic congenital syndromes associated with Wilms' tumor

Diagnostic tests	A. Laboratory assessment
	  1. Complete blood count
		A. Laboratory results
		  1. Anemia secondary to hemorrhage into tumor

	2. Urinalysis	2. Hematuria present in 20% of cases
	3. Serum chemistry profile, including SGOT, SGPT, BUN, creatinine levels	3. Elevated in the presence of extensive disease or hepatic metastasis
	B. Abdominal ultrasound	B. Initially, localized renal tumor; provides dimensions of tumor and information on the integrity of the contralateral kidney and the liver
	C. Abdominal CT or MRI	C. Improved localization of intraabdominal tumors; detects bilateral tumors and presence of tumor in the inferior vena cava
	D. Chest CT scan to assess pulmonary metastatic disease	D. Presence of metastatic tumor nodules in the lungs
	E. Chromosome analysis	E. Rare abnormalities of 11p13 or 11p15.5
	F. Echocardiography	F. Presence of tumor in right atrium from vena caval extension or prechemotherapy with doxorubicin
	G. Bone marrow biopsy	G. Anemia

BUN, Blood urea nitrogen; *CT,* computed tomography; *MRI,* magnetic resonance imaging; *SGOT,* serum glutamic oxalo-acetic transaminase; *SGPT,* serum glutamate pyruvate transaminase.
From Crom DB, Bredereck Boggs TB, Mandrell BN, Norville R: Pediatric cancers. In Miaskowski C, Buchel P (eds): Oncology Nursing: Assessment and Clinical Care. St Louis: Mosby, 1999; p 1557.

studies can further define the extent of the lesion and can identify small lesions in the opposite kidney that may be nephrogenic rests or Wilms' tumor. Regional adenopathy and extrarenal tumor extension into the perirenal fat or adjacent structures can be identified by CT or MRI.[1,50]

Plain chest x-rays or CT of the chest is indicated initially because the lung is the most common site of distant metastasis in children with Wilms' tumor. Skeletal surveys and bone scans are both recommended after the histologic diagnosis has been confirmed.

Treatment

The overall cure rate for children with Wilms' tumor is 85% using combination therapy with surgery, chemotherapy, and, for some cases, radiotherapy. However, emotional health in adult survivors appears lower than that in population norms and should be considered in long-term follow-up.[55]

Surgery. Initial therapy for most children with Wilms' tumor is radical nephrectomy via a transabdominal approach. Exploration of the contralateral kidney and abdominal cavity is done to exclude local tumor extension, liver and nodal metastases, and peritoneal seeding. Gerota's fascia is opened and the kidney is palpated and visually inspected thoroughly for evidence of a tumor or nephrogenic rests. The renal vein and inferior vena cava are palpated to exclude intravascular tumor extension. Selective sampling of suspicious nodes is done, although RPLND is not routine because of its associated complications.[50] Gentle handling throughout the procedure is mandatory to avoid tumor spillage because of the high risk of tumor growth from abdominal seeding.[56] Complications of surgery that the urology nurse must be particularly alert for include hemorrhage and small bowel obstruction.

Partial nephrectomy may be done for selected patients with renal insufficiency, a solitary kidney, or other congenital risk factors (see Box 17-2).[57] Children with bilateral Wilms' tumors are initially treated with 6 to 8 weeks of chemotherapy, followed by radionuclide studies of the kidneys to determine the feasibility of a nephron-sparing (partial) nephrectomy of one or both kidneys.[18]

Chemotherapy. Chemotherapy may be administered prior to and following surgical resection.[18] For children with early-stage disease, dactinomycin, vincristine, and doxorubicin are the agents of choice. Cyclophosphamide or several other agents may be added when managing children with higher stage tumors. Because of the rarity of the disease, an international collaborative Wilms' tumor group has defined protocols and enters every child diagnosed into the database.[57] The urologic nurse will provide parents with information about this tumor group and help clarify its important role for understanding the disease and its treatment.

Radiation. Two studies completed by the National Wilms' Tumor Study Group have demonstrated no benefit when radiotherapy is combined with chemotherapy in children with stage 1 or 2 tumors. In contrast, external beam radiation therapy has proved beneficial for children with pulmonary metastases. Preoperative irradiation combined with vincristine may be given to achieve sufficient tumor shrinkage to allow nephrectomy. Postoperative radiation therapy also may be administered to stage 3, 4, or 5 patients who did not receive it preoperatively.[50]

Late Effects of Treatment. After treatment for Wilms' tumor, numerous organ systems are subject to the late sequelae of anticancer therapy, particularly radiotherapy. Urologic nurses must be aware of the potential problems that these children and their parents may face as they grow into adulthood. Radiation places children and adolescents at risk of musculoskeletal problems (e.g., scoliosis and soft tissue),[58] hypogonadism and temporary azoospermia in boys,[59] ovarian failure, and risk of adverse pregnancy outcomes.[60] Moreover, an increased incidence of secondary malignant neoplasms, especially in children who have undergone radiotherapy, has been observed.[61] Finally, there is a risk of congestive heart failure in children who have been treated with anthracyclines such as daunomycin.[62] In addition to acute cardiotoxicity of anthracyclines, cardiac failure may develop many years after treatment.[63] Similar findings have been noted in long-term follow-up of children with treated rhabdomyosarcoma. Approximately 30% will experience progression or relapse; secondary neoplasms may be related to high doses of chemotherapy or radiotherapy.[64] The Intergroup Rhabdomyosarcoma Study Group suggests that relapse is dependent on various factors—histologic subtype of rhabdomyosarcoma, disease group, and stage at diagnosis.[65] The initial treatment of childhood genitourinary cancer therefore has a significant impact on long-term health outcomes.

SUMMARY

The urologic nurse plays a major role in supporting the family, caring for the child with urologic cancer, acting as a liaison between the medical staff and other healthcare professionals, and ensuring that families and children understand the imaging techniques, laboratory studies, and surgical interventions. Nursing management includes the following: assessment of coping skills, anxiety, and self-esteem; establishing realistic goals for families and children; and setting interventions based on individual needs and developmental level of the child (see box, Clinical Highlights for Advanced and Expert Practice: Nursing Management of the Child With a Urologic Malignancy).[66] Specific teaching about the risk of infection, necessity of transfusions, nutrition, and pain control is part of the nurse's role (Table 17-5).

The urologic nurse is key in assessing needs of the family and child in regard to learning about the specific disease and its evaluation and treatment, as well as helping families and children prepare for late physical and psychosocial effects of therapy once the

Clinical Highlights for Advanced and Expert Practice: Nursing Management of the Child with a Urologic Malignancy [31]

· ·

Outcome Goals

The patient and family will be able to:

- Ask for assistance.
- Participate in decision making with regard to health care, activities of daily living, and family interaction.
- Identify, cultivate, and use available resources.
- Openly communicate feelings related to disease, treatment, and prognosis.
- Identify alternative resources when present coping strategies do not provide support.

Interventions

- Recognize individual needs and developmental level of child:
  - Infant—dependent on parents' presence and support
  - Toddler—separation from parent is major issue; fear of bodily injury and pain; loss of control related to loss of routine, physical restriction, and dependency; benefits from play therapy
  - Preschooler—parents' presence of primary importance; fear of mutilation related to surgery or injections; hospital viewed as punishment or rejection, treatment seen as punishment or hostile; benefits from play therapy
  - School-age child—concerned with lack of body control and mastery; anxiety handled through knowledge
  - Adolescent—focus is on peers and separation from them and family; hospital, treatment a threat to independence; anxiety handled through knowledge and participating in decision making
- Determine patient's and family's learning needs and knowledge levels pertaining to specific disease process, treatment modalities, and diagnostic testing.
- Assess patient's and family's views and beliefs about cancer.
- Observe patient's and family's coping mechanisms.
- Assess cultural background and belief systems.
- Assess readiness of patient and family to learn.
- Determine what patient and family believe is important for them to know.
- Provide and discuss information related to specific type of cancer, diagnostic testing, and treatment.
- Teach about emotional reactions to cancer and possible developmental regression.
- Initiate referrals to other health team members—child life therapy, physical therapy, dietitian, and social services.
- Promote normalcy through attending in-hospital classroom, maintaining schoolwork, and providing opportunities for play and recreation.
- Foster maintenance of peer relationships and reentry into the community through school reentry intervention and continued contact although hospitalized or at home.

Patient Teaching Priorities

Pediatric Cancers

Assess patient's and family's learning needs for:

- Specific disease process (e.g., Wilms' tumor, rhabdomyosarcoma, neuroblastoma)
- Specific diagnostic testing (e.g., arteriography, bone marrow biopsy, MRI)
- Specific treatment modalities (e.g., chemotherapy, radiation therapy, surgery)

Assess and monitor developmental and psychosocial responses to cancer.

Initiate referrals to multidisciplinary healthcare team—physical therapist, dietitian, social services, occupational therapist, rehabilitation services, and school system.

child is considered cured. The urologic nurse should assess and monitor the child and family for adjustment in response to the cancer diagnosis and treatment. Mood changes and difficulties in peer relationships, particularly with adolescents, are common during treatment.[67] Many families and children will benefit from peer support and counseling groups.

Finally, support for parents and caregivers must not be overlooked. Having a child with cancer places an emotional and financial burden on families

TABLE 17-5 Potential Complications for the Child Undergoing Cancer Treatment

COMPLICATION	DESCRIPTION
Risk of infection	The risk of infection is increased by altered mucosal and skin barriers, compromised immunity, and malnutrition. There is a particular risk of mucocutaneous and systemic *Candida*, viral infections such as herpes simplex, varicella zoster, cytomegalovirus, and Epstein-Barr, and protozoal infections with *Pneumocystis jiroveci* (formerly called *P. carinii*). *Note:* There is broad agreement that no child should receive vaccinations within 1 year of completing chemotherapy.
Blood product transfusion	In addition to immunosuppression caused by failure of white cell production, cytotoxics also inhibit red cell and platelet production. Patients will usually require platelet and red cell transfusions.
Nutrition	Malnutrition is a common problem in children with cancer. Dietary counseling and selection of high-protein and high-calorie food choices is recommended. Nausea following chemotherapy treatments has greatly decreased as a result of current available antiemetic agents.
Analgesia	Special care must be taken to assess pain in small children who are unable to express themselves verbally. Careful psychological preparation and administration of adequate analgesia are required prior to treatment procedures.

that can be challenging. Parents describe never having enough time to meet their own needs or the needs of their other children, skipping meals, and feeling guilty when they do consider their own needs. The financial burden is significant, with wage loss or even job loss occurring because of the extensive time away from work. In one study, parents were asked what they found the most helpful when caring for their child with cancer.[68] They overwhelmingly identified receiving accurate, carefully delivered information to themselves and their children from healthcare providers as the most helpful way to be prepared for what to expect. Parents also valued emotional support from family, friends, and healthcare providers. They found household assistance and child care extremely valuable, and identified even minor financial assistance with parking or transportation as helping with the burden of extra cost.[68] Finally, parents and children require support with coping and adjusting as the child becomes an adolescent and then an adult survivor of childhood cancer.[69] Box 17-3 lists websites that may be of benefit to families and children as they struggle when dealing with cancer diagnosis, treatment, and ongoing care.

BOX 17-3 Web Resources for Parents*

http://www.cancer.gov/cancer_information (explains the disease, ongoing clinical trials, new treatments; for healthcare professionals and parents)

http://www.cancer.org (American Cancer Society)

http://www.cancer.ca (Canadian Cancer Society)

http://www.patientcenters.com (publications and resources on childhood cancer)

http://pdqsearch@icicc.nic.nih.gov (National Institutes of Health)

http://www.acor.org (Association of Cancer Online Resources)

*All retrieved March 1, 2008.

REFERENCES

1. Park JR, Eggert A, Caron H: Neuroblastoma: Biology, prognosis, and treatment. Pediatric Clinics of North America, 2008; 55:97-120.
2. Friedman GK, Castleberry RP: Changing trends of research and treatment in infant neuroblastoma. Pediatric Blood & Cancer, 2007; 49(7 Suppl):1060-5.
3. Gurney JG, Smith MA, Ross JA: Cancer among infants. Retrieved October 1, 2007 from http://seer.cancer.gov/publications/childhood/infant.pdf.
4. Cotterill SJ, Parker L, More L, Craft AW: Neuroblastoma: changing incidence and survival in young people aged 0-24 years. A report from the North England Young Persons' Malignant Disease Registry. Medical and Pediatric Oncology, 2001; 36:231-4.

5. Canadian Cancer Society/National Cancer Institute of Canada: New cases and age-standardized cancer incidence rates and deaths and age-standardized cancer mortality rates by histologic cell type for children and youth aged 0-19 years, Canada, 1999-2003. In Canadian Cancer Society/National Cancer Institute of Canada: Canadian Cancer Statistics 2007. Toronto: Author, 2007; p 68.

6. De Roos AJ, Teschke K, Savitz DA, Poole C, Grufferman S, Pollock BH, et al: Parental occupational exposures to electromagnetic fields and radiation and the incidence of neuroblastoma in offspring. Epidemiology, 2001; 12:508-17.

7. De Roos AJ, Olshan AF, Teschke K, Poole C, Savitz DA, Blatt J, et al: Parental occupational exposures to chemicals and incidence of neuroblastoma in offspring. American Journal of Epidemiology, 2001; 154:106-14.

8. Longo L, Panza E, Schena F, Seri M, Devoto M, Romeo G, Bini C, Pappalardo G, Tonini GP, Perri P: Genetic predisposition to familial neuroblastoma: identification of two novel genomic regions at 2p and 12p. Human Heredity, 2007; 63(3-4):205-11.

9. Hiyama E, Hiyama K, Ohtsu K, Yamaoka H, Fukuba I, Matsuura Y, et al: Biological characteristics of neuroblastoma with partial deletion in the short arm of chromosome 1. Medical and Pediatric Oncology, 2001; 36:67-74.

10. Brodeur GM, Look AT, Shimada H, Hamilton VM, Maris JM, Hann HW, et al: Biological aspects of neuroblastomas identified by mass screening in Quebec. Medical and Pediatric Oncology, 2001; 36:157-9.

11. French AE, Grant R, Weitzman S, Ray JG, Vermeulen MJ, Sung L, et al: Folic acid food fortification is associated with a decline in neuroblastoma. Clinical Pharmacology and Therapeutics, 2003; 74(3):288-94.

12. Daniels JL, Olsnan AF: Re. Breast-feeding and neuroblastoma, USA and Canada. Cancer Causes and Control, 2003; 14(3):300.

13. Henry MC, Tashjian DB, Breuer CK: Neuroblastoma update. Current Opinion in Oncology, 2005; 17(1):19-23.

14. Shimada H, Ambros IM, Dehner LP, Joshi VV, Roald B: Terminology and morphologic criteria of neuroblastic tumors: recommendations by the International Neuroblastoma Pathology Committee. Cancer, 1999; 86:349-63.

15. Yoneda A, Oue T, Imura M, Inoue M, Yagi K, Kawa K, et al: Observation of untreated patients with neuroblastoma detected by mass screening: a 'wait and see' pilot study. Medical and Pediatric Oncology, 2001; 36:160-2.

16. Trahair TN, Vowels MR, Johnston K, Cohn RJ, Russell SJ, Neville KA, Carroll S, Marshall GM: Long-term outcomes in children with high-risk neuroblastoma treated with autologous stem cell transplantation. Bone Marrow Transplant, 2007; 40(8):741-6.

17. Parise IZ, Haddad BR, Cavalli LR, Pianovski MA, Maggio EM, Parise GA, et al: Neuroblastoma in southern Brazil: an 11-year study. Journal of Pediatric Hematology/Oncology, 2006; 28(2):82-7.

18. Kim S, Chung MD: Pediatric solid malignancies: neuroblastoma and Wilms' tumor. Surgical Clinics of North America, 2006;469-87.

19. De Bernardi B, Pianca C, Pistamiglio P, Veneselli E, Viscardi E, Pession A, et al: Neuroblastoma with symptomatic spinal cord compression at diagnosis: treatment and results with 76 cases. Journal of Clinical Oncology, 2001; 19:183-90.

20. Ara T, DeClerck YA: Mechanisms of invasion and metastasis in human neuroblastoma. Cancer Metastasis Review, 2006; 25(4):645-57.

21. Suita S, Stephen L: Gans overseas lecture. Mass screening for neuroblastoma in Japan: lessons learned and future directions. Journal of Pediatric Surgery, 2002:949-54.

22. Schilling FH, Spix C, Berthold F, Erttmann R, Fehse N, Hero B, et al: Neuroblastoma screening at one year of age. New England Journal of Medicine, 2002; 346:1047-53.

23. Roberts S, Creamer K, Shoupe B, Flores Y, Daniel R: Unique management of stage 4S neuroblastoma complicated by massive hepatomegaly: case report and review of the literature. Journal of Pediatric Hematology/Oncology, 2002; 24:142-4.

24. Leavey PJ, Odom LF, Poole M, McNeely L, Tyson RW, Haase GM: Intra-operative radiation therapy in pediatric neuroblastoma. Medical and Pediatric Oncology, 1997; 28:424-8.

25. Kushner BH, Wolden S, LaQuaglia MP, Kramer K, Verbel D, Heller D, et al: Hyperfractionated low-dose radiotherapy for high-risk neuroblastoma after intensive chemotherapy and surgery. Journal of Clinical Oncology, 2001; 19:2821-8.

26. Grupp SA, Cohn SL, Wall D, Reynolds CP: Hematopoietic Stem Cell Transplant Discipline and the Neuroblastoma Disease Committee, Children's Oncology Group: Collection, storage, and infusion of stem cells in children with high-risk neuroblastoma: saving for a rainy day. Pediatric Blood and Cancer, 2006; 46(7):719-22.

27. Hug EB, Nevinny-Stickel M, Fuss M, Miller DW, Schaefer RA, Slater JD: Conformal proton radiation treatment for retroperitoneal neuroblastoma: introduction of a novel technique. Medical and Pediatric Oncology, 2001; 37:36-41.

28. Martin KA, Hatch DA, Furness PD III, Lovell MA, Odom LF, Kurzrock EA: Long-term urological complications in survivors younger than 15 months of advanced stage abdominal neuroblastoma. Journal of Urology, 2001; 166:1455-8.

29. Dorlands Illustrated Medical Dictionary. 31st edition. Philadelphia: Saunders, 2007; p 1662.

30. National Cancer Institute: Childhood rhabdomyosarcoma. Retrieved October 1, 2007 from http://www.cancer.gov/cancertopics/pdq/treatment/childrhabdomyosarcoma/ healthprofessional.

31. Toro JR, Travis LB, Wu HJ, Zhu K, Fletcher CD, Devesa SS: Incidence patterns of soft tissue sarcomas, regardless of primary site, in the surveillance, epidemiology and end results program, 1978-2001: An analysis of 26,758 cases. International Journal of Cancer, 2006; 119(12):2922-30.

32. Kaefer M, Rink RC: Genitourinary rhabdomyosarcoma. Treatment options. Urologic Clinics of North America, 2000; 27:471-87.

33. Crist W, Gehan EA, Ragab AH, Dickman PS, Donaldson SS, Fryer C, et al: The Third Intergroup Rhabdomyosarcoma Study. Journal of Clinical Oncology, 1995; 13:610-30.

34. Ruymann FB, Grovas AC: Progress in the diagnosis and treatment of rhabdomyosarcoma and related soft tissue sarcomas. Cancer Investigation, 2000; 18:223-41.

35. Stiller CA, Draper GJ: Epidemiology of cancer in children. In Voute PA (ed): Cancer in Children: Clinical Management, 5th edition. Oxford: Oxford University Press, 2005; pp 1-16.

36. Nishi M, Hatae Y: Epidemiology of malignant neoplasms in soft tissue during childhood. Journal of Experimental and Clinical Cancer Research, 2004; 23(3):437-40.

37. American Cancer Society: Cancer reference information, 2006. Retrieved October 1, 2007 from http://www.cancer.org/docroot/CRI/content/CRI_2_4_1X_ What_are_the_key_statistics_for_rhabdomyosarcoma_53.asp?sitearea=.

38. La Quaglia M, Heller G, Ghavimi F, Casper ES, Vlamis V, Hajdu S, et al: The effect of age at diagnosis on outcome in rhabdomyosarcoma. Cancer, 1994; 73:109-17.

39. Li FP, Fraumeni JF: Rhabdomyosarcoma in children: epidemiologic study and identification of a familial cancer syndrome. Journal of National Cancer Institute, 1969; 43:1365-75.

40. Malkin D, Li FP, Strong LC, Fraumeni JF Jr, Nelson CE, Kim DH, et al: Germ line p53 mutations in a familial syndrome of breast cancer, sarcomas, and other neoplasms. Science, 1990; 250:1233-8.

41. Rudnik-Schoneborn S, Anhuf D, Koscielniak E, Zerres K: Alveolar rhabdomyosarcoma in infantile spinal muscular atrophy: coincidence or predisposition? Neuromuscular Disorders, 2005; 15(1):45-7.

42. Hays DM, Raney RB, Lawrence W Jr, Tefft M, Soule EH, Crist WM, et al: Primary chemotherapy in the treatment of children with bladder-prostate tumors in the Intergroup Rhabdomyosarcoma Study (IRS-II). Journal of Pediatric Surgery, 1982; 17:812-20.

43. Wexler LH, Meyer WH, Helman LJ: Rhabdomyosarcoma and the undifferentiated sarcomas. In Pizzo PA, Poplack DG (eds): Principles and Practice of Pediatric Oncology, 5th edition. Philadelphia: Lippincott, Williams & Wilkins, 2006; pp 991-1001.

44. Lawrence W Jr, Gehan EA, Hays DM, Beltangady M, Maurer HM: Prognostic significance of staging factors of the UICC staging system in childhood rhabdomyosarcoma: a report from the Intergroup Rhabdomyosarcoma Study (IRS-II). Journal of Clinical Oncology, 1987; 5:46-54.

45. Breitfeld PP, Meyer WH: Rhabdomyosarcoma: new windows of opportunity. Oncologist, 2005; 10(7):518-27.

46. Völker T, Denecke T, Steffen I, Misch D, Schönberger S, Plotkin M, Ruf J, Furth C, Stöver B, Hautzel H, Henze G, Amthauer H: Positron emission tomography for staging of pediatric sarcoma patients: results of a prospective multicenter trial. Clinical Oncology, 2007; 1;25(34):5435-41.

47. Navid F, Santana VM, Billups CA, Merchant TE, Furman WL, Spunt SL, et al: Concomitant administration of vincristine, doxorubicin, cyclophosphamide, ifosfamide, and etoposide for high-risk sarcomas: the St. Jude Children's Research Hospital experience. Cancer, 2006; 106(8):1846-56.

48. Trobs RB, Krauss M, Geyer C, Tannapfel A, Korholz D, Hirsch W: Surgery in infants and children with testicular and paratesticular tumours: a single centre experience over a 25-year-period. Klinische Padiatrie, 2007; 219:146-51.

49. Fukuzawa R, Reeve AE: Molecular pathology and epidemiology of nephrogenic rests and Wilms tumors. Journal of Pediatric Hematology/Oncology, 2007; 29:589-94.

50. McHugh K: Renal and adrenal tumours in children. Cancer Imaging, 2007; 7:41-51.

51. Bonaiti-Pellie C, Chompret A, Tournade MF, Hochez J, Moutou C, Zucker JM, et al: Genetics and epidemiology of Wilms' tumor: the French Wilms' tumor study. Medical and Pediatric Oncology, 1992; 20:284-91.

52. Dome JS, Perlman EJ, Ritchey ML, Coppes MJ, Kalapurakal J, Grundy PE: Renal tumors. In Pizzo PA, Poplack DG (eds): Principles and Practice of Pediatric Oncology, 5th edition. Philadelphia: Lippincott Williams & Wilkins, 2006; pp 905-32.

53. Crom DB, Bredereck Boggs TB, Mandrell BN, Norville R: Pediatric cancers. In Miaskowski C, Buchel P (eds): Oncology Nursing: Assessment and Clinical Care. St Louis: Mosby, 1999; pp 1525-83.

54. Castellino SM, McLean TW: Pediatric genitourinary tumors. Current Opinion in Oncology, 2007; 19:248-53.

55. Nathan PC, Ness KK, Greenberg ML, Hudson M, Wolden S, Davidoff A, et al: Health-related quality of life in adult survivors of childhood Wilms' tumor or neuroblastoma: a report from the childhood cancer survivor study. Pediatric Blood and Cancer, 2007; 49:704-15.

56. Ahmed HU, Arya M, Tsiouris A, Sellaturay SV, Shergill IS, Duffy PG, et al: An update on the management of Wilms' tumour. European Journal of Surgical Oncology, 2007; 33:824-31.

57. Coppes MJ, Egeler RM: Genetics of Wilms' tumor. Seminars in Urologic Oncology, 1999; 17:2-10.

58. Oliver JH, Gluck G, Gledhill RB, Chavalier L: Musculoskeletal deformities following treatment of Wilms' tumor. Canadian Medical Association Journal, 1978; 119:459-64.

59. Blumenfeld Z, Haim N: Prevention of gonadal damage during cytotoxic therapy. Annals of Medicine, 1997; 29:199-206.

60. Li FP, Gimbrere K, Gelber RD, Sallan SE, Flamant F, Green DM, Meadows AT, et al: Outcome of pregnancy in survivors of Wilms' tumor. Journal of the American Medical Association, 1987; 257:216-9.

61. Kovalic JJ, Thomas PR, Beckwith JB, Feusner JH, Norkool PA: Hepatocellular carcinoma as second malignant neoplasms in successfully treated Wilms' tumor patients. A National Wilms' Tumor Study report. Cancer, 1991; 67:342-44.

62. Gilladoga AC, Manuel C, Tan CT, Wollner N, Sternberg SS, Murphy ML: The cardiotoxicity of adriamycin and daunomycin in children. Cancer, 1976; 37:1070-8.

63. Scully RE, Lipshultz SE: Anthracycline cardiotoxicity in long-term survivors of childhood cancer. Cardiovascular Toxicology, 2007; 7:122-8.

64. Scaradavou A, Heller G, Sklar CA, Ren L, Ghavimi F: Second malignant neoplasms in long-term survivors of childhood rhabdomyosarcoma. Cancer, 1995; 76:1860-7.

65. Chui CH, Billups CA, Pappo AS, Rao BN, Spunt SL: Predictors of outcome in children and adolescents with rhabdomyosarcoma of the trunk—the St Jude Children's Research Hospital experience. Journal of Pediatric Surgery, 2005; 40:1691-5.

66. Klassen A, Raina P, Reineking S, Dix D, Pritchard S, O'Donnell M: Developing a literature base to understand the caregiving experience of parents of children with cancer: A systematic review of factors related to parental health and well-being. Supportive Care in Cancer, 2007; 15:807-18.

67. Brody AC, Simmons LA: Family resiliency during childhood cancer: The father's perspective. Journal of Pediatric Oncology Nursing, 2007; 24:152-65.

68. James K, Keegan-Wells D, Hinds PS, Kelly KP, Bond D, Hall B, et al: The care of my child with cancer: parents' perceptions of caregiving demands. Journal of Pediatric Oncology Nursing, 2002; 19:218-28.

69. Sharp LK, Kinahan KE, Didwania A, Stolley M: Quality of life in adult survivors of childhood cancer. Journal of Pediatric Oncology Nursing, 2007; 24:220-6.

CHAPTER
18
Surgical Procedures
....

Surgery represents both physical and psychological challenges that are interpreted differently and provoke variable coping responses in infants, children, and adolescents. Coping responses are influenced by the type of surgical procedure, preoperative testing and physical preparation, postoperative management (especially hospitalization), and involvement of parents or guardians.[1] Special challenges facing the pediatric patient undergoing urologic surgery include issues related to informed consent, including assent from minor children, whenever feasible. In addition, preoperative education must be tailored to meet the needs of the child and parents and should involve siblings and other family members, whenever indicated. Physical preparation also incorporates knowledge of the physical needs of the infant or child, such as age-adjusted NPO schedules, personal hygiene and grooming issues prior to surgery, and tailoring preoperative procedures, including bowel preparation, transportation to and from the operative suite, and arrangements allowing the presence of one or more parent or care provider in preoperative holding areas. Fears and anxieties should be acknowledged, particularly when facing urologic surgery involving the reproductive system or external genitalia, because these procedures may provoke fear of mutilation in boys and girls.[1]

Postoperative management also must be tailored based on age and familial context, particularly when hospitalization, with its associated fears of separation from family and home, is necessary. Pain management is a special challenge when managing infants or children, who lack adult physical maturity and sophistication when seeking pain relief from care providers.[2] When caring for infants, the nurse must set aside myths about the infant's inability to experience pain.[3] When managing a toddler or preschooler, the urologic nurse must tease out expressions of fear and frustration from behavior meant to indicate incisional pain, renal colic, or bladder spasm.

The development and use of instruments such as the Oucher or Wong-Baker Faces Pain Rating Scale help nurses identify pain and evaluate reduction in pain with appropriate analgesia and nonpharmacologic comfort measures.[4] When managing older children or adolescents, the Visual Analog Scale used for adults may be applied, but a Color Analog, Oucher, or Wong-Baker Faces Pain Rating Scale may be indicated for certain patients.

With the exception of a modest but growing body of evidence focusing on the assessment and management of pain in children,[2] literature review has revealed a surprising paucity of research concerning children's perceptions or experiences of surgery and subsequent recovery. Research has shown that in most cases, the presence of one or both parents tends to diminish anxiety in the child.[5-7] Clinical experience has also demonstrated that very anxious parents can unwittingly exacerbate anxiety and fear in their child. However, we have found that gentle counseling concerning the effect of their anxiety, provided in a supportive and nonthreatening manner, combined with repeated explanations to the child concerning the reason for procedures and their necessity, helps parents provide reassurance and comfort to their child, even during uncomfortable or anxiety-provoking interventions.

Even less is known about the long-term effects of surgery on academic performance and emotional state. LaMontague and colleagues[8] have demonstrated that orthopedic surgery in adolescents causes distress that provokes avoidance and/or coping strategies, which persist for at least 6 months following the procedure. Mintzer and co-workers[9] found evidence of significant posttraumatic stress disorder, including reexperiencing, avoidance behaviors, feelings of detachment from others, sense of a foreshortened future, irritability, and increased arousal in 16% of a group of 104 adolescents who had undergone organ transplantation, including 39 who underwent kidney transplantation. However, no studies were found that examine long-term recovery in children or adolescents undergoing urologic procedures.

UPPER URINARY TRACT PROCEDURES

Surgical reconstruction of the upper urinary tracts may be necessary to relieve obstructive uropathy associated with congenital defects of the urinary system. Common anomalies associated with obstruction that may require surgical intervention include ureteropelvic junction (UPJ) obstruction, megaureter, and ureterocele.

Pyeloplasty and Endopyelotomy

The indications for surgery and techniques for repairing UPJ obstruction have evolved over the past several decades. At the dawn of the twenty-first century, open surgical or endoscopic techniques are used to relieve UPJ obstruction. The dismembered pyeloplasty remains the predominant open surgical technique because of several advantages: (1) it can be used for both extrinsic and intrinsic cases; (2) it preserves anomalous vessels; (3) it allows optimal repositioning of the UPJ for transport of urine to the lower urinary tracts; and (4) it allows reduction of an enlarged renal pelvis.[10] An anterior subcostal posterior lumbotomy or flank incision is created, each muscle layer is carefully split, and Gerota's fascia is entered, exposing a lateral view of the kidney. The renal pelvis, UPJ, and proximal ureter are identified and a traction suture is placed to minimize the need for handling the ureter. Dismemberment of the UPJ is completed by spatulating it on the opposite side of the retention suture. The pelvis may be reduced in size, if indicated, and reanastomosed to the proximal ureter, leaving a ureteral stent or small feeding tube to ensure adequate drainage. In one series of 103 children, dismembered pyeloplasty reestablished adequate upper tract urine flow in 89% of patients and renal function in 87%. It remains the gold standard to which other techniques are compared (Figure 18-1).

Endoscopic management initially used balloon dilation techniques to enlarge the UPJ, but this technique has been replaced by the Acucise device (Applied Medical, Rancho Santa Margarita, Calif).[11] The Acucise device contains a monopolar electrosurgical cutting wire and a balloon. The balloon serves to define the area of stenosis, deliver the wire to the tissue to be incised, and tamponade bleeding after the incision is made. The procedure is performed under fluoroscopic guidance via a retrograde approach. A guidewire is placed under ureteroscopic and radiographic guidance and the 6-French device is passed over the guidewire until radiopaque balloon markers straddle the stenotic area. The balloon is inflated with a small volume of contrast material and the position of the cutting wire confirmed radiographically (Figure 18-2). The balloon is further inflated and the cutting wire used to relive UPJ obstruction, resulting in extravasation. Potential advantages of endoscopic endopyelotomy include avoidance of a surgical incision and reduced incisional pain and recovery time. Disadvantages include the need for prolonged drainage via a ureteral stent for approximately 6 weeks and the possible need to replace the stent during this period or remove it, usually under some form of anesthesia. A Penrose drain is left in place initially to drain urine until the ureter heals. Success rates, even in carefully selected patients, are lower than those reported for open pyeloplasty and vary from 48% to 85%.[11] However, these findings must be carefully weighed against the less invasive nature of the procedure, particularly when applied to carefully selected patients.

Alternative methods to the Acucise endopyelotomy include antegrade endopyelotomy and laparoscopic dismembered pyeloplasty. Antegrade endopyelotomy is feasible in adolescents and older children. Percutaneous access is gained via a calyx and a 10-French tract is established. Potential advantages to the antegrade approach include the ability to use cold knife, electrocautery, or a laser in addition to the Acucise device to ensure adequate relief from UPJ obstruction while controlling bleeding.

Laparoscopic pyeloplasty uses a four-port retroperitoneal approach to achieve access to the kidney and its collecting system.[12] A working space is created by insufflation with an appropriate gas, usually carbon dioxide (CO_2), and two trocars are used to identify the UPJ and perform a dismembered pyeloplasty. In experienced hands, results from laparoscopic dismembered pyeloplasty have been reported to be comparable to those achieved by open surgery, without the operative morbidity associated with an open surgical approach.[13]

Robotic assistance may provide an attractive alternative to traditional laparoscopic techniques.[14]

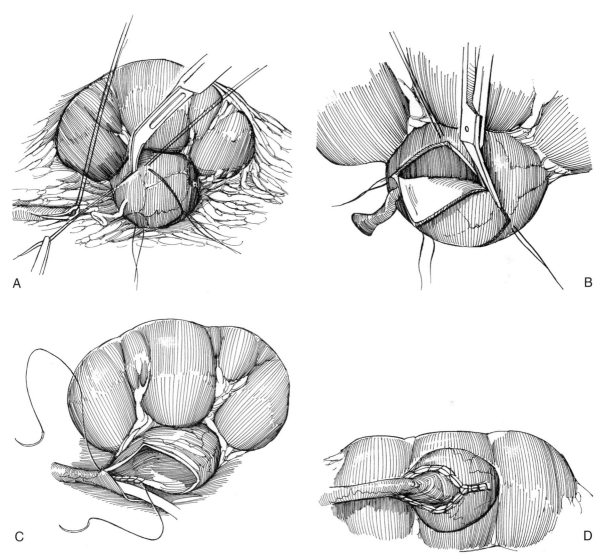

Fig. 18-1 Dismembered pyeloplasty. **A, B,** A diamond-shaped incision is made and the renal pelvis size reduced to ensure more efficient drainage from upper to lower urinary tract. **C, D,** Following removal of excessive tissue, a ureteral stent or feeding tube is inserted into the ureter and the ureter closed in a fashion that provides unobstructed flow from the renal pelvis to proximal ureter. (From Hinman F: Atlas of Urologic Surgery, 2nd edition. Philadelphia: Saunders, 1998; pp 915, 916.)

A case series of 50 children managed by robotic-assisted dismembered laparoscopy reported persistent relief from UPJ obstruction in 90% of patients.[15] Operative time averaged just over 2 hours, but the range extended from 60 to 330 minutes. Intraoperative blood loss averaged 40 ml and 95% of patients were discharged on postoperative day 1. A retrospective study has compared eight children who underwent robotic-assisted laparoscopic dismembered pyeloplasty with eight age-matched children who underwent open surgery.[16] The children who underwent robotic-assisted laparoscopic pyeloplasty had shorter hospital stays, required fewer pain medications, and had outcomes comparable to those undergoing surgery. Nevertheless, their operative times were longer. A prospective comparison completed in 2006 has revealed that robotic-assisted laparoscopic dismembered pyeloplasty costs 1.7 times that required for laparoscopic pyeloplasty.[17] Nevertheless, these data must be interpreted with

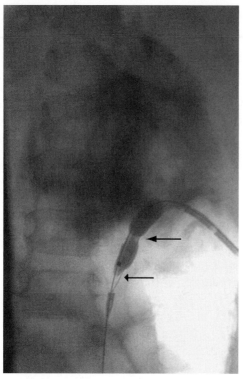

Fig. 18-2 Acucise ballon being inflated across the ureteropelvic junction narrowing. Note waist present in ballon (*upper arrow*) and cutting wire positioned laterally (*lower arrow*). (From Wein AJ, Kavoussi LR, Peters CA, Novick AC, Partin AW [eds]: Campbell-Walsh Urology, 9th edition. Philadelphia: Saunders, 2007; p 3375)

some caution, because a significant portion of the expense arose from differences in procedural length, and all the surgeons involved described themselves as "experienced laparoscopists." Given that many urologists do not frequently perform surgery using laparoscopic techniques, this difference may be affected or even negated if this cost comparison is repeated using surgeons with less familiarity or training in laparoscopy.

Complications. Complications associated with pyelostomy include urinary tract infection, prolonged drainage of urine from the Penrose drain, and urinoma. Bleeding during the procedure or postoperative hematuria may occur, occasionally requiring a blood transfusion. Stent migration with loss of adequate urinary drainage from the affected upper urinary tract may occur, leading to persistence or exacerbation of hydronephrosis.[18,19]

Preparation for Surgery. Advances in imaging techniques have increased the frequency with which UPJ obstruction and hydronephrosis are diagnosed and our understanding of their natural history and long-term implications to renal function.[20] Although prenatal ultrasonography has greatly increased the known prevalence of UPJ obstruction, long-term follow-up of these children has revealed that not all cases benefit as a result of aggressive intervention. As a result, endopyelotomy or laparoscopic or open pyeloplasty are limited to cases in which UPJ obstruction is associated with the following: (1) bothersome or clinically relevant symptoms of obstruction; (2) impaired renal function in the presence of bilateral obstruction or a solitary kidney; (3) evidence of progressive renal function impairment in unilateral UPJ obstruction; or (4) development of complicating factors, such as stones, upper urinary tract infection, or secondary hypertension.

Although an ultrasound typically leads to the diagnoses of UPJ obstruction and associated hydronephrosis, other imaging studies should be completed to determine the type of obstruction (extrinsic versus intrinsic) and differential renal function (renal function in each kidney). An intravenous pyelogram (excretory urogram) may be obtained to determine the anatomic characteristics of the obstructive lesion and provide an overall assessment of its impact on renal function. A radionuclide study also may be performed, particularly in the infant or young child. The radionuclide scan is useful because it provides a good assessment of differential renal function and the likelihood that intervention will result in a clinically relevant improvement in overall renal function, particularly if a kidney is nonvisualized on excretory urography. Preoperative preparation also includes careful consideration of the optimal timing of surgical intervention, particularly when UPJ obstruction and hydronephrosis are discovered on prenatal ultrasonography or during early infancy.[20]

In addition to these considerations, preoperative preparation focuses on the choice of procedure. Although newer approaches such as endopyelotomy are less invasive, they are also associated with lower success rates.[20] Until the collective experience with various newer techniques matures and appropriate randomized clinical trials are completed, the potential advantages and disadvantages associated with each procedure must be thoroughly discussed to ensure that an informed consent to surgery is obtained.

Postoperative Care. Postoperative management is profoundly influenced by the surgical technique and surgeon's preference. The principal goals of care include maintenance of drainage from the affected kidney, healing of the reconstructed UPJ and surgical incision (if present), and care of drains or internal stents.

Open pyeloplasty. The patient and family are advised that open surgery, such as the dismembered pyeloplasty, requires 2 to 3 hours. The urologic nurse should consult with the urologist to determine which drainage devices may be left in place following the procedure. An indwelling catheter is left in place for several days and removed prior to discharge from hospital. A Penrose drain may be left in the incision, which will provide a modest volume of reddish-brown exudate; it is removed 1 to 2 days after drainage ceases, often about 7 days postoperatively. A nephrostomy tube also may be placed during surgery. It typically remains in place for 7 to 10 days; removal is based on the results of a nephrostogram that demonstrates patency of the reconstructed UPJ and the absence of any extravasation.[20] Even in the presence of these findings, many pediatric urologists will clamp the nephrostomy tube and postpone removal for 12 to 24 hours to ensure that no flank pain, fever, or leakage around the tube develops.

Alternatively, an internal ureteral stent may be placed to ensure drainage across the affected UPJ.[21] Similar to nephrostomy tubes, ureteral stents are typically left in place for 7 to 10 days. In some cases, a ureteral stent may remain in place for as long as 6 weeks following surgery, depending on the individual procedure and surgeon's preference. The critical advantage of the indwelling ureteral stent is its ability to maintain patency while the reconstructed UPJ heals. Disadvantages of the presence of a ureteral stent include bothersome lower urinary tract symptoms, hematuria, and discomfort associated with its presence. If a ureteral stent is not left in place, the patient is monitored for persistent urinary drainage from the Penrose drain, lasting for 7 to 10 days or longer, or for recurrent drainage after the external drain has been removed. If persistent or recurrent drainage is observed, the physician is informed and a ureteral stent is placed to promote complete healing of the UPJ.

Pain is typically managed by a caudal or epidural nerve block and an epidural catheter may be left in place for approximately 48 hours. Intravenous or caudal morphine may be administered to younger children or infants and a patient-controlled analgesia (PCA) pump may be used for older children. The older child is then switched to oral analgesic medications as soon as feasible. Prophylactic antimicrobials are usually administered during the immediate postoperative period.

Although most infants or children who undergo open pyeloplasty remain in the hospital for approximately 3 to 5 days, a critical pathway has been reported, designed to achieve discharge after a single night in hospital.[22] After undergoing open dismembered pyeloplasty, a ureteral stent, Penrose or similar perinephric drain, and indwelling urethral catheter are placed. The child is sent to the regular unit for recovery, oral fluids are held until the following morning, and the child remains on strict bedrest for the remainder of the operative evening. The indwelling catheter is removed the following morning and the patient begins a regular diet. The child is maintained on a strict 2-hour toileting schedule and ambulation begun. The patient is discharged after lunch provided the following outcomes have been achieved: (1) urination has occurred more than once without suprapubic discomfort or urinary incontinence; (2) a regular diet is tolerated; (3) pain can be managed by oral analgesics; (4) the child is able to ambulate; and (5) parents state that they are comfortable taking the infant or child home. This protocol was implemented on a consecutive series of 26 patients (including 15 infants) undergoing open pyeloplasty; 92% were successfully discharged on postoperative day.[1]

Laparoscopic pyeloplasty. Postoperative pain is lessened and hospital discharge usually occurs earlier following a laparoscopic pyeloplasty. Nevertheless, postoperative pain following a laparoscopic pyeloplasty may be more intense than that seen with other laparoscopic procedures and opioid analgesics are typically required during the immediate postoperative period. However, some researchers have found that ketorolac, a nonsteroidal anti-inflammatory drug, provides an effective alternative to narcotic analgesics without compromising renal function in infants or very young children.[23] Management of drainage devices is similar to that described for open pyeloplasty. Patients and families are also counseled about the presence of residual CO_2 in the abdomen that may be associated with perceptions of bloating or shoulder pain until the CO_2 is absorbed.

Endopyelotomy. The patient is typically managed in an outpatient surgical area for 12 to 24 hours.[20,24] An indwelling catheter is placed during the procedure and typically removed the following morning or within 1 or 2 days. Prophylactic antibiotics may be administered for 1 to 5 days following the procedure. An internal ureteral stent is inserted and left in place for approximately 1 month, depending on the patient's postoperative course and surgeon preference.

Robotic-assisted pyeloplasty. Multiple aspects of postoperative management resemble those for laparoscopic pyeloplasty including urinary drainage, aggressive pain management, rapid progression from clear liquids to solid foods, early ambulation, and counseling about management of drains and ureteral stents in the home care setting.[25] Counseling and reassurance are given when the child or infant has a distended abdomen and/or abdominal or shoulder discomfort from CO_2 infused into the abdomen.

Patient Teaching Highlights. The patient and/or family are taught to care for external drains and to observe the incision for signs of urinary drainage indicating extravasation. Specifically, they are taught to change dressings at drainage sites, empty urine bags, and monitor the drain for patency and character of the urine. Parents are advised to contact the urologist or urologic nurse if the child develops a fever of 100.5° F (38° C) or higher. The child and family may be counseled to avoid showering or bathing in a tub filled with water for 3 days and avoid soaking incision sites for as long as 2 weeks.[25] Particular emphasis is placed on the importance of adhering to appointments that include follow-up imaging studies to ensure adequate drainage from the affected kidney and the absence of postoperative complications. Imaging studies may be performed within 2 months and reevaluated every 6 to 12 months during the first 2 years following pyeloplasty or endopyelotomy.

Megaureter

Surgical management of a megaureter is limited to selected patients with associated obstruction or urinary stasis and clinically relevant symptoms.

Regardless of whether megaureter is associated with obstruction, surgical management consists of ureteral tailoring via excision or plication to enable more effective ureteral peristalsis and drainage of urine from the upper to lower urinary tracts. In addition, as noted in Chapter 12, megaureter may be associated with an aperistaltic, obstructing distal segment that may require excision; ureteral reimplantation is generally required.

Two techniques are typically used to reduce the caliber of the ureter. Plication reduces ureteral diameter by infolding its walls to form a smaller lumen[26] (Figure 18-3). A potential advantage of plication is the ability to preserve ureteral vascularity readily or reverse the surgery if vascular compromise is suspected. However, plication is limited to moderately dilated ureters smaller than 1.75 cm in diameter to avoid excessive redundancy.[27] Tapering reduces ureteral diameter by excision of the redundant ureter while carefully preserving adequate ureteral diameter and vascularity. Tapering is completed to the level of the proximal ureter; its proximal portion is reimplanted into the bladder, often using a transtrigonal technique in combination with tapering or plication, as indicated. Tapering may be combined with extravesical ureteral reimplantation when indicated; the success rate of this combined procedure is approximately 86%.[28]

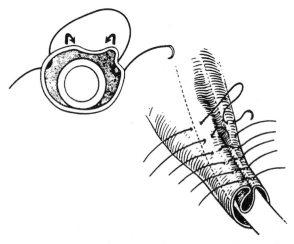

Fig. 18-3 Ureteral plication reduces internal diameter by infolding the redundant ureter (*arrows*). (From Walsh P, Retik AB, Vaughan ED, Wein AJ [eds]: Campbell's Urology, 8th edition. Philadelphia: Saunders, 2002; p 2107.)

Ureterocele

As noted in Chapter 12, ureteroceles are associated with various other defects, so that no single surgical approach is adequate for managing its sequelae. Instead, surgery is individualized for each child based on the results of a detailed urologic evaluation, including imaging studies and laboratory analysis of renal function and obstruction. The goals of surgery are to preserve renal function and urinary continence, prevent obstruction and infection, prevent reflux nephropathy, and minimize surgical morbidity.[29] Because of individual variability, a number of taxonomies have been proposed to assist the pediatric urologist in making surgical decisions about the management of ureteroceles (Table 18-1).[30-33] Additional factors affecting the surgical management of a ureterocele include the context of its diagnosis, incidental detection via imaging study or purposeful evaluation because of symptoms, presence and extent of upper urinary tract obstruction, and presence of vesicoureteral reflux (VUR). When detected incidentally, the timing of intervention is carefully weighed; it is based on considerations of damage to the growing kidney versus morbidity associated with a significant surgical procedure during early life.

The ureterocele may be incised using a cystoscope, a procedure sometimes called unroofing. If the ureterocele is contained entirely within the bladder (intravesical), a single incision is created at the lowest level feasible above the bladder neck. If the ureterocele involves the bladder neck or extends into the urethra, two incisions are created, one in the lowest level above the bladder neck and another in the urethral segment. An alternative is to create a larger longitudinal incision for the ectopic ureterocele. Incisions are created by a Bugbee electrode, metal stylet or ureteric catheter, or potassium titanyl phosphate laser.

An incision may be undertaken initially because it requires only a very short anesthetic time, avoids a cutaneous incision, and can be accomplished on an outpatient basis. Disadvantages include residual VUR, which affects almost 100% of patients undergoing extensive unroofing,[34,35] although its incidence can be reduced by puncturing or limiting the incision. Endoscopic management of ureterocele has evolved over the past several decades; creation of a single simple incision provided only limited success (0%-33%), but double puncture of the cystocele with fulguration of the anterior and posterior walls has raised the success rate to 90%, with a residual reflux rate of 47%.[36]

A number of alternatives may be used for managing ureterocele, including upper pole heminephrectomy without lower urinary tract reconstruction, upper pole heminephrectomy with lower urinary tract reconstruction, and total nephroureterectomy. Upper pole nephrectomy may be undertaken when the segment of the kidney that drains into the ureterocele contributes less than 10% to total renal function, is found to be dysplastic or scarred, and there is low-grade or no VUR. In some patients, heminephrectomy provides a definitive repair or delays reconstruction until the risks associated with surgery and anesthesia have subsided.

Upper pole heminephrectomy with lower urinary tract reconstruction is sometimes called a combined approach or complete reconstruction.[29,33] It requires

TABLE 18-1 Taxonomies for Classifying Ureteroceles

TAXONOMY	GRADE OR TYPE	DESCRIPTION
Stephens (1968)[30]	Stenotic	Narrow orifice within bladder vesicle
	Sphincteric	Wide orifice within proximal urethra or at bladder neck
	Sphincterostenotic	Narrow orifice within proximal urethra or at bladder neck
	Cecoureterocele	Blind-ending canal (cecal) ureterocele that extends down the urethra
American Academy of Pediatrics (1984)[32]	Intravesical	Contained entirely within bladder vesicle
	Ectopic	Some portions located at bladder neck or urethra
Churchill (1992)[31]	Grade 1	Ureterocele segment alone affected
	Grade 2	Both segments of one kidney affected
	Grade 3	Both kidneys affected

two incisions, a flank incision to complete a hemi-nephrectomy and a lower abdominal incision for excision of the ureterocele and reimplantation of the ipsilateral lower pole ureter, possibly combined with reimplantation of the contralateral ureter. The principal indication is an older child with no renal function in the upper pole of the affected kidney combined with higher grade VUR into the ipsilateral and/or contralateral ureter.

Total nephroureterectomy is sometimes indicated for children with massive lower pole VUR and damage to the entire affected kidney. This approach is reserved for children with significant complications associated with their ureterocele, such as infection or stones.

URETERAL REIMPLANTATION FOR VESICOURETERAL REFLUX

Surgical management of VUR is reserved for children who cannot be adequately managed by more conservative means, such as watchful waiting and suppressive antimicrobial therapy. Although the decision to proceed with a surgical repair of reflux must be individualized, common indications include the following: (1) breakthrough urinary tract infection (UTI) despite prophylactic antimicrobial therapy; (2) poor adherence to medical therapy; (3) very high-grade VUR, especially when combined with parenchymal scarring; (4) failure of renal growth, renal function deterioration, or formation of new renal scars; (5) VUR in girls that persists after full linear growth is achieved; and (6) reflux coexisting with a congenital anomaly affecting the ureterovesical junction.[26] Various surgical techniques may be used to correct VUR; the predominant approaches are open surgery and endoscopic injection of bulking agents.

Open Surgery

Various open surgical techniques have been described. Collectively, they are referred to as ureteral reimplantation or ureteroneocystostomy because all require tunneling the ureter through the trigone or bladder wall in a manner that provides adequate length and muscular backing to prevent retrograde movement of urine from the lower to upper urinary tracts. The ureterovesical junction may be approached using an intravesical, extravesical, or combined approach, based on the position of the new submucosal tunnel in relation to its original location.[26,37]

Table 18-2 lists common intravesical approaches to ureteroneocystostomy, and Figure 18-4 illustrates basic principles of intravesical ureteroneocystostomy.

Several extravesical techniques have also been described. These methods are often selected because of their technical simplicity, especially when operating on a single refluxing urinary tract. The Lich-Gregoir technique requires dissection along the lateral bladder wall.[26,37] Using electrocautery, the detrusor muscle is divided down to the level of the bladder mucosa from an extravesical approach, beginning at the tunica serosa and proceeding inward toward the vesicle. A 3-cm trough is created to the level of the mucosa and the ureter is laid into this defect in a tunneled fashion. The surgeon takes care to orient the ureter along its natural course and to avoid medial placement of the tunnel, which could lead to ureteral kinking as the bladder fills with urine (Figure 18-5). Detrusorrhaphy arose as a modification of the Lich-Gregoir procedure. For this procedure, the ureter is located via an extravesical approach and its insertion into the detrusor is identified. An incision is made around the point of the ureter's insertion. The orifice of the ureter is moved distally about 1 cm toward the bladder neck and placed into the trough created by the detrusor muscle incision.

Potential advantages to extravesical approaches include a more rapid return of bowel function when compared with intravesical approaches, reduced postoperative pain, fewer bladder spasms, and quicker hospital discharge. Disadvantages include a reported risk for subsequent lower urinary tract dysfunction associated with ureteral kinking and bladder distention.[38]

When a bilateral repair is indicated, a transvesical approach may be preferred, such as the Politano-Leadbetter procedure.[26] A transverse incision is created just above the symphysis pubis and the bladder is opened at its midline. The ureters are then reimplanted from an intravesical perspective. In 1975 Cohen used the intravesical approach but reimplanted the ureters transtrigonally to ensure a nonrefluxing tunnel. The Cohen transtrigonal technique has been described as the most widely used procedure in the United States.[26] Although the intravesical approach continues to be widely performed, a prospective, randomized clinical trial comparing an intravesical technique (Politano-Leadbetter) with an extravesical

TABLE 18-2 Intravesical Surgical Approaches for Ureteral Reimplantation[26,37]

TECHNIQUE	DESCRIPTION
Politano-Leadbetter	The intravesical technique requires a small suprapubic incision. The bladder is opened at the midline and one or both ureters are carefully dissected with minimal tissue handling. A mucosal tunnel is developed and the ureters are brought through the tunnel posteriorly (a step sometimes described as blind) and feeding tubes are inserted through the newly created intravesical ureters to ensure patency.
Cohen cross-trigonal	A small suprapubic incision is created and one or both ureters are mobilized. In contrast to the Politano-Leadbetter technique, one or two submucosal tunnels are created that cross the trigone and the ureters are tunneled through these tunnels. This procedure is preferred for patients undergoing bladder neck reconstruction because it allows reimplantation well above the bladder neck. A potential disadvantage is the difficulty created when attempting to catheterize the ureters using a retrograde technique.
Glen-Anderson	This procedure also yields a cross-trigonal tunnel but the ureter remains in its original hiatus, theoretically limiting the risk of kinking and obstruction. The incision and initial approach are similar to those of the Politano-Leadbetter technique. Results are optimal in patients with adequate distance between bladder neck and ureterovesical junction to allow creation of an adequate submucosal tunnel.
Gil-Vernet	This technique uses a similar approach to that of the Politano-Leadbetter technique but the ureters are advanced across the trigone, thus relying on muscular activity in the transmural ureter to correct reflux. Optimal results are obtained when attempting to prevent reflux in the child with unilateral reflux and a pathologic appearance to the contralateral ureterovesical junction. Comparatively poor results are noted when the technique is applied to older children and those with higher grade reflux.

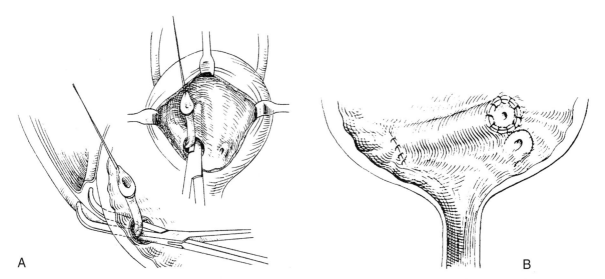

A

B

Fig. 18-4 Intravesical ureteroneocystostomy (ureteral reimplantation). **A,** Intravesical approaches require the surgeon to open the bladder vesicle, free the intravesical ureters, and reimplant them in a fashion that provides an adequate submucosal tunnel to prevent VUR. **B,** The Cohen cross-trigonal and Glenn-Anderson techniques tunnel the ureters across the trigone to prevent VUR. (From Walsh P, Retik AB, Vaughan ED, Wein AJ [eds]: Campbell's Urology, 8th edition. Philadelphia: Saunders, 2002; pp 2083; 2086.)

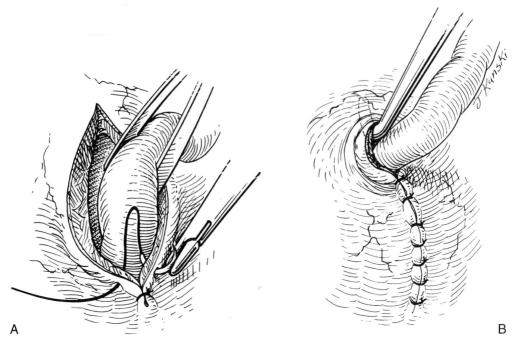

Fig. 18-5 Extravesical ureteroneocystostomy (ureteral reimplantation). **A,** Extravesical techniques require the surgeon to create a 3-cm trough without entering the bladder's vesicle. **B,** The ureter is laid into the trough, which is closed to provide greater resistance to VUR. Care is taken to orient the ureter along its natural course and to avoid medial placement and kinking as the bladder fills. (From Walsh P, Retik AB, Vaughan ED, Wein AJ [eds]: Campbell's Urology, 8th edition. Philadelphia: Saunders, 2002; p 2089.)

approach (Lich-Gregoir)[39] has provided evidence that children managed by an extravesical approach may experience reduced hematuria, postoperative pain, and fewer bladder spasms as compared with those managed by an intravesical technique; success rates exceeding 95% were maintained.

The Paquin technique combines elements of extravesical and intravesical procedures.[26] It uses an extravesical approach to mobilize the ureter and an intravesical approach for reimplantation. It has not gained widespread use in North America.

Although success rates vary, the most popular intravesical approaches ablate VUR in more than 90% of refluxing ureters.[26,37] Similarly, more recent modifications of extravesical ureteroneocystostomy have achieved success in 93% of patients, although combined approaches have reported success rates of up to 96%.

Laparoscopic Techniques

A number of surgeons have reported case series demonstrating the feasibility of intravesical and extravesical techniques via a laparoscopic approach.

Several case series have focused on a laparoscopic approach using the Lich-Gregoir extravesical technique.[40,41] Case series have also demonstrated the feasibility of a laparoscopic cross-trigonal Cohen procedure,[42] a frequently performed intravesical technique. However, technical difficulties associated with laparoscopy, as well as the development of endoscopic submucosal injection procedures, have limited its clinical application.

Endoscopic Subureteric Injection Procedures

Suburethral bulking agents have been successfully injected into the urethral mucosa to enhance sphincteric competence and treat stress urinary incontinence in children and adults (see Chapter 11). Partly based on these clinical experiences, pediatric urologists have explored the possibility of injecting bulking agents under the mucosa of the ureterovesical junction to enhance closure during bladder filling and storage and prevent reflux (Figure 18-6). The first method described in the urologic literature used polytetrafluoroethylene (Teflon) paste and was labeled the STING

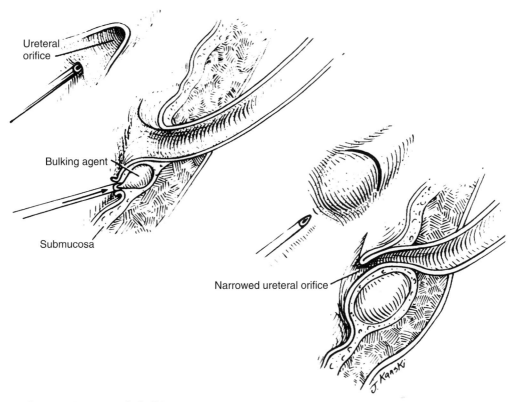

Fig. 18-6 Subureteric injection of a bulking agent. (From Walsh P, Retik AB, Vaughan ED, Wein AJ [eds]: Campbell's Urology, 8th edition. Philadelphia: Saunders, 2002; p 2092.)

procedure.[43] It is comparatively simple; cystoscopy is used to visualize the ureterovesical junction and a needle-tipped stent is introduced through the working port of the catheter without removing the telescope.[26,37] The needle is inserted several millimeters under the mucosa at a 6 o'clock position and the bulking agent is slowly injected until a bulge appears. The needle is kept in place for an addition 30 to 60 seconds to ensure that the bulking agent does not extrude through the mucosa. Only a small volume of bulking substance is required, usually from 0.1 to 0.3 ml.

Although the technique for subureteric injection is straightforward, final consensus concerning the optimal bulking agent has not been reached.[44] Teflon paste, polyvinyl alcohol, detachable membrane devices, bovine collagen, bladder muscle cells, polydimethylsiloxane (Microplastique), and autologous chondrocytes have been used as bulking agents.

More recently, a dextranomer–hyaluronic acid copolymer agent (Deflux) has become the first such material approved for clinical use by the U.S. Food and Drug Administration (FDA). Deflux consists of dextranomer microspheres suspended in a high-molecular-weight sodium hyaluronic acid solution. With adequate experience, the procedure requires about 15 minutes, and a single injection resolves VUR in 68% to 72% of refluxing ureters.[45] The success rate rises to 97% after two injections and approaches 100% after three procedures. Similar to the use of Teflon paste, injection of the material causes a local inflammatory response, but this has not led to adverse clinical outcomes. Although the success rates of subureteric injections are lower than those achieved by open surgical methods, they remain popular because of reduced complication rates, technical ease, and the ability to spare children prolonged antibiotic prophylaxis.[46]

Complications. Postoperative edema, subtrigonal bleeding, mucus plugs, blood clots, bladder spasm, or surgical correction may lead to obstruction in some cases.[26] Symptoms, including acute abdominal pain, nausea, and vomiting, usually occur 1 to 2 weeks following surgery. Some cases are transient and resolve without treatment, but a few will require placement of a nephrostomy tube or ureteral stent. Complete obstruction may occur later and is usually associated with ischemia. Transient obstruction associated with hydronephrosis and/or renal insufficiency has been reported in women who underwent Politano-Leadbetter ureteroneocystostomy as girls,[47] possibly because of kinking during pregnancy.

VUR occurs in 6% to 16% of contralateral ureters, but it is typically transient and seldom requires aggressive management. Persistent VUR in the ureter undergoing reimplantation is an unusual complication following open surgery. It may be attributable to technical errors, ureteral dilation, or persistent voiding dysfunction.[26] However, although untreated voiding dysfunction may be associated with an increased risk for recurrence of VUR or recurrent febrile or afebrile UTI, the success of ureteroneocystostomy remains high, particularly when voiding dysfunction is treated with a combination of antimuscarinic agents and behavioral interventions.[48]

As noted, endoscopic subureteric injection therapy is associated with a higher incidence of recurrent or persistent VUR. Nevertheless, it remains an attractive option because it does not require open surgery, a cutaneous incision, and the associated morbidity and complications. In a review of 650 ureters undergoing the STING procedure in 402 children between 1986 and 1993, no cases of transient persistent obstruction leading to hydronephrosis or renal insufficiency were identified.[49] Reflux nephropathy progressed unabated in 4.4% of treated kidneys, despite successful resolution of VUR. No adverse events were linked to local inflammation or migration of Teflon particles. A review of 180 children treated with Deflux between 2001 and 2003 revealed contralateral VUR in 5% and persistent reflux in 28% of patients.[50] Although local migration of the material occurred in 61%, it was not associated with adverse outcomes or obstruction.

Preparation for Surgery. The families of children undergoing open surgical repair are advised that a 3- to 4-day hospital course is anticipated.[51]

The urine is evaluated within 1 week of the procedure and any evidence of infection is managed with antimicrobial therapy to reduce the risk of complications associated with surgical reconstruction of infected, inflamed, and friable mucosa. Children undergoing subureteric injection may require a skin sensitivity test, depending on the bulking agent.

Children undergoing subureteric injections are usually managed on an outpatient basis. Parents are counseled that the procedure will require 15 to 30 minutes and that the child will be transferred to a postanesthesia care unit for a brief stay.

Postoperative Care. The child undergoing open surgery will return to the floor with an indwelling catheter and possibly ureteral stents. High fluid intake is maintained for 24 to 48 hours to minimize the risk for blood clot formation and promote urinary drainage. The nurse should expect the child's urine to be grossly bloody during the immediate postoperative period, but it is expected to clear gradually over a 2- to 3-day period. Urine output is frequently monitored for volume, character, and presence of clots. The patency of the catheter must be maintained and the physician promptly notified if excessive passage of blood clots or catheter occlusion is suspected. The surgical dressing is removed 1 to 2 days postoperatively and the urethral catheter on day 2 or 3. The ureteral stent is also removed during the early postoperative period, usually by the end of day 3.

One study has compared the postoperative course and length of stay of 300 children undergoing ureteroneocystostomy for VUR. Of these, 76 were managed with indwelling catheters but 224 had the catheters removed before returning to the postoperative ward.[52] Children who were managed without an indwelling catheter experienced shorter hospital stays than those managed using traditional methods. Despite the absence of the catheter, no statistically significant differences were observed based on rate of obstruction, readmission to hospital, or the amount of ketorolac or oxybutynin required for bladder spasm. Further study is clearly indicated, but these results provide some evidence that the indwelling catheter may not be a necessary component of the initial postoperative management of the child undergoing ureteroneocystostomy.

Causes of postoperative pain include the cutaneous incision and bladder spasm. Morphine may be administered for pain via a PCA pump. Ketorolac may be used in conjunction with morphine; a randomized clinical trial demonstrated its efficacy in reducing incisional pain and its ability to prevent or inhibit bladder spasms.[53] In addition, a single-dose caudal injection of bupivacaine may be administered to relieve immediate postoperative pain.[54] Intravesical morphine has also been recommended. A randomized clinical trial involving 80 children compared intravesical morphine with placebo (infused saline) given in addition to normal analgesia, but it failed to demonstrate significant pain relief during the first 48 hours following surgery.[55] In addition to a therapeutic role for ketorolac, bladder spasm pain may be alleviated by the administration of an antimuscarinic such as oxybutynin and avoidance of irritating substances, such as caffeine.

Postoperative management for the child undergoing subureteric injection uses many of the same broad principles used for the patient undergoing a cystoscopic procedure. The parents are advised that the child may experience transient confusion or dizziness associated with anesthesia. Rest is encouraged following the procedure, but the child can resume normal activities on the following day. Fluid intake is strongly encouraged, but caffeinated beverages are avoided in favor of water, juice, Popsicles, and soup. Children may experience difficulty voiding or bladder spasms that are usually relieved by allowing the child to soak in a tub of warm water. The child should be encouraged to urinate into the tub if discomfort leads to difficulty initiating micturition. Parents are also taught to contact the physician or urologic nurse if the child experiences a fever higher than 101° F (38.3° C), bladder spasms that become worse or fail to diminish within 24 hours, or a complete inability to urinate.

AUGMENTATION CYSTOPLASTY

Augmentation cystoplasty incorporates a segment of the gastrointestinal tract into the bladder to enlarge its capacity, increase bladder wall compliance, and diminish or abolish overactive detrusor contractions (Figure 18-7). In children, the most common indication for augmentation enterocystoplasty is hostile neurogenic bladder dysfunction, characterized by a reduced capacity, low bladder wall compliance, and/or bladder outlet obstruction. Underlying causes include myelodysplasia, sacral agenesis, VATER syndrome (*v*ertebral defects, imperforate *a*nus, *t*racheo*e*sophageal fistula, *r*adial and renal dysplasia), pelvic tumors, classic exstrophy, posterior urethral valves, and cloacal deformities. Another indication for augmentation enterocystoplasty is intractable detrusor overactivity (refractory to all forms of conservative or pharmacologic management) caused by spinal cord tumor, injury, or vascular malformation. Indications affecting adults and children include tubercular cystitis and severe chemotherapy- or radiotherapy-induced cystitis.

Multiple segments of the gastrointestinal tract may be used to augment bladder size, including the small bowel, cecum, sigmoid colon, and stomach.[56] Each segment offers potential advantages and disadvantages depending on the patient's age, size and medical history, underlying cause, and surgeon's experience and preference. For example, the stomach was once widely used for augmentation procedures because it avoided the metabolic acidosis associated with large and small bowel segments, reduced susceptibility to infection, and was postulated to potentiate long-term renal growth and overall growth in children. However, gastrocystoplasty is no longer widely performed because of observed long-term disadvantages associated with incorporation of the stomach into the bladder, including the hematuria-dysuria syndrome. The small bowel remains popular for augmentation procedures because it is easily accessed, has very high compliance when properly reconstructed, and produces less mucus than large bowel segments. Disadvantages associated with use of the small bowel include metabolic acidosis and loss of resorptive surface in the gastrointestinal system that may lead to long-term deficiencies of vitamin B_{12} and folate. The large bowel is also widely used because it is easily accessed during surgery, it provides good compliance when adequately detubularized, and its use makes it easier to create nonrefluxing tunnels for ureteral reimplantation as needed. Disadvantages include lack of availability in patients who have undergone pelvic radiation therapy, metabolic acidosis, and a risk for spontaneous or trauma-related rupture.

Regardless of the bowel segment selected, preservation of the bowel's vascular supply, detubularization of the bowel segment, and creation of a maximal intravesical surface area in accordance with Laplace's law are critical to the long-term success of bladder augmentation surgery.[56] Four major steps are common to all augmentation procedures: (1) an adequate segment of the gastrointestinal tract is isolated from the stomach or fecal stream and the

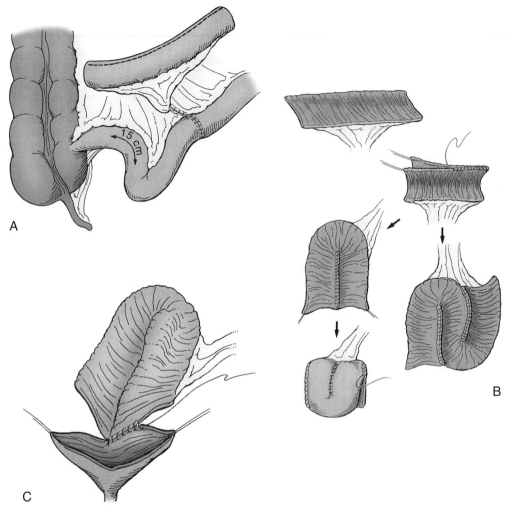

Fig. 18-7 Augmentation enterocystoplasty. **A,** The bladder is bivalved in preparation for anastomosis and augmentation with a segment of bowel or stomach. **B,** A segment of the gastrointestinal system is isolated from the fecal stream, detubularized, and brought down to the bladder with its vascular supply intact. **C,** The bladder and bowel are anastomosed, beginning at the posterior aspect. (From Wein AJ, Kavoussi LR, Peters CA, Novick AC, Partin AW [eds]: Campbell-Walsh Urology, 9th edition. Philadelphia: Elsevier, 2007; p 3674.)

remaining bowel reanastomosed; (2) the isolated segment is cut along its antimesenteric border and folded into a U, W, or S shape, a procedure called detubularization; (3) the bladder is bivalved to create a clam configuration; and (4) the detubularized bowel is anastomosed to the opened bladder.

Two alternatives to augmentation enterocystoplasty are ureterocystoplasty or autoaugmentation. Ureterocystoplasty is highly desirable but rarely feasible; it requires a massively dilated ureter (megaureter) attached to a nonfunctioning or poorly functioning kidney. Similar to enterocystoplasty, the ureter is detubularized, folded into a U-shaped pouch, and anastomosed to the bivalved bladder. Significant advantages of the procedure include incorporation of the ureter, which is lined with urothelium; this is a mucosal structure designed to contain urine without producing excessive mucus or absorbing any of its luminal components. In addition, ureterocystoplasty avoids the need to interrupt the gastrointestinal tract, with its associated short- and long-term sequelae and complications.

Autoaugmentation enlarges bladder capacity by incising the dome of the bladder while leaving its mucosa intact to form a large, wide-mouthed diverticulum. Similar to the ureterocystoplasty, this technique offers the potentially significant advantage of avoiding the need for interrupting the gastrointestinal tract. Unfortunately, long-term experience has demonstrated that scarring or fibrosis of the diverticulum limits bladder capacity and compliance, which outweighs its potential advantage.[56]

Depending on the situation, augmentation enterocystoplasty may be combined with ureteroneocystostomy to correct VUR, a Mitrofanoff procedure to promote atraumatic intermittent catheterization and preserve urethral continence, and a suburethral sling or artificial urinary sphincter to promote urethral continence.[56] Laparoscopic approaches have been described for augmentation enterocystoplasty,[57] but most surgeons continue to perform this complex procedure using open surgical techniques.[56,58]

Despite the need for ongoing intermittent catheterization and regular irrigation, long-term follow-up studies have clearly demonstrated that a properly performed augmentation enterocystoplasty provides a durable, large-capacity, and highly compliant bladder that preserves renal function and maintains a health-related quality of life.[59-61]

Complications. The complications associated with augmentation enterocystoplasty are similar to those seen with cutaneous continent urinary diversions and neobladder; these are discussed in detail in Chapter 11. Briefly, they include metabolic acidosis associated with hypokalemia, hypomagnesemia, and hyperammonemia. Vitamin B_{12} or folate deficiency is most likely to occur when the distal ileum is incorporated. Mucus production may be significant, particularly when the sigmoid colon is incorporated, leading to a risk for calculi and incomplete emptying caused by clogging of the catheter. Regardless of the segment selected for enterocystoplasty, compliance of the augmented bladder and urinary incontinence associated with bolus contractions may occur when adequate detubularization is not accomplished during the original procedure.

Although rare, approximately 30 cases of cancer in augmented bladders have been reported[60] as well as two cases of malignancies associated with gastrocystoplasty.[62] Most are adenocarcinomas involving the urothelium and arising from fibrotic bladders in patients with tubercular cystitis. The risk for malignancy has been attributed to chronic inflammation and metaplasia caused by nitrosamines, a known carcinogen, found in augmented bladders with chronic bacterial colonization.[60,63] Dyer and colleagues[62] have investigated a possible role for intravesical therapy using short-chain fatty acids to reduce the inflammation and subsequent risk for malignancy associated with incorporation of an intestinal segment into the urinary stream.

Bladder rupture has been found to occur spontaneously or as the result of trauma in approximately 5% of cases over a 5-year period.[56,64] Risk factors identified during a retrospectively analysis of a group of 17 children who underwent augmentation using stomach, large bowel, and small bowel included the following: (1) use of a bowel segment—the highest risk was associated with use of the stomach and the lowest when small bowel was used; and (2) irregular intermittent catheterization schedule.[64] Incorporation of the cecum into an augmentation has been associated with chronic diarrhea that is sometimes severe.

A retrospective review of 144 patients with a median follow-up of 112 months has suggested that simultaneous performance of an augmentation enterocystoplasty and artificial urinary sphincter may increase the risk for infection of the implant.[65] This increased risk appears to affect patients during the first postoperative years but it subsequently disappears, suggesting that bacterial colonization and inflammation of the diverted intestinal segment may be associated with seeding of the artificial urinary sphincter.

Bladder calculi occur in as many as 50% of patients with augmentation enterocystoplasties, particularly when the ileum or small bowel is incorporated.[66] Daily irrigation with 30 to 60 ml of normal saline has been suggested as a preventive strategy.

Preparation for Surgery. It is essential that preoperative counseling includes education about the need to manage the augmented bladder by ongoing and regular clean intermittent catheterization and bladder irrigation. A bowel preparation is completed immediately prior to surgery. For children, bowel preparation typically includes 2 days of a clear liquid diet and mechanical bowel cleansing within 24 hours of the procedure using bisacodyl (Dulcolax) tablets or suppository and/or polyethylene glycol–electrolyte solution (GoLYTELY).

An aggressive preparation is particularly important for the child with a neurogenic bladder, because constipation and neurogenic bowel dysfunction often impair the efficiency of fecal evacuation. Hydration must be maintained during aggressive bowel preparation, and parenteral fluid support may be needed for the infant or child undergoing aggressive bowel preparation for augmentation enterocystoplasty.[58]

A sample for urine culture should be obtained several days prior to surgery and any bacteriuria eradicated with appropriate antibiotics. Treatment of a urinary tract infection or bacteriuria is particularly important in the child with myelodysplasia and a ventriculoperitoneal shunt, because it is possible that some urine will enter into the peritoneal space during surgery. Endoscopy also may be performed immediately prior to the surgical procedure itself to evaluate the urethral outlet and ureterovesical junctions.

Postoperative Care. Postoperatively, patients will have a nasogastric tube for gastric decompression that will remain in place until bowel function returns. Fluid and electrolyte monitoring are critical, with particular attention to third-space losses. The sequestration of body fluids in a potential space is called third-spacing and is associated with intravascular volume deficit. Fluid is not lost from the body, but is unavailable for use. Initial signs and symptoms are those of volume depletion, including decreased urine output and a simultaneous increase in its specific gravity. The child may report thirst, mucous membranes will be dry, and skin turgor will be poor. The child is also likely to experience postural hypotension, tachycardia, tachypnea, and decreased capillary filling when nail beds are gently compressed. Additional symptoms will occur but vary, depending on where fluid gathers. If fluid gathers in the peritoneal space, symptoms include ascites, a feeling of abdominal fullness, shortness of breath, and an increase in abdominal girth. Fluid that gathers in the pericardial area leads to chest pain and tachycardia; excess fluid in the intrapleural space results in dyspnea, shortness of breath, and a dull response when percussing over lung fields.

A suprapubic catheter will be placed for approximately 3 weeks to ensure rapid urinary drainage, prevent bladder distention, and promote healing of the bowel to bladder anastomosis. Continuous drainage is often followed by a clamping routine to stretch the augmented bladder gradually. Initially, catheter irrigation with normal saline will be required at least three times daily. As capacity increases and oral hydration is maintained, irrigations may be decreased to once daily. However, because of the risk of obstruction or calculus formation, ongoing daily irrigation is strongly recommended. The suprapubic catheter is removed once intermittent catheterization is successfully underway or, in rare cases, when spontaneous voiding occurs.

Adequate fluid intake is important to assist with mucus evacuation and to reduce the risk of urine supersaturation and calculus formation. Long-term follow-up often includes ultrasonography or possibly radionuclide renal scanning at 6 and 12 months postoperatively. Urodynamic testing may be completed to evaluate bladder capacity and compliance and to determine the presence, frequency, and amplitude of bolus contractions. As with ileal conduit or continent diversion, serum electrolyte, blood urea nitrogen (BUN), and creatinine levels and urinalysis results are followed over time. Because of the liver's considerable ability to store vitamin B_{12}, serum levels should be measured over a period of at least 2 years to determine whether supplementation will be required.

Patient Teaching Highlights. The child and at least one family member or regular care provider must be able to catheterize the child and perform bladder irrigation. Postoperative counseling also emphasizes the need for ongoing assessment for metabolic acidosis (or alkalosis if a gastrocystoplasty is completed), vitamin B_{12} deficiency, or chronic bowel elimination disorders. The family is taught the signs and symptoms of bladder rupture and the need to seek care immediately.

TISSUE ENGINEERING, BLADDER AUGMENTATION, AND BLADDER REPLACEMENT

Tissue engineering is a potentially valuable new technology that combines genetic engineering of cells with chemical engineering to create new tissue, including skin, bone, bladder mucosa, vaginal mucosa, and renal parenchyma.[67,68] Rather than using a segment of bowel to augment the bladder, tissue engineering techniques can be used to create a bladder wall that contains urothelium, submucosa, and muscle cells. Atala and coworkers[69] have obtained autologous cells from a group of eight children with myelodysplasia and hostile neurogenic bladder dysfunction via biopsy. These cells were cultured and placed on biodegradable scaffolds of collagen or a composite of collagen and polyglycolic acid. After 7 to 8 weeks of growth, the engineered tissue constructs were used to perform cystoplasty surgery. Subjects were treated with antibiotics for 7 days to ensure a sterile urinary tract. The bladder was opened to form a clam cystoplasty and the engineered tissue was anastomosed to the endogenous bladder with polyglycolic sutures and fibrin glue. The bladder was drained via a urethral catheter and a silicone drain was placed in the retroperitoneal cavity. Nasogastric drainage was not required because the gastrointestinal tract was not interrupted, and most of the subjects were able to resume a normal diet within 24 hours of surgery.

Although still investigational, this procedure offers several significant advantages when compared with traditional augmentation enterocystoplasty. In addition to avoiding the postoperative recovery, pain, and ileus involved with harvesting bowel for use in the urinary system, it also avoids multiple long-term effects including malignancy, bladder calculi, excessive mucus production, and metabolic disorders associated with a shortened gastrointestinal tract. More studies must be done before existing techniques can be considered safe and effective for routine clinical use, but tissue engineering offers a novel and potentially revolutionary method of reconstructing the urinary tract in children and adults with neurogenic bladder dysfunction that threatens renal function or produces long-term intractable incontinence.

HYPOSPADIAS

The severity of hypospadias varies significantly, based on its location along the penile shaft and the presence of associated defects, such as a chordee with penile curvature. Proximal hypospadias adversely affects urination and fertility function, and the need for surgical reconstruction is apparent. However, distal lesions (subcoronal or proximal glanular defects) are more prevalent, produce a less apparent defect, which may not be noticeable in some uncircumcised men, and are less likely to produce significant voiding symptoms.[70] These observations, combined with knowledge of the sequelae and complications associated with hypospadias surgery, have led some to question whether mild distal lesions routinely justify surgical correction.

Arguments supporting the need for surgical correction include the frequency of circumcision in North America, leading to greater awareness of the defect, frequency of an abnormal appearance of the foreskin in uncircumcised males, presence of a transverse web of tissue just distal to the urethral meatus, which often leads to a spraying urinary stream, and the significant risk for ventral penile curvature. Limited clinical evidence has supported the hypothesis that an unrepaired hypospadias associated with a visible genital defect tends to produce lower social skills, a greater tendency to internalize problems, and worse school performance when compared with children with repaired defects.[71] Insufficient evidence exists to determine the long-term psychological, psychosocial, and sexual impact of distal hypospadias and how these outcomes are affected by early surgical intervention.

Therefore, the decision to undertake surgical correction is necessarily based on the location of the defect, presence of associated defects, and clinical judgment as to whether urinary or reproductive function is likely to be impaired unless surgical repair is completed. When a decision to pursue surgical repair is reached, the timing of surgery must be carefully considered. A number of factors enter into this decision, including likely psychological responses to penile surgery, technical aspects of the surgery, and anesthetic-related considerations. Surgery is normally completed in male infants between 6 and 12 months of age,[72] although repair may occur as early as 3 months in full-term deliveries or at 5 months for premature infants when an early repair is deemed desirable.

Various surgical techniques have been used for hypospadias repair. However, advances in our understanding of the pathophysiology of hypospadias and extensive surgical experience have led to a consensus that four principles must be taken into account whenever a surgical repair is undertaken:
1. The tissue distal to the hypospadiac meatus comprises the urethral plate.
2. This urethral plate is rarely the cause of penile bending,
3. It should be incorporated into the surgical repair because it reduces the risk for postoperative complications,

4. The plate can usually be tubularized without resorting to additional skin flaps, provided a dorsal relaxing midline incision is made.

The selection of specific surgical techniques for hypospadias repair often occurs intraoperatively.[73] A primary surgical repair begins with preservation of the urethral plate and degloving the penis to correct any associated chordee. A meatal advancement glanuloplasty (MAGPI) procedure (Figure 18-8) requires a circumferential procedure 6 to 8 mm proximal to the corona of the glans penis. A longitudinal incision from the distal edge of the meatus is then created and extended to the groove of the distal glans. The incised edges are approximated in a manner that provides a rounded appearance and normally located meatus. The tubularized incised plate urethroplasty (TIP) uses a midline relaxing incision from within the meatus to the end of the urethral plate, thus reducing the risk for meatal stenosis. It is preferred when a hypospadias defect produces a flat urethral plate as compared with the deeply grooved plate seen in many cases. An onlay flap or tubularized preputial flap may be incorporated into the surgical repair of a distal hypospadias defect when severe penile curvature requires transection of the urethral plate or the plate is not sufficiently widened despite an adequate dorsal relaxing incision. A transverse island tube repair also may be used as a one-stage option for boys with proximal hypospadias.

Two-stage procedures may provide better results in some male infants with severe curvature and proximal defects necessitating transection of the urethral plate. During stage 1 of the procedure, penile curvature is corrected, the dorsal foreskin is split to the level of the corona, and the flaps are advanced ventrally to provide skin that will be used in the second stage of the procedure to complete tubularization to the level of the distal meatus. Stage 2 is usually completed 6 to 12 months later. Parallel longitudinal incisions are created and the urethral plate is incised along its midpoint. The resulting tissue is used to create a fully tubularized neourethra. Although this approach is limited to a small number of complex cases, the apparent disadvantage of a two-stage procedure must be carefully weighed against advantages such as a superior cosmetic result, better correction of penile curvature, and lower risk of surgical complications.

Long-term data on voiding and sexual function in male patients who have undergone hypospadias repair

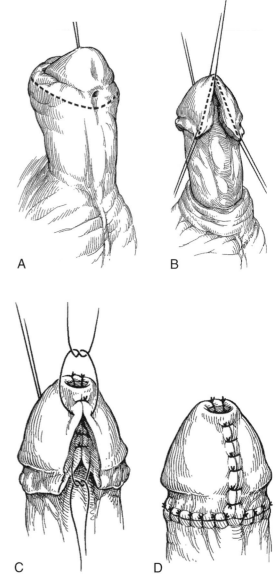

Fig. 18-8 Meatoplasty and glanuloplasty (MAGPI) procedure for distal hypospadias defects. **A,** Circumferential and longitudinal incisions are made. **B,** The ventral edge of the meatus is pulled distally. **C,** The reconstructed glans is closed with deep sutures. **D,** The resulting urethra extends to the distal meatus. (From Walsh P, Retik AB, Vaughan ED, Wein AJ [eds]: Campbell's Urology, 8th edition. Philadelphia: Saunders, 2002; p 2307.)

are sparse, and they continue to evolve as techniques of surgical repair advance. One study compared sexual function in 57 men who underwent hypospadias repair with a group of 60 age-matched controls.[74] It revealed equivalent libido and erectile function in both groups, but patients who had undergone hypospadias repairs reported impaired ejaculation function. In addition, they masturbated less often, were less sexually active, and reported a smaller number of sexual partners than age-matched controls.

Complications. The most common complication of surgical repair is a urethrocutaneous fistula, which occurs in approximately 2% of patients undergoing the TIP procedure, 0% to 12% of those managed by a MAGPI procedure,[75-77] 5% to 17% of boys managed with an onlay or tubularized preputial flap, and 5% of those with two-stage repairs.[73] Inadequate vascular supply to reconstructed tissue is thought to contribute to meatal stenosis, which occurs in less than 5%, and urethral stricture, which is seen about 6%.[73] Other less common complications include urethral diverticula associated with postvoid dribbling, recurring penile curvature, wound dehiscence, and scarring. Hair growth into the urethra occurs in approximately 0.2% of patients.[78] Clinical experience and some evidence have suggested that surgeon experience and repetition are important factors that influence not only efficacy rates, but also the risk for subsequent complications.[79]

Preparation for Surgery. In addition to the preparation typical for any open surgical procedure, the perineal skin must be carefully inspected for signs of severe perineal dermatitis or candidal infection, which must be treated before surgery can proceed. As noted, hypospadias repair usually occurs between 6 and 12 months of age. Therefore, informed consent and preoperative counseling focus on the parents or caregivers. The purpose of the surgery and expectations about the anticipated postoperative course are reviewed. Depending on institutional policies, one parent may accompany the child to the surgical area and remain with the child during anesthesia induction.[51] The parents are advised that the child is expected to struggle during early stages of induction, followed by relaxation as the anesthetic takes effect.

Postoperative Care. Most infants who undergo single-stage primary repair of a distal hypospadias defect are managed in an outpatient setting, although boys who require more extensive surgery or a two-stage procedure may require a brief hospital admission. The child is likely to return from surgery with a urethral stent—feeding tube rather than traditional indwelling catheter—to ensure unobstructed urinary outflow. The stent drains directly into a diaper or a collection bag, depending on the age of the child, surgeon's preference, and anticipated time prior to removal. The stent is typically attached to the glans penis by one or two sutures that must be removed prior to discontinuation. Removal is from 2 to 14 days postoperatively. The urologic nurse or parents regularly monitor the tube for patency and urinary drainage for color, character, and presence of clots. Following stent removal, the child may experience anxiety or discomfort with urination; this may be relieved by allowing the child to urinate while in a tub of warm water for the first few voids. Parents are also advised to observe the stream immediately following stent removal. They should be reassured that some spraying of the stream is anticipated, but a complete inability to void or a dribbling stream is not expected and should prompt a call to the pediatric urologist or urologic nurse.

The pediatric urologist is likely to prescribe an antibiotic for several days following surgery, particularly when the urethral stent remains in place. Suppressive antimicrobial therapy is indicated because it has been found to reduce the risk for subsequent complications, including urinary tract infection, urethrocutaneous fistula, and meatal stenosis.[80]

A thin-film dressing is usually placed over the repair and removed at the first postoperative office visit or by the parents in the home setting. The dressing may fall off by itself, and parents are reassured in advance that this is not a cause for concern. However, a dressing may occasionally become partly dislodged and bunch around the base of the penis, constricting local blood flow. If bunching occurs, parents are usually advised to remove the dressing or promptly contact the pediatric urologist or urologic nurse if they cannot easily remove the dressing.

Incisional pain may be managed by a nerve block during surgery, followed by oral opioid analgesics or acetaminophen as the incision heals and pain diminishes. Parents may be taught to double-diaper the child following hypospadias surgery to protect the incision and stent and to protect the area from fecal soiling. They are reassured that a small amount of bloody discharge is common during the early postoperative period. Parents are also advised of the signs of bladder spasm in the infant—arching the back and bringing the knees to the chest in association with a rush of urine through or around the urethral stent. An antimuscarinic medication is commonly prescribed for bladder spasms, and parents are taught to observe the stent for blockage if spasms increase in frequency or are associated with little or no urine output into the diaper or drainage bag. Bathing is limited to sponge baths prior to dressing removal, and parents are taught to cleanse any fecal soiling away from the penis and stent carefully. Brisk scrubbing is avoided. Bathing in a tub is usually allowed after the surgical dressing is removed or falls off, but the parents are advised to avoid scrubbing the surgical repair directly until given specific permission by the pediatric urologist.

The older child's diet is advanced rapidly and fluid intake is encouraged, particularly while the stent remains in place. The child should be limited to quiet activity for the first several days following repair; strenuous activity is limited until cleared by the physician.

Patient Teaching Highlights. Because most infants undergoing hypospadias surgery are managed as outpatients, education focuses on the postoperative interventions discussed above. In addition to these considerations, parents or guardians are taught to observe the child for long-term complications such as urethrocutaneous fistula or meatal stenosis. Follow-up may continue until puberty, particularly if the initial defect was proximal, required a complex or staged repair, or resulted in complications such as urethrocutaneous fistula, urethral stricture, or stenosis.[77] Psychological counseling or support is occasionally indicated, particularly for the adolescent or young adult who has undergone multiple surgical repairs or has residual complications adversely affecting sexual or voiding function.

SURGERY FOR PREVIOUS FAILED HYPOSPADIAS REPAIRS

A small number of boys will experience significant complications despite one or more hypospadias repairs.[73] In these cases, all subsequent repairs should be completed by a pediatric urologist with significant experience in this highly specialized field of care. Redo repairs often incorporate onlay island flaps, preputial island flaps, oral mucosa graft urethroplasties, and similarly complex maneuvers to repair tubular defects or strictures.[81,82]

CIRCUMCISION

Circumcision is the surgical removal of the penile foreskin. It is one of the oldest surgical procedures in the world and fraught with religious, cultural, social, and personal values and beliefs that cannot be meaningfully separated from any discussion of its medical value, indications, or consequences. Refer to the box, Clinical Highlights for Advanced and Expert Practice: Controversies and Clinical Evidence Surrounding Male Circumcision—Counseling Prospective and New Parents About a Source of Continuing Controversy. This provides a brief review of clinical evidence related to benefits and harms associated with circumcision and implications for counseling potential or new parents who are considering whether their male child should undergo this procedure.[83-96]

Most circumcisions are not performed by pediatric urologists. Rather, they are more commonly performed by pediatricians, obstetricians, or family practitioners,[97] and Jewish male infants may have circumcision performed by a mohel (Hebrew, "circumciser," a person with special training in performing ritual circumcision, called a *brit milah*). Nevertheless, circumcisions are occasionally performed by a pediatric urologist and it is not uncommon for prospective or new parents to approach a urologic nurse to clarify information supporting or arguing against neonatal circumcision. Regardless of who performs the procedure, two principal roles of the urologic nurse are to ensure that adequate pain management is provided for the procedure and to ensure that parents understand that neonatal circumcision is neither medically indicated nor contraindicated. Instead, it is an elective procedure, and any decision to undertake surgery should be based on close consultation between the parents and their health care providers.

If a decision is made to proceed with circumcision, the urologic nurse should then counsel the parents about an infant's ability to perceive and experience pain and the subsequent need for pain management during circumcision. Research has clearly demonstrated that infants experience pain and that male neonates undergoing circumcision experience physiologic distress ameliorated by local anesthesia.[98] However, a study of practices related to circumcision in 1998 revealed that only 71% of pediatricians, 56% of family practitioners, and 25% of obstetricians regularly used anesthesia when performing neonatal

Clinical Highlights for Advanced and Expert Practice: Controversies and Clinical Evidence Surrounding Male Circumcision–Counseling Prospective and New Parents About a Source of Continuing Controversy

Introduction

Given its sociocultural and religious context, it does not seem surprising that circumcision is a focus of controversy throughout many parts of the world, including North America. Some groups object vehemently to the practice, claiming that it is a form of ritualistic genital mutilation and detrimental to sexual function, although others defend the procedure as socially desirable or an expression of religious faith. This clinical highlights box focuses on clinical evidence related to potential benefits and harms arising from circumcision, and provides suggestions for counseling prospective or new parents about whether they plan to have their child undergo this frequently performed procedure.

Clinical Evidence

Medical justification for circumcision centers on its role as a protective factor against certain illnesses, while research arguing against its use focuses on impairments in sexual function, complications and sequelae related to the procedure, and adverse psychosocial outcomes.

Sexual Function

Circumcision removes the protective cutaneous layer over the glans penis, leading to increased keratinization and possibly to reduced sensitivity of the penis to sexual stimulation. Limited evidence reveals no measurable differences in glanular tactile sensations in adult men.[93] Collins and colleagues[92] compared multiple indicators of sexual function in a group of 15 men undergoing elective circumcision as an adult and found no differences in libido, erectile function, ejaculatory function, or overall satisfaction with sexual function following circumcision.

Urinary Tract Infection

Mixed evidence demonstrates that uncircumcised males have a higher risk for urinary tract infection during the first year of life.[88-91] However, this must be carefully weighed against the overall risk for infections in male infants, which remains quite low.

Risk of Sexually Transmitted Disease (STD)

The glans penis in the uncircumcised male is less keratinized, moister, and warmer than that of the circumcised male, rendering it a supportive microenvironment for sexually transmitted pathogens.[87] Epidemiologic studies addressing this issue have suffered from several significant limitations, including small sample size, retrospective sampling, and/or use of STD clinics, leading to a high likelihood of sampling bias. The most consistent and powerful observations have demonstrated an association between uncircumcised men and an increased risk for genital ulcerative diseases.[91]

HIV Risk

There is growing body of evidence that suggests that HIV transmission in African males is higher in uncircumcised males.[91a] Two meta-analyses have examined the evidence from these studies. Weiss and colleagues[86] pooled data from 27 studies and concluded that male circumcision significantly reduces the risk for HIV infection in males living in Africa. Siegfried and associates[85] completed a meta-analysis of 34 studies and found a strong epidemiologic association between male circumcision and prevention of HIV infection, but they refrained from concluding that circumcision acts as a protective factor until results of ongoing randomized clinical trials have been completed.

Penile Cancer

Circumcision reduces the risk of invasive squamous cell carcinoma, but it exerts a less protective effect on penile squamous cell carcinoma in situ.[84] However, the overall risk for urinary tract infection in male infants remains small and the risk for penile cancer is slight, so neither of these arguments creates a compelling medical argument for the routine performance of circumcision.[83]

Human Papillomavirus (HPV) and Cervical Cancer

Multiple case-control studies demonstrate that circumcision reduces the risk for penile HPV infection in men and the risk for cervical cancer in their female partners.[94]

Continued

Clinical Highlights for Advanced and Expert Practice: Controversies and Clinical Evidence Surrounding Male Circumcision–Counseling Prospective and New Parents About a Source of Continuing Controversy—cont'd

Surgical Complications

Complications associated with neonatal circumcision are uncommon. Local bleeding and infection occur in less than 0.5% of all cases. The risk of complications is higher when brit milah (ritual) circumcisions are performed by a mohel[95] or when a Plastibell device is used.[96]

Counseling Prospective Parents

Although a growing body of clinical evidence demonstrates a number of potential benefits related to neonatal circumcision, none provide a sufficiently powerful argument to conclude that routine neonatal circumcision is medically indicated for male infants born in North America. The strongest arguments supporting neonatal circumcision are its potential to prevent urinary tract infection during the first year of life and genital ulcers during adulthood, which simultaneously reduces the risk for HPV-related cervical cancer in a regular female sexual partner. Nevertheless, the strength of these arguments must be carefully weighed against the low overall risks of a urinary tract infection during the first year of life. Also, it is well-known that limiting sexual partners or the regular use of condoms if engaging in sexual intercourse with multiple partners reduces the risk for both parties. The strongest medical arguments against routine neonatal circumcision include the risk of complications and the possibility of impaired sexual function.

A review of existing clinical evidence reveals that the risk of complications is small and any differences in sexual function based on the presence of a foreskin have not been detected. Therefore, the decision to have a child undergo neonatal circumcision should be based on the parents' and family's values and beliefs related to circumcision and not on mythical or emotionally charged (and insupportable) arguments for clear health benefits or psychological or physical harm.

circumcision.[97] A number of pain management techniques have been used for neonatal circumcision, including a local anesthetic cream, dorsal penile nerve block using a 1% lidocaine solution, circumferential injection of lidocaine, or allowing the infant to suck on a cloth soaked with sweet wine during ritual circumcision. A prospective, randomized, clinical trial has investigated pain associated with circumcision. Pain was measured using the Neonatal Infant Pain Scale; subjects were videotaped to maximize reliability of scoring.[99] Subjects underwent circumcision using topical anesthesia or a dorsal penile nerve block and a separate group underwent a sham procedure. Subjects managed by the dorsal penile nerve block had significantly lower pain scores than those managed with topical anesthesia.

ORCHIOPEXY

Orchiopexy is the surgical placement of a cryptorchid testis in the scrotum. Surgery remains a mainstay of treatment for cryptorchidism because failure to achieve scrotal placement of a cryptorchid testis is associated with significant risks for infertility and cancer, and because the medical alternative (hormonal stimulation) has a success rate lower than 20%. Orchiopexy achieves a success rate from 67%

to 95%, depending on the location of the testis and operative technique.[100] The procedure may be done by an open or laparoscopic technique. Regardless of the approach, the goals of surgery are to mobilize the testis and its spermatic cord, repair the patent processus vaginalis, achieve a tension-free placement of the testis within the scrotum to prevent reascent, and create a pouch within the hemiscrotum to optimize scrotal placement.

The timing of surgery is significant.[73] Research shows that significant histologic deterioration occurs in the undescended testis between the fourth and tenth years of life and that evidence of deterioration can be found as early as the end of the first year of life. Spontaneous descent is not uncommon during the first 6 months of life, but this then diminishes significantly and the chance of spontaneous descent after year 1 is almost nonexistent. Based on these considerations, the American Academy of Pediatrics recommends treatment of cryptorchidism after 6 months of age.[73]

Orchiopexy is also performed to relieve ischemia in the presence of spermatic cord and testicular torsion.[101] In this case, the goal of surgery is not to deliver a cryptorchid testis to the scrotal sac but to restore blood supply by correcting the twisting of the abdominal wall and to prevent recurrence. Because of the risk of recurrence, the contralateral testis is also fixated in the scrotum, although this maneuver does not entirely eliminate the risk for later torsion.[102]

Open Orchiopexy

Open surgery often begins with a transverse inguinal incision in a skin crease over the midinguinal canal[103] (Figure 18-9). Overlying fascial structures are opened and the distal gubernacular attachments are dissected. After the spermatic cord is mobilized to the level of the internal ring, the tunica vaginalis is opened over the testis and it is inspected for size and integrity of paratesticular structures. Additional dissection may be required to ensure complete mobility of the testis and spermatic cord, which is essential to successful and lasting placement in the scrotum. Generally, the testis is placed in the hemiscrotum within a superficial pouch of dartos fascia. A transverse midscrotal skin incision is created within a rugal skin fold, a tissue plane is developed just under this superficial incision, and the fascial window is closed with a fine absorbable suture. A prescrotal approach that uses a skin incision along the crease between the scrotal and inguinal skin is an alternative procedure for the palpable cryptorchid testis. The potential advantage to this procedure is its reportedly low complication rate.

Testes located in higher intraabdominal positions may require more extensive manipulation to achieve adequate mobilization to transfer the testis in the appropriate hemiscrotum.[103] For example, the proximal spermatic cord vessels may be freed and repositioned medially to extend spermatic cord length or a staged procedure may be undertaken. In the staged procedure, the testis is first brought to the external ring or symphysis pubis and anchored. A second procedure is then performed 6 to 12 months later to mobilize the testis and spermatic cord further and place them in the appropriate hemiscrotum.

Laparoscopic Orchiopexy

Laparoscopic technique has evolved significantly since the 1970s and it now plays a central role in assessment and management of cryptorchidism.[103] Initially, laparoscopy is used to locate the testis. Laparoscopic assessment of patients with nonpalpable testes is particularly valuable because it allows the urologist to differentiate a cryptorchid from a congenitally absent testis. If the testis is found to be within 2 cm of the internal inguinal ring, a primary laparoscopic orchiopexy is completed. Two working ports are placed just medial to the anterior superior iliac spines of the pelvic bone. The peritoneum is incised with endoscopic instruments and the testis and spermatic cord are mobilized. Techniques for mobilization differ from those used during open surgery and care is taken to prevent inadvertent torsion of the cord. Following mobilization, the testis and cord are placed in the scrotum using a dartos pouch, as described. As the ports are removed, the patient is carefully observed for bleeding. Bleeding is managed by placement of figure-of-eight ligatures and all portholes are closed to prevent herniation of the omentum. Higher placed testes can be approached using a two-stage laparoscopic approach.

Success rates for open surgery vary based on the technique used and location of the testis. An analysis of open surgical techniques in 1995 has revealed a 92% success rate for testes located below the inguinal ring, 89% for testes in the inguinal canal and 81% for intraabdominal testes.[104] The success rate for staged Fowler-Stephens repairs was 77%. Staged intraabdominal orchiopexy using laparoscopic techniques has a comparatively high success rate of 95%, and the success rate for single-stage laparoscopic orchiopexy is 86%.[103,105]

Complications. Complications include testicular retraction, scrotal hematoma, damage to the vas deferens, and postoperative torsion. Devascularization with testicular atrophy is a serious but uncommon complication, and may justify orchiectomy.[100] Complications seen with laparoscopic orchiectomy include bleeding or herniation of omentum from port sites, inadequate grounding with subsequent thermal injury, and rare cases of bowel perforation.

Preparation for Surgery. Infants or children undergoing open or laparoscopic orchiopexy may be managed as outpatients or admitted to the hospital for a brief period only, usually 23 hours or less. If the child undergoes an open procedure, the family is informed that two small incisions are anticipated, one in the inguinal area and one in the scrotum. The infant or child undergoing laparoscopic surgery will also be managed as an outpatient. Similar to open surgery, laparoscopy is performed under general anesthesia and an orogastric tube and indwelling urethral catheter are placed during the operation.

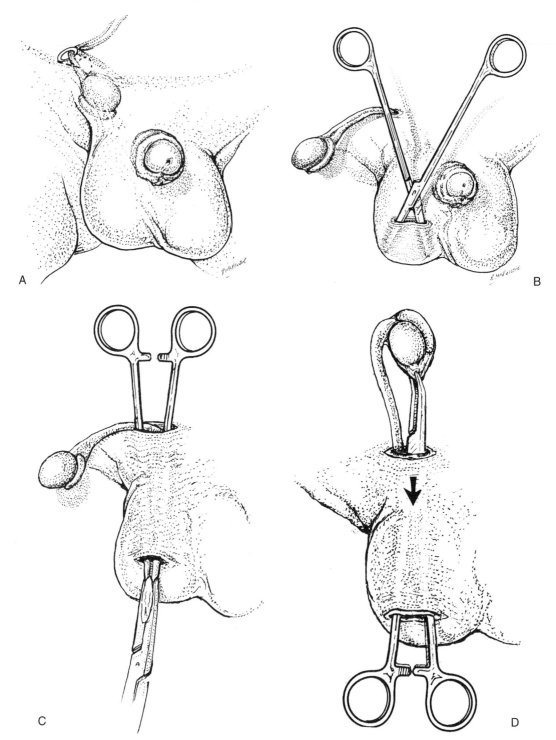

Fig. 18-9 Open orchiopexy. **A,** A small transverse incision is made in the inguinal crease. **B,** After the testis and spermatic cord are separated from the processus vaginalis, a small scrotal incision is made and a pouch is created within dartos fascia. **C,** A passage is created into the scrotum. **D,** The testis and spermatic cord are placed in the appropriate hemiscrotum. (From Walsh P, Retik AB, Vaughan ED, Wein AJ [eds]: Campbell's Urology, 8th edition. Philadelphia: Saunders, 2002; pp 2371, 2374, 2375.)

Postoperative Care. Incisional pain may occur following surgery, but it is typically mild and managed by acetaminophen alone. Bruising and swelling, particularly apparent over the scrotum, are anticipated but expected to subside within a period of 2 weeks. Parents are advised to support their child's buttocks when lifting to prevent tension and discomfort at the surgery site. Bathing is limited to a sponge bath for approximately 3 days following surgery; regular tub bathing or showering can then resume.

Parents are counseled that the child should only engage in quiet activities for about 24 hours following the procedure. Straddle toys are avoided for 1 to 2 weeks postoperatively, and strenuous play, swimming, or athletic activities such as football or gymnastics are avoided for about 2 weeks.

Patient Teaching Highlights. In addition to immediate postoperative care, education focuses on long-term issues, including the small but increased risk for subfertility and malignancy. Boys with a history of cryptorchidism are taught to perform testicular self-examination as adolescents and to remain aware of this history if they experience difficulty conceiving children as adults.

SUMMARY

Various surgical procedures are performed to correct congenital anomalies, alleviate obstructive uropathy, relieve incontinence, and prevent reflux nephropathy. The nursing management of these children focuses on education of the patient and family or care providers, psychological support of the child who may experience intense anxiety associated with manipulation of the genitourinary system, and long-term follow-up to ensure optimal urologic health and prevent unforeseen complications.

REFERENCES

1. Hockenberry MJ, Wilson D, Winkelstein ML, Kline NE: In Wong's Nursing Care of Infants and Children, 7th edition. St Louis: Mosby, 2003; pp 1110-21.
2. Franck LS: Focus. Nursing management of children's pain: current evidence and future directions for research. Nursing Times Research, 2003; 8(5):330-53.
3. Byers JF, Thornley K: Cueing into infant pain. American Journal of Maternal/Child Nursing 2004; 29(2):84-91.
4. Bishop-Kurylo D: Pediatric pain management in the emergency department. Topics in Emergency Medicine, 2002; 24(1):19-30.
5. Hall PA, Payne JF, Stack CG, Stokes MA: Parents in the recovery room:survey of parental and staff attitudes. British Medical Journal, 1995; 310(6973):163-4.
6. LaRosa-Nash PA, Murphy JM: An approach to pediatric perioperative care. Parent-present induction. Nursing Clinics of North America, 1997; 32(1):183-99.
7. Munro H, D'Errico FC: Parental involvement in perioperative anesthetic management. Journal of Perianesthesia Nursing, 2000; 15(6):397-400.
8. LaMontagne LL, Hepworth JT, Cohen F, Salisbury MH: Adolescents' coping with surgery for scoliosis: effects on recovery outcomes over time. Research in Nursing and Health, 2004; 27(4):237-53.
9. Mintzer LL, Stuber ML, Seacord D, Castaneda M, Mesrkhani V, Glover D: Traumatic stress symptoms in adolescent organ transplant recipients. Pediatrics, 2005; 115(6):1640-4.
10. Tal R, Bar-Sever Z, Livne PM: Dismembered pyeloplasty in children: a review of 5 years single center experience. International Journal of Urology, 2005; 12(12):1028-31.
11. Biyani CS, Minhas S, el Cast J, Almond DJ, Cooksey G, Hetherington JW: The role of Acucise endopyelotomy in the treatment of ureteropelvic junction obstruction. European Urology, 2002; 41(3):305-12.
12. El-Ghoneimi A, Farhat W, Bolduc S, Bagli D, McLorie G, Aigrain Y, Khoury A: Laparoscopic dismembered pyeloplasty by a retroperitoneal approach in children. BJU International, 2003; 92(1):104-8.
13. Moon DA, El-Shazly MA, Chang CM, Gianduzzo TR, Eden CG: Laparoscopic pyeloplasty: evolution of a new gold standard. Urology, 2006; 67(5):932-6.
14. Bentas W, Wolfram M, Brautigam R, Probst M, Beecken WD, Jonas D, Binder J: Da Vinci robot-assisted Anderson-Hynes dismembered pyeloplasty: technique and 1 year follow-up. World Journal of Urology, 2003; 21(3):133-8.
15. Patel V: Robotic-assisted laparoscopic dismembered pyeloplasty. Urology, 2005; 66(1):45-9.
16. Yee DS, Shanberg AM, Duel BP, Rodriguez E, Eichel L, Rajpoot D: Initial comparison of robotic-assisted laparoscopic versus open pyeloplasty in children. Urology, 2006; 67(3):599-602.
17. Link RE, Bhayani SB, Kavoussi LR: A prospective comparison of robotic and laparoscopic pyeloplasty. Annals of Surgery, 2006; 243(4):486-91.
18. Nicholls G, Hrouda D, Kellett MJ, Duffy PG: Endopyelotomy in the symptomatic older child. BJU International, 2001; 87(6):525-7.
19. Schwartz BF, Stoller ML: Complications of retrograde balloon cautery endopyelotomy. Journal of Urology, 1999; 162(5):1594-8.
20. Hsu TH, Streem SB, Kakada SY: Management of upper urinary tract obstruction. In Wein AJ, Kavoussi LR, Novick AC, Partin AW, Peters CA (eds): Campbell-Walsh Urology, 9th edition. Philadelphia: Saunders, 2007; pp 1227-73.
21. Chandrasekharam VV: Is retrograde stenting more reliable than antegrade stenting for pyeloplasty in infants and children? Urology, 2005; 66(6):1301-4.
22. Piedrahita YK, Palmer JS: Is one-day hospitalization after open pyeloplasty possible and safe? Urology, 2006; 67(1):181-4.
23. Chow GK, Fabrizio MD, Steer T, Potter SR, Jarrett TW, Gelman S, Kavoussi LR: Prospective double-blind study of effect of ketorolac administration after laparoscopic urologic surgery. Journal of Endourology, 2001; 15(2):171-4.
24. Aslan P, Preminger GM: Retrograde balloon cautery incision of ureteropelvic junction obstruction. Urologic Clinics of North America, 1998; 25(2):295-304.
25. Francis P, Winfield, HN: Care of the patient undergoing robotic-laparoscopic assisted pyeloplasty. Urology Nursing, 2006; 26(2):110-5.
26. Khoury A, Bagli DJ: Reflux and megaureter. In Wein AJ, Kavoussi LR, Novick AC, Partin AW, Peters CA (eds): Campbell-Walsh Urology, 9th edition. Philadelphia: Saunders, 2007; pp 3423-81.
27. Parrott TS, Woodard JR, Wolpert JJ: Ureteral tailoring: a comparison of wedge resection with infolding. Journal of Urology, 1990; 144(2 Pt 1):328-9.
28. DeFoor W, Minevich E, Reddy P, Polsky E, McGregor A, Wacksman J, Sheldon C: Results of tapered ureteral reimplantation

for primary megaureter: extravesical versus intravesical approach. Journal of Urology, 2004; 172(4 Pt 2):1640-3.

29. Schlussel RN, Retik AB: Ectopic ureter, ureterocele and other anomalies of the ureter. In Wein AJ, Kavoussi LR, Novick AC, Partin AW, Peters CA (eds): Campbell-Walsh Urology, 9th edition. Philadelphia: Saunders, 2007; pp 3383-3422.

30. Stephens FD: Etiology of ureteroceles and effects of ureteroceles on the urethra. British Journal of Urology, 1968; 40(4):483-7.

31. Churchill BM, Sheldon CA, McLorie GA: The ectopic ureterocele: a proposed practical classification based on renal unit jeopardy. Journal of Pediatric Surgery, 1992; 27(4):497-500.

32. Glassberg KI, Braren V, Duckett JW, Jacobs EC, King LR, Lebowitz RL, Perlmutter AD, Stephens FD: Suggested terminology for duplex systems, ectopic ureters and ureteroceles. Journal of Urology, 1984; 132(6):1153-4.

33. Shokeir AA, Nijman RJM: Ureterocele: an ongoing challenge in infancy and childhood. BJU International, 2002; 90(8):777-83.

34. King LR, Kozlowski JM, Schacht MJ: Ureteroceles in children. A simplified and successful approach to management. Journal of the American Medical Association, 1983; 249(11):1461-5.

35. Shimada K, Matsumoto F, Matsui F: Surgical treatment for ureterocele with special reference to lower urinary tract reconstruction. International Journal of Urology, 2007; 14(12):1063-7.

36. Kajbafzadeh A, Salmasi AH, Payabvash S, Arshadi H, Akbari HR, Moosavi S: Evolution of endoscopic management of ectopic ureterocele: a new approach. Journal of Urology, 2007; 177(3):1118-23.

37. Snow BW, Cartwright PC: Vesicoureteral reflux surgery. In Gillenwater JY, Grayhack JT, Howards SS, Mitchell ME (eds): Adult and Pediatric Urology, 4th edition. Philadelphia: Lippincott Williams & Wilkins, 2002; pp 2415-43.

38. Lipski BA, Mitchell ME, Burns MW: Voiding dysfunction after bilateral extravesical ureteral reimplantation. Journal of Urology, 1998; 159(3):1019-21.

39. Schwentner C, Oswald J, Lunacek A, Deibl M, Koerner I, Bartsch G, Radmayr C: Lich-Gregoir reimplantation causes less discomfort than Politano-Leadbetter technique: results of a prospective, randomized, pain scale-oriented study in a pediatric population. European Urology, 2006; 49(2):388-95.

40. Janetschek G, Radmayr C, Bartsch G: Laparoscopic ureteral anti-reflux plasty reimplantation. First clinical experience. Annales d'Urologie, 1995; 29(2):101-5.

41. Erlich RM, Gershman A, Fuchs S: Laparoscopic vesicoureteroplasty in children: initial case reports. Urology, 1994; 43(2):255.

42. Gill IS, Ponsky LE, Desai M, Kay R, Ross JH: Laparoscopic crosstrigonal Cohen ureteroneocystostomy: novel technique. Journal of Urology, 2001; 166(5):1811-4.

43. Matouschek E: New concept for the treatment of vesicoureteral reflux. Endoscopic application of teflon. Archivos Españoles de Urologia, 1981; 34(5):385-8.

44. Chertin B, Puri P: Endoscopic management of vesicoureteral reflux: does it stand the test of time? European Urology, 2002; 42(6):598-606.

45. Bartoli F, Niglio F, Gentile O, Penza R, Aceto G, Leggio S: Endoscopic treatment with polydimethylsiloxane in children with dilating vesico-ureteric reflux. BJU International, 2006; 97(4):805-8.

46. Aboutaleb H, Bolduc S, Upadhyay J, Farhat W, Bagli DJ, Khoury AE: Subureteral polydimethylsiloxane injection versus extravesical reimplantation for primary low-grade vesicoureteral reflux in children: a comparative study. Journal of Urology, 2003; 169(1):313-6.

47. Mor Y, Liebovitch I, Fridmans A, Farkas A, Jonas P, Ramon J: Late post reimplantation ureteral obstruction during pregnancy: a transient phenomenon? Journal of Urology, 2003; 170(3):845-8.

48. Barroso U Jr, Jednak R, Bethold JS, Gonzalez R: Outcome of ureteral reimplantation in children with urge syndrome. Journal of Urology, 2001; 166(3):1031-5.

49. Chaffange P, Dubois R, Bouhafs A, Valmalle AF, Dodat H: Endoscopic treatment of vesicorenal reflux in children: short- and long-term results of polytetrafluoroethylene (Teflon) injections. Progres en Urologie, 2001; 11(3):546-51.

50. Kirsch AJ, Rerez-Rayfield MR, Sherz HC: Minimally invasive treatment of vesicoureteral reflux with endoscopic injection of dextranomer/hyaluronic acid copolymer: the children's hospitals of Atlanta experience. Journal of Urology, 2003; 170:211-5.

51. Ellsworth PI, Cendron M, McCullough MF: Surgical management of vesicoureteral reflux. AORN Journal, 2000; 71(3):498-524.

52. Duong DT, Parekh DJ, Pope JC 4th, Adams MC, Brock JW 3rd: Ureteroneocystostomy without urethral catheterization shortens hospital stay without compromising postoperative success. Journal of Urology, 2003; 170(4 Pt 2):1570-3.

53. Park JM, Houck CS, Sethna NF, Sullivan LJ, Atala A, Borer JG, Cilento BG, Diamond DA, Peters CA, Retik AB, Bauer SB: Ketorolac suppresses postoperative bladder spasms after pediatric ureteral reimplantation. Anesthesia and Analgesia, 2000; 91(1):11-5.

54. Merguerian PA, Sutters KA, Tang E, Kaji D, Chang B: Efficacy of continuous epidural analgesia versus single-dose caudal analgesia in children after intravesical ureteroneocystostomy. Journal of Urology, 2004; 172(4 Pt 2):1621-5.

55. El-Ghoneimi A, Deffarges C, Hankard R, Jean-Eudes F, Aigrain Y, Jacqz-Aigrain E: Intravesical morphine analgesia is not effective after bladder surgery in children: results of a randomized double-blind study. Journal of Urology, 2002; 168(2):694-7.

56. Mitchell ME, Plaire JC: Augmentation enterocystoplasty. In Gillenwater JY, Grayhack JT, Howards SS, Mitchell ME (eds): Adult and Pediatric Urology, 4th edition. Philadelphia: Lippincott Williams & Wilkins, 2002; pp 2445-59.

57. Gill IS, Rackely RR, Meraney AM, Marcello PW, Snug PT: Laparoscopic enterocystoplasty. Urology, 2000; 55(2):178-81.

58. Adams MC, Joseph DB: Urinary tract reconstruction in children. In Wein AJ, Kavoussi LR, Novick AC, Partin AW, Peters CA (eds): Campbell-Walsh Urology, 9th edition. Philadelphia: Saunders, 2007; pp 3656-3702.

59. Quek ML, Ginsberg DA: Long-term urodynamics follow-up of bladder augmentation for neurogenic bladder. Journal of Urology, 2003:195-8.

60. Venn S, Mundy T: Bladder reconstruction: urothelial augmentation, trauma, fistula. Current Opinion in Urology, 2002; 12:201-3.

61. Chartier-Kastler EJ, Mongiat-Artus P, Bitker MO, Chancellor MB, Richard F, Denys P: Long-term results of augmentation cystoplasty in spinal cord injury patients. Spinal Cord, 2000; 38(8):490-4.

62. Dyer JP, Featherstone JM, Solomon LZ, Crook TJ, Cooper AJ, Malone PS: The effect of short-chain fatty acids butyrate, propionate, and acetate on urothelial cell kinetics in vitro: potential therapy in augmentation cystoplasty. Pediatric Surgery International, 2005; 21(7):521-6.

63. Barrington JW, Fulford S, Griffiths D, Stephenson TP: Tumors in bladder remnant after enterocystoplasty. Journal of Urology, 1997; 157(2):482-6.

64. DeFoor W, Tackett L, Minevich E, Wacksman J, Sheldon C: Risk factors for spontaneous perforation after augmentation enterocystoplasty. Urology, 2003; 62(4):737-41.

65. Catto JW, Natarajan V, Tophill PR: Simultaneous augmentation cystoplasty is associated with earlier rather than increased artificial urinary sphincter infection. Journal of Urology, 2005; 173(4):1237-41.

66. DeFoor W, Minevich E, Reddy P, Sekhon D, Polsky E, Wacksman J, Sheldon C: Bladder calculi after augmentation cystoplasty: risk factors and prevention strategies. Journal of Urology, 2004; 172(5 Pt 1):1964-6.

67. Hodges SJ, Atala A: Initial clinical results of the bioartificial kidney containing human cells in ICU patients with acute renal failure. Current Urology Reports, 2006; 7(1):41-2.

68. Atala A: Technology insight: Applications of tissue engineering and biological substitutes in urology. Nature Clinical Practice Urology, 2005; 2(3):143-9.

69. Atala A, Bauer SB, Soker S, Yoo JJ, Retik AB: Tissue-engineered autologous bladders for patients needing cystoplasty. Lancet, 2006; 367(9518):1241-6.

70. Fichtner J, Filipas D, Mottrie AM, Voges GE, Hohenfellner R: Analysis of meatal location in 500 men: wide variation questions need for meatal advancement in all pediatric anterior hypospadias cases. Journal of Urology, 1995; 154(2 Pt 2):833-4.

71. Mieusset R, Soulie M: Hypospadias: psychosocial, sexual and reproductive consequences in adult life. Journal of Andrology, 2005; 26(2):153-68.

72. American Academy of Pediatrics: Timing of elective surgery on the genitalia of male children with particular reference to the risks, benefits, and psychological effects of surgery and anesthesia. Pediatrics, 1996; 97(4):590-4.

73. Shukla AR, Patel RP, Canning DA: Hypospadias. Urologic Clinics of North America, 2004; 31(3):445-60.

74. Bubanj TB, Perovic SV, Milicevic RM, Jovcic SB, Marjanovic ZO, Djordjevic MM: Sexual behavior and sexual function of adults after hypospadias surgery: a comparative study. Journal of Urology, 2004; 171(5):1876-9.

75. Watanabe K, Ogawa A, Kiyono M, Yoneyama T, Muraishi O: Results of one-stage hypospadias repair. Nippon Hinyokika Gakkai Zasshi. Japanese Journal of Urology, 1994; 85(11):1656-63.

76. Bondonny JM, Barthaburu D, Vergnes P: Glandular and penile hypospadias. Elements of the abnormality. Therapeutic implications and results from a study of 135 protocols. Annales d'Urologie, 1984; 18(1):21-7.

77. Marrocco G, Vallascani S, Fiocca G, Calisti A: Hypospadia surgery: a 10-year review. Pediatric Surgery International, 2004; 20:200-3.

78. Obaidullah, Aslam M: Ten-year review of hypospadias surgery from a single center. British Journal of Plastic Surgery, 2005; 58(6):780-9.

79. Horowitz M, Salzhauer E: The 'learning curve' in hypospadias surgery. BJU International, 2006; 97(3):593-6.

80. Meir DB, Levine PM: Is prophylactic antimicrobial treatment necessary after hypospadias repair? Journal of Urology, 2004; 171(6 Part 2):2621-2.

81. Nelson CP, Bloom DA, Kinast R, Wei JT, Park JM: Patient-reported sexual function after oral mucosa graft urethroplasty for hypospadias. Urology, 2005; 66(5):1086-90.

82. Bar-Yosef Y, Binyamini J, Matzkin H, Ben-Chaim J: Salvage Mathieu urethroplasty: reuse of local tissue in failed hypospadias repair. Urology, 2005; 65(6):1212-5.

83. Fetus and Newborn Committee, Canadian Pediatric Society: Neonatal circumcision revisited. Canadian Medical Association Journal, 1996; 154:769-80.

84. Schoen EJ, Oehrli M, Colby C, Machin G: The highly protective effect of newborn circumcision against invasive penile cancer [abstract]. Pediatrics, 2000; 105:627-8.

85. Siegfried N, Muller M, Volmink J, Deeks J, Egger M, Low N, Weiss H, Walker S, Williamson P: Male circumcision for prevention of heterosexual acquisition of HIV in men. Cochrane Database of Systematic Reviews, 2003; (3)CD003362.

86. Weiss HA, Quigley MA, Hayes RJ. Male circumcision and risk of HIV infection in sub-Saharan Africa: a systematic review and meta-analysis. AIDS, 2000; 14:2261-70.

87. Fleiss PM, Hodges FM, Van Howe RS: Immunological functions of the human prepuce. Sexually Transmitted Infections, 1998; 74(5):364-7.

88. Crain EF, Gershel JC: Urinary tract infections in febrile infants younger than 8 weeks of age. Pediatrics, 1990; 86(3):363-7.

89. Wiswell TE, Smith FR, Bass JW: Decreased incidence of urinary tract infections in circumcised male infants. Pediatrics, 1985; 75(5):901-3.

90. Herzog LW: Urinary tract infections and circumcision. A case-control study. American Journal of Diseases of Children, 1989; 143(3):348-50.

91. Alanis MC, Lucidi RS: Neonatal circumcision: a review of the world's oldest and most controversial operation. Obstetrical and Gynecological Survey, 2004; 59(5):379-95.

91a. Shaffer DN, Bautista CT, Sateren WB, Sawe FK, Kiplangat SC, Miruka AO, Renzullo PO, Scott PT, Robb ML, Michael NL, Birx DL: The protective effect of circumcision on HIV incidence in rural low-risk men circumcised predominantly by traditional circumcisers in Kenya: two-year follow-up of the Kericho HIV Cohort Study. Journal of Acquired Immune Deficiency Syndromes, 2007; 45(4):371-9.

92. Collins S, Upshaw J, Rutchik S, Ohannessian C, Ortenberg J, Albertsen P: Effects of circumcision on male sexual function: debunking a myth? Journal of Urology, 2002; 167(5):2111-2.

93. Masters WH, Johnson VE: Human Sexual Response. Boston: Little, Brown, 1966.

94. Castellsague X, Bosch FX, Munoz N, Meijer CJ, Shah KV, de Sanjose S, Eluf-Neto J. Ngelangel CA, Chicareon S, Smith JS, Herrero R, Moreno V, Franceschi S, International Agency for Research on Cancer Multicenter Cervical Cancer Study Group: Male circumcision, penile human papillomavirus infection, and cervical cancer in female partners. New England Journal of Medicine, 2002; 346(15):1105-12.

95. Cohen HA, Drucker MM, Vainer S, Ashkenasi A, Amir J, Frydman M, Varsano I: Postcircumcision urinary tract infection. Clinical Pediatrics, 1992; 31(6):322-4.

96. Gee WF, Ansell JS: Neonatal circumcision: a ten-year overview with comparison of the Gomco clamp and the Plastibell device. Pediatrics, 1976; 58(6):824-7.

97. Stang HJ, Snellman LW: Circumcision practice patterns in the United States. Pediatrics, 1998; 101(6):E5.

98. Williamson PS, Williamson ML: Physiologic stress reduction by a local anesthetic during newborn circumcision. Pediatrics, 1983; 71(1):36-40.

99. Garry DJ. Swoboda E. Elimian A. Figueroa R: A video study of pain relief during newborn male circumcision. Journal of Perinatology, 2006; 26(2):106-10.

100. Schenk FX, Bellinger MF. Abnormalities of the testis and scrotum and their management. In Wein AJ, Kavoussi LR, Novick AC, Partin AW, Peters CA (eds): Campbell-Walsh Urology, 9th edition. Philadelphia: Saunders, 2007; pp 3761-98.

101. Woodard JR: Neonatal and perinatal emergencies. In Walsh PC, Gittes RF, Perlmutter AD, Stamey TA (eds): Campbell's Urology, 5th edition. Philadelphia: Saunders, 1986; pp 2217-2243.

102. Mor Y, Pinthus JH, Nadu A, Raviv G, Golomb J, Winkler H, Ramon J: Testicular fixation following torsion of the spermatic cord—does it guarantee prevention of recurrent torsion events? Journal of Urology, 2006; 175(1):171-4.

103. Strand WR, Bloom DB: Pediatric endourology. In Gillenwater JY, Grayhack JT, Howards SS, Mitchell ME (eds): Adult and Pediatric Urology, 4th edition, Philadelphia: Lippincott Williams & Wilkins, 2002; pp 2719-2760.

104. Docimo SG, Moore RG, Adams J, Kavoussi LR: Laparoscopic orchiopexy for the high palpable undescended testis: preliminary experience. Journal of Urology, 1995; 154(4):1513-5.

105. Samadi AA, Palmer LS, Franco I: Laparoscopic orchiopexy: report of 203 cases with review of diagnosis, operative technique, and lessons learned. Journal of Endourology, 2003; 17(6):365-8.

Index

··································

Page numbers followed by *b* indicate box, *f* indicate
figure, and *t* indicate table.

487